BURTON'S

Microbiology

for the

Health Sciences

TENTH EDITION

Paul G. Engelkirk, PhD, MT(ASCP), SM(NRCM)

Microbiology Consultant and Co-Founder
Biomedical Educational Services (Biomed Ed)
Round Rock, Texas

Janet Duben-Engelkirk, EdD, MT(ASCP)

Biotechnology/Education Consultant and Co-Founder
Biomedical Educational Services (Biomed Ed)
Round Rock, Texas

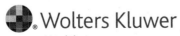

. Wolters Kluwer

Health

Philadelphia • Baltimore • New York • London
Buenos Aires • Hong Kong • Sydney • Tokyo

Acquisitions Editor: Michael Nobel
Product Manager: Paula C. Williams
Marketing Manager: Shauna Kelley
Production Project Manager: Priscilla Crater
Designer: Terry Mallon
Manufacturing Coordinator: Margie Orzech
Compositor: S4Carlisle Publishing Services

Tenth Edition

© 2015 Wolters Kluwer Health
2001 Market Street
Philadelphia, PA 19103 USA
LWW.com

© 2011 Lippincott Williams & Wilkins, a Wolters Kluwer business, © 2007 Lippincott Williams & Wilkins, © 2004 Lippincott Williams & Wilkins, © 2000 Lippincott Williams & Wilkins, © 1996 Lippincott-Raven, © 1992, 1988, 1983, 1979 JB Lippincott Co.

Printed in China

Library of Congress Cataloging-in-Publication Data
ISBN 978-1-4511-8632-1
Cataloging-in-Publication data available on request from the Publisher.

DISCLAIMER

Care has been taken to confirm the accuracy of the information present and to describe generally accepted practices. However, the authors, editors, and publisher are not responsible for errors or omissions or for any consequences from application of the information in this book and make no warranty, expressed or implied, with respect to the currency, completeness, or accuracy of the contents of the publication. Application of this information in a particular situation remains the professional responsibility of the practitioner; the clinical treatments described and recommended may not be considered absolute and universal recommendations.

The authors, editors, and publisher have exerted every effort to ensure that drug selection and dosage set forth in this text are in accordance with the current recommendations and practice at the time of publication. However, in view of ongoing research, changes in government regulations, and the constant flow of information relating to drug therapy and drug reactions, the reader is urged to check the package insert for each drug for any change in indications and dosage and for added warnings and precautions. This is particularly important when the recommended agent is a new or infrequently employed drug.

Some drugs and medical devices presented in this publication have Food and Drug Administration (FDA) clearance for limited use in restricted research settings. It is the responsibility of the health care provider to ascertain the FDA status of each drug or device planned for use in their clinical practice.

To purchase additional copies of this book, call our customer service department at **(800) 638-3030** or fax orders to **(301) 223-2320**. International customers should call **(301) 223-2300**.

Visit Lippincott Williams & Wilkins on the Internet: **http://www.lww.com**. Lippincott Williams & Wilkins customer service representatives are available from 8:30 am to 6:00 pm, EST.

9 8 7 6 5 4 3 2 1

Dedicated to our parents,
teachers, mentors, colleagues,
and friends who have encouraged
and helped us to fulfill our dreams.

About the Authors

Paul G. Engelkirk, PhD, MT(ASCP), SM(NRCM), is a retired professor of biological sciences from the Science Department at Central Texas College in Killeen, Texas, where he taught introductory microbiology for 12 years. Before joining Central Texas College, he was an associate professor at the University of Texas Health Science Center in Houston, Texas, where he taught diagnostic microbiology to medical laboratory science students for 8 years. Prior to his teaching career, Dr. Engelkirk served 22 years as an officer in the U.S. Army Medical Department, supervising various immunology, clinical pathology, and microbiology laboratories in Germany, Vietnam, and the United States. He retired from the Army with the rank of Lieutenant Colonel.

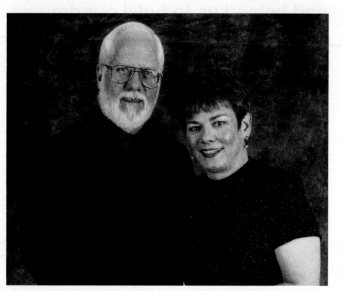

Dr. Engelkirk received his bachelor's degree in biology from New York University and his master's and doctorate degrees (both in microbiology and public health) from Michigan State University. He received additional medical technology and tropical medicine training at Walter Reed Army Hospital in Washington, D.C., and specialized training in anaerobic bacteriology, mycobacteriology, and virology at the Centers for Disease Control and Prevention in Atlanta, Georgia.

Dr. Engelkirk is an author of four microbiology textbooks, 10 additional book chapters, five medical laboratory-oriented self-study courses, and many scientific articles. He also served for 14 years as coeditor of four separate newsletters for clinical microbiology laboratory personnel. Dr. Engelkirk has been engaged in various aspects of clinical microbiology for over 50 years and is a past president of the Rocky Mountain Branch of the American Society for Microbiology. He and his wife, Janet, currently provide biomedical educational services through their consulting business, Biomedical Educational Services (Biomed Ed), located in Round Rock, Texas. Dr. Engelkirk's hobbies include traveling, hiking, nature photography, writing, and relaxing on his back deck.

Janet Duben-Engelkirk, EdD, MT(ASCP), has over 40 years of experience in clinical laboratory science and higher education. She received her bachelor's degrees in biology and medical technology and her master's degree in technical education from the University of Akron. She obtained her doctorate in allied health education and administration from a combined program at the University of Houston and Baylor College of Medicine in Houston, Texas.

Dr. Duben-Engelkirk began her career in clinical laboratory science education teaching students "on the bench" in a medical center hospital in Akron, Ohio. She then became Senior Education Coordinator and Associate Professor for the Clinical Laboratory Science Program at the University of Texas Health Science Center at Houston, where she taught clinical chemistry and related subjects for 12 years. In 1992, Dr. Duben-Engelkirk assumed the position of Director of Allied Health and Clinical Laboratory Science Education at Scott and White Hospital in Temple, Texas, wherein her responsibilities included teaching microbiology and clinical chemistry. In 2006, Dr. Duben-Engelkirk assumed the position of chair of the biotechnology department at the Texas Bioscience Institute and Temple College, where she was responsible for curriculum development and administration of the biotechnology degree programs. As a result of her efforts, the college received the prestigious Bellwether Award for innovative programs or practices. She and her husband, Paul, are currently co-owners of a biomedical educational consulting business.

Dr. Duben-Engelkirk was coeditor of a widely used clinical chemistry textbook and has coauthored three microbiology textbooks with Paul (clinical anaerobic bacteriology; laboratory diagnosis of infectious diseases; and this book). She has authored or coauthored numerous book chapters, journal articles, self-study courses, newsletters, and other educational materials over the course of her career.

Dr. Duben-Engelkirk has received many awards during her career, including Outstanding Young Leader in Allied Health, the American Society for Clinical Laboratory Science's Omicron Sigma Award for outstanding service, and Teaching Excellence Awards. Her professional interests include instructional technology, computer-based instruction, and distance education. Dr. Duben-Engelkirk enjoys traveling, reading, writing, music, yoga, movies, hiking, and photography.

Microbiology—the study of microbes—is a fascinating subject that impacts our daily lives in numerous ways. Microbes live on us and in us and virtually everywhere around us. They are vital in many industries. Microbes are essential for the cycling and recycling of elements such as carbon, oxygen, and nitrogen, and provide most of the oxygen in our atmosphere. They are used to clean up toxic wastes. Microbes are used in genetic engineering and gene therapy. And, of course, many microbes cause disease. In recent years, the public has been bombarded with news reports about microbe-associated medical problems such as swine flu, bird flu, severe acute respiratory syndrome (SARS), hantavirus pulmonary syndrome, flesh-eating bacteria, mad cow disease, superbugs, black mould in buildings, West Nile virus, bioterrorism, anthrax, smallpox, food recalls as a result of *Escherichia coli* and *Salmonella* contamination, and epidemics of meningitis, hepatitis, influenza, tuberculosis, whooping cough, and diarrheal diseases.

Written for Healthcare Professionals

Burton's Microbiology for the Health Sciences has been written primarily for nurses and other healthcare professionals. This book provides students of these professions with vital microbiology information that will enable them to carry out their duties in an informed, safe, and efficient manner, and protect themselves and their patients from infectious diseases. It is appropriate for use in any introductory microbiology course, as it contains all of the concepts and topics recommended by the American Society for Microbiology for such courses. Unlike many of the lengthy introductory microbiology texts on the market, *all* of the material in this book can be covered in a typical undergraduate microbiology course.

Chapters of special importance to students of the healthcare professions include those dealing with disinfection and sterilization (Chapter 8), antibiotics and other antimicrobial agents (Chapter 9), epidemiology and public health (Chapter 11), healthcare-associated infections and infection control (Chapter 12), how infectious diseases are diagnosed (Chapter 13), how microbes cause disease Chapter 14), how our bodies protect us from pathogens and infectious diseases (Chapters 15 and 16), and the major viral, bacterial, fungal, and parasitic diseases of humans (Chapters 17 through 21).

New to the Tenth Edition

The most obvious changes in the tenth edition are an increased number of full-color illustrations and improvement of the artwork. The book is divided into eight major sections, containing a total of 21 chapters. Each chapter contains a Chapter Outline, Learning Objectives, Self-Assessment Exercises, and information about the contents on thePoint. Interesting historical information, in the form of "Historical Notes," is spread throughout the book and is presented in appropriate chapters. Information summarizing important bacterial pathogens has been relocated from an appendix to Chapter 19. There are more Case Studies than in the ninth edition, and these, along with their answers, are located in the book rather than on thePoint. The number of Critical Thinking questions has been increased and are located on thePoint.

Student-Friendly Features

The authors have made every attempt to create a student-friendly book. The book can be used by all types of students, including those with little or no science background and mature students returning to school after an absence of several years. It is written in a clear and concise manner. It contains more than 50 Study Aid boxes, which explain difficult concepts and similar-sounding terms. Key points are highlighted. New terms are defined in the text and are included in a Glossary at the back of the book.

Answers to Self-Assessment Exercises contained in the book can be found in Appendix A. Appendix C contains useful formulas for conversion of one type of unit to another (e.g., Fahrenheit to Celsius and vice versa). Because Greek letters are commonly used in microbiology, the Greek alphabet can be found in Appendix D.

Additional Resources

Burton's Microbiology for the Health Sciences, 10th edition, includes additional resources for both instructors and students that are available on the book's companion Web site at http://thePoint.lww.com/Engelkirk10e.

Instructor Resources

Approved adopting instructors will be given access to the following additional resources:

- Image Bank
- Test Generator
- Lesson Plans
- PowerPoint Slides
- Clinical Microbiology Laboratory Procedures Manual

- Guidelines for Handling Microorganisms in the Teaching Laboratory
- Instructor's Guide
  - Answers to Critical Thinking Questions
  - Laboratory Activities

Student Resources

Students who have purchased *Burton's Microbiology for the Health Sciences, 10th edition*, have access to the following additional resources:

- Animations covering various topics in the text
- Interactive Quiz Bank
- Student Guide
  - Additional Self-Assessment Exercises for each chapter
  - Lists of new terms in each chapter
  - Review of Key Points
  - Special "A Closer Look," "Increase Your Knowledge," and "Critical Thinking" sections to provide additional insight as well as interesting facts on selected topics from the text
- Appendix 1: Microbial Intoxications
- Appendix 2: Phyla and Medically Important Genera Within the Domain *Bacteria*
- Appendix 3: Basic Chemistry Concepts
- Appendix 4: Responsibilities of the Clinical Microbiology Laboratory
- Appendix 5: Clinical Microbiology Procedures
- Appendix 6: Preparing Solutions and Dilutions

Purchasers of the text can access the resources online at the *Burton's Microbiology for the Health Sciences, 10th edition*, Web site at http://thePoint.lww.com/Engelkirk10e. See the inside front cover of this text for more details, including the passcode you will need to gain access to the Web site.

To Our Readers

As you will discover, the concise nature of this book makes each sentence significant. Thus, you will be intellectually challenged to learn each new concept as it is presented. It is our hope that you will enjoy your study of microbiology and be motivated to further explore this exciting field, especially as it relates to your occupation. Many students who have used this textbook in their introductory microbiology course have gone on to become infection control nurses, epidemiologists, medical laboratory professionals, and microbiologists.

Our Thanks

We are deeply indebted to the late **Gwen Burton, Ph.D.**—sole author of the first four editions of this book and coauthor of the next four. Her spirit lives on in the pages of this, the tenth edition. We can only hope that she would be as proud of what her creation has become as we are. We are also grateful to all of the Lippincott Williams & Wilkins people who helped with the editing and publication of this book, including Paula Williams, Product Development Editor; Michael Nobel, Acquisitions Editor; Leah Thomson, Marketing Manager; Priscilla Crater, Production Project Manager; and Terry Mallon, Designer.

Paul G. Engelkirk, PhD, MT(ASCP), SM(NRCM)
Janet Duben-Engelkirk, EdD, MT(ASCP)

In today's health careers, a thorough understanding of microbiology is more important than ever. *Burton's Microbiology for the Health Sciences, Tenth Edition*, not only provides the conceptual knowledge you will need but also teaches you how to apply it. This User's Guide introduces you to the features and tools of this innovative textbook. Each feature is specifically designed to enhance your learning experience, preparing you for a successful career as a health professional.

Chapter Opener Features

The features that open each chapter are an introduction to guide you through the remainder of the lesson.

Chapter Outline

Serves as a "roadmap" to the material ahead.

Learning Objectives

Highlight important concepts—helping you to organize and prioritize learning.

Introduction

Familiarizes you with the material covered in the chapter.

Chapter Features

The following features appear throughout the body of the chapter. They are designed to hone critical thinking skills and judgment, build clinical proficiency, and promote comprehension and retention of the material.

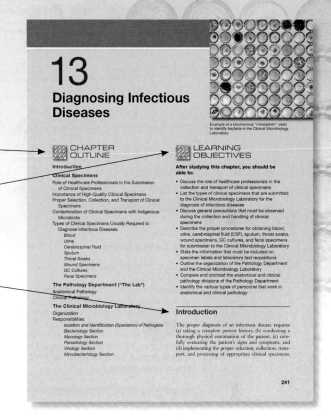

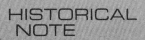

Historical Note Boxes

Provide insight into the history and development of microbiology and healthcare.

SPOTLIGHTING

Phlebotomists

As stated in the American Medical Association's Health Care Careers Directory (available under "Education," "Health Service Careers Directory" at http://www.ama-assn .org), "Phlebotomists collect, transport, handle, and process blood specimens for analysis; identify and select equipment, supplies, and additives used in blood collection; and understand factors that affect specimen collection procedures and test results. Recognizing the importance of specimen collection in the overall patient care system, phlebotomists adhere to infection control and safety policies and procedures. They practice safe blood collection and handling techniques that protect patients from injury, safeguard themselves from accidents, and produce high-quality specimens while demonstrating compassion for the patient. Phlebotomists monitor quality control within predetermined limits while demonstrating professional conduct, stress management, and communication skills with patients, peers, and other healthcare personnel as well as with the public." Information concerning educational requirements and programs, certification, and salary is available at the AMA Web site.

Spotlighting Boxes

These are a new feature spotlighting healthcare careers.

STUDY AID

The Central Dogma

The term "dogma" usually refers to a basic or fundamental doctrinal point in religion or philosophy. Francis Crick's use of the term "Central Dogma" refers to the most fundamental process of molecular biology—the flow of genetic information within a cell. Although originally referred to as the one gene–one protein hypothesis, it is now known that a particular gene may code for one or more proteins.

Study Aid Boxes

Summarize key information, explain difficult concepts, and differentiate similar-sounding terms.

CLINICAL PROCEDURE

CCMS Urine Collection Procedure for Female Patients

Purpose: To instruct a female in how to properly collect a CCMS urine specimen.
Equipment: Requisition, specimen label, sterile urine container, special sterile antiseptic wipes, and copy of written instructions.

Step	Rationale
1. Wash hands thoroughly.	Aids in infection control and helps avoid contamination of the site while cleaning.
2. Remove the lid of the container, being careful not to touch the inside of the cover or the container.	The lid and container must remain sterile for accurate interpretation of results.
3. Stand in a squatting position over the toilet.	Facilitates cleaning and downward flow of urine.
4. Separate the folds of skin around the urinary opening.	Allows proper cleaning of the area.

Clinical Procedure Boxes

Set forth step-by-step instructions for common procedures.

Something To Think About

These boxes contain information that will stimulate students to ponder interesting possibilities.

SOMETHING TO THINK ABOUT

"In addition to diagnosing infections caused by well-established pathogens, clinical microbiologists uncover new pathogens, acting as sentinels for possible epidemics. They also provide statistical and clinical information regarding pathogens on the scene and spur demands on research to create novel diagnostic tools. In fact, development of such tools is taking place so swiftly that, in not too many years, the practice of clinical microbiology may well become unrecognizable. Not only is the use of nucleic acid-based techniques expected to expand, but other sophisticated techniques such as mass spectrometry will make microbiological diagnoses ever more rapid and accurate."

Schaechter E. The excitement of clinical microbiology. *Microbe*. 2013;8:11–14.

Key Points

Help you pinpoint the main ideas of the text.

chemistry as part of a microbiology course. The reason why chemistry is an important component of a microbiology course is the answer to the question, "What exactly is a microorganism?" A cellular microbe can be thought of as a "bag" of chemicals that interact with each other in various ways. Even the bag itself is composed of chemicals. Everything a microorganism is and does relates to chemistry. The various ways microorganisms function and survive in their envi-

> Cells can be thought of as "bags" of chemicals. Even the bags themselves are composed of chemicals.

Self-Assessment Exercises

Help you gauge your understanding of what you have learned.

Self-Assessment Exercises

After studying this chapter, answer the following multiple-choice questions.

1. Molecules of extrachromosomal DNA are also known as:
   a. Golgi bodies
   b. lysosomes
   c. plasmids
   d. plastids

2. A bacterium possessing a tuft of flagella at one end of its cell would be called what kind of bacterium?
   a. amphitrichous
   b. lophotrichous
   c. monotrichous
   d. peritrichous

ON thePoint

- Terms Introduced in This Chapter
- Review of Key Points
- Spotlighting: Asexual versus Sexual Reproduction; Life Cycles; Eukaryotic Cell Reproduction (Mitosis and Meiosis)
- The Origin of Mitochondria and Chloroplasts
- Increase Your Knowledge
- Critical Thinking
- Additional Self-Assessment Exercises

On thePoint Boxes

Directs you to additional content and exercises for review on thePoint. Included are the following features that help reinforce and review the material covered in the book.

Reviewers

Dr. Patrick Godfrey
Microbiology Department
Prairie State College
Chicago Heights, Illinois

Robert Leunk, PhD
Associate Professor
Department of Biological Sciences
Grand Rapids Community College
Grand Rapids, Michigan

Suzanne Long, MS
Professor
Biology Department
Monroe Community College
Rochester, New York

Mark Pilgrim, PhD
Assistant Professor
Biology Department
Lander University
Greenwood, South Carolina

Veronica Riha, PhD
Associate Professor
Biology Department
Madonna University
Livonia, Michigan

Patricia Sjolie, MS
Instructor
Science Department
MSCTC-Fergus Falls
Perham, Minnesota

David Wartell, MS
Sr. Instructional Technology Specialist/Adjunct Faculty
Biology Department
Harrisburg Area Community College
Harrisburg, Pennsylvania

Contents

Section V   Environmental and Applied Microbiology

Section VI   Microbiology within Healthcare Facilities

Section VII   Pathogenesis and Host Defense Mechanisms

1

Microbiology — The Science

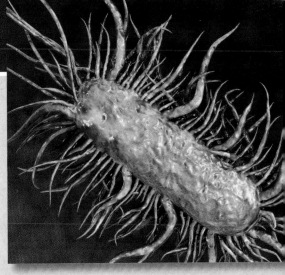

Artist rendering of an *Escherichia coli (E. coli)* bacterial cell, one of the most thoroughly studied of all microbes.

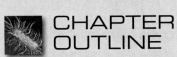

CHAPTER OUTLINE

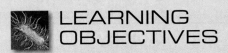

LEARNING OBJECTIVES

After studying this chapter, you should be able to:

- Define microbiology, pathogen, nonpathogen, and opportunistic pathogen
- Differentiate between acellular microbes and microorganisms and list several examples of each
- List several reasons why microbes are important (e.g., as a source of antibiotics)
- Explain the relationship between microbes and infectious diseases
- Differentiate between infectious diseases and microbial intoxications

- List some of the contributions of Leeuwenhoek, Pasteur, and Koch to microbiology
- Differentiate between biogenesis and abiogenesis
- Explain the germ theory of disease
- Outline Koch's Postulates and cite some circumstances in which they may not apply
- Discuss two medically related fields of microbiology

Introduction

Welcome to the fascinating world of microbiology, where you will learn about creatures so small that the vast majority cannot be seen with the naked eye. In this chapter, you will discover the effects that these tiny creatures have on our daily lives, the ecosystems, and the environment around us, and why knowledge of them is of great importance to healthcare professionals. You will learn that some of them are our friends, whereas others are our enemies. You are about to embark on an exciting journey. Enjoy the adventure!

What Is Microbiology?

The study of microbiology is essentially an advanced biology course. Ideally, students taking microbiology will have some background in biology. Although **biology** is the study of *living* organisms (from *bios*, referring to living organisms, and *logy*, meaning "the study of"), microbiology includes the study of certain nonliving entities as well as certain living organisms. Collectively, these nonliving entities and living organisms

> Microbiology is the study of microbes. With only rare exceptions, individual microbes can be observed only with the use of various types of microscopes.

1

The two major categories of microbes are called acellular microbes (also called infectious particles) and cellular microbes (also called microorganisms). Acellular microbes include viruses and prions. Cellular microbes include all bacteria, all archaea, all protozoa, some algae, and some fungi.

are called **microbes**. *Micro* means very small—anything so small that it must be viewed with a **microscope** (an optical instrument used to observe very small objects). Therefore, **microbiology** can be defined as the *study of microbes*. With only rare exceptions (described in Chapter 4), individual microbes can be observed only with the use of various types of microscopes. Microbes are said to be *ubiquitous*, meaning they are virtually everywhere.

The various categories of microbes include viruses, bacteria, archaea, protozoa, and certain types of algae and fungi (Fig. 1-1). These categories of microbes are discussed in detail in Chapters 4 and 5. Because most scientists do not consider viruses to be living organisms, they are often referred to as "acellular microbes" or "infectious particles" rather than microorganisms.

Your first introduction to microbes may have been when your mother warned you about "germs" (Fig. 1-2). Although not a scientific term, germs are the microbes that cause disease. Your mother worried that you might become infected with these types of microbes. Disease-causing microorganisms are technically known as **pathogens** (also referred to as infectious agents) (Table 1-1). Actually, only about

Microbes that cause disease are known as pathogens. Those that do not cause disease are called nonpathogens.

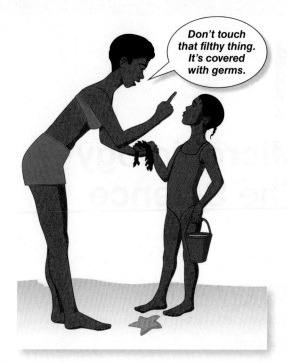

Don't touch that filthy thing. It's covered with germs.

Figure 1-2. "Germs." In all likelihood, your mother was your first microbiology instructor. Not only did she alert you to the fact that there were "invisible" critters in the world that could harm you, she also taught you the fundamentals of hygiene—like hand washing.

3% of known microbes are capable of causing disease (i.e., only about 3% are pathogenic). Thus, the vast majority of known microbes are **nonpathogens**—microbes that do not cause disease. Some nonpathogens are beneficial to us, whereas others have no effect on us at all. In newspapers and on television, we read and hear more about pathogens than we do about nonpathogens, but in this book you will learn about both categories—the microbes that help us ("microbial allies") and those that harm us ("microbial enemies").

Why Study Microbiology?

Although they are very small, microbes play significant roles in our lives. Listed below are a few of the many reasons to take a microbiology course and to learn about microbes:

- We have, living on and in our bodies (e.g., on our skin and in our mouths and intestinal tract), approximately 10 times as many microbes as the total number of cells (i.e., epithelial cells, nerve cells, muscle cells, etc.) that make up our bodies (10 trillion cells × 10 = 100 trillion microbes). It has been estimated

The microbes that live on and in the human body are referred to as our indigenous microbiota.

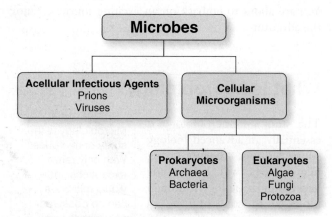

Figure 1-1. Acellular and cellular microbes. Acellular microbes (also known as infectious particles) include prions and viruses. Cellular microbes include the less complex **prokaryotes** (organisms composed of cells that lack a true nucleus, such as archaea and bacteria) and the more complex **eukaryotes** (organisms composed of cells that contain a true nucleus, such as algae, protozoa, and fungi). Prokaryotes and eukaryotes are discussed more fully in Chapter 3.

Table 1-1 Pathogens

Category	Examples of Diseases They Cause
Algae	A very rare cause of infections, but they can cause intoxications (which result from ingestion of toxins)
Bacteria	Anthrax, botulism, cholera, diarrhea, diphtheria, ear and eye infections, food poisoning, gas gangrene, gonorrhea, hemolytic uremic syndrome (HUS), intoxications, Legionnaires disease, leprosy, Lyme disease, meningitis, plague, pneumonia, spotted fever, scarlet fever rickettsiosis, staph infections, strep throat, syphilis, tetanus, tuberculosis, tularemia, typhoid fever, typhus, urethritis, urinary tract infections, whooping cough
Fungi	Allergies, cryptococcosis, histoplasmosis, intoxications, meningitis, pneumonia, thrush, tinea (ringworm) infections, yeast vaginitis
Protozoa	African sleeping sickness, amebic dysentery, babesiosis, Chagas disease, cryptosporidiosis, diarrhea, giardiasis, malaria, meningoencephalitis, pneumonia, toxoplasmosis, trichomoniasis
Viruses	AIDS, "bird flu," certain types of cancer, chickenpox, cold sores (fever blisters), common cold, dengue, diarrhea, encephalitis, genital herpes infections, German measles, hantavirus pulmonary syndrome (HPS), hemorrhagic fevers, hepatitis, infectious mononucleosis, influenza, measles, meningitis, monkeypox, mumps, pneumonia, polio, rabies, severe acute respiratory syndrome (SARS), shingles, smallpox, "swine flu," warts, yellow fever

that perhaps as many as 500 to 1,000 different species of microbes live on and in us. Collectively, these microbes are known as our **indigenous microbiota** (or human microbiome or human bioneme)[a] and, for the most part, they are of benefit to us. For example, the indigenous microbiota inhibit the growth of pathogens in those areas of the body where they live by occupying space, depleting the food supply, and secreting materials (waste products, toxins, antibiotics, etc.) that may prevent or reduce the growth of pathogens. Indigenous microbiota are discussed more fully in Chapter 10.

- Some of the microbes that colonize (inhabit) our bodies are known as **opportunistic pathogens** (or *opportunists*). Although these microbes usually do not cause us any problems, they have the potential to cause infections if they gain access to a part of our anatomy where they do not belong. For example, a bacterium called *Escherichia coli* (*E. coli*) lives in our intestinal tracts. This organism does not cause us any harm as long as it remains in our intestinal tract, but can cause disease if it gains access to our urinary bladder, bloodstream, or a wound. Other opportunistic pathogens strike when a person becomes run-down, stressed out, or debilitated (weakened) as a result of some disease or condition. Thus, opportunistic pathogens can be thought of as microbes awaiting the opportunity to cause disease.

> Opportunistic pathogens do not cause disease under ordinary conditions, but have the potential to cause disease should the opportunity present itself.

- Microbes are essential for life on this planet as we know it. For example, some microbes produce oxygen by the process known as **photosynthesis** (discussed in Chapter 7). Actually, microbes contribute more oxygen to our atmosphere than do plants. Thus, organisms that require oxygen—humans, for example—owe a debt of gratitude to the algae and cyanobacteria (a group of photosynthetic bacteria) that produce oxygen.

- Many microbes are involved in the decomposition of dead organisms and the waste products of living organisms. Collectively, these microbes are referred to as **decomposers** or **saprophytes**. Decomposition is the process by which substances are broken down into simpler forms of matter. By definition, a saprophyte is an organism that lives on dead or decaying organic matter. Imagine living in a world with no decomposers. Not a pleasant thought! Saprophytes aid in fertilization by returning inorganic nutrients to the soil. They break down dead and dying organic materials (plants and animals) into nitrates, phosphates, and other chemicals necessary for the growth of plants (Fig. 1-3).

- Some microbes are capable of decomposing industrial wastes (oil spills, for example). Thus, we can use microbes—genetically engineered microbes, in some cases—to clean up after ourselves. The use of microbes in this manner is called **bioremediation**, a topic discussed in more detail in Chapter 10. **Genetic engineering** is discussed briefly in a following section and more fully in Chapter 7.

- Many microbes are involved in elemental cycles, such as the carbon, nitrogen, oxygen, sulfur, and phosphorous cycles. In the nitrogen cycle, certain bacteria convert nitrogen gas in the air to ammonia in the soil. Other soil bacteria then convert the ammonia to nitrites and nitrates. Still other bacteria convert the nitrogen in nitrates to nitrogen gas, thus completing the cycle (Fig. 1-4). Knowledge of these microbes is important to farmers who practice crop rotation to

---

[a]Use of the older terms "normal flora" and "indigenous microflora" is discouraged because "flora" refers to plants. Microbes are *not* plants.

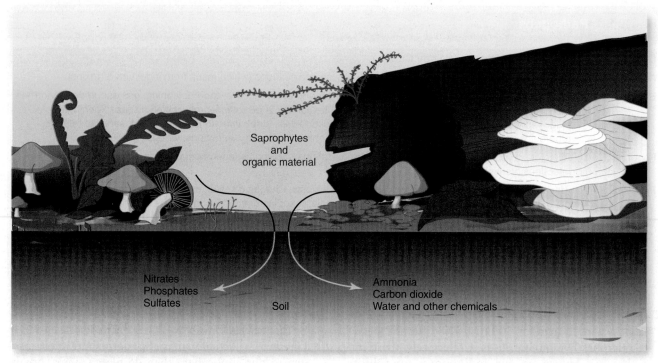

Figure 1-3. Saprophytes. Saprophytes break down dead and decaying organic material into inorganic nutrients in the soil.

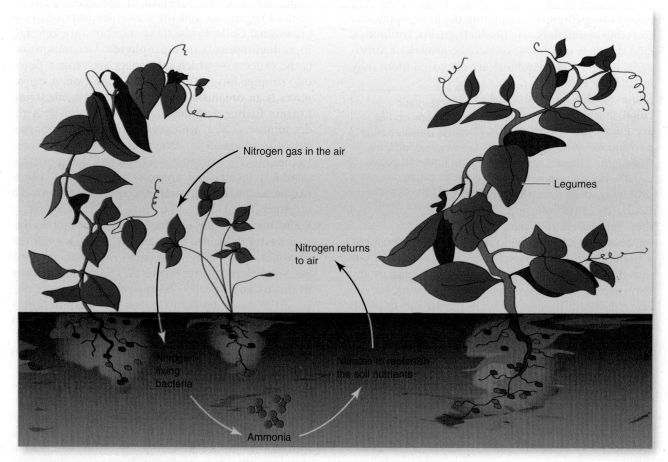

Figure 1-4. Nitrogen fixation. Nitrogen-fixing bacteria that live on or near the roots of legumes convert free nitrogen from the air into ammonia in the soil. Nitrifying bacteria then convert the ammonia into nitrites and nitrates, which are nutrients used by plants.

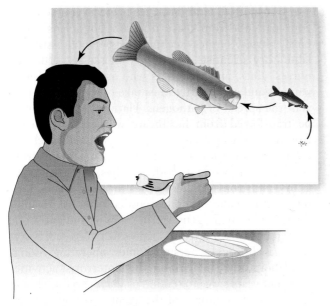

Figure 1-5. Food chain. Tiny living organisms such as bacteria, algae, microscopic aquatic plants (e.g., phytoplankton), and microscopic aquatic animals (e.g., zooplankton) are eaten by larger animals, which in turn are eaten by still larger animals, etc., until an animal in the chain is consumed by a human. Humans are at the top of the food chain.

replenish nutrients in their fields and to gardeners who keep compost pits as a source of natural fertilizer. In both cases, dead organic material is broken down into inorganic nutrients (e.g., nitrates and phosphates) by microbes. The study of the relationships between microbes and the environment is called **microbial ecology**. Microbial ecology and the nitrogen cycle are discussed more fully in Chapter 10.

- Algae and bacteria serve as food for tiny animals. Then, larger animals eat the smaller creatures, and so on. Thus, microbes serve as important links in food chains (Fig. 1-5). Microscopic organisms in the ocean, collectively referred to as **plankton**, serve as the starting point of many food chains. Tiny marine plants and algae are called **phytoplankton**, whereas tiny marine animals are called **zooplankton**.

- Some microbes live in the intestinal tracts of animals, where they aid in the digestion of food and, in some cases, produce substances that are of value to the host animal. For example, the *E. coli* bacteria that live in the human intestinal tract produce vitamins K and B_1, which are absorbed and used by the human body. Although termites eat wood, they cannot digest wood. Fortunately for them, termites have cellulose-eating protozoa in their intestinal tracts that break down the wood that the termites consume into smaller molecules that the termites can use as nutrients.

- Many microbes are essential in various food and beverage industries, whereas others are used to produce certain enzymes and chemicals (Table 1-2). The use of living organisms or their derivatives to make or modify useful products or processes is called **biotechnology**, an exciting and timely topic that is discussed more fully in Chapter 10.

- Some bacteria and fungi produce antibiotics that are used to treat patients with infectious diseases. By definition, an **antibiotic** is a substance produced by a microbe that is effective in killing or inhibiting the growth of other microbes. The use of microbes in the antibiotic industry is an example of biotechnology. Production of antibiotics by microbes is discussed in Chapter 9.

- Microbes are essential in the field of genetic engineering. In genetic engineering, a gene or genes from one organism (e.g., from a bacterium, a human, an animal, or a plant) is/are inserted into a bacterial or yeast cell. Because a gene contains the instructions for the production of a gene product (usually a protein), the cell that receives a new gene can now produce whatever product is coded for by that gene; so too can all of the cells that arise from the original cell. Microbiologists have engineered bacteria and yeasts to produce a variety of useful substances, such as insulin, various types of growth hormones, interferons, and materials for use as vaccines. Genetic engineering is discussed more fully in Chapter 7.

- For many years, microbes have been used as "cell models." The more the scientists learned about the

Category	Examples
Foods	Acidophilus milk, bread, butter, buttermilk, chocolate, coffee, fish sauces, green olives, kimchi (from cabbage), meat products (e.g., country-cured hams, sausage, salami), pickles, poi (fermented taro root), sauerkraut, sour cream, sourdough bread, soy sauce, various cheeses (e.g., cottage cheese, cream cheese, cheddar, Swiss, Limburger, Camembert, Roquefort, and other blue cheeses), vinegar, yogurt
Alcoholic beverages	Ale, beer, brandy, sake (rice wine), rum, sherry, vodka, whiskey, wine
Chemicals	Acetic acid, acetone, butanol, citric acid, ethanol, formic acid, glycerol, isopropanol, lactic acid
Antibiotics	Amphotericin B, bacitracin, cephalosporins, chloramphenicol, cycloheximide, cycloserine, erythromycin, griseofulvin, kanamycin, lincomycin, neomycin, novobiocin, nystatin, penicillin, polymyxin B, streptomycin, tetracycline

Table 1-2 Products Requiring Microbial Participation in the Manufacturing Process

structure and functions of microbial cells, the more they learned about cells in general. The intestinal bacterium *E. coli* is one of the most studied of all microbes. By studying *E. coli*, scientists have learned a great deal about the composition and inner workings of cells, including human cells.

- Finally, we come to diseases. Microbes cause two categories of diseases: infectious diseases and microbial intoxications (Fig. 1-6). An **infectious disease** results when a pathogen colonizes the body and subsequently causes disease. A **microbial intoxication** results when a person ingests a *toxin* (poisonous substance) that has been produced by a microbe. Of the two categories, infectious diseases cause far more illnesses and deaths. Infectious diseases are the leading cause of death in the world and the third leading cause of death in the United States (after heart disease and cancer). Worldwide, infectious diseases cause about 50,000 deaths per day, with the majority of deaths occurring in developing countries. Anyone pursuing a career in a healthcare profession must be aware of infectious diseases, the pathogens that cause them, the sources of the pathogens, how these diseases

> Pathogens cause two major types of diseases: infectious diseases and microbial intoxications.

are transmitted, and how to protect yourself and your patients from these diseases. Physicians' assistants, nurses, surgical technologists, dental assistants, laboratory scientists, respiratory therapists, orderlies, nurses' aides, and all others who are associated with patients and patient care must take precautions to prevent the spread of pathogens. Harmful microbes may be transferred from healthcare workers to patients; from patient to patient; from contaminated mechanical devices, instruments, and syringes to patients; from contaminated bedding, clothes, dishes, and food to patients; and from patients to healthcare workers, hospital visitors, and other susceptible persons. To limit the spread of pathogens, sterile, aseptic, and antiseptic techniques (discussed in Chapter 12) are used everywhere in hospitals, nursing homes, operating rooms, and laboratories. In addition, the bioterrorist activities of recent years serve to remind us that everyone should have an understanding of the agents (pathogens) that are involved and how to protect ourselves from becoming infected. Bioterrorist and biological warfare agents are discussed in Chapter 11. Additional information about microbial intoxications can be found in Appendix 1 on thePoint: "Microbial Intoxications."

First Microorganisms on Earth

Perhaps you have wondered how long microbes have existed on Earth. Scientists tell us that Earth was formed about 4.5 billion years ago and, for the first 800 million to 1 billion years of Earth's existence, there was no life on this planet. Fossils of primitive microbes (as many as 11 different types) found in ancient sandstone formations in northwestern Australia date back to about 3.5 billion years ago. By comparison, animals and humans are relative newcomers. Animals made their appearance on Earth between 900 and 650 million years ago (there is some disagreement in the scientific community about the exact date), and, in their present form, humans (*Homo sapiens*) have existed for only the past 100,000 years or so. Candidates for the first microbes on Earth are archaea and cyanobacteria; these types of microbes are discussed in Chapter 4.

Infectious Disease	Microbial Intoxication
A pathogen colonizes a person's body.	A pathogen produces a toxin in vitro.
The pathogen causes a disease.	A person ingests the toxin. The toxin causes a disease.
This type of disease is known as an infectious disease.	This type of disease is known as a microbial intoxication.
Examples: • MRSA infection • Gas gangrene	Examples: • Staphylococcal food poisoning • Foodborne botulism

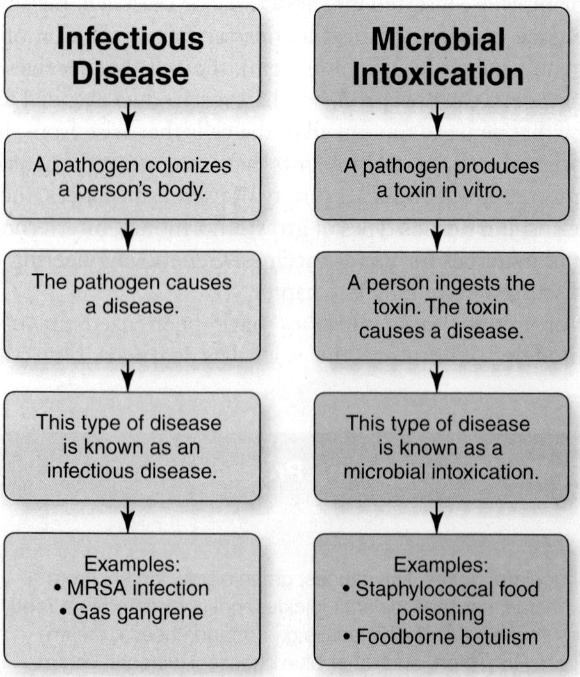

Figure 1-6. The two categories of diseases caused by pathogens. Infectious diseases result when a pathogen colonizes (inhabits) the body and subsequently causes disease. Microbial intoxications result when a person ingests a toxin (poisonous substance) that has been produced by a pathogen in vitro (outside the body). MRSA, methicillin-resistant *Staphylococcus aureus*.

Earliest Known Infectious Diseases

In all likelihood, infectious diseases of humans and animals have existed for as long as humans and animals have inhabited the planet. We know that human pathogens have existed for thousands of years because damage caused by them has been observed in the bones and internal organs of mummies and early human fossils. By studying mummies, scientists have learned that bacterial diseases, such as tuberculosis, leprosy, and syphilis, malaria, hepatitis, and parasitic worm infections, such as schistosomiasis, dracunculiasis (guinea worm infection), hookworm, and fluke and tapeworm infections, have been around for a very long time.

The earliest known account of a "pestilence" occurred in Egypt about 3180 BC. This may represent the first recorded epidemic, although words such as *pestilence* and *plague* were used without definition in early writings. Around 1900 BC, near the end of the Trojan War, the Greek army was decimated by an epidemic of what is thought to have been bubonic plague. The Ebers papyrus, describing epidemic fevers, was discovered in a tomb in Thebes, Egypt; it was written around 1500 BC. A disease thought to be smallpox occurred in China around 1122 BC. Epidemics of plague occurred in Rome in 790, 710, and 640 BC, and in Greece around 430 BC.

In addition to the diseases already mentioned, there are early accounts of rabies, anthrax, dysentery, smallpox, ergotism, botulism, measles, typhoid fever, typhus fever, diphtheria, and syphilis. The syphilis story is quite interesting. It made its first appearance in Europe in 1493. Many people believe that syphilis was carried to Europe by Native Americans who were brought to Portugal by Christopher Columbus. The French called syphilis the *Neapolitan disease*; the Italians called it the *French or Spanish disease*; and the English called it the *French pox*. Other names for syphilis were Spanish, German, Polish, and Turkish pocks. The name "syphilis" was not given to the disease until 1530.

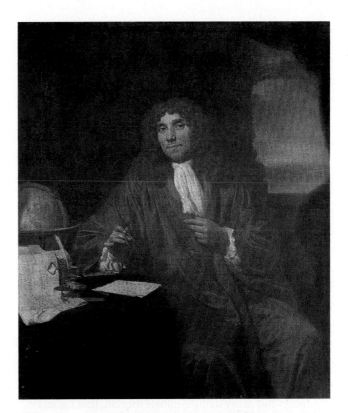

Figure 1-7. Portrait of Anton van Leeuwenhoek by Jan Verkolje. (Courtesy of Wikipedia.)

Pioneers in the Science of Microbiology

Bacteria and protozoa were the first microbes to be observed by humans. It then took about 200 years before a connection was established between microbes and infectious diseases. Among the most significant events in the early history of microbiology were the development of microscopes, bacterial staining procedures, techniques that enabled microorganisms to be cultured (grown) in the laboratory, and steps that could be taken to prove that specific microbes were responsible for causing specific infectious diseases. During the past 400 years, many individuals contributed to our present understanding of microbes. Three early microbiologists are discussed in this chapter; others are discussed at appropriate points throughout the book.

Anton van Leeuwenhoek (1632–1723)

Because Anton van Leeuwenhoek was the first person to see live bacteria and protozoa, he is sometimes referred to as the "Father of Microbiology," the "Father

of Bacteriology," and the "Father of Protozoology."[b] Interestingly, Leeuwenhoek was not a trained scientist. At various times in his life, he was a fabric merchant, a surveyor, a wine assayer, and a minor city official in Delft, Holland. As a hobby, he ground tiny glass lenses, which he mounted in small metal frames, thus creating what today are known as **single-lens microscopes** or **simple microscopes**. During his lifetime, he made more than 500 of these microscopes. Leeuwenhoek's fine art of grinding lenses that would magnify an object to 200 to 300 times its size was lost at his death because he had not taught this skill to anyone during his lifetime. In one of the hundreds of letters that he sent to the Royal Society of London, he wrote:

> My method for seeing the very smallest animalcules I do not impart to others; nor how to see very many animalcules at one time. This I keep for myself alone.

Apparently, Leeuwenhoek had an unquenchable curiosity, as he used his microscopes to examine almost anything he could get his hands on (Fig. 1-7). He examined

---

[b]Although Leeuwenhoek was probably the first person to see live protozoa, he may not have been the first person to observe protozoa. Many scholars believe that Robert Hooke (1635–1703), an English physician, was the first person to observe and describe microbes, including a fossilized protozoan and two species of live microfungi.

scrapings from his teeth, water from ditches and ponds, water in which he had soaked peppercorns, blood, sperm, and even his own diarrheal stools. In many of these specimens, he observed various tiny living creatures, which he called "animalcules." He recorded his observations in the form of letters, which he sent to the Royal Society of London. The following passage is an excerpt from one of those letters (*Milestones in Microbiology*, edited by Thomas Brock. American Society for Microbiology, Washington, DC, 1961):

> Tho my teeth are kept usually very clean, nevertheless when I view them in a Magnifying Glass, I find growing between them a little white matter as thick as wetted flower. . . . I therefore took some of this flower and mixt it . . . with pure rain water wherein were no Animals. and then to my great surprize perceived that the aforesaid matter contained very many small living Animals, which moved themselves very extravagantly. . . . The number of these Animals in the scurf of a mans Teeth, are so many that I believe they exceed the number of Men in a kingdom. For upon the examination of a small parcel of it, no thicker than a Horse-hair, I found too many living Animals therein, that I guess there might have been 1000 in a quantity of matter no bigger than the 1/100 part of a sand.

Leeuwenhoek's letters finally convinced scientists of the late 17th century of the existence of microbes. Leeuwenhoek never speculated on their origin, nor did he associate them with the cause of disease. Such relationships were not established until the work of Louis Pasteur and Robert Koch in the late 19th century.

The following quote is from Paul de Kruif's book, *Microbe Hunters*, Harcourt Brace, 1926:

> [Leeuwenhoek] had stolen and peeped into a fantastic sub-visible world of little things, creatures that had lived, had bred, had battled, had died, completely hidden from and unknown to all men from the beginning of time. Beasts these were of a kind that ravaged and annihilated whole races of men ten million times larger than they were themselves. Beings these were, more terrible than fire-spitting dragons or hydra-headed monsters. They were silent assassins that murdered babes in warm cradles and kings in sheltered places. It was this invisible, insignificant, but implacable—and sometimes friendly—world that Leeuwenhoek had looked into for the first time of all men of all countries.

Once scientists became convinced of the existence of tiny creatures that could not be observed with the naked eye, they began to speculate on their origin. On the basis of observation, many of the scientists of that time believed that life could develop spontaneously from inanimate substances, such as decaying corpses, soil, and

swamp gases. The idea that life can arise spontaneously from nonliving material is called the theory of spontaneous generation or **abiogenesis**. For more than two centuries, from 1650 to 1850, this theory was debated and tested. Following the work of others, Louis Pasteur (discussed later) and John Tyndall (discussed in Chapter 3) finally disproved the theory of spontaneous generation and proved that life can only arise from preexisting life. This is called the theory of **biogenesis**, first proposed by a German scientist named Rudolf Virchow in 1858. Note that the theory of biogenesis does not speculate on the *origin* of life, a subject that has been discussed and debated for hundreds of years.

Louis Pasteur (1822–1895)

Louis Pasteur (Fig. 1-8), a French chemist, made numerous contributions to the newly emerging field of microbiology, and, in fact, his contributions are considered by many people to be the foundation of the science of microbiology and a cornerstone of modern medicine. Listed below are some of his most significant contributions:

• While attempting to discover why wine becomes contaminated with undesirable substances, Pasteur

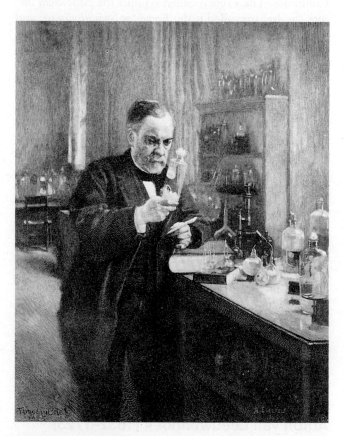

Figure 1-8. Pasteur in his laboratory. A 1925 wood engraving by Timothy Cole. (From Zigrosser C. *Medicine and the Artist* [Ars Medica]. New York: Dover Publications, Inc.; 1970. With permission from the Philadelphia Museum of Art.)

discovered what occurs during alcoholic fermentation (discussed in Chapter 7). He also demonstrated that different types of microbes produce different fermentation products. For example, yeasts convert the glucose in grapes to ethyl alcohol (ethanol) by fermentation, but certain contaminating bacteria, such as *Acetobacter*, convert glucose to acetic acid (vinegar) by fermentation, thus, ruining the taste of the wine.

- Through his experiments, Pasteur dealt the fatal blow to the theory of spontaneous generation.
- Pasteur discovered forms of life that could exist in the absence of oxygen. He introduced the terms "aerobes" (organisms that require oxygen) and "anaerobes" (organisms that do not require oxygen).
- Pasteur developed a process (today known as pasteurization) to kill microbes that were causing wine to spoil—an economic concern to France's wine industry. **Pasteurization** can be used to kill pathogens in many types of liquids. Pasteur's process involved heating wine to 55°C[c] and holding it at that temperature for several minutes. Today, pasteurization is accomplished by heating liquids to 63°C to 65°C for 30 minutes or to 73°C to 75°C for 15 seconds. It should be noted that pasteurization does not kill *all* of the microbes in liquids—just the pathogens.
- Pasteur discovered the infectious agents that caused the silkworm diseases that were crippling the silk industry in France. He also discovered how to prevent such diseases.
- Pasteur made significant contributions to the germ theory of disease—the theory that specific microbes cause specific infectious diseases. For example, anthrax is caused by a specific bacterium (*Bacillus anthracis*), whereas tuberculosis is caused by a different bacterium (*Mycobacterium tuberculosis*).
- Pasteur championed changes in hospital practices to minimize the spread of disease by pathogens.
- Pasteur developed vaccines to prevent chicken cholera, anthrax, and swine erysipelas (a skin disease). It was the development of these vaccines that made him famous in France. Before the vaccines, these diseases were decimating chickens, sheep, cattle, and pigs in that country—a serious economic problem.
- Pasteur developed a vaccine to prevent rabies in dogs and successfully used the vaccine to treat human rabies. (See the following Historical Note.)

To honor Pasteur and continue his work, especially in the development of a rabies vaccine, the Pasteur Institute was created in Paris in 1888. It became a clinic for rabies treatment, a research center for infectious diseases, and a teaching center. Many scientists who studied under

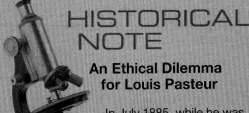

HISTORICAL NOTE

An Ethical Dilemma for Louis Pasteur

In July 1885, while he was developing a vaccine that would prevent rabies in dogs, Louis Pasteur faced an ethical decision. A 9-year-old boy, named Joseph Meister, had been bitten 14 times on the legs and hands by a rabid dog. At the time, it was assumed that virtually anyone who was bitten by a rabid animal would die. Meister's mother begged Pasteur to use his vaccine to save her son. Pasteur was a chemist, not a physician, and thus was not authorized to treat humans. Also, his experimental vaccine had never been administered to a human being. Nonetheless, 2 days after the boy had been bitten, Pasteur injected Meister with the vaccine in an attempt to save the boy's life. The boy survived, and Pasteur realized that he had developed a rabies vaccine that could be administered to a person after he or she had been infected with rabies virus.

Pasteur went on to make important discoveries of their own and create a vast international network of Pasteur Institutes. The first of the foreign institutes was founded in Saigon, Vietnam, which is today known as Ho Chi Minh City. One of the directors of that institute was Alexandre Emile Jean Yersin—a former student of Robert Koch and Louis Pasteur—who, in 1894, discovered the bacterium that causes plague.

Robert Koch (1843–1910)

Robert Koch (Fig. 1-9), a German physician, made numerous contributions to the science of microbiology. Some of them are listed here:

- Koch made many significant contributions to the germ theory of disease. For example, he proved that the anthrax bacillus (*B. anthracis*), which had been discovered earlier by other scientists, was truly the causative agent of anthrax. He accomplished this using a series of scientific steps that he and his colleagues had developed; these steps later became known as Koch's Postulates (described later in this chapter).
- Koch discovered that *B. anthracis* produces spores, capable of resisting adverse conditions.
- Koch developed methods of fixing, staining, and photographing bacteria.

---

[c]"C" is an abbreviation for Celsius. Although Celsius is also referred to as centigrade, Celsius is preferred. Formulas for converting Celsius to Fahrenheit and vice versa can be found in Appendix C ("Useful Conversions").

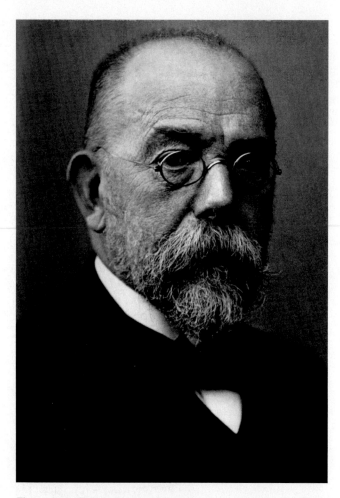

Figure 1-9. Robert Koch. (Courtesy of www.wpclipart.com.)

- Koch developed methods of cultivating bacteria on solid media. One of Koch's colleagues, R.J. Petri, invented a flat glass dish (now known as a **Petri dish**) in which to culture bacteria on solid media. It was Frau Hesse—the wife of another of Koch's colleagues—who suggested the use of agar (a polysaccharide obtained from seaweed) as a solidifying agent. These methods enabled Koch to obtain pure cultures of bacteria. The term **pure culture** refers to a condition in which only one type of organism is growing on a solid culture medium or in a liquid culture medium in the laboratory; no other types of organisms are present. Petri dishes containing agar are still used to culture bacteria and fungi in laboratories.
- Koch discovered the bacterium (*M. tuberculosis*) that causes tuberculosis and the bacterium (*Vibrio cholerae*) that causes cholera.
- Koch's work on tuberculin (a protein derived from *M. tuberculosis*) ultimately led to the development of a skin test valuable in diagnosing tuberculosis.

Koch's Postulates

During the mid- to late-1800s, Koch and his colleagues established an experimental procedure to prove that a specific microbe is the cause of a specific infectious disease. This scientific procedure, published in 1884, became known as **Koch's Postulates** (Fig. 1-10).

Koch's Postulates (paraphrased):

1. A particular microbe must be found in all cases of the disease and must not be present in healthy animals or humans.
2. The microbe must be isolated from the diseased animal or human and grown in pure culture in the laboratory.
3. The same disease must be produced when microbes from the pure culture are inoculated into healthy susceptible laboratory animals.
4. The same microbe must be recovered from the experimentally infected animals and grown again in pure culture.

After completing these steps, the microbe is said to have fulfilled Koch's Postulates and has been proven to be the cause of that particular infectious disease. Koch's Postulates not only helped to prove the germ theory of disease, but also gave a tremendous boost to the development of microbiology by stressing laboratory culture and identification of microbes.

Exceptions to Koch's Postulates

Circumstances do exist in which Koch's Postulates cannot be fulfilled. Examples of such circumstances are as follows:

- To fulfill Koch's Postulates, it is necessary to grow (culture) the pathogen in the laboratory (in vitro[d]) in or on artificial culture media. However, certain pathogens will not grow on artificial media. Such pathogens include viruses, rickettsias (a category of bacteria), chlamydias (another category of bacteria), and the bacteria that cause leprosy and syphilis. Viruses, rickettsias, and chlamydias are called *obligate intracellular pathogens* (or *obligate intracellular parasites*) because they can survive and multiply only within living host cells. Such organisms can be grown in cell cultures (cultures of living human or animal cells of various types), embryonated chicken eggs, or certain animals (referred to as laboratory animals). In the laboratory, the leprosy bacterium (*Mycobacterium leprae*) is propagated in armadillos, and the spirochetes of syphilis (*Treponema pallidum*) grow well in the testes of rabbits and chimpanzees. Microbes having complex and demanding nutritional requirements are said to be **fastidious** (meaning fussy). Although certain fastidious organisms can be grown in the laboratory by adding special mixtures of vitamins, amino acids, and other nutrients to the culture media, others cannot be grown in the laboratory because no

---

[d]As used in this book, the term **in vitro** refers to something that occurs *outside* the living body, whereas the term **in vivo** refers to something that occurs *within* the living body. In vitro often refers to something that occurs in the laboratory.

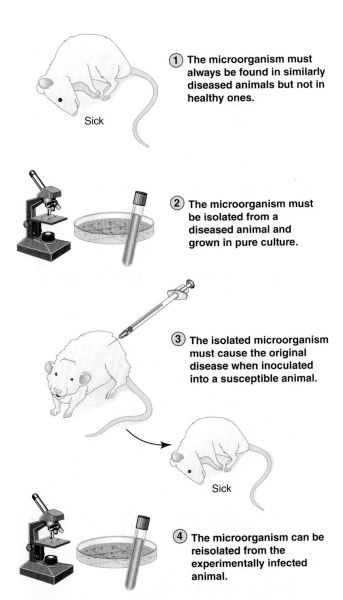

① **The microorganism must always be found in similarly diseased animals but not in healthy ones.**

Sick

② **The microorganism must be isolated from a diseased animal and grown in pure culture.**

③ **The isolated microorganism must cause the original disease when inoculated into a susceptible animal.**

Sick

④ **The microorganism can be reisolated from the experimentally infected animal.**

Figure 1-10. Koch's Postulates: proof of the germ theory of disease.

one has discovered what ingredient(s) to add to the medium to enable them to grow.

• To fulfill Koch's Postulates, it is necessary to infect laboratory animals with the pathogen being studied. However, many pathogens are species-specific, meaning that they infect only one species of animal. For example, some pathogens that infect humans will infect *only* humans. Thus, it is not always possible to find a laboratory animal that can be infected with a pathogen that causes human disease. Because human volunteers are difficult to obtain and ethical considerations limit their use, the researcher may only be able to observe the changes caused by the pathogen in human cells that can be grown in the laboratory (called cell cultures).

• Some diseases, called **synergistic infections** or **polymicrobial infections**, are caused not by one particular microbe, but by the combined effects of two or more

different microbes. Examples of such infections include acute necrotizing ulcerative gingivitis (ANUG; also known as "trench mouth") and bacterial vaginosis. It is very difficult to reproduce such synergistic infections in the laboratory.

• Another difficulty that is sometimes encountered while attempting to fulfill Koch's Postulates is that certain pathogens become altered when grown in vitro. Some become less pathogenic, whereas others become nonpathogenic. Thus, they will no longer infect animals after being cultured on artificial media.

It is also important to keep in mind that not all diseases are caused by microbes. Many diseases, such as rickets and scurvy, result from dietary deficiencies. Some diseases are inherited because of an abnormality in the chromosomes, as in sickle cell anemia. Others, such as diabetes, result from malfunction of a body organ or system. Still others, such as cancer of the lungs and skin, are influenced by environmental factors. However, all infectious diseases are caused by microbes, as are all microbial intoxications.

> All infectious diseases and microbial intoxications are caused by microbes.

Careers in Microbiology

A **microbiologist** is a scientist who studies microbes. He or she might have a bachelor's, master's, or doctoral degree in microbiology.

There are many career fields within the science of microbiology. For example, a person may specialize in the study of just one particular category of microbes. A **bacteriologist** is a scientist who specializes in **bacteriology**—the study of the structure, functions, and activities of bacteria. Scientists specializing in the field of **phycology** (or algology) study the various types of algae and are called **phycologists** (or algologists). **Protozoologists** explore the area of **protozoology**—the study of protozoa and their activities. Those who specialize in the study of fungi, or **mycology**, are called **mycologists**. **Virology** encompasses the study of viruses and their effects on living cells of all types. **Virologists** and cell biologists may become genetic engineers who transfer genetic material (deoxyribonucleic acid or DNA) from one cell type to another. Virologists may also study prions and viroids, acellular infectious agents that are even smaller than viruses (discussed in Chapter 4).

Other career fields in microbiology pertain more to applied microbiology, that is, how a knowledge of microbiology can be applied to different aspects of society, medicine, and industry. (Two medically related career fields are discussed here; other microbiology career fields are discussed on thePoint.) The scope of microbiology has broad, far-reaching effects on humans and their environment.

Medical and Clinical Microbiology

Medical microbiology is an excellent career field for individuals having interests in medicine and microbiology. The field of medical microbiology involves the study of pathogens, the diseases they cause, and the body's defenses against disease. This field is concerned with epidemiology, transmission of pathogens, disease-prevention measures, aseptic techniques, treatment of infectious diseases, immunology, and the production of vaccines to protect people and animals against infectious diseases. The complete or almost complete eradication of diseases like smallpox and polio, the safety of modern surgery, and the successful treatment of victims of infectious diseases are attributable to many technological advances in this field. A branch of medical microbiology, called **clinical microbiology** or **diagnostic microbiology**, is concerned with the laboratory diagnosis of infectious diseases of humans. This is an excellent career field for individuals with interests in laboratory sciences and microbiology. Diagnostic microbiology and the clinical microbiology laboratory are discussed in Chapter 13.

ON thePoint

- Terms Introduced in This Chapter
- Review of Key Points
- Spotlighting Additional Careers in Microbiology
- Increase Your Knowledge
- Critical Thinking
- Additional Self-Assessment Exercises

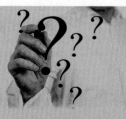

Self-Assessment Exercises

After studying this chapter, answer the following multiple-choice questions.

1. Which of the following individuals is considered to be the "Father of Microbiology?"
   a. Anton van Leeuwenhoek
   b. Louis Pasteur
   c. Robert Koch
   d. Rudolf Virchow

2. The microbes that usually live on or in a person are collectively referred to as:
   a. germs
   b. indigenous microbiota
   c. nonpathogens
   d. opportunistic pathogens

3. Microbes that live on dead and decaying organic material are known as:
   a. indigenous microbiota
   b. parasites
   c. pathogens
   d. saprophytes

4. The study of algae is called:
   a. algaeology
   b. botany
   c. mycology
   d. phycology

5. The field of parasitology (see thePoint) involves the study of which of the following types of organisms?
   a. arthropods, bacteria, fungi, protozoa, and viruses
   b. arthropods, helminths, and certain protozoa
   c. bacteria, fungi, and protozoa
   d. bacteria, fungi, and viruses

6. Rudolf Virchow is given credit for proposing which of the following theories?
   a. abiogenesis
   b. biogenesis
   c. germ theory of disease
   d. spontaneous generation

7. Which of the following microbes are considered obligate intracellular pathogens?
   a. chlamydias, rickettsias, *Mycobacterium leprae*, and *Treponema pallidum*
   b. *M. leprae* and *T. pallidum*
   c. *M. tuberculosis* and viruses
   d. rickettsias, chlamydias, and viruses

8. Which of the following statements is true?
   a. Koch developed a rabies vaccine
   b. Microbes are ubiquitous
   c. Most microbes are harmful to humans
   d. Pasteur conducted experiments that proved the theory of abiogenesis

9. Which of the following are even smaller than viruses?
   a. chlamydias
   b. prions and viroids
   c. rickettsias
   d. cyanobacteria

10. Which of the following individuals introduced the terms "aerobes" and "anaerobes?"
    a. Anton van Leeuwenhoek
    b. Louis Pasteur
    c. Robert Koch
    d. Rudolf Virchow

2

Viewing the Microbial World

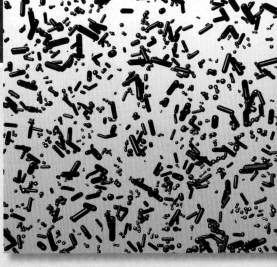

Gram-positive (blue) and Gram-negative (red) bacteria as they would appear when observed using a compound light microscope.

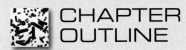

CHAPTER OUTLINE

Introduction

Using the Metric System to Express the Sizes of Microbes

Microscopes
Simple Microscopes
Compound Microscopes
Electron Microscopes
Atomic Force Microscopes

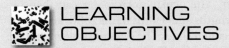

LEARNING OBJECTIVES

After studying this chapter, you should be able to:

- Explain the interrelationships among the following metric system units of length: centimeters, millimeters, micrometers, and nanometers
- State the metric units used to express the sizes of bacteria, protozoa, and viruses
- Compare and contrast the various types of microscopes, to include simple microscopes, compound light microscopes, electron microscopes, and atomic force microscopes

Introduction

Microbes are very tiny. But how tiny are they? In most cases, some type of microscope is required to see them; thus, microbes are said to be *microscopic*. Various types of microscopes are discussed in this chapter. The metric system will be discussed first, however, because metric system units of length are used to express the sizes of microbes and the resolving power of optical instruments.

Using the Metric System to Express the Sizes of Microbes

In microbiology, metric units (primarily micrometers and nanometers) are used to express the sizes of microbes. The basic unit of length in the metric system, the meter (m), is equivalent to approximately 39.4 inches (in) and is, therefore, about 3.4 in longer than a yard. A meter may be divided into 10 (10^1) equally spaced units called **decimeters**; or 100 (10^2) equally spaced units called **centimeters**; or 1,000 (10^3) equally spaced units called **millimeters**; or 1 million (10^6) equally spaced units called **micrometers**; or 1 billion (10^9) equally spaced units called **nanometers**. Interrelationships among these units are shown in Figure 2-1. Formulas that can be used to convert inches into centimeters, millimeters, etc. can be found in Appendix C ("Useful Conversions") at the back of the book.

It should be noted that the old terms *micron* (μ)[a] and *millimicron* (mμ) have been replaced by the terms *micrometer* (μm) and *nanometer* (nm), respectively. An *angstrom* (Å) is 0.1 nm. Using this scale, human red blood cells are about 7 μm in diameter.

The sizes of bacteria and protozoa are usually expressed in terms of micrometers. For example, a typical spherical bacterium (**coccus**; pl., **cocci**) is approximately 1 μm in diameter.

> The sizes of bacteria are expressed in micrometers, whereas the sizes of viruses are expressed in nanometers.

[a]The Greek letter μ is pronounced "mew." Greek letters are frequently used in science, including the science of microbiology. To aid students who are unfamiliar with the Greek alphabet, Appendix D contains the complete Greek alphabet.

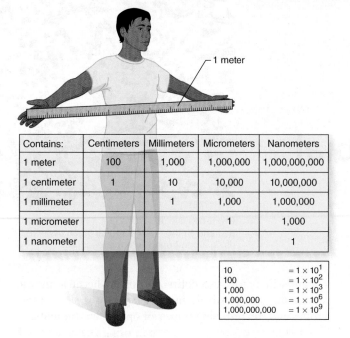

Contains:	Centimeters	Millimeters	Micrometers	Nanometers
1 meter	100	1,000	1,000,000	1,000,000,000
1 centimeter	1	10	10,000	10,000,000
1 millimeter		1	1,000	1,000,000
1 micrometer			1	1,000
1 nanometer				1

10	$= 1 \times 10^1$
100	$= 1 \times 10^2$
1,000	$= 1 \times 10^3$
1,000,000	$= 1 \times 10^6$
1,000,000,000	$= 1 \times 10^9$

Figure 2-1. Representations of metric units of measure and numbers.

About seven cocci could fit side by side across a human red blood cell. If the head of a pin was 1 mm (1,000 μm) in diameter, then 1,000 cocci could be placed side by side on the pinhead. A typical rod-shaped bacterium (**bacillus**; pl., **bacilli**) is about 1 μm wide × 3 μm long, although some bacilli are shorter, and some form very long filaments. The sizes of viruses are expressed in terms of nanometers. Most of the viruses that cause human disease range in size from about 10 to 300 nm, although some (e.g., Ebola virus, a cause of hemorrhagic fever) can be as long as 1,000 nm (1 μm). Some very large protozoa reach a length of 2,000 μm (2 mm).

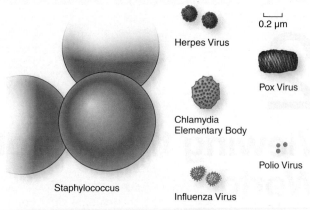

Figure 2-2. The relative sizes of *Staphylococcus* and *Chlamydia* bacteria and several viruses. Poliovirus is one of the smallest viruses that infect humans. (Redrawn from Winn WC Jr, Allen S, Janda W, et al. *Koneman's Color Atlas and Textbook of Diagnostic Microbiology*. 6th ed. Philadelphia, PA: Lippincott Williams & Wilkins; 2006.)

In the microbiology laboratory, the sizes of cellular microbes are measured using an ocular micrometer, a tiny ruler within the eyepiece (ocular) of the compound light microscope (described later). Before it can be used to measure objects, however, the ocular micrometer must first be calibrated, using a measuring device called a **stage micrometer**. Calibration must be performed for each of the objective lenses to determine the distance between the marks on the ocular micrometer. The ocular micrometer can then be used to measure lengths and widths of microbes and other objects on the specimen slide. The sizes of some microbes are shown in Figure 2-2 and Table 2-1.

> An ocular micrometer is used to measure the dimensions of objects being viewed with a compound light microscope.

Table 2-1	**Relative Sizes of Microbes**		

Microbe or Microbial Structure	Dimension(s)	Approximate Size (μm)
Viruses (most)	Diameter	0.01–0.3
Bacteria		
Cocci (spherical bacteria)	Diameter	Average = 1
Bacilli (rod-shaped bacteria)	Width × length	Average = 1 × 3
	Filaments (width)	1
Fungi		
Yeasts	Diameter	3–5
Septate hyphae (hyphae containing cross-walls)	Width	2–15
Aseptate hyphae (hyphae without cross-walls)	Width	10–30
Pond water protozoa		
Chlamydomonas	Length	5–12
Euglena	Length	35–55
Vorticella	Length	50–145
Paramecium	Length	180–300
Volvox[a]	Diameter	350–500
Stentor[a]	Length (when extended)	1,000–2,000

[a]These organisms are visible with the unaided human eye.

Microscopes

The human eye, a telescope, a pair of binoculars, a magnifying glass, and a microscope can all be thought of as various types of optical instruments. A **microscope** is an optical instrument that is used to observe tiny objects, often objects that cannot be seen at all with the unaided human eye (the "naked eye"). Each optical instrument has a limit as to what can be seen using that instrument. This limit is referred to as the **resolving power** or **resolution** of the instrument. Resolving power is discussed in more detail later in this chapter. Table 2-2 contains the resolving powers for various optical instruments.

Simple Microscopes

A **simple microscope** is defined as a microscope containing only one magnifying lens. Actually, a magnifying glass could be considered a simple microscope. Images seen when using a magnifying glass usually appear about 3 to 20 times larger than the object's actual size. During the late 1600s, Anton van Leeuwenhoek, who was discussed in Chapter 1, used simple microscopes to observe many tiny objects, including bacteria and protozoa (Fig. 2-3). Because of his unique ability to grind glass lenses, scientists believe that Leeuwenhoek's simple microscopes had a maximum magnifying power of about ×300 (300 times).

Compound Microscopes

A **compound microscope** is a microscope that contains more than one magnifying lens. Although the first person to construct and use a compound microscope is not known with certainty, Hans Jansen and his son Zacharias are often given

> A simple microscope contains only one magnifying lens, whereas a compound microscope contains more than one magnifying lens.

credit for being the first (see the following "Historical Note"). Compound light microscopes usually magnify objects about 1,000 times. Photographs taken through the lens system of compound microscopes are called **photomicrographs**.

Because visible light (from a built-in light bulb) is used as the source of illumination, the compound microscope is also referred to as a **compound light microscope**. It is the wavelength of visible light (approximately 0.45 µm) that limits the size of objects that can be seen using the compound light microscope. When using the compound light microscope, objects cannot be seen if they are smaller than half of the wavelength of visible light (i.e., smaller than about 0.225 µm). A compound light microscope is shown in Figure 2-5, and the functions of its various components are described in Table 2-3.

The compound light microscopes used in today's laboratories contain two magnifying lens systems. Within

---

Table 2-2	**Characteristics of Various Types of Microscopes**		
Type	**Resolving Power**	**Useful Magnification**	**Characteristics**
Brightfield	0.2000 µm	×1,000	Used to observe morphology of microorganisms such as bacteria, protozoa, fungi, and algae in living (unstained) and nonliving (stained) state Objects are observed against a bright background Cannot observe microbes less than 0.2 µm in diameter or thickness, such as spirochetes and viruses
Darkfield	0.2000 µm	×1,000	Unstained organisms are observed against a dark background Useful for examining thin spirochetes Slightly more difficult to operate than brightfield
Phase-contrast	0.2000 µm	×1,000	Can be used to observe unstained living microorganisms
Fluorescence	0.2000 µm	×1,000	Fluorescent dye attached to organism Primarily an immunodiagnostic technique (immunofluorescence) Used to detect microbes in cells, tissues, and clinical specimens
TEM	0.0002 mm (0.2 nm)	×200,000	Specimen is viewed on a screen Excellent resolution Allows examination of cellular and viral ultrastructure Specimen is nonliving Reveals internal features of thin specimens
SEM	0.0200 mm (20 nm)	×10,000	Specimen is viewed on a screen Gives the illusion of depth (three dimensions) Useful for examining surface features of cells and viruses Specimen is nonliving Resolution is less than that of TEM

immediately above the object to be viewed. The four objectives used in most laboratory compound light microscopes are ×4, ×10, ×40, and ×100 objectives. As shown in Table 2-4, total magnification is calculated by multiplying the magnifying power of the ocular (×10) by the magnifying power of the objective that you are using.

The ×4 objective is rarely used in microbiology laboratories. Usually, specimens are first observed using the ×10 objective. Once the specimen is in focus, the high-power or "high-dry" objective is then swung into position. This lens can be used to study algae, protozoa, and other large microorganisms. However, the oil-immersion objective (total magnification = ×1,000) must be used to study bacteria, because they are so tiny. To use the oil-immersion objective, a drop of immersion oil must first be placed between the specimen and the objective; the immersion oil reduces the scattering of light and ensures that the light will enter the oil-immersion lens. The oil-immersion objective cannot be used without immersion oil. Oil is not required when using the other objectives.

For optimal observation of the specimen, the light must be properly adjusted and focused. The condenser, located beneath the stage, focuses light onto the specimen, adjusts the amount of light, and shapes the cone of light entering the objective. Generally, the higher the magnification, the more light that is needed.

As magnification is increased, the amount of light striking the object being examined must also be increased.

> Total magnification of the compound light microscope is calculated by multiplying the magnifying power of the ocular lens by the magnifying power of the objective being used.

the eyepiece or ocular is a lens called the **ocular lens**; it usually has a magnifying power of ×10. The second magnifying lens system is in the objective, which is positioned

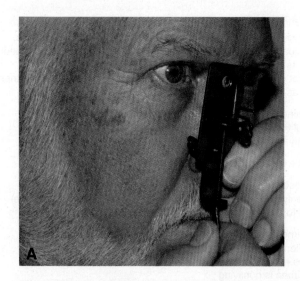
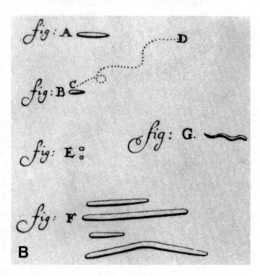

Figure 2-3. Leeuwenhoek's microscopes. A. Leeuwenhoek's microscopes were very simple devices. Each had a tiny glass lens, mounted in a brass plate. The specimen was placed on the sharp point of a brass pin, and two screws were used to adjust the position of the specimen. The entire instrument was about 3 to 4 in long. It was held very close to the eye. (Courtesy of Biomed Ed, Round Rock, TX.) **B.** Although his microscopes had a magnifying capability of only around ×200 to ×300, he was able to create remarkable drawings of different types of bacteria that he observed. (From Volk WA, Gebhardt BM, Hammarskjold ML, et al. *Essentials of Medical Microbiology*. 5th ed. Philadelphia, PA: Lippincott-Raven; 1996.)

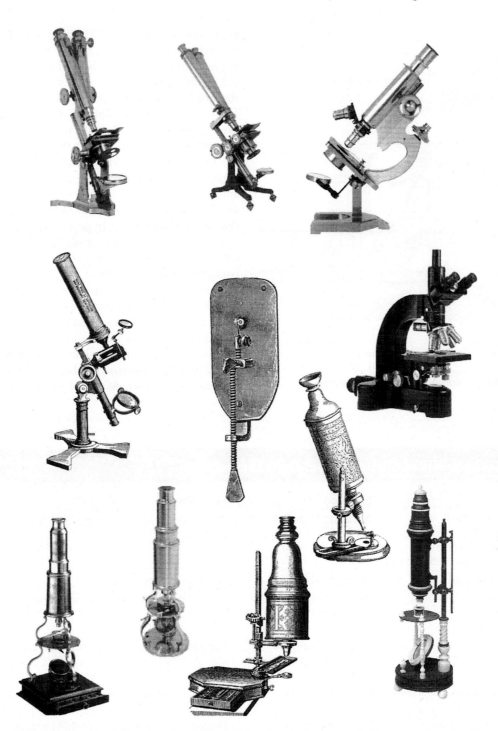

Figure 2-4. A simple Leeuwenhoek microscope (center), surrounded by examples of early compound light microscopes.

There are three correct ways to accomplish this: (a) by opening the iris diaphragm in the condenser, (b) by opening the field diaphragm, and (c) by increasing the intensity of light being emitted from the microscope's light bulb, by turning the rheostat knob clockwise. Turning the knob that raises and lowers the condenser is an *incorrect* way to adjust lighting.

Magnification alone is of little value unless the enlarged image possesses increased detail and clarity. Image clarity depends on the microscope's resolving power (or resolution), which is the ability of the lens system to distinguish between two adjacent objects. If two objects are moved closer and closer together, there comes a point when the objects are so close together that the lens system can no longer resolve them as two separate objects (i.e., they are so close together that they

> The resolving power or resolution of an optical instrument is its ability to distinguish between two adjacent objects. The resolving power of the unaided human eye is 0.2 mm.

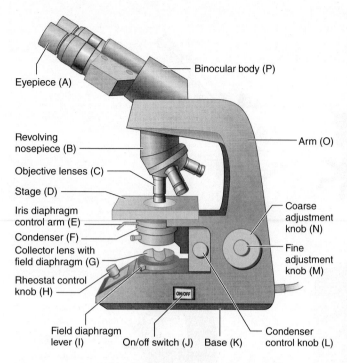

Eyepiece (A)

Binocular body (P)

Revolving
nosepiece (B)

Arm (O)

Objective lenses (C)

Stage (D)

Iris diaphragm
control arm (E)

Coarse
adjustment
knob (N)

Condenser (F)

Collector lens with
field diaphragm (G)

Fine
adjustment
knob (M)

Rheostat control
knob (H)

ON/OFF

Field diaphragm
lever (I)   On/off switch (J)   Base (K)

Condenser
control knob (L)

Figure 2-5. A modern compound light microscope.

appear to be one object). That distance between them, at which they cease to be seen as separate objects, is referred to as the resolving power of the optical instrument. Knowing the resolving power of an optical instrument also defines the smallest object that can be seen with that instrument. For example, the resolving power of the unaided human eye is approximately 0.2 mm. Thus, the unaided human eye is unable to see objects smaller than 0.2 mm in diameter.

The resolving power of the compound light microscope is approximately 1,000 times better than the resolving power of the unaided human eye. In practical terms, this means that objects can be examined with the compound microscope that are as much as 1,000 times smaller than the smallest objects that can be seen with the unaided human eye. Using a compound light microscope, we can see objects down to about 0.2 μm in diameter.

> The resolving power of the compound light microscope is approximately 0.2 μm, which is approximately one half the wavelength of visible light.

Additional magnifying lenses could be added to the compound light microscope, but this would not increase the resolving power. As stated earlier, as long as visible

Table 2-3 Components of the Compound Light Microscope

Component	Location	Function
(A) Ocular lens (also known as an eyepiece); a monocular microscope has one; a binocular microscope (such as shown in Figure 2-5) has two	At the top of the microscope	The ocular lens is a ×10 magnifying lens
(B) Revolving nosepiece	Above the stage	Holds the objective lenses
(C) Objective lenses	Held in place above the stage by the revolving nosepiece	Used to magnify objects placed on the stage
(D) Stage	Directly beneath the nosepiece and objective lenses	Flat surface on which the specimen is placed
Stage adjustment knobs (not shown in Figure 2-5)	Beneath the stage	Used to move the stage and microscope slide
(E) Iris diaphragm control arm	On the condenser	Used to adjust the amount of light passing through the condenser
(F) Condenser	Beneath the stage	Contains a lens system that focuses light onto the specimen
(G) Collector lens with field diaphragm	Beneath the condenser	Controls the amount of light entering the condenser
(H) Rheostat control knob	Front side of the base	Controls the amount of light emitted from the light source
(I) Field diaphragm lever	Attached to the field diaphragm	Used to adjust the amount of light passing through the collector lens
(J) On/off switch	On the side of the base	Turns the light source on and off
(K) Base		Contains the light source
(L) Condenser control knob	Beneath and behind the condenser	Used to adjust the height of the condenser
(M and N) Fine and coarse adjustment knobs	On the arm of the microscope near the base	Used to focus the objective lenses

Component	Location	Function
(O) Arm		Supports the binocular body and the revolving nosepiece; held with one hand when carrying the microscope, with the other hand beneath the base to support the weight of the microscope
(P) Binocular body		Holds the ocular lenses in their proper locations

Letters within parentheses refer to parenthesized letters in Figure 2-5.

light is used as the source of illumination, objects smaller than half of the wavelength of visible light cannot be seen. Increasing magnification without increasing the resolving power is called **empty magnification**. It does no good to increase magnification without increasing resolving power.

Because objects are observed against a bright background (or "bright field") when using a compound light microscope, that microscope is sometimes referred to as a **brightfield microscope**. If the regularly used condenser is replaced with what is known as a darkfield condenser, illuminated objects are seen against a dark background (or "dark field"), and the microscope has been converted into a **darkfield microscope**. In the clinical microbiology laboratory, darkfield microscopy is routinely used to diagnose primary syphilis (the initial stage of syphilis). The etiologic (causative) agent of syphilis—a spiral-shaped bacterium, named *Treponema pallidum*—cannot be seen with a brightfield microscope because it is thinner than 0.2 µm and, therefore, is beneath the resolving power of the compound light microscope. *T. pallidum* can be seen using a darkfield microscope, however, much in the same way that you can "see" dust particles in a beam of sunlight. Dust particles are actually beneath the resolving power of the unaided eye and, therefore, cannot really be seen. What you see in the beam is sunlight being reflected off the dust particles. With the darkfield microscope, laboratory technologists do not really see the treponemes—they see the light being reflected off the bacteria, and that light is easily seen against the dark background (Fig. 2-6).

> When using a brightfield microscope, a person observes objects against a bright background. When using a darkfield microscope, a person observes illuminated objects against a dark background.

Other types of compound microscopes include phase-contrast microscopes and fluorescence microscopes. **Phase-contrast microscopes** can be used to observe unstained living microorganisms. Because the light refracted by living cells is different from the light refracted by the surrounding medium, contrast is increased, and the organisms are more easily seen. **Fluorescence microscopes** contain a built-in ultraviolet (UV) light source. When UV light strikes certain dyes and pigments, these substances emit a longer wavelength light, causing them to glow against a dark background (Fig. 2-7). Fluorescence microscopy is often used in immunology laboratories to demonstrate that antibodies stained with a fluorescent dye have combined with specific antigens; this is a type of immunodiagnostic procedure. (Immunodiagnostic procedures are described in Chapter 16.)

Electron Microscopes

Although extremely small infectious agents, such as rabies and smallpox viruses, were known to exist, they could not be seen until the electron microscope was developed. It should be noted that electron microscopes cannot be used to observe living organisms. Organisms are killed during the specimen-processing procedures. Even if they were not, they would be unable to survive in the vacuum created within the electron microscope.

Electron microscopes use an electron beam as a source of illumination and magnets to focus the beam. Because the wavelength of electrons traveling in a vacuum is much shorter than the wavelength of visible light—about 100,000 times shorter—electron microscopes have a much greater resolving power than compound light microscopes. There are two types of electron microscopes: transmission electron microscopes (TEMs) and scanning electron microscopes (SEMs).

	Table 2-4	**Magnifications Achieved Using the Compound Light Microscope**

Objective	Total Magnification Achieved When the Objective Is Used in Conjunction with a ×10 Ocular Lens
×4 (scanning objective)	×40
×10 (low-power objective)	×100
×40 (high-dry objective)	×400
×100 (oil-immersion objective)	×1,000

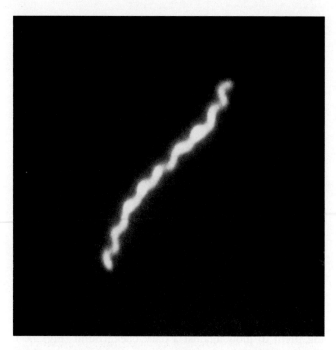

Figure 2-6. Spiral-shaped *T. pallidum* bacterium. The causative agent of syphilis, as seen by darkfield microscopy. (Courtesy of the Centers for Disease Control and Prevention [CDC].)

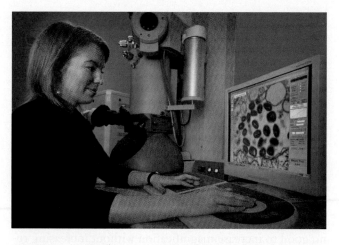

Figure 2-8. A CDC intern using a TEM. (Courtesy of Cynthia Goldsmith, James Gathany, and the CDC.)

A **TEM** (Fig. 2-8) has a tall column, at the top of which an electron gun fires a beam of electrons downward. When an extremely thin specimen (less than 1 μm thick) is placed into the electron beam, some of the electrons are transmitted through the specimen, and some are blocked. An image of the specimen is produced on a phosphor-coated screen at the bottom of the microscope's column. The object can be magnified up to approximately 1 million times. Thus, using a TEM, a magnification is achieved that is about 1,000 times greater than the maximum magnification achieved using a compound light microscope. Even very tiny microbes (e.g.,

viruses) can be observed using a TEM (Fig. 2-9). Because thin sections of cells are examined, transmission electron microscopy enables scientists to study the internal structure of cells. Special staining procedures are used to increase contrast between different parts of the cell. The first TEMs were developed during the late 1920s and early 1930s, but it was not until the early 1950s that electron microscopes began to be used routinely to study cells.

> The resolving power of a TEM is approximately 0.2 nm, which is about 1 million times better than the resolving power of the unaided human eye and 1,000 times better than the resolving power of the compound light microscope.

An **SEM** (Fig. 2-10) has a shorter column, and instead of being placed into the electron beam, the specimen is placed at the bottom of the column. Electrons that bounce off the surface of the specimen are captured by detectors, and an image of the specimen appears on

Figure 2-7. Photomicrograph of *T. pallidum* spirochetes using immunofluorescence. A fluorescent dye is first attached to anti-*T. pallidum* antibodies. The antibodies are then attached to the surface of the bacteria. When examined under UV light, the fluorescent dye emits a greenish light. (Courtesy of Russell and the CDC.)

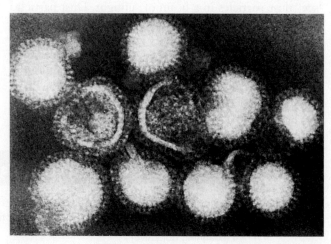

Figure 2-9. Transmission electron micrograph of influenza virus A. (From Winn WC Jr, Allen S, Janda W, et al. *Koneman's Color Atlas and Textbook of Diagnostic Microbiology*. 6th ed. Philadelphia, PA: Lippincott Williams & Wilkins; 2006.)

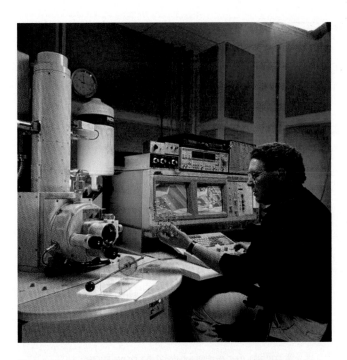

Figure 2-10. Scanning electron microscope. (Courtesy of Jim Yost and the National Renewable Energy Institute.)

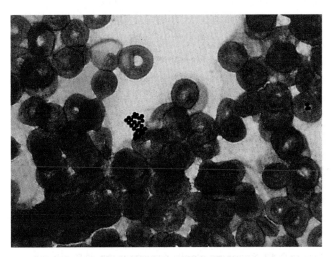

Figure 2-11. A grapelike cluster of blue-stained *S. aureus* bacteria and red blood cells, as seen by light microscopy. (From Marler LM, Siders JA, Allen SD. *Direct Smear Atlas*. Philadelphia, PA: Lippincott Williams & Wilkins; 2001.)

SEMs have a resolving power of about 20 nm—about 100 times less than the resolving power of TEMs.

a monitor. SEMs are used to observe the outer surfaces of specimens (i.e., surface detail). Although the resolving power of SEMs (about 20 nm) is not quite as good as the resolving power of TEMs (about 0.2 nm), it is still possible to observe extremely tiny objects using an SEM. SEMs became available during the late 1960s.

Both types of electron microscopes have built-in camera systems. The photographs taken using TEM and SEM

Photographs taken using compound light microscopes are called photomicrographs. Those taken using TEMs and SEMs are called transmission electron micrographs and scanning electron micrographs, respectively.

are called **transmission electron micrographs** and **scanning electron micrographs**, respectively. They are black and white images. If you ever see electron micrographs in color, they have been artificially colorized. Figures 2-11 to 2-13 show the differences in magnification and detail between photomicrographs and electron micrographs. Note that Figures 2-11 to 2-13 all depict *Staphylococcus aureus* bacteria, but each of these photographs was made using a different type of microscope. Refer back to Table 2-2 for the characteristics of various types of microscopes.

Atomic Force Microscopes

Neither TEMs nor SEMs enable scientists to observe live microbes because of the required specimen-processing

procedures and subjection of the specimens to a vacuum. Atomic force microscopy (AFM) enables scientists to observe living cells at extremely high magnification and resolution under physiological conditions. Using AFM, it is possible to observe single live cells in aqueous solutions where dynamic physiological processes can be observed

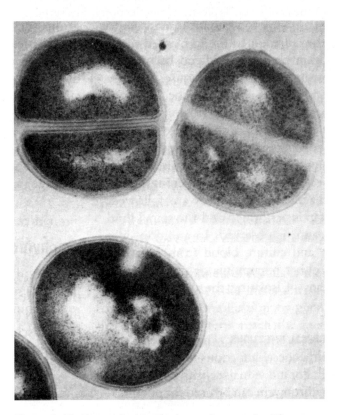

Figure 2-12. Transmission electron micrograph of *S. aureus* showing *S. aureus* cells in various stages of binary fission. (From Volk WA, Gebhardt BM, Hammarskjold ML, et al. *Essentials of Medical Microbiology*. 5th ed. Philadelphia, PA: Lippincott-Raven; 1996.)

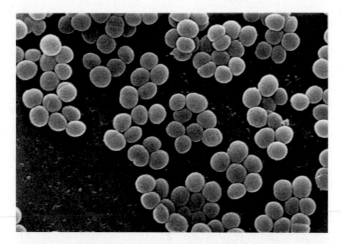

Figure 2-13. Scanning electron micrograph of *S. aureus*. (Courtesy of Janice Carr, Matthew J. Arduino, and the CDC.)

in real time. Unlike the SEM, which provides a two-dimensional image of a sample, the AFM provides a true three-dimensional surface profile.

Figure 2-14 is a diagrammatic representation of an AFM. A silicon or silicon nitride cantilever having a sharp tip (probe) at its end is used to scan the specimen surface. When the tip is brought in proximity to a sample surface, forces between the tip and the sample lead to a deflection of the cantilever. Typically, the deflection is measured using a laser spot reflected from the top surface of the cantilever into an array of photodiodes, creating an image on a monitor screen. Additional information regarding AFM can be found using an Internet search engine.

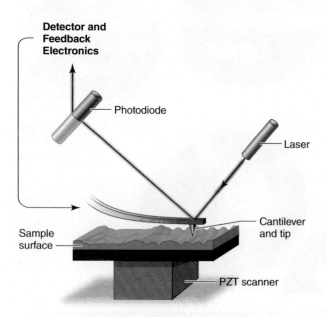

Figure 2-14. Atomic force microscope. See text for details. PZT, lead zirconate titanate. (Courtesy of Askewmind and Wikipedia.)

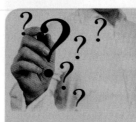

ON thePoint

- Terms Introduced in This Chapter
- Review of Key Points
- Increase Your Knowledge
- Critical Thinking
- Additional Self-Assessment Exercises

Self-Assessment Exercises

After studying this chapter, answer the following multiple-choice questions.

1. A millimeter is equivalent to how many nanometers?
   a. 1,000
   b. 10,000
   c. 100,000
   d. 1,000,000

2. Assume that a pinhead is 1 mm in diameter. How many spherical bacteria (cocci), lined up side by side, would fit across the pinhead? (Hint: Use information from Table 2-1.)
   a. 100
   b. 1,000
   c. 10,000
   d. 100,000

3. What is the length of an average rod-shaped bacterium (bacillus)?
   a. 3 µm
   b. 3 nm
   c. 0.3 mm
   d. 0.03 mm

4. What is the total magnification when using the high-power (high-dry) objective of a compound light microscope equipped with a ×10 ocular lens?
   a. 40
   b. 50
   c. 100
   d. 400

5. How many times better is the resolution of the transmission electron microscope than the resolution of the unaided human eye?
   a. 1,000
   b. 10,000
   c. 100,000
   d. 1,000,000

6. How many times better is the resolution of the transmission electron microscope than the resolution of the compound light microscope?
   a. 100
   b. 1,000
   c. 10,000
   d. 100,000

7. How many times better is the resolution of the transmission electron microscope than the resolution of the scanning electron microscope?
   a. 100
   b. 1,000
   c. 10,000
   d. 100,000

8. The limiting factor of any compound light microscope (i.e., the thing that limits its resolution to 0.2 μm) is the:
   a. number of condenser lenses it has
   b. number of magnifying lenses it has
   c. number of ocular lenses it has
   d. wavelength of visible light

9. Which of the following individuals is given credit for developing the first compound microscope?
   a. Anton van Leeuwenhoek
   b. Hans Jansen
   c. Louis Pasteur
   d. Robert Hooke

10. A compound light microscope differs from a simple microscope in that the compound light microscope contains more than one:
    a. condenser lens
    b. magnifying lens
    c. objective lens
    d. ocular lens

3

Cell Structure and Taxonomy

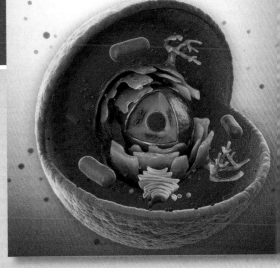

Cut-away illustration of a eukaryotic cell.

 ## CHAPTER OUTLINE

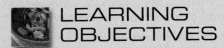 ## LEARNING OBJECTIVES

After studying this chapter, you should be able to:

- Explain what is meant by the cell theory (see Historical Note: Cells)
- State the contributions of Hooke, Schleiden and Schwann, and Virchow to the study of cells
- Cite one function for each of the following parts of a eukaryotic cell: cell membrane, nucleus, ribosomes, Golgi complex, lysosomes, mitochondria, plastids, cytoskeleton, cell wall, flagella, and cilia
- Cite a function for each of the following parts of a bacterial cell: cell membrane, chromosome, cell wall, capsule, flagella, pili, and endospores
- Compare and contrast plant, animal, and bacterial cells
- Define the following terms: genus, specific epithet, and species
- Describe the Five-Kingdom and Three-Domain Systems of Classification

Introduction

Recall from Chapter 1 that there are two major categories of microbes: **acellular microbes** (also called **infectious particles**) and **cellular microbes** (also called **microorganisms**). In this chapter, you will learn about the structure of microorganisms. Because they are so small, very little detail concerning their structure can be determined using the compound light microscope. Our knowledge of the ultrastructure of microbes has been gained through the use of electron microscopes. Ultrastructure refers to the very detailed views of cells that are beyond the resolving power of the compound light microscope. Also discussed in this chapter are the ways in which microbes

25

and their cells reproduce and how microorganisms are classified.

In biology, a **cell** is defined as the fundamental unit of any living organism because, like the total organism, the cell exhibits the basic characteristics of life. A cell obtains food (nutrients) from the environment to produce energy for metabolism and other activities. **Metabolism** refers to all of the chemical reactions that occur within a cell (see Chapter 7 for a detailed discussion of metabolism and metabolic reactions). Because of its metabolism, a cell can grow and reproduce. It can respond to stimuli in its environment such as light, heat, cold, and the presence of chemicals. A cell can mutate (change genetically) as a result of accidental changes in its genetic material—the **deoxyribonucleic acid** (DNA) that makes up the genes of its chromosomes—and, thus, can become better or less suited to its environment. As a result of these genetic changes, the mutant organism may be better adapted for survival and development into a new **species** (pl., **species**) of organism.

Bacterial cells exhibit all the characteristics of life, although they do not have the complex system of membranes and *organelles* (tiny organ-like structures) found in the more advanced single-celled organisms. These less complex cells, which include *Bacteria* and *Archaea*, are called **prokaryotes** or **prokaryotic cells**. The more complex cells, containing a true nucleus and many membrane-bound organelles, are called **eukaryotes** or **eukaryotic cells**. Eukaryotes include such organisms as algae, protozoa, fungi, plants, animals, and humans. Some microorganisms are prokaryotic, some are eukaryotic, and some (e.g., viruses) are not cells at all (Fig. 3-1).

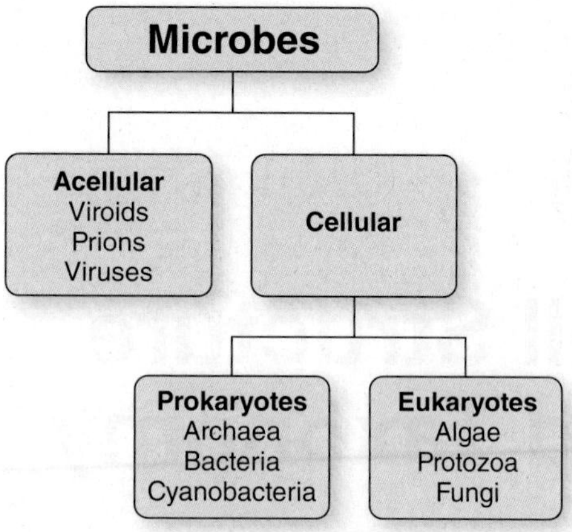

Figure 3-1. Acellular and cellular microbes. Acellular microbes include viroids, prions, and viruses. Cellular microbes include the less complex prokaryotes (archaea and bacteria) and the more complex eukaryotes (some algae, all protozoa, and some fungi).

Eukaryotic cells possess a true nucleus, whereas prokaryotic cells do not.

Viruses appear to be the result of regressive or reverse evolution. They are composed of only a few genes protected by a protein coat, and sometimes may contain one or a few enzymes. Viruses depend on the energy and metabolic machinery of a host cell to reproduce. Because viruses are acellular (not composed of cells), they are placed in a completely separate category. They are discussed in detail in Chapter 4.

For those in the health professions, it is important to learn differences in the structure of various cells, not only for identification purposes, but also to understand differences in their metabolism. These factors must be known before one can determine or explain why antimicrobial agents (drugs) attack and destroy pathogens, but do not harm human cells.

Cytology, the study of the structure and function of cells, has developed during the past 75 years with the aid of the electron microscope and sophisticated biochemical research. Many books have been written about the details of these tiny functional factories—cells—but only a brief discussion of their structure and activities is presented here.

Eukaryotic Cell Structure

Eukaryotes (*eu* = true; *karyo* refers to a nut or nucleus) are so named because they have a true nucleus, in that their DNA is enclosed by a nuclear membrane. Most animal and plant cells are 10 to 30 µm in diameter, about 10 times larger than most prokaryotic cells. Figure 3-2 illustrates a typical

HISTORICAL NOTE

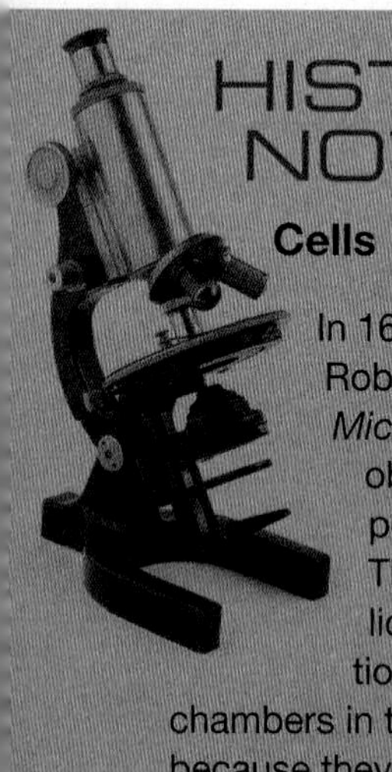

Cells

In 1665, an English physicist named Robert Hooke published a book, entitled *Micrographia*, containing descriptions of objects he had observed using a compound light microscope that he had made. These objects included molds, rusts, fleas, lice, fossilized plants and animals, and sections of cork. He referred to the small empty chambers in the structure of cork as "cells," probably because they reminded him of the bare rooms (called cells) in a monastery. He was the first person to use the term *cells* in this manner. Around 1838 to 1839, a German botanist named Matthias Schleiden and a German zoologist named Theodor Schwann concluded that all plant and animal tissues were composed of cells; this later became known as the **cell theory**. Then, in 1858, the German pathologist Rudolf Virchow proposed the theory of *biogenesis*—that life can arise only from preexisting life, and, therefore, that cells can arise only from preexisting cells. Biogenesis does not address the issue of the origin of life on Earth, a complex topic about which much has been written.

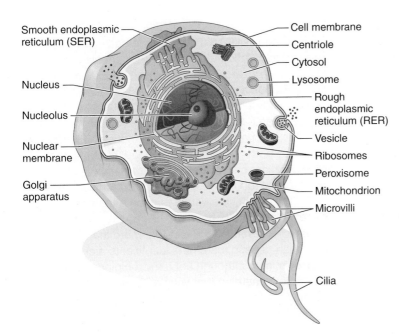

Figure 3-2. **A typical eukaryotic animal cell.** (Redrawn from Cohen BJ. *Memmler's The Human Body in Health and Disease*. 11th ed. Philadelphia, PA: Lippincott Williams & Wilkins; 2009.)

not. The **nucleus** (pl., **nuclei**) controls the functions of the entire cell and can be thought of as the "command center" of the cell. The nucleus has three components: nucleoplasm, chromosomes, and a nuclear membrane.

Nucleoplasm (a type of **protoplasm**) is the gelatinous matrix or base material of the nucleus. The **chromosomes** are embedded or suspended in the nucleoplasm.

> A "true nucleus" consists of nucleoplasm, chromosomes, and a nuclear membrane.

The membrane that serves as a "skin" around the nucleus is called the **nuclear membrane**; it contains holes (nuclear pores) through which large molecules can enter and exit the nucleus.

Eukaryotic chromosomes consist of linear DNA molecules and proteins (histones and nonhistone proteins).[a] **Genes** are located along the

eukaryotic animal cell. This illustration is a composite of most of the structures that might be found in the various types of human body cells. Figure 3-3 shows a transmission electron micrograph of an actual yeast cell. A discussion of the functional parts of eukaryotic cells can be better understood by keeping the illustrated structures in mind.

Cell Membrane

The cell is enclosed and held intact by the *cell membrane*, which is also referred to as the plasma, cytoplasmic, or cellular membrane. Structurally, it is a mosaic composed of large molecules of proteins and phospholipids (certain types of fats). The cell membrane is like a "skin" around the cell, separating the contents of the cell from the outside world. The cell membrane regulates the passage of nutrients, waste products, and secretions into and out of the cell. Because the cell membrane has the property of *selective permeability*, only certain substances may enter and leave the cell. The cell membrane is similar in structure and function to all of the other membranes that are found in eukaryotic cells.

> Cell membranes have selective permeability, meaning that they allow only certain substances to pass through them.

Nucleus

As previously mentioned, the primary difference between prokaryotic and eukaryotic cells is that eukaryotic cells possess a "true nucleus," whereas prokaryotic cells do

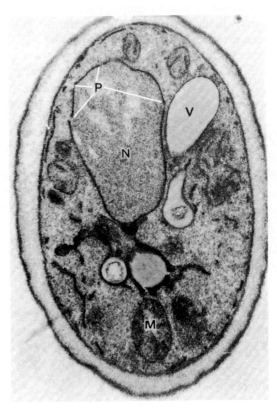

Figure 3-3. **Cross section through a yeast cell.** The cross section shows the nucleus (N) with nuclear pores (P), mitochondrion (M), and vacuole (V). The cytoplasm is surrounded by the cell membrane. The thick outer portion is the cell wall. (From Lechavalier HA, Pramer D. *The Microbes*. Philadelphia, PA: JB Lippincott; 1970.)

---

[a]Histones are positively charged, low-molecular-weight proteins found in eukaryotic cell nuclei. They act as spools around which DNA winds. This winding enables the compaction necessary to fit the large genomes of eukaryotes inside cell nuclei. A compacted DNA molecule is about 40,000 times shorter than the non compacted molecule.

DNA molecules. Although genes are sometimes described as "beads on a string," each bead (gene) is actually a particular segment of the DNA molecule. Each gene contains the genetic information that enables the cell to produce one or more **gene products**. Most gene products are proteins, but some genes code for the production of two types of **ribonucleic acid** (RNA): ribosomal ribonucleic acid (rRNA) and transfer ribonucleic acid (tRNA) molecules (discussed in Chapter 6). The organism's complete collection of genes is referred to as that organism's **genotype** (or **genome**). To understand more about how genes control the activities of the entire organism, refer to Chapters 6 and 7.

> An organism's complete collection of genes is referred to as its genotype or genome.

The number and composition of chromosomes and the number of genes on each chromosome are characteristic of the particular species of organism. Different species have different numbers and sizes of chromosomes. Human diploid cells, for example, have 46 chromosomes (23 pairs), each consisting of thousands of genes. It has been estimated that the human genome consists of between 20,000 and 25,000 genes.[b]

SOMETHING TO THINK ABOUT

According to findings of the Human Genome Project, humans possess between 20,000 and 25,000 genes. How does this compare with the genome size of other organisms? It has been reported that the animal with the largest genome is a tiny aquatic crustacean called a water flea (*Daphnia pulex*), with about 31,000 genes.[c] But what about other organisms? Examples reported by the Human Genome Project[d] and Wikipedia[e] include the bacterium *Haemophilus influenzae* (1,700), *Escherichia coli* (3,200), *Cryptosporidium* parasites (~4,000), a red alga (~5,300), a malarial parasite (~5,300), bakers' yeast (~6,000), other fungi (from ~2,000 to ~11,800), a green alga (~8,000), a mosquito (~13,600), a fruit fly (13,600), a roundworm (19,000), a mouse (~25,000 genes), a puffer fish (from 22,000 to 29,000), a wild mustard plant called *Arabidopsis thaliana* (25,000), rice (from 32,000 to 50,000), and a cottonwood tree (~45,500). Isn't it interesting that the genomes of certain plants are larger than the human genome? Equally interesting is the fact that more than 97% of human genetic material is identical to a chimpanzee's, and, although not a microbiology topic, it might be something that you would like to learn more about by using a Search Engine.

When observed using a transmission electron microscope, a dark (electron dense) area can be seen in the nucleus. This area is called the **nucleolus**; it is here that rRNA molecules are manufactured. The rRNA molecules then exit the nucleus and become part of the structure of ribosomes (discussed later in this chapter).

Cytoplasm

Cytoplasm (a type of protoplasm) is a semifluid, gelatinous, nutrient matrix. Within the cytoplasm are found insoluble storage granules and various cytoplasmic organelles, including endoplasmic reticulum, ribosomes, Golgi complexes, mitochondria, centrioles, microtubules, lysosomes, and other membrane-bound vacuoles. Each of these organelles has a highly specific function, and all of the functions are interrelated to maintain the cell and allow it to properly perform its activities. The cytoplasm is where most of the cell's metabolic reactions occur. The semifluid portion of the cytoplasm, excluding the granules and organelles, is sometimes referred to as the *cytosol*.

Endoplasmic Reticulum

The **endoplasmic reticulum** (ER) is a highly convoluted system of membranes that are interconnected and arranged to form a transport network of tubules and flattened sacs within the cytoplasm. Much of the ER has a rough, granular appearance when observed by transmission electron microscopy and is designated as **rough endoplasmic reticulum** (RER). This rough appearance is caused by the many *ribosomes* attached to

---

[b]Although the Human Genome Project was completed in 2003, the exact number of genes encoded by the human genome is still unknown. The reason for the uncertainty is that the various predictions are derived from different computational methods and gene-finding programs. Defining a gene is problematic for a number of reasons, including (1) small genes can be difficult to detect, (2) one gene can code for several protein products, (3) some genes code only for RNA, and (4) two genes can overlap. Even with improved genome analysis, computation alone is insufficient to generate an accurate gene number. Gene predictions must be verified by labor-intensive work in the laboratory before the scientific community can reach any real consensus. (From http://www.ornl.gov/hgmis.)

[c]http://earthsky.org/earth

[d]www.ornl.gov/sci/techresources/Human_Genome/faq/compgen.shtml

[e]http://en.wikipedia.org/wiki/List_of_sequenced_ eukaryotic_genomes

the outer surface of the membranes. ER to which ribosomes are not attached is called **smooth endoplasmic reticulum** (SER).

Ribosomes

Eukaryotic ribosomes are 18 to 22 nm in diameter. They consist mainly of rRNA and protein and play an important part in the synthesis (manufacture) of proteins. Clusters of ribosomes (called **polyribosomes** or **polysomes**), held together by a molecule of messenger RNA (mRNA), are sometimes observed by electron microscopy.

> Within a cell, ribosomes are the sites of protein synthesis.

Each eukaryotic ribosome is composed of two subunits—a large subunit (the 60S subunit) and a small subunit (the 40S subunit)—that are produced in the nucleolus. The subunits are then transported to the cytoplasm where they remain separate until such time as they join together with an mRNA molecule to initiate protein synthesis (Chapter 6). When united, the 40S and 60S subunits form an 80S ribosome. (The "S" refers to Svedberg units, and 40S, 60S, and 80S are sedimentation coefficients. A sedimentation coefficient expresses the rate at which a particle or molecule moves in a centrifugal field; it is determined by the size and shape of the particle or molecule.)

Most of the proteins released from the ER are not mature. They must undergo further processing in an organelle known as a Golgi complex before they are able to perform their functions within or outside of the cell.

Golgi Complex

A **Golgi complex**, also known as a Golgi apparatus or Golgi body, connects or communicates with the ER. This stack of flattened, membranous sacs completes the transformation of newly synthesized proteins into mature, functional ones and packages them into small, membrane-enclosed vesicles for storage within the cell or export outside the cell (exocytosis or secretion). Golgi complexes are sometimes referred to as "packaging plants."

> Golgi complexes can be considered "packaging plants."

Lysosomes and Peroxisomes

Lysosomes are small (about 1-μm diameter) vesicles that originate at the Golgi complex. They contain lysozyme and other digestive enzymes that break down foreign material taken into the cell by *phagocytosis* (the engulfing of large particles by amebas and certain types of white blood cells called **phagocytes**). These enzymes also aid in breaking down worn out parts of the cell and may destroy the entire cell by a process called **autolysis** if the cell is damaged or deteriorating. Lysosomes are found in all eukaryotic cells.

Peroxisomes are membrane-bound vesicles in which hydrogen peroxide is both generated and broken down. Peroxisomes contain the enzyme catalase, which catalyzes (speeds up) the breakdown of hydrogen peroxide into water and oxygen. Peroxisomes are found in most eukaryotic cells, but are especially prominent in mammalian liver cells.

Mitochondria

The energy necessary for cellular function is provided by the formation of high-energy phosphate molecules such as adenosine triphosphate (ATP). ATP molecules are the major energy-carrying or energy-storing molecules within cells. **Mitochondria** (sing., **mitochondrion**) are referred to as the "power plants," "powerhouses," or "energy factories" of the eukaryotic cell, because this is where most of the ATP molecules are formed by cellular respiration. During this process, energy is released from glucose molecules and other nutrients to drive other cellular functions (see Chapter 7). The number of mitochondria in a cell varies greatly depending on the activities required of that cell. Mitochondria are about 0.5 to 1 μm in diameter and up to 7 μm in length. Many scientists believe that mitochondria and chloroplasts arose from bacteria living within eukaryotic cells (see "The Origin of Mitochondria and Chloroplasts" on thePoint.

> Mitochondria can be considered "power plants" or "energy factories" within a cell.

Plastids

Plant cells contain both mitochondria and another type of energy-producing organelle, called a plastid. **Plastids** are membrane-bound structures containing various photosynthetic pigments; they are the sites of photosynthesis. **Chloroplasts**, one type of plastid, contain a green, photosynthetic pigment called chlorophyll. Chloroplasts are found in plant cells and algae. **Photosynthesis** is the process by which light energy is used to convert carbon dioxide and water into carbohydrates and oxygen (Chapter 7). The chemical bonds in the carbohydrate molecules represent stored energy. Thus, photosynthesis is the conversion of light energy into chemical energy.

> Within certain types of cells, plastids are the sites of photosynthesis.

Cytoskeleton

Present throughout the cytoplasm is a system of fibers, collectively known as the **cytoskeleton**. The three types of cytoskeletal fibers are microtubules, microfilaments (actin filaments), and intermediate filaments. All three types serve to strengthen, support, and stiffen the cell, and give the cell its shape. In addition to their structural roles, microtubules and microfilaments are essential for various activities, such as cell division, contraction, motility (see the section on flagella and cilia), and the movement of chromosomes within the cell. **Microtubules** are slender, hollow tubules composed of spherical protein subunits called *tubulins*.

Cell Wall

Some eukaryotic cells contain *cell walls*—external structures that provide rigidity, shape, and protection (Fig. 3-4). Eukaryotic cell walls, which are much simpler in structure than prokaryotic cell walls, may contain cellulose, pectin, lignin, chitin, and some mineral salts (usually found in algae). The cell walls of algae contain a polysaccharide—*cellulose*—that is not found in the cell walls of any other microorganisms. Cellulose is also found in the cell walls of plants. The cell walls of fungi contain a polysaccharide—*chitin*—that is not found in the cell walls of any other microorganisms. Chitin, which is similar in structure to cellulose, is also found in the exoskeletons of beetles and crabs.

Flagella and Cilia

Some eukaryotic cells (e.g., spermatozoa and certain types of protozoa and algae) possess relatively long, thin structures called **flagella** (sing., **flagellum**). Such cells are said to be flagellated or motile; flagellated protozoa are called flagellates. The whipping motion of the flagella enables flagellated cells to "swim" through liquid environments; flagella are said to be whip-like. Flagella are referred to as organelles of locomotion (cell movement). Flagellated cells may possess one flagellum or two or more flagella. **Cilia** (sing., **cilium**) are also organelles of locomotion, but they tend to be shorter (more hair-like), thinner, and more numerous than flagella. Cilia can be found on some species of protozoa (called ciliates) and on certain types of cells in our bodies (e.g., the ciliated epithelial cells that line the respiratory tract). Unlike flagella, cilia tend to beat with a coordinated, rhythmic

movement. Eukaryotic flagella and cilia, which contain an internal "9 + 2" arrangement of microtubules (Fig. 3-5), are structurally more complex than bacterial flagella.

Prokaryotic Cell Structure

Prokaryotic cells are about 10 times smaller than eukaryotic cells. A typical *E. coli* cell is about 1 μm wide and 2 to 3 μm long. Structurally, *prokaryotes* are very simple cells when compared with eukaryotic cells, and yet they are able to perform the necessary processes of life. Reproduction of prokaryotic cells is by *binary fission*—the simple division of one cell into two cells, after DNA replication (Chapter 6) and the formation of a separating membrane and cell wall. All bacteria are prokaryotes, as are the archaea.

Embedded within the cytoplasm of prokaryotic cells are a chromosome, ribosomes, and other cytoplasmic particles (Fig. 3-6). Unlike eukaryotic cells, the cytoplasm of prokaryotic cells is not filled with internal membranes. The cytoplasm is surrounded by a cell membrane, a cell wall (usually), and sometimes a capsule or slime layer. These latter three structures make up the bacterial cell envelope. Depending on the particular species of bacterium, flagella, pili

> Motile eukaryotic cells possess either flagella or cilia.

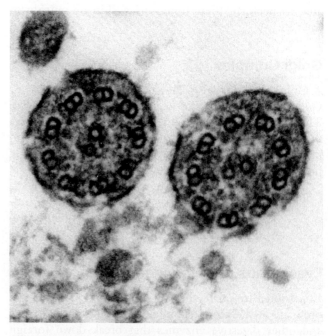

Figure 3-5. Cilia. A transmission electron micrograph showing cross sections of mouse respiratory cilia. Note the 9 + 2 arrangement of microtubules within each cilium: two single microtubules in the center, surrounded by nine doublet microtubules. (Courtesy of Louisa Howard and remf.dartmouth. edu/images.)

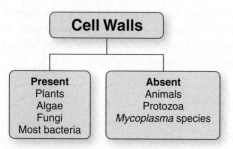

Figure 3-4. Presence or absence of a cell wall in various types of cells. *Mycoplasma* is a genus of bacteria.

In cyanobacteria and other photosynthetic bacteria (bacteria that convert light energy into chemical energy), infoldings of the cell membrane contain chlorophyll and other pigments that serve to trap light energy for photosynthesis. However, prokaryotic cells do not have complex internal membrane systems similar to the ER and Golgi complex of eukaryotic cells. Prokaryotic cells do not contain any membrane-bound organelles or vesicles.

Chromosome

The prokaryotic chromosome usually consists of a single, long, supercoiled, circular DNA

> Bacterial cells possess only one chromosome, whereas eukaryotic cells may possess many.

molecule, which serves as the control center of the bacterial cell. It is capable of duplicating itself, guiding cell division, and directing cellular activities. A prokaryotic cell contains neither nucleoplasm nor a nuclear membrane. The chromosome is suspended or embedded in the cytoplasm. The DNA-occupied space within a bacterial cell is sometimes referred to as the bacterial nucleoid.

The thin and tightly folded chromosome of *E. coli* is about 1.5 mm (1,500 µm) long and only 2 nm wide. Because a typical *E. coli* cell is about 2 to 3 µm long, its chromosome is approximately 500 to 750 times longer than the cell itself—quite a packaging feat! Bacterial chromosomes contain between 575 and 55,000 genes, depending on the species. Each gene codes for one or more gene products (enzymes, other proteins, and rRNA and tRNA molecules). In comparison, the chromosomes within a human cell contain between 20,000 and 25,000 genes.

Small, circular molecules of double-stranded DNA that are not part of the chromosome (referred to as **extrachromosomal DNA** or **plasmids**) may also be present in the cytoplasm of prokaryotic cells (Fig. 3-7). A plasmid may contain anywhere from fewer than 10 genes to several hundred genes. A bacterial cell may not contain any plasmids, or it may contain one plasmid, multiple copies of the same plasmid, or more than one type of plasmid (i.e., plasmids containing different genes). (Additional information about bacterial plasmids is found in Chapter 7.) Plasmids have also been found in yeast cells.

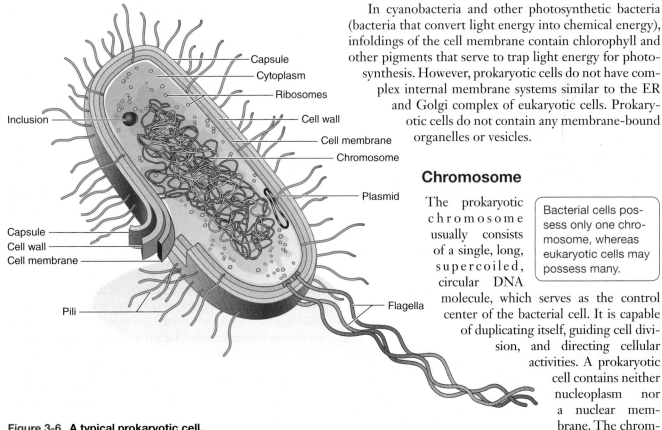

Figure 3-6. A typical prokaryotic cell.

(description follows), or both may be observed outside the cell envelope, and a spore may sometimes be seen within the cell.

Cell Membrane

Enclosing the cytoplasm of a prokaryotic cell is the cell membrane (also known as the plasma, cytoplasmic, or cellular membrane). This membrane is similar in structure and function to the eukaryotic cell membrane. Chemically, the cell membrane consists of proteins and phospholipids, which are discussed further in Chapter 6. Being selectively permeable, the membrane controls which substances may enter or leave the cell. It is flexible and so thin that it cannot be seen with a compound light microscope. However, it is frequently observed in transmission electron micrographs of bacteria.

Many enzymes are attached to the cell membrane, and various metabolic reactions take place there. Some scientists believe that inward foldings of the cell membranes—called **mesosomes**—are where cellular respiration takes place in bacteria. This process is similar to that which occurs in the mitochondria of eukaryotic cells, in which nutrients are broken down to produce energy in the form of ATP molecules. On the other hand, some scientists think that mesosomes are nothing more than artifacts created during the processing of bacterial cells for electron microscopy.

Cytoplasm

The semiliquid cytoplasm of prokaryotic cells consists of water, enzymes, dissolved oxygen (in some bacteria), waste products, essential nutrients, proteins,

Bacterium

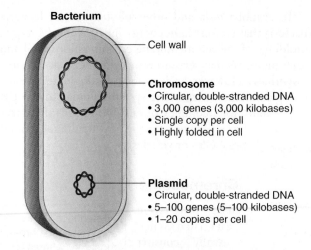

- Cell wall
- **Chromosome**
  - Circular, double-stranded DNA
  - 3,000 genes (3,000 kilobases)
  - Single copy per cell
  - Highly folded in cell
- **Plasmid**
  - Circular, double-stranded DNA
  - 5–100 genes (5–100 kilobases)
  - 1–20 copies per cell

Figure 3-7. A typical bacterial genome. The hypothetical bacterial cell illustrated here possesses a chromosome containing 3,000 genes and a plasmid containing 5 to 100 genes. (Redrawn from Harvey RA et al. Lippincott's Illustrated Reviews. *Microbiology*. 3rd ed. Philadelphia, PA: Lippincott Williams & Wilkins; 2013.)

> A bacterial cell may not contain any plasmids, or it may contain one plasmid, multiple copies of the same plasmid, or more than one type of plasmid.

carbohydrates, and lipids—a complex mixture of all the materials required by the cell for its metabolic functions. There is some evidence to suggest that bacterial cytoplasm contains a cytoskeletal structure similar to that of eukaryotic cells.

STUDY AID

Beware of Similar Sounding Words

A **plasmid** is a small, circular molecule of double-stranded DNA. It is referred to as extrachromosomal DNA because it is not part of the chromosome. Plasmids are found in most bacteria. A **plastid** is a cytoplasmic organelle, found only in certain eukaryotic cells (e.g., algae and plants). Plastids are the sites of photosynthesis.

Cytoplasmic Particles

Within the bacterial cytoplasm, many tiny particles have been observed. Most of these are ribosomes, often occurring in clusters called polyribosomes or polysomes (*poly* meaning many). Prokaryotic ribosomes are smaller than eukaryotic ribosomes, but their function is the same—they are the sites of protein synthesis. A 70S prokaryotic ribosome is composed of a 30S subunit and a 50S

subunit. It has been estimated that there are about 15,000 ribosomes in the cytoplasm of an *E. coli* cell.

Cytoplasmic granules occur in certain species of bacteria. These may be stained by using a suitable stain, and then identified microscopically. The granules may consist of starch, lipids, sulfur, iron, or other stored substances.

Bacterial Cell Wall

The rigid exterior cell wall that defines the shape of bacterial cells is chemically complex. Thus, the structure of bacterial cell walls is quite different from the relatively simple structure of eukaryotic cell walls, although they serve the same functions—providing rigidity, strength, and protection. The main constituent of most bacterial cell walls is a complex macromolecular polymer known as peptidoglycan (also known as murein), consisting of many polysaccharide chains linked together by small peptide (protein) chains (Fig. 3-8). Peptidoglycan is only found in bacteria. The thickness of the cell wall and its exact composition vary with the species of bacteria. The cell walls of certain bacteria, called **Gram-positive bacteria** (to be explained in Chapter 4), have a thick layer of peptidoglycan combined with teichoic acid and lipoteichoic acid molecules (Fig. 3-9). The cell walls of **Gram-negative bacteria** (also explained in Chapter 4) have a much thinner layer of peptidoglycan, but this layer is covered with a complex layer of lipid macromolecules, usually referred to as the outer membrane, as shown in Figure 3-9. These macromolecules are discussed in Chapter 6. Although most bacteria have cell walls, bacteria in the genus *Mycoplasma* do not. Archaea (described in Chapter 4) have cell walls, but their cell walls do not contain peptidoglycan.

Some bacteria lose their ability to produce cell walls, transforming into tiny variants of the same species, referred to as **L-form** or **cell wall–deficient** (CWD) bacteria. Over 50 different species of bacteria are capable of transforming into CWD bacteria, some of which

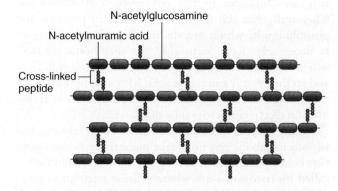

N-acetylglucosamine

N-acetylmuramic acid

Cross-linked peptide

Figure 3-8. Structure of peptidoglycan. The peptidoglycan (murein) layer in a bacterial cell is a crystal lattice. Polysaccharide chains consisting of two alternating amino sugars are attached to a short peptide chain. Some of the peptide chains of one polysaccharide chain are cross-linked to peptide chains of another polysaccharide chain, thus producing a three-dimensional lattice structure. (Redrawn from Engleberg NC, et al. *Schaechter's Mechanisms of Microbial Disease*. 5th ed. Philadelphia, PA: Lippincott Williams & Wilkins; 2013.)

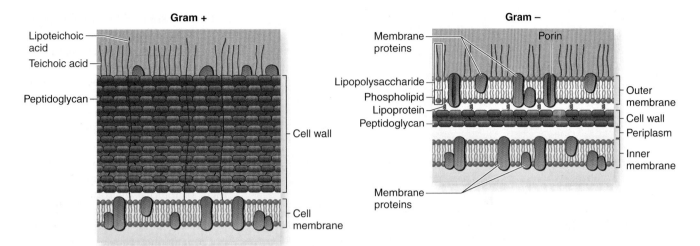

Figure 3-9. Differences between Gram-negative and Gram-positive cell walls. The relatively thin Gram-negative cell wall contains a thin layer of peptidoglycan, an outer membrane, and lipopolysaccharide (LPS). The thicker Gram-positive cell wall contains a thick layer of peptidoglycan and teichoic and lipoteichoic acids. (From Engleberg NC, et al. *Schaechter's Mechanisms of Microbial Disease*. 5th ed. Philadelphia, PA: Lippincott Williams & Wilkins; 2013.)

> Most bacteria possess cell walls. Exceptions include CWD and bacteria in the genus *Mycoplasma*.

might be responsible for chronic diseases such as chronic fatigue syndrome, Lyme disease, rheumatoid arthritis, and sarcoidosis. Clinicians are often unaware that CWD bacteria are present in their patients because they will not grow under standard laboratory conditions; they must be cultured in a different medium and at a different temperature than typical bacteria.

Glycocalyx (Slime Layers and Capsules)

Some bacteria have a thick layer of material (known as glycocalyx) located outside their cell wall. **Glycocalyx** is a slimy, gelatinous material produced by the cell membrane and secreted outside of the cell wall. There are two types of glycocalyx. One type, called a **slime layer**, is not highly organized and is not firmly attached to the cell wall. It easily detaches from the cell wall and drifts away. Bacteria in the genus *Pseudomonas* produce a slime layer, which sometimes plays a role in diseases caused by *Pseudomonas* species. Slime layers enable certain bacteria to glide or slide along solid surfaces, and seem to protect bacteria from antibiotics and desiccation.

> Depending on the species, bacterial cells may or may not be surrounded by glycocalyx. The two types of glycocalyx are slime layers and capsules.

The other type of glycocalyx, called a **capsule**, is highly organized and firmly attached to the cell wall. Capsules usually consist of polysaccharides, which may be combined with lipids and proteins, depending on the bacterial species. Knowledge of the chemical composition of capsules is useful in differentiating among different types of bacteria within a particular species; for example,

different strains of the bacterium *H. influenzae*, a cause of meningitis and ear infections in children, are identified by their capsular types. A vaccine, called Hib vaccine, is available for protection against disease caused by *H. influenzae* capsular type b. Other examples of encapsulated bacteria are *Klebsiella pneumoniae*, *Neisseria meningitidis*, and *Streptococcus pneumoniae*.

Capsules can be detected using a capsule staining procedure, which is a type of *negative stain*. The bacterial cell and background become stained, but the capsule remains unstained (Fig. 3-10). Thus, the capsule appears as an unstained halo around the bacterial cell. Antigen–antibody tests (described in Chapter 16) may be used to identify specific strains of bacteria possessing unique capsular molecules (antigens).

Encapsulated bacteria usually produce colonies on nutrient agar that are smooth, mucoid, and glistening; they are referred to as **S-colonies**. Nonencapsulated bacteria tend to grow as dry, rough colonies, called **R-colonies**. Capsules serve an antiphagocytic function, protecting the encapsulated bacteria from being phagocytized (ingested) by phagocytic white blood cells. Thus, encapsulated bacteria are able to survive longer in the human body than nonencapsulated bacteria.

> Bacterial capsules serve an antiphagocytic function, meaning that they protect encapsulated bacteria from being phagocytized by white blood cells.

Flagella

Flagella (sing., **flagellum**) are thread-like, protein appendages that enable bacteria to move. Flagellated bacteria are said to be motile, whereas nonflagellated

> Motile bacteria usually possess flagella. Bacteria never possess cilia.

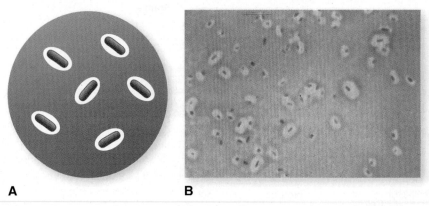

A   **B**

Figure 3-10. Capsule staining. A. Drawing illustrating the results of the capsule staining technique. **B.** Photomicrograph of encapsulated bacteria that have been stained using the capsule staining technique. The capsule staining is an example of a negative staining technique. Note that the bacterial cells and the background stain, but the capsules do not. The capsules are seen as unstained "halos" around the bacterial cells. (**[B]** From Winn WC Jr, et al. *Koneman's Color Atlas and Textbook of Diagnostic Microbiology*. 6th ed. Philadelphia, PA: Lippincott Williams & Wilkins; 2006.)

bacteria are usually nonmotile. Bacterial flagella are about 10 to 20 nm thick; too thin to be seen with the compound light microscope.

The number and arrangement of flagella possessed by a certain species of bacterium are characteristic of that species and can, thus, be used for classification and identification purposes (Fig. 3-11). Bacteria possessing flagella over their entire surface (perimeter) are called **peritrichous bacteria**. Bacteria with a tuft of flagella at one end are described as being **lophotrichous bacteria,** whereas those having one or more flagella at each end are said to be **amphitrichous bacteria**. Bacteria possessing a single polar flagellum are described as **monotrichous bacteria**. In the laboratory, the number of flagella that a cell possesses and their locations on the cell can be determined using what is known as

a flagella stain. The stain adheres to the flagella, making them thick enough to be seen under the microscope (Fig. 3-12).

Bacterial flagella consist of three, four, or more threads of protein (called **flagellin**) twisted like a rope. Thus, the structures of bacterial flagella and eukaryotic flagella are quite different. You will recall that eukaryotic flagella (and cilia) contain a complex arrangement of internal microtubules, which run the length of the membrane-bound flagellum. Bacterial flagella do not contain microtubules, and their flagella are not membrane-bound. Bacterial flagella arise from a basal body in the cell membrane and project outward through the cell wall and capsule (if present), as was shown in Figure 3-6.

Some **spirochetes** (spiral-shaped bacteria) have two flagella-like fibrils called **axial filaments**, one attached to each end of the bacterium. These axial filaments extend toward each other, wrap around the organism between the layers of the cell wall, and overlap in the midsection of the cell. As a result of its axial filaments, spirochetes can move in a spiral, helical, or inchworm manner.

Pili (Fimbriae)

Pili (sing., **pilus**) or **fimbriae** (sing., **fimbria**) are hair-like structures, most often observed on Gram-negative bacteria. They are composed of polymerized protein molecules called pilin. Pili are much thinner than flagella, have a rigid structure, and are not associated with motility. These tiny appendages arise from the cytoplasm and extend through the plasma membrane, cell wall, and capsule (if present). There are two types of pili: one type merely enables bacteria to adhere or attach to surfaces; the other type (called a **sex pilus**) facilitates transfer of genetic material from one bacterial cell to another following attachment of the cells to each other.

The pili that merely enable bacteria to anchor themselves to surfaces (e.g., tissues within the human body) are usually quite numerous (Fig. 3-13). In some species of bacteria, piliated strains (those possessing pili) are able to cause diseases such as urethritis and cystitis, whereas nonpiliated strains (those not

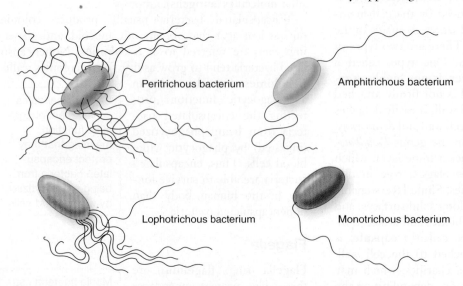

Peritrichous bacterium

Amphitrichous bacterium

Lophotrichous bacterium

Monotrichous bacterium

Figure 3-11. Flagellar arrangement. The four basic types of flagellar arrangement on bacteria: peritrichous, flagella all over the surface; lophotrichous, a tuft of flagella at one end; amphitrichous, one or more flagella at each end; monotrichous, one flagellum.

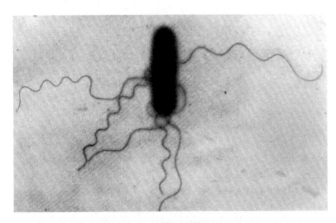

Figure 3-12. *Salmonella* cells, showing peritrichous flagella. *Salmonella* is a bacterial genus. The cells were stained using a flagella stain. (Courtesy of the CDC.)

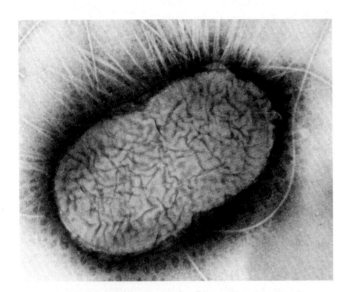

Figure 3-13. *Proteus vulgaris* cell, possessing numerous short, straight pili and several longer, curved flagella; the cell is undergoing binary fission. *P. vulgaris* is a bacterial species. (From Volk WA, et al. *Essentials of Medical Microbiology.* 5th ed. Philadelphia, PA: Lippincott-Raven; 1996.)

possessing pili) of the same organisms are unable to cause these diseases.

> Pili are organelles of attachment. That is, they enable bacteria to adhere to surfaces.

A bacterial cell possessing a sex pilus (called a **donor cell**)—and the cell only possesses one sex pilus—is able to attach to

> A sex pilus facilitates the transfer of genetic material from one bacterial cell (the donor cell) to another (the recipient cell).

another bacterial cell (called a recipient cell) by means of the sex pilus. Genetic material (usually in the form of a plasmid) is then transferred from the donor cell to the recipient cell—a process known as **conjugation** (described more fully in Chapter 7).

Spores (Endospores)

A few genera of bacteria (e.g., *Bacillus* and *Clostridium*) are capable of forming thick-walled spores as a means of survival when their moisture or nutrient supply is low. Bacterial spores are referred to as **endospores**, and the process by which they

> Endospores enable bacteria to survive in adverse conditions, such as temperature extremes, desiccation, and lack of nutrients.

are formed is called **sporulation**. During sporulation, a copy of the chromosome and some of the surrounding cytoplasm becomes enclosed in several thick protein coats. Spores are resistant to heat, cold, drying, and most chemicals. Spores have been shown to survive for many years in soil or dust, and some are quite resistant to disinfectants and boiling. When the dried spore lands on a moist, nutrient-rich surface, it germinates, and a new vegetative bacterial cell (a cell capable of growing and dividing) emerges. Germination of a spore may be compared with germination of a seed. However, in bacteria, spore formation is related to the survival of the bacterial cell, not to reproduction. Usually, only one spore is produced in a bacterial cell and it germinates into only one vegetative bacterium. In the laboratory, endospores can be stained using what is known as a spore stain. Once a particular bacterium's endospores are stained, the laboratory technologist can determine whether the organism is producing terminal or subterminal spores. A terminal spore is produced at the very end of the bacterial cell, whereas a subterminal spore is produced elsewhere in the cell (Fig. 3-14). Where a spore is being produced within the cell and whether or not it causes a swelling of the cell serve as clues to the identity of the organism.

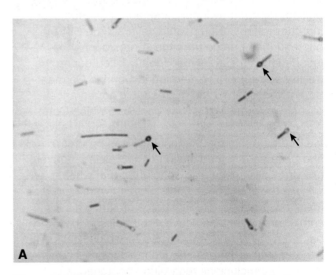

A

Figure 3-14. Terminal and subterminal spores. A. Gram-stained *Clostridium tetani* bacteria, revealing terminal spores (*arrows*). *C. tetani* causes the disease known as tetanus. (Courtesy of Dr. Holdeman and the CDC.) Continued on next page

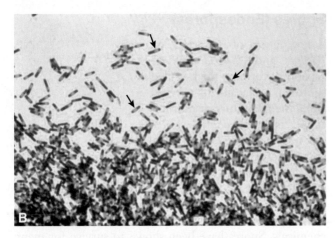

Figure 3-14. Continued. **B.** Gram-stained *Clostridium difficile* bacteria, revealing subterminal spores (the light areas within the cells). *C. difficile* causes a diarrheal disease. (Courtesy of Dr. Gilda Jones and the CDC.)

HISTORICAL NOTE

The Discovery of Endospores

While performing spontaneous generation experiments in 1876 and 1877, a British physicist named John Tyndall concluded that certain bacteria exist in two forms: a form that is readily killed by simple boiling (i.e., a heat-labile form), and a form that is not killed by simple boiling (i.e., a heat-stable form). He developed a fractional sterilization technique, known as *tyndallization*, which successfully killed both the heat-labile and heat-stable forms. Tyndallization involves boiling, followed by incubating, and then reboiling; these steps are repeated several times. The bacteria that emerge from the spores during the incubation steps are subsequently killed during the boiling steps. In 1877, Ferdinand Cohn, a German botanist, described the microscopic appearance of the two forms of the "hay bacillus," which Cohn named *Bacillus subtilis*. He referred to small refractile bodies within the bacterial cells as "spores" and observed the conversion of spores into actively growing cells. Cohn also concluded that when they were in the spore phase, the bacteria were heat resistant. Today, bacterial spores are known as *endospores*, whereas active, metabolizing, growing bacterial cells are referred to as vegetative cells. The experiments of Tyndall and Cohn supported Louis Pasteur's conclusions regarding spontaneous generation and dealt the final death blow to that theory.

Summary of Structural Differences between Prokaryotic and Eukaryotic Cells

Eukaryotic cells contain a true nucleus, whereas prokaryotic cells do not. Eukaryotic cells are divided into plant and animal types. Animal cells do not have a cell wall, whereas plant cells have a simple cell wall, usually containing cellulose. Cellulose, a type of polysaccharide, is a rigid polymer of glucose (polymers and polysaccharides are described in Chapter 6). Prokaryotic cells have complex cell walls consisting of proteins, lipids, and polysaccharides. Eukaryotic cells contain membranous structures (such as ER and Golgi complexes) and many membrane-bound organelles (such as mitochondria and plastids). Prokaryotic cells possess no membranes other than the cell membrane that encloses the cytoplasm. Eukaryotic ribosomes (referred to as 80S ribosomes) are larger and denser than those found in prokaryotes (70S ribosomes). The fact that 70S ribosomes are found in the mitochondria and chloroplasts of eukaryotes may indicate that these structures were derived from parasitic prokaryotes during their evolutionary development. Other differences between prokaryotic and eukaryotic cells are listed in Table 3-1.

> Eukaryotic cells contain numerous membranes and membrane-bound structures. The only membrane possessed by a prokaryotic cell is its cell membrane.

Reproduction of Organisms and Their Cells

Reproduction (referring to the manner in which organisms reproduce) and cell reproduction (referring to the process by which individual cells reproduce) are complex topics, which can only be briefly discussed in a book of this size. The following topics are discussed briefly on thePoint:

- asexual versus sexual reproduction
- life cycles
- eukaryotic cell reproduction (mitosis and meiosis)

Prokaryotic Cell Reproduction

Prokaryotic cell reproduction is quite simple when compared with eukaryotic cell division. Prokaryotic cells reproduce by a process known as *binary fission*, in which one cell (the parent cell) splits in half to become two daughter cells (Fig. 3-15). Before a prokaryotic cell

Table 3-1   Comparison between Eukaryotic and Prokaryotic Cells

| | Eukaryotic Cells | | Prokaryotic Cells |
	Plant type	Animal type	
Biologic distribution	All plants, fungi, and algae	All animals and protozoa	All bacteria
Nuclear membrane	Present	Present	Absent
Membranous structures other than cell membranes	Present	Present	Generally absent except for mesosomes and photosynthetic membranes
Microtubules	Present	Present	Absent
Cytoplasmic ribosomes (density)	80S	80S	70S
Chromosomes	Composed of DNA and proteins	Composed of DNA and proteins	Composed of DNA alone
Flagella or cilia	When present, have a complex structure	When present, have a complex structure	When present, flagella have a simple twisted protein structure; prokaryotic cells do not possess cilia
Cell wall	When present, of simple chemical constitution; usually contains cellulose	Absent	Of complex chemical constitution, containing peptidoglycan
Photosynthesis (chlorophyll)	Present	Absent	Present in cyanobacteria and some other bacteria

> Bacterial cells reproduce by binary fission—one cell splits in half to become two cells (known as daughter cells).

can divide in half, its chromosome must be duplicated (a process known as DNA replication; discussed in Chapter 6), so that each daughter cell will possess the same genetic information as the parent cell (Fig. 3-16).

The time it takes for binary fission to occur (i.e., the time it takes for one prokaryotic cell to become two cells) is called the **generation time**. The generation time varies from one bacterial species to another and also depends on the growth conditions (e.g., pH, temperature, and availability of nutrients). In the laboratory (in vitro), under ideal conditions, *E. coli* has a generation time of about 20 minutes—the number of cells will double every 20 minutes. Bacterial generation times range from as short as 10 minutes to as long as 24 hours, or even longer in some cases.

> The length of time it takes for one bacterial cell to split into two cells is referred to as the organism's generation time.

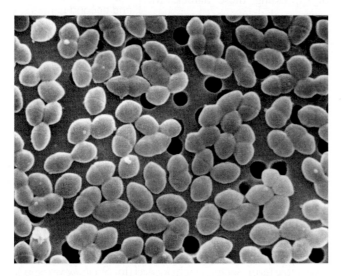

Figure 3-15. A scanning electron micrograph showing *Enterococcus* bacteria, many of which are in the process of binary fission. (Courtesy of Janice Haney Carr and the CDC.)

Taxonomy

According to *Bergey's Manual of Systematic Bacteriology* (described in Chapter 4 and on thePoint), **taxonomy** (the science of classification of living organisms) consists of three separate but interrelated areas: classification, nomenclature, and identification. *Classification* is the arrangement of organisms into taxonomic groups (known as **taxa** [sing., **taxon**]) on the basis of similarities or relationships. Taxa include kingdoms or domains, divisions or phyla, classes, orders, families, genera, and species. Closely related organisms (i.e., organisms having similar characteristics) are

Parent cell

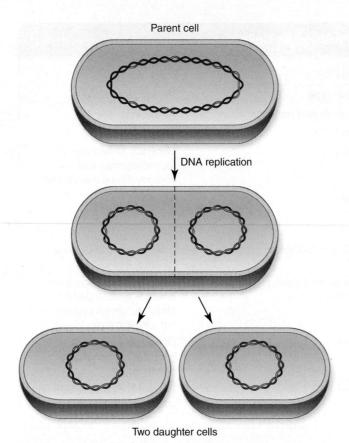

DNA replication

Two daughter cells

Figure 3-16. Binary fission. Note that DNA replication must occur prior to the actual splitting (fission) of the parent cell. (An animated version of this figure can be found on thePoint.)

placed into the same taxon. *Nomenclature* is the assignment of names to the various taxa according to international rules. *Identification* is the process of determining whether an isolate belongs to one of the established, named taxa or represents a previously unidentified species.

When attempting to identify an organism that has been isolated from a clinical specimen, laboratory technologists are very much like crime scene investigators or detectives. They gather "clues" (characteristics, attributes, properties, and traits) about the organism until they have sufficient clues to identify (speciate) the organism. In most cases, the clues that have been gathered will match the characteristics of an established species. (Note: throughout this book, the term "to identify an organism" means to learn the organism's species name—i.e., to speciate it.) An organism's complete collection of physical characteristics is known as the organism's phenotype.

> An organism's complete collection of genes is referred to as the organism's genotype or genome. An organism's complete collection of physical characteristics is known as the organism's phenotype.

Microbial Classification

Since Aristotle's time, scientists have attempted to name and classify living organisms in a meaningful way, based on their appearance and behavior. Thus, the science of taxonomy was established, based on the binomial system of nomenclature developed in the 18th century by the Swedish scientist Carolus Linnaeus. In the binomial system, each organism is given two names (e.g., *Homo sapiens* for humans). The first name is the **genus** (pl., **genera**), and the second name is the **specific epithet**. The first and second names together are referred to as the *species*.

Because written reference is often made to genera and species, biologists throughout the world have adopted a standard method of expressing these names. To express the genus, capitalize the first letter of the word and underline or italicize the whole word—for example, *Escherichia*. To express the species, capitalize the first letter of the genus name (the specific epithet is not capitalized) and then underline or italicize the entire species name—for example, *Escherichia coli*. Frequently, the genus is designated by a single-letter abbreviation; in the example just given, *E. coli* indicates the species. In an essay or article about *Escherichia coli*, *Escherichia* would be spelled out the first time the organism is mentioned; thereafter, the abbreviated form, *E. coli*, could be used. The abbreviation "sp." is used to designate a single species, whereas the abbreviation "spp." is used to designate more than one species.

> In the binomial system of nomenclature, the first name (e.g., *Escherichia*) is the genus, and the second name (e.g., *coli*) is the specific epithet. When used together, the first and second names (e.g., *Escherichia coli*) are referred to as a species.

In addition to the proper scientific names for bacteria, acceptable terms such as staphylococci (for *Staphylococcus* spp.), streptococci (for *Streptococcus* spp.), clostridia (for *Clostridium* spp.), pseudomonads (for *Pseudomonas* spp.), mycoplasmas (for *Mycoplasma* spp.), rickettsias (for *Rickettsia* spp.), and chlamydias (for *Chlamydia* spp.) are commonly used. Nicknames and slang terms frequently used within hospitals are GC and gonococci (for *Neisseria gonorrhoeae*), meningococci (for *N. meningitidis*), pneumococci (for *S. pneumoniae*), staph (for *Staphylococcus* or staphylococcal), and strep (for *Streptococcus* or streptococcal). It is common to hear healthcare workers using terms such as meningococcal meningitis, pneumococcal pneumonia, staph infection, and strep throat.

Quite often, bacteria are named for the disease that they cause (see Table 3-2 for examples). In a few cases, bacteria are misnamed. For example, *H. influenzae* does not cause influenza, which is a respiratory disease caused by influenza viruses.

Organisms are categorized into larger groups based on their similarities and differences. It should be noted that the classification of living organisms is a complex and controversial subject.

In 1969, Robert H. Whittaker proposed a Five-Kingdom System of Classification, in which all organisms are placed into five kingdoms:

- Bacteria and archaea are in the Kingdom Prokaryotae (or Monera)
- Algae and protozoa are in the Kingdom Protista (organisms in this kingdom are referred to as **protists**)
- Fungi are in the Kingdom Fungi
- Plants are in the Kingdom Plantae
- Animals are in the Kingdom Animalia (Although humans are in the Kingdom Animalia, in this book, the word "animals" refers to animals other than humans.)

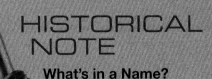

HISTORICAL NOTE

What's in a Name?

Sometimes, bacteria and other microorganisms are named for the person who discovered the organism. An interesting example is the name of the plague bacillus. The bacterium that causes plague was discovered in 1894 by Alexandre Emile Jean Yersin (1863–1943), a French bacteriologist of Swiss descent, who worked for many years at various Pasteur Institutes in Vietnam. Yersin originally named the organism *Bacillus pestis*, but in 1896 the name was changed to *Pasteurella pestis*, to honor Louis Pasteur, with whom Yersin had studied. Then, many years later, taxonomists changed the name to *Yersinia pestis* to honor Yersin—the person who discovered the organism. Other genera named for bacteriologists include *Bordetella* (Jules Bordet), *Escherichia* (Theodore Escherich), *Neisseria* (Albert Ludwig Neisser), and *Salmonella* (Daniel Elmer Salmon).

Table 3-2 Examples of Bacteria Named for the Diseases That They Cause[a]

Bacterium	Disease
Bacillus anthracis	Anthrax
Chlamydophila pneumoniae	Pneumonia
Chlamydophila psittaci	Psittacosis ("parrot fever")
Chlamydia trachomatis	Trachoma
Clostridium botulinum	Botulism
Clostridium tetani	Tetanus
Corynebacterium diphtheriae	Diphtheria
Francisella tularensis	Tularemia ("rabbit fever")
Klebsiella pneumoniae	Pneumonia
Mycobacterium leprae	Leprosy (Hansen disease)
Mycobacterium tuberculosis	Tuberculosis
Mycoplasma pneumoniae	Pneumonia
Neisseria gonorrhoeae	Gonorrhea
Neisseria meningitidis	Meningitis
Streptococcus pneumoniae	Pneumonia
Vibrio cholerae	Cholera

[a]In some cases, these bacteria cause more than one disease.

Viruses are not included in the Five-Kingdom System of Classification because they are not living cells; they are acellular. Note that four of the five kingdoms consist of eukaryotic organisms. Each kingdom consists of divisions or phyla, which, in turn, are divided into classes, orders, families, genera, and species (Table 3-3). In some cases, species are subdivided into subspecies, their names consisting of a genus, a specific epithet, and a subspecific epithet (abbreviated "ssp."); an example would be *H. influenzae* ssp. *aegyptius*, the most common cause of "pinkeye." Although Whittaker's Five-Kingdom System of Classification has been a popular classification system for the past 30 or so years, not all scientists agree with it; other taxonomic classification schemes exist. For example, some scientists do not agree that algae and protozoa should be placed into the same kingdom, and in some classification schemes, protozoa are placed into a subkingdom of the Animal Kingdom.

In the late 1970s, Carl R. Woese (see the following "Historical Note") devised a Three-Domain System of Classification, which is gaining in popularity among scientists. The Three-Domain System of Classification is based on differences in the structure of certain rRNA molecules among organisms in the three domains. In this Three-Domain System, there are two domains of prokaryotes (*Archaea* and *Bacteria*) and one domain, called *Eucarya* or *Eukarya*, which includes all eukaryotic organisms. Note that the domain names are italicized.

Table 3-3 Comparison of Human and Bacterial Classification

	Human being	*Escherichia coli* (a medically important Gram-negative bacillus)[a]	*Staphylococcus aureus* (a medically important Gram-positive coccus)[a]
Kingdom (Domain)	Animalia (*Eukarya*)	Prokaryotae (*Bacteria*)	Prokaryotae (*Bacteria*)
Phylum	Chordata	Proteobacteria	Firmicutes
Class	Mammalia	Gammaproteobacteria	Bacilli
Order	Primates	Enterobacteriales	Bacillales
Family	*Hominidae*	*Enterobacteriaceae*	*Staphylococcaceae*
Genus	*Homo*	*Escherichia*	*Staphylococcus*
Species (a species has two names; the first name is the genus, and the second name is the specific epithet)	*Homo sapiens*	*Escherichia coli*	*Staphylococcus aureus*

[a]Based on *Bergey's Manual of Systematic Bacteriology*. vol 1. 2nd ed. New York, NY: Springer-Verlag; 2001. A bacillus is a rod-shaped bacterium. A coccus is a spherical-shaped bacterium.

Archaea comes from *archae*, meaning "ancient." Although members of the Domain *Archaea* have been referred to in the past as archaebacteria and archaeobacteria (meaning ancient bacteria), these names have fallen out of favor because the **archaea** are so different from bacteria. Similarly, organisms in the Domain *Bacteria* have, at times, been referred to as eubacteria, meaning "true" bacteria, but are now usually referred to simply as **bacteria**. Domain *Archaea* contains 2 phyla, and Domain *Bacteria* contains 23.

The Domain *Eukarya* is divided into four kingdoms: Kingdom Protista or Protoctista (algae and protozoa); Kingdom Plantae; Kingdom Fungi; Kingdom Animalia.

Perhaps taxonomists will someday combine the Three-Domain System and the Five-Kingdom System, producing either a Six-Kingdom System (Bacteria, Archaea, Protista, Fungi, Plantae, and Animalia) or a Seven-Kingdom System (Bacteria, Archaea, Algae, Protozoa, Fungi, Plantae, and Animalia).

HISTORICAL NOTE

Carl R. Woese

During the 1970s, a molecular biologist named Carl Woese and his colleagues at the University of Illinois shook up the scientific community by developing a system of classifying organisms that was based on the sequences of nucleotide bases in their ribosomal RNA (rRNA) molecules.

They demonstrated that prokaryotic organisms can be divided into two major groups (referred to as domains), based on differences in their rRNA sequences, and that the rRNA from these two groups differed from the rRNA of eukaryotic organisms. Although this system of classification was not widely accepted at first, Woese's Three-Domain System of Classification has become the classification system most favored by microbiologists.

Evolution and the Tree of Life

Although evolutionary biology is a complex and controversial topic, many scientists believe that life on Earth originated and then evolved from what is commonly referred to as the last universal common ancestor (LUCA)[f] approximately 3.5 to 3.9 billion years ago. A popular theory is that highly energetic chemical reactions produced self-replicating molecules (such as RNA) around 4 billion years ago, which led to the assembly of simple cells, and then about a half billion years later, the LUCA existed.

Prokaryotes inhabited Earth from approximately 3 to 4 billion years ago, and eukaryotic cells emerged between 1.6 and 2.7 billion years ago. It is thought that certain bacterial cells were engulfed by eukaryotic cells, leading to a cooperative association known as endosymbiosis. Some endosymbiotic bacteria evolved into mitochondria,

[f]LUCA is also referred to as the last universal ancestor (LUA), the cenancestor, and the most recent common ancestor (MRCA).

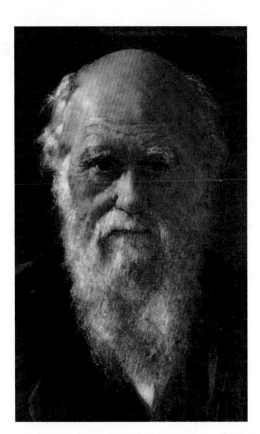

Figure 3-17. Charles Darwin. (Courtesy of Sciencebuzz.org.)

whereas others (the photosynthetic cyanobacteria) evolved into chloroplasts.

The current "tree of life" (Fig. 3-18) consists of three major domains of organisms, each of which arose separately from an ancestor with poorly developed genetic machinery, often called a progenote.

Determining Relatedness among Organisms

How do scientists determine how closely related one organism is to another? The most widely used technique for gauging diversity or relatedness is called

[g]An alternate theory, known as intelligent design, argues that "certain features of the universe and of living things are best explained by an intelligent cause, not an undirected process such as natural selection" (as defined by the Discovery Institute). The intelligent design theory implies the existence of a "designer" or "creator." According to Wikipedia, "intelligent design is seen as a pseudoscience in the scientific community, because it lacks empirical support, supplies no tentative hypotheses, and resolves to describe natural history in terms of scientifically untestable supernatural causes."

[h]Refers to the *HMS Beagle*, the ship upon which Darwin sailed in the 1830s, during which time he was developing his theory of evolution by natural selection.

rRNA sequencing. Ribosomes are made up of two subunits: a small subunit and a large subunit. The small subunit contains only one RNA molecule, which is referred to as the "small subunit rRNA" or SSUrRNA. The SSUrRNA in prokaryotic ribosomes is a 16S rRNA molecule, whereas the SSUrRNA in eukaryotes is an 18S rRNA molecule. (The "S" in 16S and 18S refers to Svedberg units, which were discussed earlier.) The gene that codes for the 16S rRNA molecule contains about 1,500 DNA nucleotides, whereas the gene that codes for the 18S rRNA molecule contains about 2,000 nucleotides. The sequence of nucleotides in the gene that codes for the 16S rRNA molecule is called the 16s rDNA sequence. To determine "relatedness," researchers compare the sequence of nucleotide base pairs in the gene, rather than comparing the actual SSUrRNA molecules. If the 16S rDNA sequence of one prokaryotic organism is quite similar to the 16S rDNA sequence of another prokaryotic organism, then the organisms are closely related. The less similar the 16S rDNA sequences in prokaryotes (or the 18S rDNA sequences in eukaryotes), the less related are the organisms. For example, the 18S rDNA sequence of a human is much more similar to the 18S rDNA sequence of a chimpanzee than to the 18S rDNA sequence of a fungus.

Phylogenetic Tree of Life

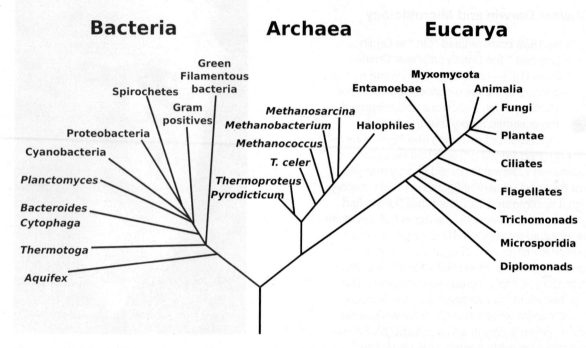

Figure 3-18. The Phylogenetic Tree of Life. The exact relationships of the three domains are still being debated, as is the position of the root of the tree. (A discussion of all of the various branches on the tree of life is beyond the scope of this book. Students wishing to learn more about the branches should utilize an Internet Search Engine.) (Courtesy of NASA and Wikimedia.)

rRNA can be used not only for taxonomic purposes, but also in the clinical microbiology laboratory to identify pathogens. Microorganisms are identified by comparing the rRNA gene sequences that are recovered from clinical specimens to sequences contained in high-quality reference databanks.

ON thePoint

- Terms Introduced in This Chapter
- Review of Key Points
- A Closer Look: Asexual versus Sexual Reproduction; Life Cycles; Eukaryotic Cell Reproduction (Mitosis and Meiosis)
- The Origin of Mitochondria and Chloroplasts
- Increase Your Knowledge
- Critical Thinking
- Additional Self-Assessment Exercises

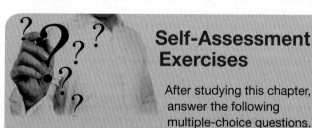

Self-Assessment Exercises

After studying this chapter, answer the following multiple-choice questions.

1. Molecules of extrachromosomal DNA are also known as:
   a. Golgi bodies
   b. lysosomes
   c. plasmids
   d. plastids

2. A bacterium possessing a tuft of flagella at one end of its cell would be called what kind of bacterium?
   a. amphitrichous
   b. lophotrichous
   c. monotrichous
   d. peritrichous

3. One way in which an archaean would differ from a bacterium is that the archaean would possess no:
   a. DNA in its chromosome
   b. peptidoglycan in its cell walls
   c. ribosomes in its cytoplasm
   d. RNA in its ribosomes

4. Some bacteria stain Gram-positive and others stain Gram-negative as a result of differences in the structure of their:
   a. capsule
   b. cell membrane
   c. cell wall
   d. ribosomes

5. Of the following, which one is *not* found in prokaryotic cells?
   a. cell membrane
   b. chromosome
   c. mitochondria
   d. plasmids

6. The Three-Domain System of Classification is based on differences in which of the following molecules?
   a. mRNA
   b. peptidoglycan
   c. rRNA
   d. tRNA

7. Which of the following is in the correct sequence?
   a. Kingdom, Class, Division, Order, Family, Genus
   b. Kingdom, Division, Class, Order, Family, Genus
   c. Kingdom, Division, Order, Class, Family, Genus
   d. Kingdom, Order, Division, Class, Family, Genus

8. Which one of the following is never found in prokaryotic cells?
   a. flagella
   b. capsule
   c. cilia
   d. ribosomes

9. The semipermeable structure controlling the transport of materials between the cell and its external environment is the:
   a. cell membrane
   b. cell wall
   c. cytoplasm
   d. nuclear membrane

10. In eukaryotic cells, what are the sites of photosynthesis?
    a. mitochondria
    b. plasmids
    c. plastids
    d. ribosomes

4

Microbial Diversity

Part 1: Acellular and Prokaryotic Microbes

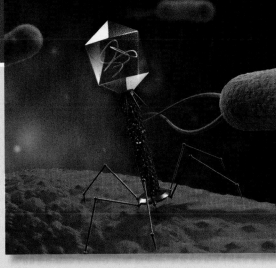

Artist rendering of a bacteriophage on the surface of a bacterial cell.

 CHAPTER OUTLINE

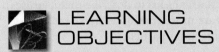 **LEARNING OBJECTIVES**

After studying this chapter, you should be able to:

- Describe the characteristics used to classify viruses (e.g., DNA vs. RNA)
- List five specific properties of viruses that distinguish them from bacteria
- List at least three important viral diseases of humans
- Discuss differences between viroids and prions, and the diseases they cause
- List various ways in which bacteria can be classified
- State the three purposes of fixation
- Define the terms diplococci, streptococci, staphylococci, tetrad, octad, coccobacilli, diplobacilli, streptobacilli, and pleomorphism
- Define the terms obligate aerobe, microaerophile, facultative anaerobe, aerotolerant anaerobe, obligate anaerobe, and capnophile
- State key differences among rickettsias, chlamydias, and mycoplasmas
- Identify several important bacterial diseases of humans
- State several ways in which archaea differ from bacteria

Introduction

Imagine the excitement that Anton van Leeuwenhoek experienced as he gazed through his tiny glass lenses and became the first person to see live microbes. In the years that have followed his eloquently written late 17th-century to early 18th-century accounts of the bacteria and protozoa that he observed, tens of thousands of microbes have been discovered, described, and classified. In this chapter and the next, you will be introduced to the diversity of form and function that exists in the microbial world.

As you will recall, microbiology is the study of microbes, most of which are too small to be seen by the naked eye. Microbes can be divided into those that are truly cellular (bacteria, archaea, algae, protozoa, and fungi) and those that are acellular (viruses, viroids, and prions). The cellular microorganisms can be subdivided into those that are prokaryotic (bacteria and archaea) and those that are eukaryotic (algae, protozoa, and fungi). For a variety of reasons, acellular microorganisms are not considered by most scientists to be living organisms. Thus, rather than using the term microorganisms to describe them, viruses, viroids, and prions are more correctly referred to as acellular microbes or infectious particles.

Acellular Microbes

Viruses

Complete virus particles, called *virions*, are very small and simple in structure. Most viruses range in size from 10 to 300 nm in diameter, although some—like Ebola virus—can be up to 1 µm in length. The smallest virus is about the size of the large hemoglobin molecule of a red blood cell. Scientists were unable to see viruses until electron microscopes were invented in the 1930s. The first photographs of viruses were obtained in 1940. A negative staining procedure, developed in 1959, revolutionized the study of viruses, making it possible to observe unstained viruses against an electron-dense, dark background.

> Viruses are extremely small. They are observed using electron microscopes.

No type of organism is safe from viral infections; viruses infect humans, animals, plants, fungi, protozoa, algae, and bacterial cells (Table 4-1). Many human diseases are caused by viruses (refer back to Table 1-1). Many of the viruses that infect humans are shown in Figure 4-1. Some viruses—called oncogenic viruses or oncoviruses—cause specific types of cancer, including human cancers such as lymphomas, carcinomas, and some types of leukemia.

> Viruses are not alive. To replicate, viruses must invade live host cells.

Viruses are said to have five specific properties that distinguish them from living cells:

- The vast majority of viruses possess *either* DNA or RNA, unlike living cells, which possess both.
- They are unable to replicate (multiply) on their own; their replication is directed by the viral nucleic acid once it has been introduced into a host cell.
- Unlike cells, they do not divide by binary fission, mitosis, or meiosis.
- They lack the genes and enzymes necessary for energy production.
- They depend on the ribosomes, enzymes, and metabolites ("building blocks") of the host cell for protein and nucleic acid production.

A typical virion consists of a genome of either DNA or RNA, surrounded by a *capsid* (protein coat), which is composed of many small protein units called *capsomeres* (or capsomers). Together, the nucleic acid and the capsid are referred to as the nucleocapsid (Fig. 4-2). Some viruses (called enveloped viruses) have an outer envelope composed of lipids and polysaccharides (Fig. 4-3). Bacterial viruses may also have a tail, sheath, and tail fibers. There are no ribosomes for protein synthesis or sites of energy production; hence, the virus must

> Except in very rare cases, a particular virus contains either DNA or RNA—not both.

> The simplest of human viruses consists of nothing more than nucleic acid surrounded by a protein coat (the capsid). The capsid plus the enclosed nucleic acid are referred to as the nucleocapsid.

Table 4-1 Relative Sizes and Shapes of Some Viruses

Viruses	Nucleic Acid Type	Shape	Size Range (nm)
Animal viruses			
Vaccinia	DNA	Complex	200 × 300
Mumps	RNA	Helical	150–250
Herpes simplex	DNA	Polyhedral	100–150
Influenza	RNA	Helical	80–120
Retroviruses	RNA	Helical	100–120
Adenoviruses	DNA	Polyhedral	60–90
Retroviruses	RNA	Polyhedral	60–80
Papovaviruses	DNA	Polyhedral	40–60
Polioviruses	RNA	Polyhedral	28
Plant viruses			
Turnip yellow mosaic	RNA	Polyhedral	28
Wound tumor	RNA	Polyhedral	55–60
Alfalfa mosaic	RNA	Polyhedral	18 × 36–40
Tobacco mosaic	RNA	Helical	18 × 300
Bacteriophages			
T2	DNA	Complex	65 × 210
L	DNA	Complex	54 × 194
F_x-174	DNA	Complex	25

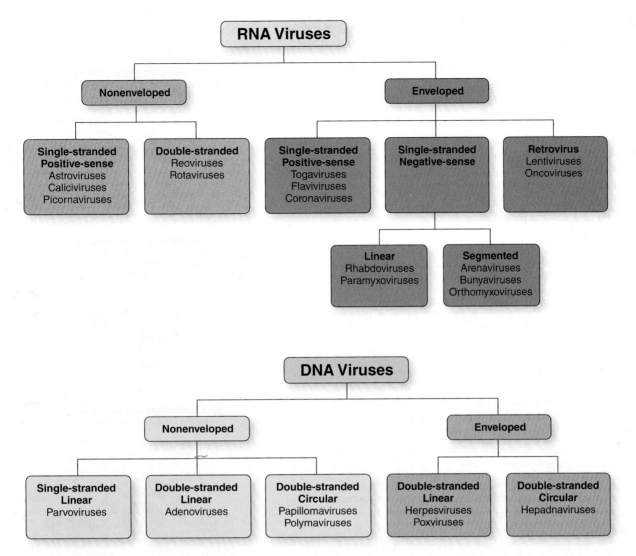

RNA Viruses

- **Nonenveloped**
  - **Single-stranded Positive-sense**
    Astroviruses
    Caliciviruses
    Picornaviruses
  - **Double-stranded**
    Reoviruses
    Rotaviruses
- **Enveloped**
  - **Single-stranded Positive-sense**
    Togaviruses
    Flaviviruses
    Coronaviruses
  - **Single-stranded Negative-sense**
    - **Linear**
      Rhabdoviruses
      Paramyxoviruses
    - **Segmented**
      Arenaviruses
      Bunyaviruses
      Orthomyxoviruses
  - **Retrovirus**
    Lentiviruses
    Oncoviruses

DNA Viruses

- **Nonenveloped**
  - **Single-stranded Linear**
    Parvoviruses
  - **Double-stranded Linear**
    Adenoviruses
  - **Double-stranded Circular**
    Papillomaviruses
    Polymaviruses
- **Enveloped**
  - **Double-stranded Linear**
    Herpesviruses
    Poxviruses
  - **Double-stranded Circular**
    Hepadnaviruses

Figure 4-1. Some of the viruses that infect humans. Note that some viruses contain RNA, whereas others contain DNA, and that the nucleic acid that they possess may either be single- or double-stranded. Within the host cell, single-stranded positive-sense RNA functions as messenger RNA (mRNA), whereas single-stranded negative-sense RNA serves as a template for the production of mRNA. Some of the viruses possess an envelope, whereas others do not. (Redrawn from Engleberg NC, et al. *Schaechter's Mechanisms of Microbial Diseases.* 4th ed. Philadelphia, PA: Lippincott Williams & Wilkins; 2007.)

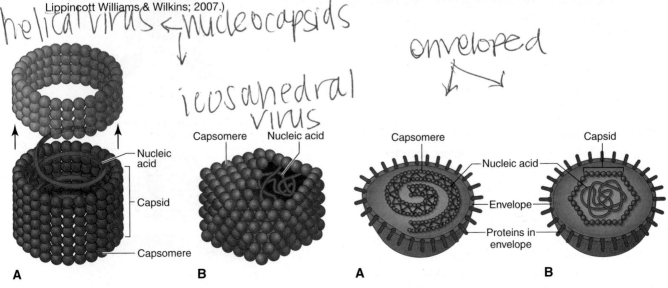

Figure 4-2. Viral nucleocapsids. A. Nucleocapsid of a helical virus. **B.** Nucleocapsid of an icosahedral virus. (From Harvey RA, et al. *Lippincott's Illustrated Reviews: Microbiology.* 3rd ed. Philadelphia, PA: Lippincott Williams & Wilkins; 2013.)

Figure 4-3. Enveloped viruses. A. Enveloped helical virus. **B.** Enveloped icosahedral virus. (Redrawn from Harvey RA, et al. *Lippincott's Illustrated Reviews: Microbiology.* 3rd ed. Philadelphia, PA: Lippincott Williams & Wilkins; 2013.)

invade and take over a functioning cell to produce new virions.

Viruses are classified by the following characteristics:

a. type of genetic material (either DNA or RNA),
b. shape of the capsid,
c. number of capsomeres,
d. size of the capsid,
e. presence or absence of an envelope,
f. type of host that it infects,
g. type of disease it produces,
h. target cell, and
i. immunologic or antigenic properties.

There are four categories of viruses based on the type of genome they possess. The genome of most viruses is either double-stranded DNA or single-stranded RNA, but a few viruses possess single-stranded DNA or double-stranded RNA. Viral genomes are usually circular molecules, but some are linear (having two ends). Capsids of viruses have various shapes and symmetry. They may be polyhedral (many sided), helical (coiled tubes), bullet shaped, spherical, or a complex combination of these shapes. Polyhedral capsids have 20 sides or facets; geometrically, they are referred to as icosahedrons. Each facet consists of several capsomeres; thus, the size of the virus is determined by the size of each facet and the number of capsomeres in each. Frequently, the envelope around the capsid makes the virus appear spherical or irregular in shape in electron micrographs. The envelope is acquired by certain animal viruses as they escape from the nucleus or cytoplasm of the host cell by budding (Figs. 4-4 and 4-5). In other words, the envelope is derived from either the host cell's nuclear membrane or cell membrane. Apparently, viruses are then able to alter these membranes by adding protein fibers, spikes, and knobs that enable the virus to recognize the next host cell to be invaded. A list of some viruses, their characteristics, and diseases they cause is presented in Table 4-2. Sizes of some viruses are depicted in Figure 4-6.

Origin of Viruses

Viruses have probably existed for as long as bacteria and archaea have existed. But where did they come from? This is an intriguing question and one that has been debated by scientists for many years. Three major theories have emerged to explain the origin of viruses.

1. The "coevolution theory": viruses originated in the primordial soup and coevolved with bacteria and archaea. This hypothesis has few supporters.
2. The "retrograde evolution theory": viruses evolved from free-living prokaryotes that invaded other living organisms, and gradually lost functions which were provided by the host cell. This theory has little support.
3. The "escaped gene theory": viruses are pieces of host cell RNA or DNA that have escaped from living cells, and are no longer under cellular control. Of the three

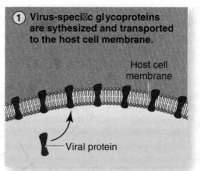

① Virus-specific glycoproteins are sythesized and transported to the host cell membrane.

Host cell membrane

Viral protein

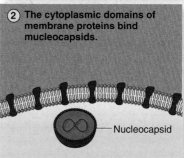

② The cytoplasmic domains of membrane proteins bind mucleocapsids.

Nucleocapsid

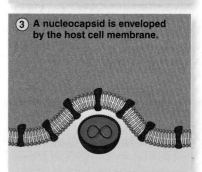

③ A nucleocapsid is enveloped by the host cell membrane.

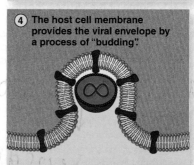

④ The host cell membrane provides the viral envelope by a process of "budding".

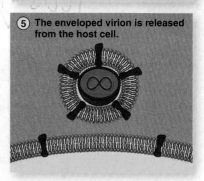

⑤ The enveloped virion is released from the host cell.

Figure 4-4. Virus particle becoming enveloped in the process of budding from a host cell. (Redrawn from Harvey RA, et al. *Lippincott's Illustrated Reviews: Microbiology*. 3rd ed. Philadelphia, PA: Lippincott Williams & Wilkins; 2013.)

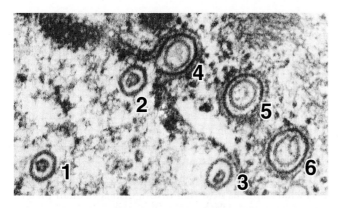

Figure 4-5. Herpesviruses acquiring their envelopes as they leave a host cell's nucleus by budding. 1–3. Viruses within the nucleus. **4.** Virus in the process of leaving the nucleus by budding. **5, 6.** Viruses that have already acquired their envelopes. (From Volk WA, et al. *Essentials of Medical Microbiology*. 5th ed. Philadelphia, PA: Lippincott-Raven; 1996.)

theories, this is currently the most widely accepted explanation for the origin of viruses.

The question of whether viruses are alive or not depends on one's definition of life and, thus, is not an easy question to answer. However, most scientists agree that viruses lack most of the basic features of cells; thus, they consider viruses to be nonliving entities.

> Because they are not composed of cells, viruses are not considered to be living organisms. They are referred to as acellular microbes or infectious particles.

Bacteriophages

The viruses that infect bacteria are known as *bacteriophages* (or simply, *phages*). Like all viruses, they are obligate intracellular pathogens, in that they must enter a cell

Table 4-2	Selected Important Groups of Viruses and Viral Diseases		
Virus Type	**Viral Characteristics**	**Virus**	**Disease**
Poxviruses	Large, brick shape with envelope, dsDNA	Variola	Smallpox
		Vaccinia	Cowpox
Polyoma–papilloma	dsDNA, polyhedral	Papillomavirus	Warts
		Polyomavirus	Some tumors, some cancer
Herpesvirus	Polyhedral with envelope, dsDNA	Herpes simplex I	Cold sores or fever blisters
		Herpes simplex II	Genital herpes
		Herpes zoster	Shingles
		Varicella	Chickenpox
Adenovirus	dsDNA, icosahedral, with envelope		Respiratory infections, pneumonia, conjunctivitis, some tumors
Picornaviruses (the name means small RNA viruses)	ssRNA, tiny icosahedral, with envelope	Rhinovirus	Colds
		Poliovirus	Poliomyelitis
		Hepatitis types A and B	Hepatitis
		Coxsackie virus	Respiratory infections, meningitis
Reoviruses	dsRNA, icosahedral with envelope	Enterovirus	Intestinal infections
Myxoviruses	RNA, helical with envelope	Orthomyxoviruses types A and B	Influenza
		Myxovirus parotidis	Mumps
		Paramyxovirus	Measles (rubeola)
		Rhabdovirus	Rabies
Arbovirus	Arthropod-borne RNA, cubic	Mosquito-borne type B	Yellow fever
		Mosquito-borne types A and B	Encephalitis (many types)
		Tick-borne, coronavirus	Colorado tick fever
Retrovirus	dsRNA, helical with envelope	RNA tumor virus	Tumors
		HTLV	Leukemia
		HIV	AIDS

ds, double-stranded; ss, single-stranded.

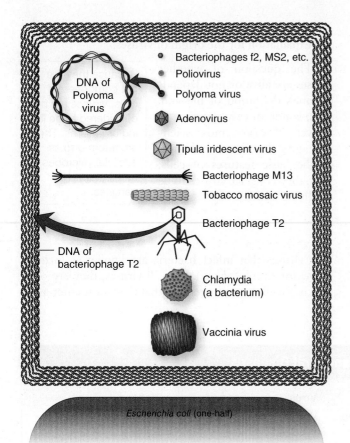

Figure 4-6. Comparative sizes of virions, their nucleic acids, and bacteria. (Redrawn from Davis BD, et al. *Microbiology* 4th ed. Philadelphia, PA: JB Lippincott. 1990.)

to replicate. There are three categories of bacteriophages, based on their shape:

- Icosahedron bacteriophages: an almost spherical shape, with 20 triangular facets; the smallest icosahedron phages are about 25 nm in diameter.
- Filamentous bacteriophages: long tubes formed by capsid proteins assembled into a helical structure; they can be up to about 900 nm long.
- Complex bacteriophages: icosahedral heads attached to helical tails; they may also possess base plates and tail fibers.

In addition to shape, bacteriophages can be categorized by the type of nucleic acid that they possess; there are single-stranded DNA phages, double-stranded DNA phages, single-stranded RNA phages, and double-stranded RNA phages. From this point, only DNA phages will be discussed.

Bacteriophages can be categorized by the events that occur after invasion of the bacterial cell: some are virulent phages, whereas others are temperate phages. Phages in either category do not actually enter the bacterial cell—rather, they inject their nucleic acid into the cell. It is what happens next that distinguishes virulent phages from temperate phages.

Virulent bacteriophages always cause what is known as the *lytic cycle*, which ends with the destruction (lysis) of the bacterial cell. For most phages, the whole process (from attachment to lysis) takes less than 1 hour. The steps in the lytic cycle are shown in Table 4-3.

> Once it enters a host cell, a virulent bacteriophage always initiates the lytic cycle, which results in the destruction of the cell.

The first step in the lytic cycle is *attachment* (adsorption) of the phage to the surface of the bacterial cell. The phage can only attach to bacterial cells that possess the appropriate receptor—a protein or polysaccharide molecule on the surface of the cell that is recognized by a molecule on the surface of the phage. Most bacteriophages are species- and strain-specific, meaning that they only infect a particular species or strain of bacteria. Those

> Bacteriophages can only attach to bacteria that possess surface molecules (receptors) that can be recognized by molecules on the phage surface.

that infect *Escherichia coli* are called coliphages. Some bacteriophages can attach to more than one species of bacterium. Figure 4-7 shows numerous bacteriophages attached to the surface of bacterial cells.

The second step in the lytic cycle is called *penetration*. In this step, the phage injects its DNA into the bacterial cell, acting much like a hypodermic needle (Fig. 4-8). From this point on, the phage DNA "dictates" what occurs within the bacterial cell. This is sometimes

Step	Name of Step	What Occurs During This Step
1	Attachment (adsorption)	The phage attaches to a protein or polysaccharide molecule (receptor) on the surface of the bacterial cell
2	Penetration	The phage injects its DNA into the bacterial cell; the capsid remains on the outer surface of the cell
3	Biosynthesis	Phage genes are expressed, resulting in the production of phage pieces or parts (i.e., phage DNA and phage proteins)
4	Assembly	The phage pieces or parts are assembled to create complete phages
5	Release	The complete phages escape from the bacterial cell by lysis of the cell

Table 4-3 **Steps in the Multiplication of Bacteriophages (Lytic Cycle)**

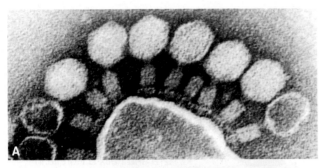

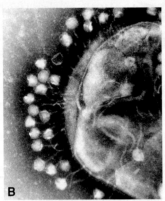

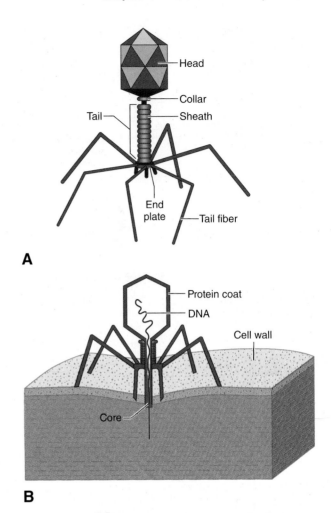

Figure 4-7. Bacteriophages. A. A partially lysed cell of a *Vibrio cholerae* bacterium, with many attached virions of phage CP-T1. (Courtesy of R.W. Taylor and J.E. Ogg, Colorado State University, Fort Collins, CO.) **B.** Numerous bacteriophages attached to a bacterial cell. (Courtesy of Dr. Graham Beards, Graham Colm, and Wikipedia.)

Figure 4-8. Bacteriophage structures. A. The bacteriophage T4 is an assembly of protein components. The head is a protein membrane with 20 facets, filled with DNA. It is attached to a tail consisting of a hollow core surrounded by a sheath and based on a spiked end plate to which six fibers are attached. **B.** Following attachment to a host cell, the sheath contracts, driving the core through the cell wall, and viral DNA enters the cell.

described as the phage DNA taking over the host cell's "machinery."

The third step in the lytic cycle is called *biosynthesis*. It is during this step that the phage genes are expressed, resulting in the production (biosynthesis) of viral pieces. It is also during this step that the host cell's enzymes (e.g., DNA polymerase and RNA polymerase), nucleotides, amino acids, and ribosomes are used to make viral DNA and viral proteins. In the fourth step of the lytic cycle, called *assembly*, the viral pieces are assembled to produce complete viral particles (virions). It is during this step that viral DNA is packaged up into capsids.

The final step in the lytic cycle, called *release*, is when the host cell bursts open and all of the new virions (about 50–1,000) escape from the cell. Thus, the lytic cycle ends with lysis of the host cell. Lysis is caused by an enzyme (referred to as an endolysin) that is coded for by a phage gene. At the appropriate time—after assembly—the appropriate viral gene is expressed, the enzyme is produced, and the bacterial cell wall is destroyed. With certain bacteriophages, a phage gene codes for an enzyme that interferes with cell wall synthesis, leading to weakness and, finally, collapse of the cell wall. The lytic cycle is summarized in Figure 4-9.

The other category of bacteriophages—*temperate phages* (also known as *lysogenic phages*)—do not immediately initiate the lytic cycle, but rather, their DNA remains integrated into the bacterial cell chromosome, generation

after generation. Temperate bacteriophages are discussed further in Chapter 7.

Bacteriophages are involved in two of the four major ways in which bacteria acquire new genetic information. These processes—called lysogenic conversion and transduction—are discussed in Chapter 7.

Because bacteriophages destroy bacteria, there has been much speculation and experimentation throughout the years regarding their use to destroy bacterial pathogens and treat bacterial infections. The earliest research of this nature was conducted in 1919, but ended when antibiotics were discovered in the 1940s. Since the emergence of multidrug-resistant bacteria ("superbugs"), research into the use of bacteriophages to treat bacterial diseases has been renewed. Additionally, bacteriophage enzymes that

> Unlike virulent bacteriophages, temperate bacteriophages do not immediately initiate the lytic cycle. Their DNA can remain integrated into the host cell's chromosome for generation after generation.

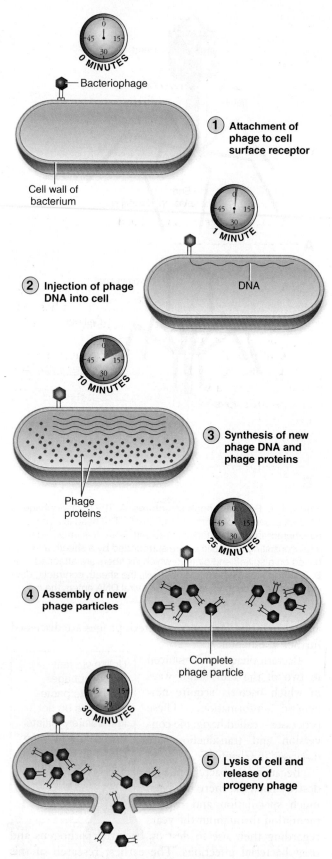

1. **Attachment of phage to cell surface receptor**

2. **Injection of phage DNA into cell**

3. **Synthesis of new phage DNA and phage proteins**

4. **Assembly of new phage particles**

5. **Lysis of cell and release of progeny phage**

Figure 4-9. Summary of the lytic process. (Redrawn from Harvey RA, et al. *Lippincott's Illustrated Reviews: Microbiology.* 3rd ed. Philadelphia, PA: Lippincott Williams & Wilkins; 2013.) (An animated version of this figure can be found on thePoint.)

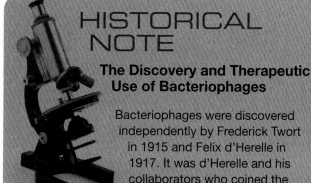

HISTORICAL NOTE

The Discovery and Therapeutic Use of Bacteriophages

Bacteriophages were discovered independently by Frederick Twort in 1915 and Felix d'Herelle in 1917. It was d'Herelle and his collaborators who coined the term "bacteriophage" (*phagein* is Greek for devour), and first used bacteriophages therapeutically. During the next 20 or so years, there were hundreds of published reports—many of which were controversial—concerning the use of bacteriophages to treat bacterial infections in humans and animals. Interest in phage therapy started to decline around the time that antibiotics were discovered. However, the emergence of multidrug-resistant bacteria has rekindled interest in phage therapy.

destroy cell walls or prevent their synthesis are currently being studied for use as therapeutic agents. Currently, phage-based treatments of patients are not authorized in the United States, but the Food and Drug Administration (FDA) has approved the use of a phage mixture to use on certain foods to prevent *Listeria* contamination. It is possible that, in the future, certain bacterial diseases will be treated using orally administered or injected pathogen-specific bacteriophages or bacteriophage enzymes.

Animal Viruses

Viruses that infect humans and animals are collectively referred to as *animal viruses.* Some animal viruses are DNA viruses; others are RNA viruses. Animal viruses may consist solely of nucleic acid surrounded by a protein coat (capsid), or they may be more complex. For example, they may be enveloped or they may contain enzymes that play a role in viral multiplication within host cells. The steps in the multiplication of animal viruses are shown in Table 4-4.

The first step in the multiplication of animal viruses is *attachment* (or adsorption) of the virus to the cell. Like bacteriophages, animal viruses can only attach to cells bearing the appropriate protein or polysaccharide receptors on their surface. Did you ever wonder why certain viruses cause infections in dogs, but not in humans, or vice versa? Did you ever wonder

> Like bacteriophages, animal viruses can only attach to and invade cells bearing appropriate surface receptors.

Table 4-4 Steps in the Multiplication of Animal Viruses

Step	Name of Step	What Occurs During This Step
1	Attachment (adsorption)	The virus attaches to a protein or polysaccharide molecule (receptor) on the surface of a host cell
2	Penetration	The entire virus enters the host cell, in some cases because it was phagocytized by the cell
3	Uncoating	The viral nucleic acid escapes from the capsid
4	Biosynthesis	Viral genes are expressed, resulting in the production of pieces or parts of viruses (i.e., viral DNA and viral proteins)
5	Assembly	The viral pieces or parts are assembled to create complete virions
6	Release	The complete virions escape from the host cell by lysis or budding

why certain viruses cause respiratory infections, whereas others cause gastrointestinal infections? It all boils down to receptors. Viruses can only attach to and invade cells that bear a receptor that they can recognize.

The second step in the multiplication of animal viruses is *penetration*, but, unlike bacteriophages, the entire virion usually enters the host cell, sometimes because the cell phagocytizes the virus (Figs. 4-10 to 4-12). This necessitates a third step that was not required for bacteriophages—*uncoating*—whereby the viral nucleic acid escapes from the capsid.

As with bacteriophages, from this point on, the viral nucleic acid "dictates" what occurs within the host cell. The fourth step is *biosynthesis*, whereby many viral pieces (viral nucleic acid and viral proteins) are produced. This step can be quite complicated, depending on what type of virus infected the cell (i.e., whether it was a single-stranded DNA virus, a double-stranded DNA virus, a single-stranded RNA virus, or a double-stranded RNA

virus). Some animal viruses do not initiate biosynthesis right away, but rather, remain latent within the host cell for variable periods. Latent viral infections are discussed in more detail in a subsequent section.

The fifth step—*assembly*—involves fitting the virus pieces together to produce complete virions. After the virus particles are assembled, they must escape from the cell—a sixth step called *release*. How they escape from the cell depends on the type of virus that it is. Some animal viruses escape by destroying the host cell, leading to cell destruction and some of the symptoms associated with infection with that particular virus. Other viruses escape the cell by a process known as budding. Viruses that escape from the host cell cytoplasm by budding become surrounded with pieces of the cell membrane,

> Animal viruses escape from their host cells by either lysis of the cell or budding. Viruses that escape by budding become enveloped viruses.

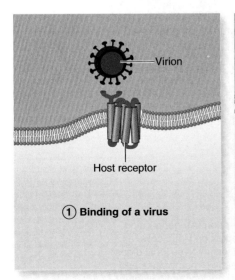
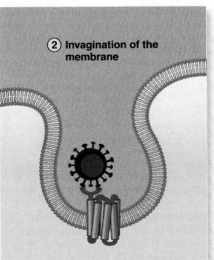
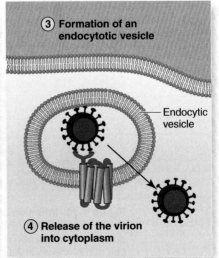

Figure 4-10. Penetration of a host cell by a nonenveloped virus via endocytosis. (Redrawn from Harvey RA, et al. *Lippincott's Illustrated Reviews: Microbiology*. 3rd ed. Philadelphia, PA: Lippincott Williams & Wilkins; 2013.)

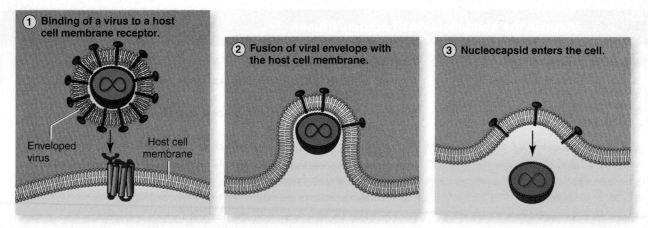

Figure 4-11. Penetration of a host cell by an enveloped virus. (Redrawm from Harvey RA, et al. *Lippincott's Illustrated Reviews: Microbiology*. 3rd ed. Philadelphia, PA: Lippincott Williams & Wilkins; 2013.)

thus becoming enveloped viruses. Whenever you encounter an enveloped virus, you know that it has escaped from its host cell by budding. The similarities and differences between bacteriophage and animal virus multiplication are summarized in Table 4-5.

Remnants or collections of viruses, called *inclusion bodies*, are often seen in infected cells and are used as a diagnostic tool to identify certain viral diseases. Inclusion bodies may be found in the cytoplasm (cytoplasmic inclusion bodies) or within the nucleus (intranuclear inclusion bodies), depending on the particular disease. In rabies, the cytoplasmic inclusion bodies in nerve cells are called *Negri bodies*. The inclusion bodies of acquired immunodeficiency syndrome (AIDS) and the Guarnieri bodies of smallpox are also cytoplasmic. Herpes and poliomyelitis

viruses cause intranuclear inclusion bodies. In each case, inclusion bodies may represent aggregates or collections of viruses. Some important human viral diseases include AIDS, chickenpox, cold sores, the common cold, Ebola virus infections, genital herpes infections, German measles, Hantavirus pulmonary syndrome, infectious mononucleosis, influenza, measles, mumps, poliomyelitis, rabies, severe acute respiratory syndrome (SARS), and viral encephalitis. In addition, all human warts are caused by viruses.

Latent Virus Infections

Herpes virus infections, such as cold sores (fever blisters), are good examples of latent virus infections. Although the infected person is always harboring the virus in nerve

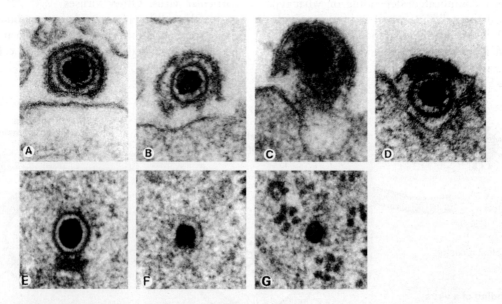

Figure 4-12. Infection of host cells by Herpes simplex virus. Adsorption **(A)**, penetration **(B–D)**, and uncoating and digestion of the capsid **(E–G)** of herpes simplex on HeLa cells, as deduced from electron micrographs of infected cell sections. Penetration involves local digestion of the viral and cellular membranes **(B, C)**, resulting in fusion of the two membranes and release of the nucleocapsid into the cytoplasmic matrix **(D)**. The naked nucleocapsid is intact in **E**, is partially digested in **F**, and has disappeared in **G**, leaving a core containing DNA and protein. (From Morgan C, et al. *J Virol*. 1968;2:507.)

Table 4-5 Similarities and Differences between Bacteriophage and Animal Virus Multiplication

Step	Bacteriophages	Animal Viruses
Attachment	Yes	Yes
Penetration	Yes, but only by the phage nucleic acid	Yes, by the entire virion
Uncoating	No (unnecessary)	Yes
Biosynthesis	Yes	Yes
Assembly	Yes	Yes
Release	Yes, by lysis of the host cell	Yes, either by budding or by lysis of the host cell

cells, the cold sores come and go. A fever, stress, or excessive sunlight can trigger the viral genes to take over the cells and produce more viruses; in the process, cells are destroyed and a cold sore develops. Latent viral infections are usually limited by the defense systems of the human body—phagocytes and antiviral proteins called interferons that are produced by virus-infected cells (discussed in Chapter 15). Shingles, a painful nerve disease that is also caused by a herpesvirus, is another example of a latent viral infection. After a chickenpox infection, the virus can remain latent in the human body for many years. Then, when the body's immune defenses become weakened by old age or disease, the latent chickenpox virus resurfaces to cause shingles.

Antiviral Agents

Antibiotics function by inhibiting certain metabolic activities within cellular pathogens, and viruses are not cells. However, for certain patients with colds and influenza, antibiotics may be prescribed in an attempt to prevent secondary bacterial infections that might follow the virus infection. In recent years, a relatively small number of chemicals—called antiviral agents—have been developed to interfere with virus-specific enzymes and virus production by either disrupting critical phases in viral cycles or inhibiting the synthesis of viral DNA, RNA, or proteins. Antiviral agents are discussed further in Chapter 9.

> It is very important for healthcare professionals to understand that antibiotics are not effective against viral infections.

> Drugs used to treat viral infections are called antiviral agents.

Oncogenic Viruses

Viruses that cause cancer are called *oncogenic viruses* or *oncoviruses*. The first evidence that viruses cause cancers came from experiments with chickens. Subsequently, viruses were shown to be the cause of various types of cancers in rodents, frogs, and cats. Although the causes of many (perhaps most) types of human cancers remain unknown, it is known that *some* human cancers are caused by viruses. Epstein–Barr virus (a type of herpes virus) causes infectious mononucleosis (not a type of cancer), but also causes three types of human cancers: nasopharyngeal carcinoma, Burkitt lymphoma, and B-cell lymphoma. Kaposi sarcoma, a type of cancer common in AIDS patients, is caused by human herpesvirus 8. Associations between hepatitis B and C viruses and hepatocellular (liver) carcinoma have been established. Human papillomaviruses (HPV; wart viruses) can cause different types of cancer, including cancers of the cervix and other parts of the genital tract. A retrovirus that is closely related to human immunodeficiency virus (HIV; the causative agent of AIDS), called human T-lymphotropic virus type 1 (HTLV-1), causes a rare type of adult T-cell leukemia. All of the mentioned oncogenic viruses, except HIV and HTLV-1, are DNA viruses. HIV and HTLV-1 are RNA viruses.

> Viruses that cause cancer are known as oncogenic viruses or oncoviruses.

Human Immunodeficiency Virus

HIV, the cause of AIDS, is an enveloped, single-stranded RNA virus[a] (Fig. 4-13). It is a member of a genus of viruses called lentiviruses, in a family of viruses called Retroviridae (retroviruses). HIV is able to attach to and invade cells bearing receptors that the virus recognizes. The most important of these receptors is designated CD4, and cells possessing that receptor are called CD4+ cells. The most important of the CD4+ cells is the helper T cell (discussed in Chapter 16); HIV infections destroy these important cells of the immune system. Macrophages also possess CD4 receptors and can, thus, be invaded by HIV. In addition, HIV is able to invade certain cells that do not possess CD4 receptors, but do possess other receptors that HIV is able to recognize.

> AIDS is caused by a single-stranded RNA virus known as HIV.

Mimivirus and Megavirus

An extremely large double-stranded DNA virus, called Mimivirus, was recovered from amebas. The virus was given the name Mimivirus because it "mimics" bacteria. It is so large that it can be observed using a standard compound light microscope. The Mimivirus particle has a 7-nm-thick capsid with a diameter of 750 nm. An array of 80- to 125-nm-long closely packed fibers project outward from the capsid surface (Fig. 4-14). Within the capsid, its DNA is surrounded by two 4-nm-thick lipid membranes. Its genome is at least 10 times larger than that of the large viruses in the smallpox family and larger than the

---

[a]The HIV virion contains two single-stranded RNA molecules.

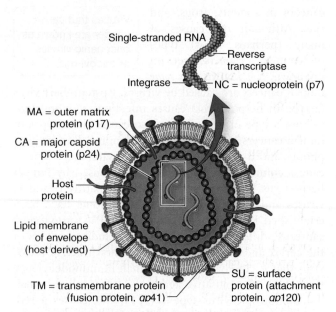

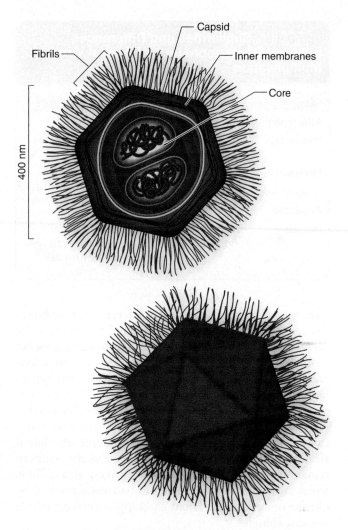

Figure 4-13. Human immunodeficiency virus. HIV is an enveloped virus, containing two identical single-stranded RNA molecules. Each of its 72 surface knobs contains a glycoprotein (designated *gp*120) capable of binding to a CD4 receptor on the surface of certain host cells (e.g., T-helper cells). The "stalk" that supports the knob is a transmembrane glycoprotein (designated *gp*41), which may also play a role in attachment to host cells. Reverse transcriptase is an RNA-dependent DNA polymerase. (Redrawn from Harvey RA, et al. *Lippincott's Illustrated Reviews: Microbiology*. 3rd ed. Philadelphia, PA: Lippincott Williams & Wilkins; 2013.)

Figure 4-14. Mimivirus structure. The Mimivirus virion consists of a double-stranded DNA core, surrounded by two lipid membranes and a protein capsid. Numerous fibrils extend outward from the capsid surface. (Courtesy of Xanthine and Wikipedia.)

genome of some of the smallest bacteria. It is thought to possess close to 1,000 genes. Some of its genes code for functions that were previously thought to be the exclusive province of cellular organisms, such as the translation of proteins and DNA repair enzymes. Mimivirus contains several genes for sugar, lipid, and amino acid metabolism. And, unlike most DNA viruses, Mimivirus contains some RNA molecules. A limited number of reports suggest that Mimivirus may be the cause of some cases of human pneumonia.

An even larger double-stranded DNA virus was discovered in a water sample collected in 2010 off the coast of Chile. It has been given the name Megavirus chilensis, although it is most often referred to simply as Megavirus (Fig. 4-15). It has the largest capsid diameter (440 nm) and largest and most complex genome of all known viruses. Its genome is predicted to encode over 1,000 different proteins; thus, it is larger than that of some bacteria. Megavirus was isolated in a French laboratory by co-cultivation with amebas. Its natural host is not known.

Plant Viruses

More than 1,000 different viruses cause plant diseases, including diseases of citrus trees, cocoa trees, rice, barley, tobacco, turnips, cauliflower, potatoes, tomatoes, and many other fruits, vegetables, trees, and grains. These diseases result in huge economic losses, estimated to be in excess of $70 billion per year worldwide. Plant viruses are usually transmitted via insects (e.g., aphids, leaf hoppers, and whiteflies); mites; nematodes (round worms); infected seeds, cuttings, and tubers; and contaminated tools (e.g., hoes, clippers, and saws).

Viroids and Prions

Although viruses are extremely small nonliving infectious agents, viroids and prions are even smaller and less complex infectious agents. *Viroids* consist of short, naked fragments of single-stranded RNA (about 300–400 nucleotides in length) that can interfere with the metabolism of plant cells and

> Viroids are infectious RNA molecules that cause a variety of plant diseases.

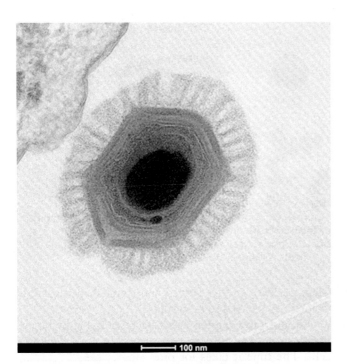

Figure 4-15. Transmission electron micrograph of Megavirus. (Courtesy of Chantal Abergel and Wikipedia.)

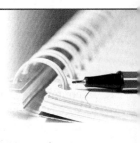

STUDY AID

Beware of Similar Sounding Terms

A **virion** is a complete viral particle (i.e., one that has all its parts, including nucleic acid and a capsid). A **viroid** is an infectious RNA molecule.

stunt the growth of plants, sometimes killing the plants in the process. They are transmitted between plants in the same manner as viruses. Plant diseases thought or known to be caused by viroids include potato spindle tuber (producing small, cracked, spindle-shaped potatoes), citrus exocortis (stunting of citrus trees), and diseases of chrysanthemums, coconut palms, and tomatoes. Thus far, no animal diseases have been discovered that are caused by viroids.

Prions (pronounced "pree-ons") are small infectious proteins that apparently cause fatal neurological diseases in animals, such as scrapie (pronounced "scrape-ee") in sheep and goats; bovine spongiform encephalopathy (BSE; "mad cow disease"); and kuru, Creutzfeldt–Jakob (C–J) disease, Gerstmann–Sträussler–Scheinker (GSS) disease, and fatal familial insomnia in humans. In fatal familial insomnia, insomnia and dementia follow difficulty sleeping. All these diseases are fatal spongiform encephalopathies, in which the brain becomes riddled with holes (sponge-like).

Similar diseases in mink, mule deer, Western white-tailed deer, elk, and cats may also be caused by prions. The name "scrapie" comes from the observation that infected animals scrape themselves against fence posts and other objects in an effort to relieve the intense pruritus (itching) associated with the disease. The disease in deer and elk is called "chronic wasting disease," in reference to the irreversible weight loss that the animals experience.

> Prions are infectious protein molecules that cause a variety of animal and human diseases.

Kuru is a disease that was once common among natives in Papua, New Guinea, where women and children ate human brains as part of a traditional burial custom (ritualistic cannibalism). If the brain of the deceased person contained prions, then persons who ate that brain developed kuru. Since the practice of ritual cannibalism was halted more than 50 years ago, kuru has nearly disappeared. Kuru, C–J, and GSS diseases involve loss of coordination and dementia. Dementia, a general mental deterioration, is characterized by disorientation and impaired memory, judgment, and intellect.

Scientists have been investigating the link between "mad cow disease" and a form of C–J disease (called variant CJD or vCJD) in humans. As of March 2011, 224 cases of vCJD had been diagnosed worldwide, including 175 in the United Kingdom; these cases probably resulted from eating prion-infected beef. The cattle may have acquired the disease through ingestion of cattle feed that contained ground-up parts of prion-infected sheep.

The 1997 Nobel Prize for Physiology or Medicine was awarded to Stanley B. Prusiner, the scientist who coined the term prion and studied the role of these proteinaceous infectious particles in disease. Of all pathogens, prions are believed to be the most resistant to disinfectants. The mechanism by which prions cause disease remains a mystery, although it is thought that prions convert normal protein molecules into nonfunctional ones by causing the normal molecules to change their shape. Many scientists remain unconvinced that proteins alone can cause disease.

In recent years, scientists have been studying possible relationships between prions and Alzheimer disease, Parkinson disease, Huntington disease, amyotrophic lateral sclerosis (ALS), some types of cancer, and type II diabetes.

The Domain *Bacteria*

Characteristics

Recall from Chapter 3 that there are two domains of prokaryotic organisms: Domain *Bacteria* and Domain *Archaea*. The bacteriologist's most important reference (sometimes referred to as the bacteriologist's "bible") is a five-volume set of books entitled *Bergey's Manual of*

Systematic Bacteriology (*Bergey's Manual* for short), which is currently being rewritten. (An outline of these volumes can be found in Appendix 2 on thePoint: "Phyla and Medically Significant Genera Within the Domain *Bacteria*.") When all five volumes have been completed, they will contain descriptions of more than 5,000 validly named species of bacteria. Some authorities believe that this number represents only from less than 1% to a few percent of the total number of bacteria that exist in nature.

According to *Bergey's Manual*, the Domain *Bacteria* contains 23 phyla, 32 classes, 5 subclasses, 77 orders, 14 suborders, 182 families, 871 genera, and 5,007 species. Organisms in this domain are broadly divided into three phenotypic categories (i.e., categories based on their physical characteristics): (a) those that are Gram-negative and have a cell wall, (b) those that are Gram-positive and have a cell wall, and (c) those that lack a cell wall. (The terms Gram-positive and Gram-negative are explained in a subsequent section of this chapter.) Using computers, microbiologists have established numerical taxonomy systems that help not only to identify bacteria by their physical characteristics, but also to establish how closely related these organisms are by comparing the composition of their genetic material and other cellular characteristics. (Note: as previously mentioned, throughout this book, the term "to identify an organism" means to learn the organism's species name [i.e., to speciate it].)

> A bacterium's Gram reaction (Gram-positive or Gram-negative), basic cell shape, and morphological arrangement of the cells are very important clues to the organism's identification.

Many characteristics of bacteria are examined to provide data for identification and classification. These characteristics include cell shape and morphological arrangement, staining reactions, motility, colony morphology, atmospheric requirements, nutritional requirements, biochemical and metabolic activities, specific enzymes that the organism produces, pathogenicity (the ability to cause disease), and genetic composition.

Cell Morphology

With the compound light microscope, the size, shape, and morphologic arrangement of various bacteria are easily observed. Bacteria vary greatly in size, usually ranging from spheres measuring about 0.2 μm in diameter to 10.0-μm-long spiral-shaped bacteria, to even longer filamentous bacteria. As previously mentioned, the average coccus is about 1 μm in diameter, and the average bacillus is about 1 μm wide × 3 μm long. Some unusually large bacteria and unusually small bacteria have also been discovered (discussed later).

There are three basic shapes of bacteria (Fig. 4-16): (a) round or spherical bacteria—the *cocci* (sing., *coccus*); (b) rectangular or rod-shaped bacteria—the *bacilli*

> The three general shapes of bacteria are round (cocci), rod-shaped (bacilli), and spiral-shaped.

Cell Shapes

Cocci

Curved and spiral-shaped

Bacilli

Figure 4-16. Categories of bacteria based on the shape of their cells. (Redrawn from Cohen BJ. *Memmler's The Human Body in Health and Disease.* 11th ed. Philadelphia, PA: Lippincott Williams & Wilkins; 2009.)

(sing., *bacillus*); and (c) curved and spiral-shaped bacteria (sometimes referred to as spirilla).

Recall from Chapter 3 that bacteria divide by binary fission—one cell splits in half to become two daughter cells. The time it takes for one cell to split into two cells is referred to as that organism's generation time. After binary fission, the daughter cells may separate completely from each other or may remain connected, forming various morphologic arrangements.

> Bacteria reproduce by binary fission. The time it takes for one bacterial cell to split into two cells is referred to as that organism's generation time.

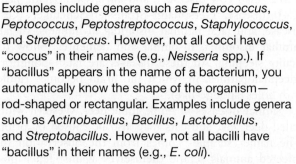

STUDY AID

Bacterial Names Sometimes Provide a Clue to Their Shape

If "coccus" appears in the name of a bacterium, you automatically know the shape of the organism—spherical. Examples include genera such as *Enterococcus*, *Peptococcus*, *Peptostreptococcus*, *Staphylococcus*, and *Streptococcus*. However, not all cocci have "coccus" in their names (e.g., *Neisseria* spp.). If "bacillus" appears in the name of a bacterium, you automatically know the shape of the organism— rod-shaped or rectangular. Examples include genera such as *Actinobacillus*, *Bacillus*, *Lactobacillus*, and *Streptobacillus*. However, not all bacilli have "bacillus" in their names (e.g., *E. coli*).

Cocci may be seen singly or in pairs (*diplococci*), chains (*streptococci*), clusters (*staphylococci*), packets of four (*tetrads*), or packets of eight (*octads*), depending on the particular species and the manner in which the cells divide (Figs. 4-17 and 4-18). Examples of medically important

Arrangement	Description	Appearance	Example	Disease
Diplococci	Cocci in pairs		*Neisseria gonorrhoeae*	Gonorrhea
Streptococci	Cocci in chains		*Streptococcus pyogenes*	Strep throat
Staphylococci	Cocci in clusters		*Staphylococcus aureus*	Boils
Tetrad	A packet of 4 cocci		*Micrococcus luteus*	Rarely pathogenic
Octad	A packet of 8 cocci		*Sarcina ventriculi*	Rarely pathogenic

Figure 4-17. Morphologic arrangements of cocci and examples of bacteria having these arrangements.

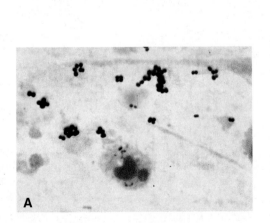
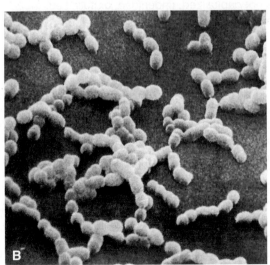

Figure 4-18. Morphologic arrangements of cocci. A. Photomicrograph of Gram-stained *Staphylococcus aureus* cells illustrating Gram-positive (blue) cocci in grapelike clusters. A pink-stained white blood cell can also be seen in the lower portion of the photomicrograph. **B.** Scanning electron micrograph of *Streptococcus mutans* illustrating cocci in chains. (**[A]** From Winn WC Jr, et al. *Koneman's Color Atlas and Textbook of Diagnostic Microbiology*. 6th ed. Philadelphia, PA: Lippincott Williams & Wilkins; 2006. **[B]** From Volk WA, et al. *Essentials of Medical Microbiology*. 5th ed. Philadelphia, PA: Lippincott-Raven; 1996.)

> Pairs of cocci are known as diplococci. Chains of cocci are known as streptococci. Clusters of cocci are known as staphylococci.

cocci include *Enterococcus* spp., *Neisseria* spp., *Staphylococcus* spp., and *Streptococcus* spp.

Bacilli (often referred to as rods) may be short or long, thick or thin, and pointed or with curved or blunt ends. They may occur singly, in pairs (*diplobacilli*), in chains (*streptobacilli*), in long filaments, or branched. Some rods are quite short, resembling elongated cocci; they are called *coccobacilli*. *Listeria monocytogenes* and *Haemophilus influenzae* are examples of coccobacilli. Some bacilli stack up next to each other, side by side in a palisade arrangement, which is characteristic of *Corynebacterium diphtheriae* (the cause of diphtheria) and organisms that resemble it in appearance (called *diphtheroids*). Examples of medically important bacilli include members of the family *Enterobacteriaceae* (e.g., *Enterobacter*, *Escherichia*, *Klebsiella*, *Proteus*, *Salmonella*, and *Shigella* spp.), *Pseudomonas aeruginosa*, *Bacillus* spp., and *Clostridium* spp.

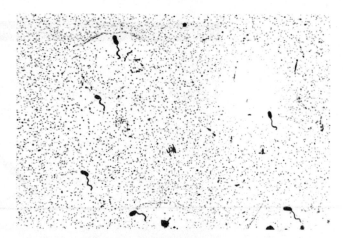

Figure 4-19. Vibrio cholerae (the causative agent of cholera) stained with a flagella stain. These curved bacteria have a single polar flagellum. (Courtesy of Dr. William A. Clark and the CDC.)

STUDY AID

Beware the Word "Bacillus"

Whenever you see the word *Bacillus*, capitalized and underlined or italicized, it is a particular genus of rod-shaped bacteria. However, if you see the word bacillus, and it is not capitalized, underlined, or italicized, it refers to any rod-shaped bacterium.

obtained from patients with primary syphilis. *Borrelia* spp., the causative agents of Lyme disease and relapsing fever, are examples of less tightly coiled spirochetes (Fig. 4-21).

Some bacteria may lose their characteristic shape because adverse growth conditions (e.g., the presence of certain antibiotics) prevent the production of normal cell walls. They are referred to as cell wall–deficient (CWD) bacteria or L-forms. Some CWD bacteria revert to their original shape when placed in favorable growth conditions, whereas others do not. Bacteria in the genus *Mycoplasma*

> A bacterial species having cells of different shapes is said to be pleomorphic.

Curved and spiral-shaped bacilli are placed into a third morphologic grouping. For example, *Vibrio* spp., such as *V. cholerae* (the causative agent of cholera) and *V. parahaemolyticus* (a causative agent of diarrhea), are curved (comma-shaped) bacilli (Fig. 4-19). Curved bacteria usually occur singly, but some species may form pairs. A pair of curved bacilli resembles a bird and is described as having a gull-wing morphology. *Campylobacter* spp. (a common cause of diarrhea) have a gull-wing morphology. Spiral-shaped bacteria are referred to as spirochetes. Different species of spirochetes vary in size, length, rigidity, and the number and amplitude of their coils. Some are tightly coiled, such as *Treponema pallidum*, the cause of syphilis, with a flexible cell wall that enables them to move readily through tissues (Fig. 4-20). Its morphology and characteristic motility—spinning around its long axis—make *T. pallidum* easy to recognize in wet preparations of clinical specimens

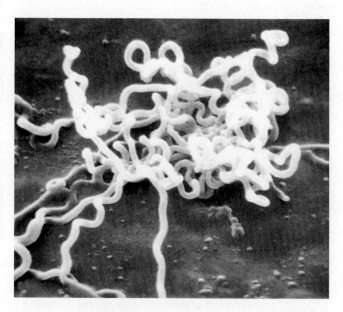

Figure 4-20. Scanning electron micrograph of *Treponema pallidum*, the bacterium that causes syphilis. (Courtesy of Dr. David Cox and the CDC.)

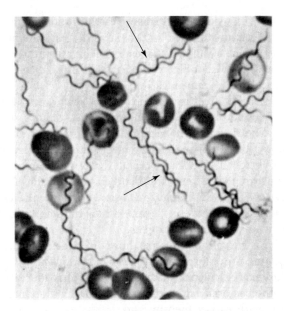

Figure 4-21. Spiral-shaped *Borrelia hermsii* (*arrows*), a cause of relapsing fever, in a stained blood smear. (From Volk WA, et al. *Essentials of Medical Microbiology*. 5th ed. Philadelphia, PA: Lippincott-Raven; 1996.)

do not have cell walls; thus, when examined microscopically, they appear in various shapes. Bacteria that exist in a variety of shapes are described as being *pleomorphic*; the ability to exist in a variety of shapes is known as *pleomorphism*. Because they have no cell walls, mycoplasmas are resistant to antibiotics that inhibit cell wall synthesis.

Staining Procedures

As they exist in nature, most bacteria are colorless, transparent, and difficult to see. Therefore, various staining methods have been devised to enable scientists to examine bacteria. In preparation for staining, the bacteria are smeared onto a glass microscope slide (resulting in what is known as a "smear"), air-dried, and then "fixed." (Methods for preparing and fixing smears are further described in Appendix 5 on thePoint: "Clinical Microbiology Laboratory Procedures.") The two most common methods of fixation are heat fixation and methanol fixation. Heat fixation is usually accomplished by passing the smear through a Bunsen burner flame. If not performed properly, excess heat can distort the morphology of the cells. Methanol fixation, which is accomplished by flooding the smear with absolute methanol for 30 seconds, is a more satisfactory fixation technique. In general, fixation serves three purposes:

1. It kills the organisms.
2. It preserves their morphology (shape).
3. It anchors the smear to the slide.

Specific stains and staining techniques are used to observe bacterial cell morphology (e.g., size, shape, morphologic arrangement, composition of cell wall, capsules, flagella, endospores).

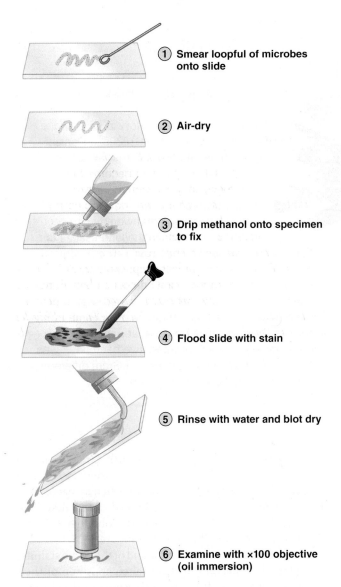

① **Smear loopful of microbes onto slide**

② **Air-dry**

③ **Drip methanol onto specimen to fix**

④ **Flood slide with stain**

⑤ **Rinse with water and blot dry**

⑥ **Examine with ×100 objective (oil immersion)**

Figure 4-22. Simple bacterial staining technique. A. With a flamed loop, smear a loopful of bacteria suspended in broth or water onto a slide. **B.** Allow slide to air-dry. **C.** Fix the smear with absolute (100%) methanol. **D.** Flood the slide with the stain. **E.** Rinse with water and blot dry with bibulous paper or paper towel. **F.** Examine the slide with the ×100 microscope objective, using a drop of immersion oil directly on the smear.

A *simple stain* is sufficient to determine bacterial shape and morphologic arrangement (e.g., pairs, chains, clusters). For this method, shown in Figure 4-22, a dye (such as methylene blue) is applied to the fixed smear, rinsed, dried, and examined using the oil immersion lens of the microscope. The procedures used to observe bacterial capsules, spores, and flagella are collectively referred to as *structural staining procedures*.

In 1883, Dr. Hans Christian Gram developed a staining technique that bears his name—the Gram stain or Gram staining procedure. The Gram stain has become the most important staining procedure in the bacteriology laboratory, because it differentiates between "Grampositive" and "Gram-negative" bacteria (these terms will

HISTORICAL NOTE

The Origin of the Gram Stain

While working in a laboratory in the morgue of a Berlin hospital in the 1880s, a Danish physician named **Hans Christian Gram** developed what was to become the most important of all bacterial staining procedures. He was developing a staining technique that would enable him to see bacteria in the lung tissues of patients who had died of pneumonia. The procedure he developed—now called the *Gram stain*—demonstrated that two general categories of bacteria cause pneumonia: some of them stained blue and some of them stained red. The blue ones came to be known as Gram-positive bacteria, and the red ones came to be known as Gram-negative bacteria. It was not until 1963 that the mechanism of Gram differentiation was explained by M.R.J. Salton.

be explained shortly). The organism's Gram reaction serves as an extremely important "clue" when attempting to learn the identity (species) of a particular bacterium. The steps in the Gram staining procedure are described in Appendix 5 on thePoint: "Clinical Microbiology Laboratory Procedures" and illustrated in Figure 4-23.

The color of the bacteria at the end of the Gram staining procedure depends on the chemical composition of their cell wall (Table 4-6). If the bacteria were not decolorized during the decolorization step, they will be blue to purple at the conclusion of the Gram staining procedure; such bacteria are said to be "Gram-positive." The thick layer of peptidoglycan in the cell walls of Gram-positive bacteria makes it difficult to remove the crystal violet–iodine complex during the decolorization step. Figures 4-24 to 4-28 depict various Gram-positive bacteria.

If, on the other hand, the crystal violet was removed from the cells during the decolorization step, and the cells were subsequently stained by the safranin (a red dye), they will be pink to red at the conclusion of the Gram staining procedure; such bacteria are said to be "Gram-negative." The thin layer of peptidoglycan in the cell walls of Gram-negative bacteria makes it easier to remove the crystal violet–iodine complex during decolorization. In

> If a bacterium is blue to purple at the end of the Gram staining procedure, it is said to be Gram-positive. If, on the other hand, it ends up being pink to red, it is said to be Gram-negative.

addition, the decolorizer dissolves the lipid in the cell walls of Gram-negative bacteria; this destroys the integrity of the cell wall and makes it much easier to remove the crystal violet–iodine complex. Figures 4-29 and 4-30 depict various Gram-negative bacteria.

Figure 4-31 illustrates the various shapes of bacteria that may be observed in a Gram-stained clinical specimen. Some strains of bacteria are consistently neither blue to purple nor pink to red after Gram staining; they are referred to as Gram-variable bacteria. Examples of Gram-variable bacteria are members of the genus *Mycobacterium*, such as *M. tuberculosis* and *M. leprae*. Refer to Table 4-7 and Figures 4-24 to 4-30 for the staining characteristics of certain pathogens.

Mycobacterium species are more often identified using a staining procedure called the *acid-fast stain*. In this procedure, carbol fuchsin (a bright red dye) is first driven into the bacterial cell using heat (usually by flooding the smear with carbol fuchsin, and then holding a Bunsen burner flame under the slide until steaming of the carbol fuchsin occurs). The heat is necessary because the cell walls of mycobacteria contain waxes, which prevent the stain from penetrating the cells. The heat softens the waxes, enabling the stain to penetrate. A decolorizing agent (a mixture of acid and alcohol) is then used in an attempt to remove the red color from the cells. Because mycobacteria are not decolorized by the acid–alcohol mixture (again owing to the waxes in

> The acid-fast stain is of value in the diagnosis of tuberculosis. Acid-fast bacteria are red at the end of the acid-fast staining procedure.

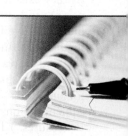

STUDY AID

A Method of Remembering a Particular Bacterium's Gram Reaction

A former student used this method to remember the Gram reaction of a particular bacterium. In her notebook, she drew two large circles. She lightly shaded in one circle, using a blue colored pencil. The other circle was lightly shaded red. Within the blue circle, she wrote the names of bacteria studied in the course that were Gram-positive. Within the red circle, she wrote the names of bacteria that were Gram-negative. She then studied the two circles. Later, whenever she encountered the name of a particular bacterium, she would remember which circle it was in. If it was in the blue circle, then the bacterium was Gram-positive. If it was in the red circle, the bacterium was Gram-negative. Clever!

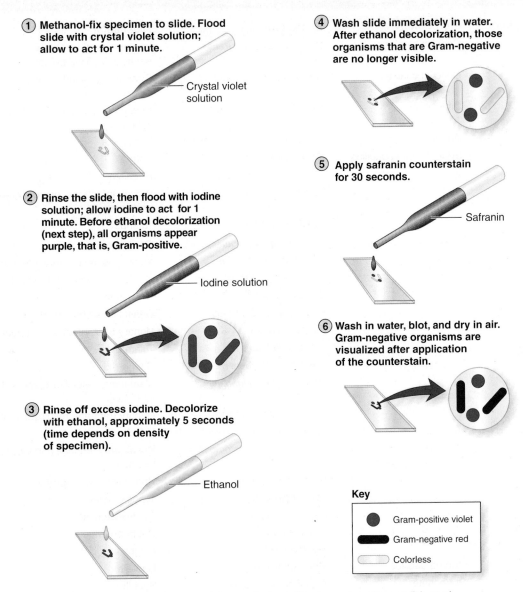

① **Methanol-fix specimen to slide. Flood slide with crystal violet solution; allow to act for 1 minute.**

Crystal violet solution

② **Rinse the slide, then flood with iodine solution; allow iodine to act for 1 minute. Before ethanol decolorization (next step), all organisms appear purple, that is, Gram-positive.**

Iodine solution

③ **Rinse off excess iodine. Decolorize with ethanol, approximately 5 seconds (time depends on density of specimen).**

Ethanol

④ **Wash slide immediately in water. After ethanol decolorization, those organisms that are Gram-negative are no longer visible.**

⑤ **Apply safranin counterstain for 30 seconds.**

Safranin

⑥ **Wash in water, blot, and dry in air. Gram-negative organisms are visualized after application of the counterstain.**

Key

⬤ Gram-positive violet

▬ Gram-negative red

⬭ Colorless

Figure 4-23. Steps in the Gram staining technique. (Redrawn from Harvey RA, et al. *Lippincott's Illustrated Reviews: Microbiology.* 3rd ed. Philadelphia, PA: Lippincott Williams & Wilkins; 2013.) (An animated version of this figure can be found on thePoint.)

their cell walls), they are said to be "acid-fast." Most other bacteria are decolorized by the acid–alcohol treatment; they are said to be non–acid-fast. The acid-fast stain is especially useful in the tuberculosis laboratory ("TB lab")

where the acid-fast mycobacteria are readily seen as red bacilli (referred to as acid-fast bacilli or AFB) against a blue or green background in a sputum specimen from a tuberculosis patient. Figure 4-32 depicts the appearance

Table 4-6 Differences between Gram-Positive and Gram-Negative Bacteria

	Gram-Positive Bacteria	Gram-Negative Bacteria
Color at the end of the Gram staining procedure	Blue to purple	Pink to red
Peptidoglycan in cell walls	Thick layer	Thin layer
Teichoic acids and lipoteichoic acids in cell walls	Present	Absent
Lipopolysaccharide in cell walls	Absent	Present

Table 4-7 Characteristics of Some Important Pathogenic Bacteria

Staining Reaction	Morphology	Bacterium	Disease(s)
Gram-positive	Cocci in clusters	*Staphylococcus aureus*	Wound infections, boils, pneumonia, septicemia, food poisoning
	Cocci in chains	*Streptococcus pyogenes*	Strep throat, scarlet fever, necrotizing fasciitis, septicemia
	Diplococci	*Streptococcus pneumoniae*	Pneumonia, meningitis, ear and sinus infections
	Bacillus	*Corynebacterium diphtheriae*	Diphtheria
	Spore-forming bacillus	*Bacillus anthracis*	Anthrax
		Clostridium botulinum	Botulism
		Clostridium perfringens	Wound infections, gas gangrene, food poisoning
		Clostridium tetani	Tetanus
Gram-negative	Diplococci	*Neisseria gonorrhoeae*	Gonorrhea
		Neisseria meningitidis	Meningitis, respiratory infections
	Bacillus	*Bordetella pertussis*	Whooping cough (pertussis)
		Brucella abortus	Brucellosis
		Chlamydia trachomatis	Genital infections, trachoma
		Escherichia coli	Urinary tract infections, septicemia
		Francisella tularensis	Tularemia
		Haemophilus ducreyi	Chancroid
		Haemophilus influenzae	Meningitis; respiratory, ear and sinus infections
		Klebsiella pneumoniae	Urinary tract and respiratory infections
		Proteus vulgaris	Urinary tract infections
		Pseudomonas aeruginosa	Respiratory, urinary, and wound infections
		Rickettsia rickettsii	Rocky Mountain spotted fever
		Salmonella typhi	Typhoid fever
		Salmonella spp.	Gastroenteritis
		Shigella spp.	Gastroenteritis
		Yersinia pestis	Plague
	Curved bacillus	*Vibrio cholerae*	Cholera
	Spirochete	*Treponema pallidum*	Syphillis
Acid-fast, Gram-variable	Branching bacilli	*Mycobacterium leprae*	Leprosy (Hansen disease)
		M. tuberculosis	Tuberculosis

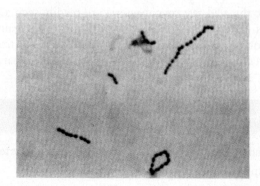

Figure 4-24. Chains of Gram-positive streptococci in a Gram-stained smear from a broth culture. (From Winn WC Jr, et al. *Koneman's Color Atlas and Textbook of Diagnostic Microbiology*. 6th ed. Philadelphia, PA: Lippincott Williams & Wilkins; 2006.)

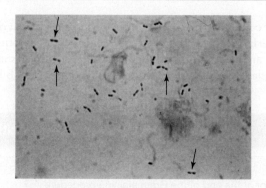

Figure 4-25. Gram-positive *Streptococcus pneumoniae* in a Gram-stained smear of a blood culture. Note the pairs of cocci, known as diplococci (*arrows*). (From Winn WC Jr, et al. *Koneman's Color Atlas and Textbook of Diagnostic Microbiology*. 6th ed. Philadelphia, PA: Lippincott Williams & Wilkins; 2006.)

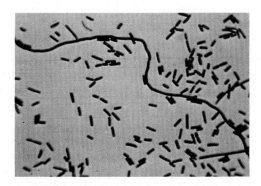

Figure 4-26. Gram-positive bacilli (*Clostridium perfringens*) in a Gram-stained smear prepared from a broth culture. Individual bacilli and chains of bacilli (streptobacilli) can be seen. (From Winn WC Jr, et al. *Koneman's Color Atlas and Textbook of Diagnostic Microbiology*. 6th ed. Philadelphia, PA: Lippincott Williams & Wilkins; 2006.)

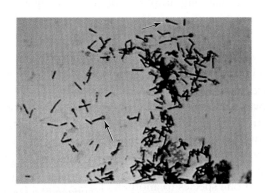

Figure 4-27. Gram-positive bacilli (*Clostridium tetani*) in a Gram-stained smear from a broth culture. Terminal spores can be seen on some of the cells (*arrows*). (From Winn WC Jr, et al. *Koneman's Color Atlas and Textbook of Diagnostic Microbiology*. 6th ed. Philadelphia, PA: Lippincott Williams & Wilkins; 2006.)

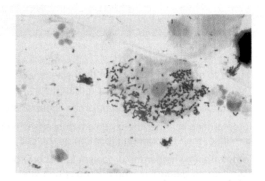

Figure 4-28. Many Gram-positive bacteria can be seen on the surface of a pink-stained epithelial cell in this Gram-stained sputum specimen. Several smaller pink-staining polymorphonuclear leukocytes can also be seen. (From Winn WC Jr, et al. *Koneman's Color Atlas and Textbook of Diagnostic Microbiology*. 6th ed. Philadelphia, PA: Lippincott Williams & Wilkins; 2006.)

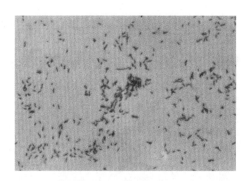

Figure 4-29. Gram-negative bacilli in a Gram-stained smear prepared from a bacterial colony. Individual bacilli and a few short chains of bacilli can be seen. (From Koneman E, et al. *Color Atlas and Textbook of Diagnostic Microbiology*. 5th ed. Philadelphia, PA: Lippincott Williams & Wilkins; 1997.)

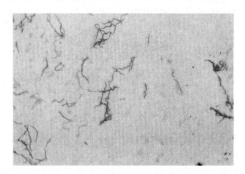

Figure 4-30. Loosely coiled Gram-negative spirochetes. *Borrelia burgdorferi* shown here, is the etiologic agent (cause) of Lyme disease. (From Winn WC Jr, et al. *Koneman's Color Atlas and Textbook of Diagnostic Microbiology*. 6th ed. Philadelphia, PA: Lippincott Williams & Wilkins; 2006.)

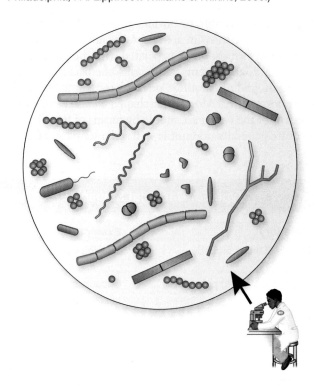

Figure 4-31. Various forms of bacteria that might be observed in Gram-stained smears. Shown here are single cocci, diplococci, tetrads, octads, streptococci, staphylococci, single bacilli, diplobacilli, streptobacilli, branching bacilli, loosely coiled spirochetes, and tightly coiled spirochetes. (See text for explanation of terms.)

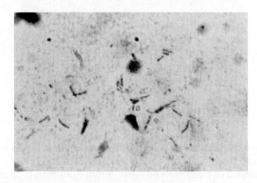

Figure 4-32. Many red acid-fast bacilli (*M. tuberculosis*) can be seen in this acid-fast stained concentrate from a digested sputum specimen. (From Koneman E, et al. *Color Atlas and Textbook of Diagnostic Microbiology.* 5th ed. Philadelphia, PA: Lippincott Williams & Wilkins; 1997.)

of mycobacteria after the acid-fast staining procedure. The acid-fast staining procedure was developed in 1882 by Paul Ehrlich—a German chemist.

The Gram and acid-fast staining procedures are referred to as *differential staining procedures* because they enable microbiologists to differentiate one group of bacteria from another (i.e., Gram-positive bacteria from Gram-negative bacteria, and acid-fast bacteria from non–acid-fast bacteria). Table 4-8 summarizes the various types of bacterial staining procedures.

Motility

If a bacterium is able to "swim," it is said to be motile. Bacteria unable to swim are said to be nonmotile. Bacterial motility is most often associated with the presence of flagella or axial filaments, although some bacteria exhibit a type of gliding motility on secreted slime. Bacteria never possess cilia. Most spiral-shaped bacteria and about one-half of the bacilli are motile by means of flagella, but cocci are generally nonmotile. A flagella stain can be used to demonstrate the presence, number, and location of flagella on bacterial cells. Various terms (e.g., monotrichous, amphitrichous, lophotrichous, peritrichous) are used to describe the number and location of flagella on bacterial cells (see Chapter 3).

Motility can be demonstrated by stabbing the bacteria into a tube of semisolid agar or by using the hanging-drop technique. Growth (multiplication) of bacteria in semisolid agar produces turbidity (cloudiness). Nonmotile organisms will grow only along the stab line (thus, turbidity will be seen only along the stab line), but motile organisms will spread away from the stab line (thus, producing turbidity throughout the medium; see Fig. 4-33). In the hanging-drop method (Fig. 4-34), a drop of a bacterial suspension is placed onto a glass coverslip. The coverslip is then inverted over a depression slide. When the preparation is examined microscopically, motile bacteria within the "hanging drop" will be seen darting around in every direction.

Colony Morphology

A single bacterial cell that lands on the surface of a solid culture medium cannot be seen, but after it divides over and over again, it produces a mound or pile of bacteria, known as a bacterial colony (Fig. 4-35). A colony contains millions of organisms. The colony morphology (appearance of the colonies) of bacteria varies from one species to another. Colony morphology includes the size, color, overall shape, elevation, and the appearance of the edge or margin of the colony. As is true for cell morphology and staining characteristics, colony features serve as important "clues" in the identification of bacteria. Size of colonies is determined

> A mound or pile of bacteria on the surface of a solid culture medium is known as a bacterial colony.

Table 4-8 | Types of Bacterial Staining Procedures

Category	Example(s)	Purpose
Simple staining procedure	Staining with methylene blue	Merely to stain the cells so that their size, shape, and morphologic arrangement can be determined
Structural staining procedures	Capsule stains	To determine whether the organism is encapsulated
	Flagella stains	To determine whether the organism possesses flagella and, if so, their number and location on the cell
	Endospore stains	To determine whether the organism is a spore former and, if so, to determine whether the spores are terminal or subterminal spores
Differential staining procedures	Gram stain	To differentiate between Gram-positive and Gram-negative bacteria
	Acid-fast stain	To differentiate between acid-fast and non–acid-fast bacteria

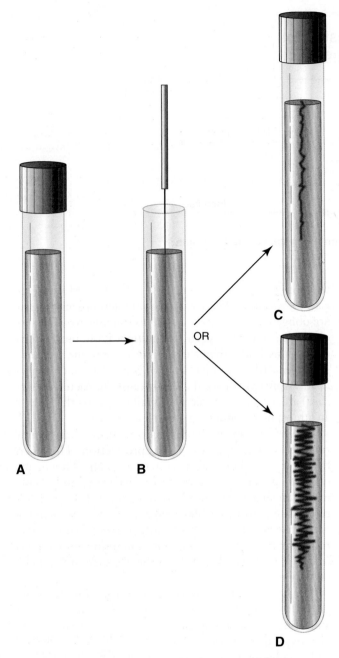

Figure 4-33. Semisolid agar method for determining motility. A. Uninoculated tube of semisolid agar. **B.** Same tube being inoculated by stabbing the inoculating wire into the medium. **C.** Pattern of growth of a nonmotile organism, after incubation. **D.** Pattern of growth of a motile organism, after incubation.

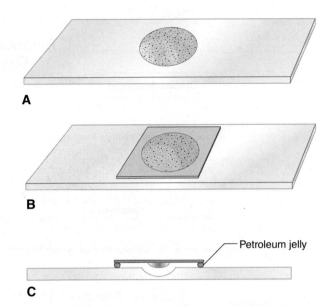

Figure 4-34. Hanging-drop preparation for study of living bacteria. A. Depression slide. **B.** Depression slide with cover glass over the depression area. **C.** Side view of hanging-drop preparation showing the drop of liquid culture medium hanging from the center of the cover glass above the depression.

carbon dioxide (CO_2). With respect to oxygen, a bacterial isolate can be classified into one of five major groups: obligate aerobes, microaerophilic aerobes (microaerophiles),

by the organism's rate of growth (generation time), and is an important characteristic of a particular bacterial species. Colony morphology also includes the results of enzymatic activity on various types of culture media, such as those shown in Figures 8-5 to 8-7 in Chapter 8.

Atmospheric Requirements

In the microbiology laboratory, it is useful to classify bacteria on the basis of their relationship to oxygen (O_2) and

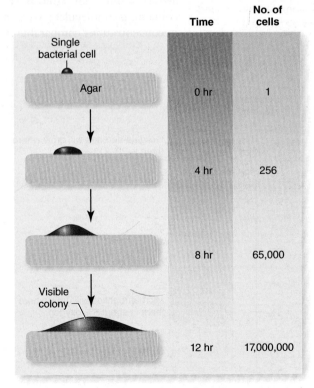

Figure 4-35. Formation of a bacterial colony on solid growth medium. In this illustration, the generation time is assumed to be 30 minutes. (Redrawn from Harvey RA, et al. *Lippincott's Illustrated Reviews: Microbiology*. 3rd ed. Philadelphia, PA: Lippincott Williams & Wilkins; 2013.)

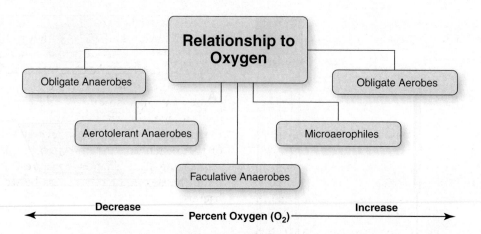

Figure 4-36. Categories of bacteria based on their relationship to oxygen.

Obligate aerobes and microaerophiles require oxygen. Obligate aerobes require an atmosphere containing about 20% to 21% oxygen, whereas microaerophiles require reduced oxygen concentrations (usually around 5% oxygen).

facultative anaerobes, aerotolerant anaerobes, and obligate anaerobes (Fig. 4-36). In a liquid medium such as thioglycollate broth (THIO), the region of the medium in which the organism grows depends on the oxygen needs of that particular species (Fig. 4-37).

To grow and multiply, *obligate aerobes* require an atmosphere containing molecular oxygen in concentrations comparable to

that found in room air (i.e., 20%–21% O_2). Mycobacteria and certain fungi are examples of microorganisms that are obligate aerobes. *Microaerophiles* (microaerophilic aerobes) also require oxygen for multiplication, but in concentrations lower than that found in room air. *Neisseria gonorrhoeae* (the causative agent of gonorrhea) and *Campylobacter* spp. (which are the major causes of bacterial diarrhea) are examples of microaerophilic bacteria that prefer an atmosphere containing about 5% oxygen.

Anaerobes can be defined as organisms that do not require oxygen for life and reproduction. However, they vary in their sensitivity to oxygen. The terms obligate anaerobe, aerotolerant anaerobe, and facultative anaerobe are used to describe the organism's relationship to molecular oxygen. An *obligate anaerobe* is an anaerobe that can grow only in an anaerobic environment (i.e., an environment containing no oxygen) (see "A Closer Look at Life in the Absence of Oxygen" on thePoint).

An *aerotolerant anaerobe* does not require oxygen, grows better in the absence of oxygen, but can survive in atmospheres containing molecular oxygen (such as air and a CO_2 incubator). The concentration of oxygen that an aerotolerant anaerobe can tolerate varies from one species to another. *Facultative anaerobes* are capable of surviving in either the presence

Obligate anaerobes, aerotolerant anaerobes, and facultative anaerobes can thrive in an atmosphere devoid of oxygen.

or the absence of oxygen; anywhere from 0% O_2 to 20% to 21% O_2. Many of the bacteria routinely isolated from clinical specimens are facultative anaerobes (e.g., members of the family *Enterobacteriaceae*, most streptococci, and most staphylococci).

Room air contains less than 1% CO_2. Some bacteria, referred to as *capnophiles* (capnophilic organisms), grow better in the laboratory in the presence of increased concentrations of

For optimum growth in the laboratory, capnophiles require an atmosphere containing 5% to 10% carbon dioxide.

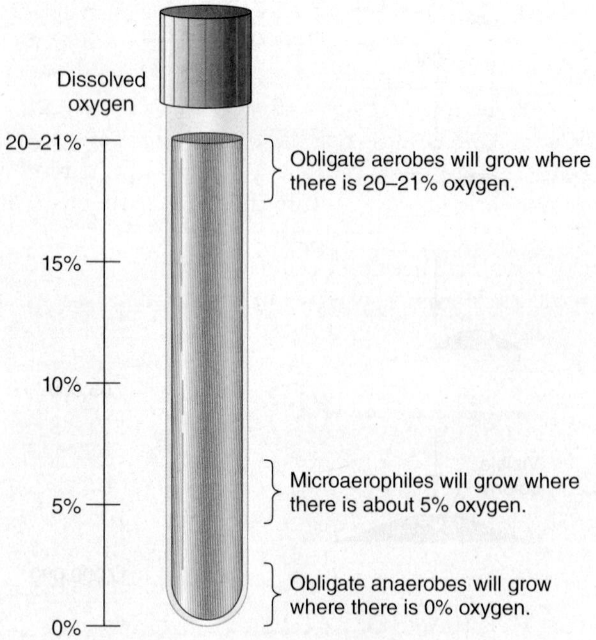

Dissolved oxygen

20–21% — Obligate aerobes will grow where there is 20–21% oxygen.

15% —

10% —

5% — Microaerophiles will grow where there is about 5% oxygen.

Obligate anaerobes will grow where there is 0% oxygen.

0% —

Figure 4-37. Culturing microorganisms in THIO. THIO contains a concentration gradient of dissolved oxygen, ranging from 20% to 21% O_2 at the top of the tube to 0% O_2 at the bottom of the tube. A bacterium will grow only in that part of the THIO containing the concentration of oxygen that it requires.

CO_2. Some anaerobes (e.g., *Bacteroides* and *Fusobacterium* species) are capnophiles, as are some aerobes (e.g., certain *Neisseria*, *Campylobacter*, and *Haemophilus* species). In the clinical microbiology laboratory, CO_2 incubators are routinely calibrated to contain between 5% and 10% CO_2.

Nutritional Requirements

All bacteria need some form of the elements carbon, hydrogen, oxygen, sulfur, phosphorus, and nitrogen for growth. Special elements, such as potassium, calcium, iron, manganese, magnesium, cobalt, copper, zinc, and uranium, are required by some bacteria. Certain microbes have specific vitamin requirements, and some need organic substances secreted by other living microorganisms during their growth. Organisms with especially demanding nutritional requirements are said to be fastidious; think of them as being "fussy." Special enriched media must be used to grow fastidious organisms in the laboratory. The nutritional needs of a particular organism are usually characteristic for that species of bacteria and sometimes serve as important clues when attempting to identify the organism. Nutritional requirements are discussed further in Chapters 7 and 8.

Biochemical and Metabolic Activities

As bacteria grow, they produce many waste products and secretions, some of which are enzymes that enable them to invade their host and cause disease. The pathogenic strains of many bacteria, such as staphylococci and streptococci, can be tentatively identified by the enzymes they secrete. Also, in particular environments, some bacteria are characterized by the production of certain gases, such as carbon dioxide, hydrogen sulfide, oxygen, or methane. To aid in the identification of certain types of bacteria in the laboratory, they are inoculated into various substrates (e.g., carbohydrates and amino acids) to determine whether they possess the enzymes necessary to break down those substrates. Learning whether a particular organism is able to break down a certain substrate serves as a clue to the identity of that organism. Different types of culture media are also used in the laboratory to learn information about an organism's metabolic activities (to be discussed in Chapter 8).

Pathogenicity

The characteristics that enable bacteria to cause disease are discussed in Chapter 14. Many pathogens are able to cause disease because they possess capsules, pili, or endotoxins (biochemical components of the cell walls of Gram-negative bacteria), or because they secrete exotoxins and exoenzymes that damage cells and tissues. Frequently, pathogenicity (the ability to cause disease) is tested by injecting the organism into mice or cell cultures. Some common pathogenic bacteria are listed in Table 4-7.

Genetic Composition

Most modern laboratories are moving toward the identification of bacteria using some type of test procedure that analyzes the organism's DNA or RNA. These test procedures are collectively referred to as molecular diagnostic procedures. The composition of the genetic material (DNA) of an organism is unique to each species. DNA probes make it possible to identify an isolate without relying on phenotypic characteristics. A DNA probe is a single-stranded DNA sequence that can be used to identify an organism by hybridizing with a unique complementary sequence on the DNA or rRNA of that organism. Also, through the use of 16S rRNA sequencing (see Chapter 3), a researcher can determine the degree of relatedness between two different bacteria.

Unique Bacteria

Rickettsias, chlamydias, and mycoplasmas are bacteria, but they do not possess all the attributes of typical bacterial cells. Thus, they are often referred to as "unique" or "rudimentary" bacteria. Because they are so small and difficult to isolate, they were formerly thought to be viruses.

Rickettsias, Chlamydias, and Closely Related Bacteria

Rickettsias and chlamydias are bacteria with a Gram-negative–type cell wall. They are obligate intracellular pathogens that cause diseases in humans and other animals. As the name implies, an obligate intracellular pathogen is a pathogen that must live within a host cell. To grow such organisms in the laboratory, they must be inoculated into embryonated chicken eggs, laboratory animals, or cell cultures. They will not grow on artificial (synthetic) culture media.

The genus *Rickettsia* was named for Howard T. Ricketts, a US pathologist; these organisms have no connection to the disease called rickets, which is the result of vitamin D deficiency. Because they appear to have leaky cell membranes, most rickettsias must live inside another cell to retain all necessary cellular substances. All diseases caused by *Rickettsia* species are arthropod-borne, meaning that they are transmitted by arthropod *vectors* (carriers); see Table 4-9.

Arthropods such as lice, fleas, and ticks transmit the rickettsias from one host to another by their bites or waste products. Diseases caused by *Rickettsia* spp. include typhus and typhus-like diseases (e.g., spotted fever rickettsiosis). All these diseases involve production of a rash. Medically important bacteria that are closely related to rickettsias include *Coxiella burnetii*, *Bartonella quintana* (formerly *Rochalimaea quintana*), *Ehrlichia* spp., and *Anaplasma* spp. *C. burnetii* (the causative agent of Q fever) is transmitted primarily by aerosols, but can be transmitted to animals by ticks. *B. quintana* is associated with trench fever (a louse-borne disease), cat scratch disease, bacteremia, and endocarditis. *Ehrlichia* and *Anaplasma* spp. cause human tick-borne diseases such as human

Human Diseases Caused by Unique Bacteria

Genus	Species	Human Disease(s)
Rickettsia	R. akari	Rickettsial pox (a mite-borne disease)
	R. prowazekii	Epidemic typhus (a louse-borne disease)
	R. rickettsii	Rocky Mountain spotted fever (a tick-borne disease)
	R. typhi	Endemic or murine typhus (a flea-borne disease)
Ehrlichia spp.	E. chaffeensis	HME
Anaplasma spp.	Anaplasma phagocytophilum	Human granulocytic ehrlichiosis
Chlamydia (and Chlamydia-like bacteria)	Chlamydophila pneumoniae	Pneumonia
	Chlamydophila psittaci	Psittacosis (a respiratory disease; a zoonosis; sometimes called "parrot fever")
	Chlamydia trachomatis	Different serotypes cause different diseases, including trachoma (an eye disease) inclusion conjunctivitis (an eye disease), nongonococcal urethritis (NGU; a sexually transmitted disease), lymphogranuloma venereum (LGV; a sexually transmitted disease)
Mycoplasma	M. pneumoniae	Atypical pneumonia
	M. genitalium	Nongonococcal urethritis (NGU)
Orientia	O. tsutsugamushi	Scrub typhus (a mite-borne disease)
Ureaplasma	U. urealyticum	Nongonococcal urethritis (NGU)

monocytic ehrlichiosis (HME) and human granulocytic anaplasmosis. *Ehrlichia* and *Anaplasma* spp. are intraleukocytic pathogens, meaning that they live within certain types of white blood cells.

The term "chlamydias" refers to *Chlamydia* spp. and closely related organisms (such as *Chlamydophila* spp.[b]). Chlamydias are referred to as "energy parasites." Although they can produce adenosine triphosphate (ATP) molecules, they preferentially use ATP molecules produced by their host cells. ATP molecules are the major energy-storing or energy-carrying molecules of cells (see Chapter 7). Chlamydias are obligate intracellular pathogens that are transferred by inhalation of aerosols or by direct contact between hosts—*not* by arthropods. Medically important chlamydias include *Chlamydia trachomatis*, *Chlamydophila pneumoniae*, and *Chlamydophila psittaci*. Different serotypes of *C. trachomatis* cause different diseases, including trachoma (the leading cause of blindness in the world), inclusion conjunctivitis (another type of eye disease), and nongonococcal urethritis (NGU; a term given to urethritis that is not caused by *Neisseria gonorrhoeae*). *C.*

> Rickettsias and chlamydias are examples of obligate intracellular organisms—organisms that can exist only *within* host cells.

pneumoniae causes a type of pneumonia, and *C. psittaci* causes a respiratory disease called psittacosis. Chlamydial diseases are listed in Table 4-9.

Mycoplasmas

Mycoplasmas are the smallest of the cellular microbes. Because they lack cell walls, they assume many shapes, from coccoid to filamentous; thus, they appear pleomorphic when examined microscopically. Sometimes they are confused with CWD forms of bacteria, described earlier; however, even in the most favorable growth media, mycoplasmas are not able to produce cell walls, which is not true for CWD bacteria. Mycoplasmas were formerly called pleuropneumonia-like organisms (PPLOs), first isolated from cattle with lung infections. They may be free-living or parasitic and are pathogenic to many animals and some plants. In humans, pathogenic mycoplasmas cause primary atypical pneumonia and genitourinary infections; some species can grow intracellularly. Because they have no cell wall, they are resistant to treatment with penicillin and other antibiotics that work by inhibiting cell wall synthesis. Mycoplasmas can be cultured on artificial media in the laboratory, where they produce tiny colonies (called "fried egg colonies") that resemble sunny-side-up fried eggs in appearance (Fig. 4-38). The absence of a cell wall prevents mycoplasmas from staining with the Gram staining

> Because *Mycoplasma* spp. do not possess cell walls, they are pleomorphic.

[b]Not all taxonomists are in agreement that *Chlamydia psittaci* and *C. pneumoniae* should have been reclassified as *Chlamydophila* spp.

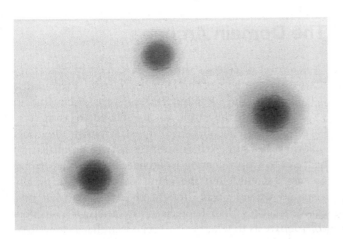

Figure 4-38. The "fried egg" appearance of *Mycoplasma* colonies on an agar medium. (Courtesy of Dr. E. Arum, Dr. N. Jacobs, and the CDC.)

procedure. Diseases caused by mycoplasmas and a closely related organism (*Ureaplasma urealyticum*) are shown in Table 4-9.

STUDY AID

"Strains" versus "Serotypes"

Within a given species, there are usually different *strains*. For example, there are many different strains of *E. coli*. If the *E. coli* that has been isolated from Patient X is producing an enzyme that is not being produced by the *E. coli* from Patient Z, the two *E. coli* isolates are considered to be different strains. Or, if one isolate of *E. coli* is resistant to ampicillin (an antibiotic), and the other *E. coli* isolate is susceptible to ampicillin, then these isolates are considered to be different strains of *E. coli*. Also, there are usually different *serotypes* (sometimes called serovars) within a given species. Serotypes of an organism differ from each other as a result of differences in their surface molecules (surface antigens). Sometimes, as is true for *C. trachomatis* and *E. coli*, different serotypes of a given species cause different diseases.

Especially Large and Especially Small Bacteria

The size of a typical coccus (e.g., a *Staphylococcus aureus* cell) is 1 µm in diameter. A typical bacillus (e.g., an *E. coli* cell) is about 1.0 µm wide × 3.0 µm long, although some bacilli are long thin filaments—up to about 12 µm in length or even longer—but still only about 1 µm wide. Thus, most bacteria are microscopic, requiring the use of a microscope to be seen.

STUDY AID

Beware of Similar Sounding Names

Do not confuse *Mycoplasma* with *Mycobacterium*. Each is a genus of bacteria. The unique thing about *Mycoplasma* spp. is that they lack cell walls. The unique thing about *Mycobacterium* spp. is that they are acid-fast.

Perhaps the largest of all bacteria—large enough to be seen with the unaided human eye—is *Thiomargarita namibiensis*, a colorless, marine, sulfide-oxidizing bacterium. Single spherical cells of *T. namibiensis* are 100 to 300 µm, but may be as large as 750 µm (0.75 mm). In terms of size, comparing a *T. namibiensis* cell to an *E. coli* cell would be like comparing a blue whale to a newly born mouse. Other marine sulfide-oxidizing bacteria in the genera *Beggiatoa* and *Thioploca* are also especially large, having diameters from 10 µm to more than 100 µm. Although *Beggiatoa* and *Thioploca* form filaments, *Thiomargarita* cells do not.

Another relatively enormous bacterium, named *Epulopiscium fishelsonii*, has been isolated from the intestines of the reef surgeonfish; this bacillus is about 80 µm wide × 600 µm (0.6 mm) long. *Epulopiscium* cells are about five times longer than eukaryotic *Paramecium* cells.[c] The volume of an *Epulopiscium* cell is about a million times greater than the volume of a typical bacterial cell. Spore-forming bacteria called metabacteria, found in the intestines of herbivorous rodents, are closely related to *Epulopiscium*, but they reach lengths of only 20 to 30 µm Although shorter than *Epulopiscium*, metabacteria are much longer than most bacteria.

At the other end of the spectrum, there are especially tiny bacteria called *nanobacteria*. Their sizes are expressed in nanometers because these bacteria are less than 1 µm in diameter; hence the name, nanobacteria. In some cases, they are as small as 20 nm in diameter. Nanobacteria have been found in soil, minerals, ocean water, human and animal blood, human dental calculus (plaque), arterial plaque, and even rocks (meteorites) of extraterrestrial origin. The existence of nanobacteria is controversial, however. Many scientists believe that these tiny structures were formed by geological, rather than biological, processes. They feel that nanobacteria are smaller than the minimum possible size for a living cell.

Photosynthetic Bacteria

Photosynthetic bacteria include purple bacteria, green bacteria, and cyanobacteria (erroneously referred to in

---

[c]*Paramecium* is a genus of freshwater protozoa.

the past as blue-green algae). Although all three groups use light as an energy source, they do not all carry out photosynthesis in the same way. For example, purple and green bacteria (which, in some cases, are not actually those colors) do not produce oxygen, whereas cyanobacteria do. Photosynthesis that produces oxygen is called *oxygenic photosynthesis*, whereas photosynthesis that does not produce oxygen is called *anoxygenic photosynthesis*.

> Photosynthetic bacteria are bacteria capable of converting light energy into chemical energy. Cyanobacteria are examples of photosynthetic bacteria.

In photosynthetic eukaryotes (algae and plants), photosynthesis takes place in plastids, which were discussed in Chapter 3. In cyanobacteria, photosynthesis takes place on intracellular membranes known as thylakoids. Thylakoids are attached to the cell membrane at various points and are thought to represent invaginations of the cell membrane. Attached to the thylakoids, in orderly rows, are numerous phycobilisomes—complex protein pigment aggregates where light harvesting occurs.

Many scientists believe that cyanobacteria were the first organisms capable of carrying out oxygenic photosynthesis and, thus, played a major part in the oxygenation of the atmosphere. Fossil records reveal that cyanobacteria were already in existence 3.3 to 3.5 billion years ago. Photosynthesis is discussed further in Chapter 7. Cyanobacteria vary widely in shape; some are cocci, some are bacilli, and others form long filaments.

When appropriate conditions exist, cyanobacteria in pond or lake water will overgrow, creating a water bloom—a "pond scum" that resembles a thick layer of bluish green (turquoise) oil paint. The conditions include a mild or no wind, a balmy water temperature (15°–30°C), a water pH of 6 to 9, and an abundance of the nutrients nitrogen and phosphorous in the water. Many cyanobacteria are able to convert nitrogen gas (N_2) from the air into ammonium ions (NH_4^+) in the soil or water; this process is known as *nitrogen fixation* (Chapter 10).

Some cyanobacteria produce toxins (poisons), such as neurotoxins (which affect the central nervous system), hepatotoxins (which affect the liver), and cytotoxins (which affect other types of cells). These cyanotoxins can cause disease and even death in wildlife species and humans that consume contaminated water. Many scientists are concerned that rising global temperatures ("global warming") will lead to increases in cyanobacterial populations and concurrent increases in cyanotoxins. Additional information about these cyanotoxins can be found in Appendix 1 on thePoint: "Microbial Intoxications."

> Some cyanobacteria produce toxins (called cyanotoxins) that can cause disease and even death in animals and humans.

The Domain *Archaea*

Prokaryotic organisms thus far described in this chapter are all members of the Domain *Bacteria*. Prokaryotic organisms in the Domain *Archaea* were discovered in 1977. Although they were once referred to as archaebacteria (or archaeobacteria), most scientists now feel that there are sufficient differences between archaea and bacteria to stop referring to archaea as bacteria. *Archae* means "ancient," and the name *archaea* was originally assigned when it was thought that these prokaryotes evolved earlier than bacteria. Now, there is considerable debate as to whether bacteria or archaea came first. Genetically, even though they are prokaryotes, archaea are more closely related to eukaryotes than they are to bacteria; some possess genes otherwise found only in eukaryotes. Many scientists believe that bacteria and archaea diverged from a common ancestor relatively soon after life began on this planet. Later, the eukaryotes split off from the archaea.

According to *Bergey's Manual of Systematic Bacteriology*, the Domain *Archaea* contains 2 phyla, 8 classes, 12 orders, 21 families, 69 genera, and 217 species. Archaea vary widely in shape; some are cocci, some are bacilli, and others form long filaments. Many, but not all, archaea are "extremophiles," in the sense that they live in extreme environments, such as extremely acidic, alkaline, hot, cold, or salty environments, or environments where there is extremely high pressure (Table 4-10).

Some live at the bottom of the ocean in and near thermal vents, where, in addition to heat and salinity, there is extreme pressure. Other archaea, called methanogens, produce methane, which is a flammable gas. Although virtually all archaea possess cell walls, their cell walls contain no peptidoglycan. In contrast, all bacterial cell walls contain peptidoglycan. The 16S rRNA

> Many archaea are extremophiles, meaning that they live in extreme environments; e.g., environments that are extremely hot, dry, or salty.

Table 4-10 Examples of Extremophiles

Type of Extreme Environment	Name Given to These Types of Extremophiles
Extremely acidic	Acidophiles
Extremely alkaline	Alkaliphiles
Extremely hot	Thermophiles
Extremely cold	Psychrophiles
Extremely salty	Halophiles
Extremely high pressure	Piezophiles (formerly barophiles)

sequences of archaea are quite different from the 16S rRNA sequences of bacteria. The 16S rRNA sequence data suggest that archaea are more closely related to eukaryotes than they are to bacteria. You will recall from Chapter 3 that differences in rRNA structure form the basis of the Three-Domain System of Classification.

ON thePoint

- Terms Introduced in This Chapter
- Review of Key Points
- A Closer Look at Life in the Absence of Oxygen
- Increase Your Knowledge
- Critical Thinking
- Additional Self-Assessment Exercises

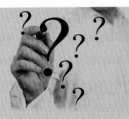

Self-Assessment Exercises

After studying this chapter, answer the following multiple-choice questions.

1. Which one of the following steps occurs during the multiplication of animal viruses, but not during the multiplication of bacteriophages?
   a. assembly
   b. biosynthesis
   c. penetration
   d. uncoating

2. Which one of the following diseases or groups of diseases is not caused by prions?
   a. certain plant diseases
   b. chronic wasting disease of deer and elk
   c. Creutzfeldt–Jacob disease of humans
   d. "mad cow disease"

3. Most prokaryotic cells reproduce by:
   a. binary fission
   b. budding
   c. gamete production
   d. spore formation

4. The group of bacteria that lack rigid cell walls and take on irregular shapes is:
   a. chlamydias
   b. mycobacteria
   c. mycoplasmas
   d. rickettsias

5. At the end of the Gram staining procedure, Gram-positive bacteria will be:
   a. blue to purple
   b. green
   c. orange
   d. pink to red

6. Which one of the following statements about rickettsias is false?
   a. Diseases caused by rickettsias are arthropod-borne
   b. Rickets is caused by a *Rickettsia* species
   c. *Rickettsia* species cause typhus and typhus-like diseases
   d. Rickettsias have leaky membranes

7. Which one of the following statements about *Chlamydia* and *Chlamydophila* spp. is false?
   a. They are obligate intracellular pathogens
   b. They are considered to be "energy parasites"
   c. The diseases they cause are all arthropod-borne
   d. They are considered to be Gram-negative bacteria

8. Which one of the following statements about cyanobacteria is false?
   a. Although cyanobacteria are photosynthetic, they do not produce oxygen as a result of photosynthesis
   b. At one time, cyanobacteria were called blue-green algae
   c. Some cyanobacteria are capable of nitrogen fixation
   d. Some cyanobacteria are important medically because they produce toxins

9. Which one of the following statements about archaea is false?
   a. Archaea are more closely related to eukaryotes than they are to bacteria
   b. Both archaea and bacteria are prokaryotic organisms
   c. Some archaea live in extremely hot environments
   d. The cell walls of archaea contain a thicker layer of peptidoglycan than the cell walls of bacteria

10. An organism that does not require oxygen, grows better in the absence of oxygen, but can survive in atmospheres containing some molecular oxygen is known as a(n):
    a. aerotolerant anaerobe
    b. capnophile
    c. facultative anaerobe
    d. microaerophile

5

Microbial Diversity

Part 2: Eukaryotic Microbes

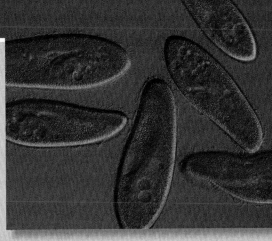

Paramecium, a nonpathogenic pond water protozoan.

CHAPTER OUTLINE

LEARNING OBJECTIVES

After studying this chapter, you should be able to:

- Compare and contrast the differences between algae, protozoa, and fungi (e.g., photosynthetic ability, chitin in cell walls)
- Explain what is meant by a "red tide" (i.e., what causes it) and its medical significance

- List the four major categories of protozoa and their most important differentiating characteristics (e.g., their mode of locomotion)
- Define the terms pellicle, cytostome, and stigma
- List five major infectious diseases of humans that are caused by protozoa and five that are caused by fungi
- Define and state the importance of phycotoxins and mycotoxins
- Explain the differences between aerial and vegetative hyphae, septate and aseptate hyphae, and sexual and asexual spores
- Explain the major difference between a lichen and a slime mould

Introduction

Acellular and prokaryotic microbes were described in Chapter 4. This chapter describes the eukaryotic microbes, which include some species of algae, all protozoa, some species of fungi, all lichens, and all slime moulds. Scientists have not yet determined when the first eukaryotic organisms appeared on Earth.

> Eukaryotic microbes include some species of algae and fungi, and all protozoa, lichens, and slime moulds.

Algae

Characteristics and Classification

Algae (sing., *alga*) are photosynthetic, eukaryotic organisms that, together with protozoa, are classified in the second kingdom (Protista) of the Five-Kingdom System of Classification. Collectively, they are referred to as protists. Not all taxonomists agree, however, that algae and

Table 5-1 Similarities and Differences between Algae and Plants

	Algae	Plants
Eukaryotic	Yes	Yes
Photosynthetic	Yes	Yes
Cells contain chlorophyll	Yes	Yes
Use carbon dioxide as an energy source	Yes	Yes
Store energy in the form of starch	Yes	Yes
Composed of roots, stems, and leaves	No	Most (bryophytes, such as mosses, are the exception)
Cell walls contain cellulose	Most (exceptions include diatoms and dinoflagellates; *Euglena* and *Volvox* do not have cell walls)	Yes
Method of reproduction	Both asexual and sexual	Sexual
Contain a vascular system to transport internal fluids	No	Most (mosses and other bryophytes are avascular)

> Algae and protozoa are referred to as protists because they are in the kingdom Protista.

protozoa should be combined in the same kingdom.[a] The study of algae is called phycology (or algology), and a person who studies algae is called a phycologist (or algologist).

All algal cells consist of cytoplasm, a cell wall (usually), a cell membrane, a nucleus, plastids, ribosomes, mitochondria, and Golgi bodies. In addition, some algal cells have a *pellicle* (a thickened cell membrane), a *stigma* (a light-sensing organelle, also known as an eyespot), and flagella. Although they are not plants, algae are more plantlike than protozoa (see Table 5-1 for similarities and differences between algae and plants). Algae lack true roots, stems, and leaves.

Algae range in size from tiny, unicellular, microscopic organisms[b] (e.g., diatoms, dinoflagellates, desmids) to large, multicellular, plantlike seaweeds (e.g., kelp; Table 5-2). Thus, not all algae are microorganisms. Algae may be arranged in colonies or strands and are found in freshwater and salt water, in wet soil, and on wet rocks. Algae produce their energy by photosynthesis, using energy from the sun, carbon dioxide, water, and inorganic nutrients from the soil to build cellular material. However, a few species use organic nutrients, and others

survive with very little sunlight. Most algal cell walls contain cellulose, a polysaccharide not found in the cell walls of any other microorganisms. Depending on the types of photosynthetic pigments they possess, algae are classified as green, golden (or golden brown), brown, or red.

Diatoms are tiny, usually unicellular algae that live in both freshwater and seawater. They are important members of the phytoplankton. Diatoms have silicon dioxide in their cell walls; thus, they have cell walls made of glass. Deposits of diatoms are used to make diatomaceous earth, which is used in filtration systems, insulation, and abrasives. Because of their attractive, geometric, and varied appearance, diatoms are quite interesting to observe microscopically (Fig. 5-1).

Dinoflagellates are microscopic, unicellular, flagellated, often photosynthetic algae. Like diatoms, they are important members of the phytoplankton, producing much of the oxygen in our atmosphere and serving as important links in food chains. Some dinoflagellates produce light and, for this reason, are sometimes referred to as fire algae. Dinoflagellates are responsible for what are known as "red tides" (discussed in Appendix 1: "Microbial Intoxications" on thePoint).

Green algae include desmids, *Spirogyra*, *Chlamydomonas*, *Volvox*, and *Euglena*, all of which can be found in pond water (Fig. 5-2). Desmids are unicellular algae, some of which resemble a microscopic banana. *Spirogyra* is an example of a filamentous alga, often producing long green strands in pond water. *Chlamydomonas* is a unicellular, biflagellated alga, containing one chloroplast and a stigma.

> Algae considered to be microorganisms include diatoms, dinoflagellates, desmids, and species of *Chlamydomonas*, *Euglena*, *Spirogyra*, and *Volvox*.

---

[a]In some classification schemes, algae are treated as a separate kingdom called Chromista.

[b]A tiny green alga, which is sometimes as small as 1.0 μm in diameter, named *Ostreococcus tauri*, is one of the smallest eukaryotes ever discovered. It contains one chloroplast, one mitochondrion, and one Golgi body. Tiny eukaryotes that range in size from 0.2 to 2 μm in diameter are collectively known as picoeukaryotes. They are smaller than some prokaryotes.

Table 5-2 Characteristics of Algae

Phylum (and Common Name)	Structural Arrangement	Predominant Color	Photosynthetic Pigments[a]	Habitat
Bacillariophyta (diatoms)	Unicellular	Olive brown	Chlorophyll *c*, carotenoids, xanthophylls	Freshwater and seawater
Chlorophyta (green algae)	Unicellular and multicellular	Green	Chlorophyll *b*, carotenoids	Freshwater (predominantly) and seawater
Chrysophyta (golden algae)	Unicellular	Golden olive	Chlorophyll *c*, carotenoids, xanthophylls	Freshwater
Dinoflagellata (dinoflagellates)	Unicellular	Brown	Chlorophyll *c*, carotenoids, xanthophylls	Freshwater and seawater
Euglenophyta (*Euglena* spp. and closely related organisms)	Unicellular	Green	Chlorophyll *b*, carotenoids, xanthophylls	Freshwater
Phaeophyta (brown algae)	Multicellular seaweeds	Olive brown	Chlorophyll *c*, carotenoids, xanthophylls	Seawater; most commonly, cold environments
Rhodophyta (red algae)	Multicellular seaweeds	Red to black	Chlorophyll *d* (in some), carotenoids, phycobilins	Seawater (predominantly) and freshwater; most commonly, tropical environments

[a] In addition to chlorophyll a, which is possessed by all algae. Carotenoids are yellow-orange; chlorophylls are greenish; phycobilins are red and blue; and xanthophylls are brownish.

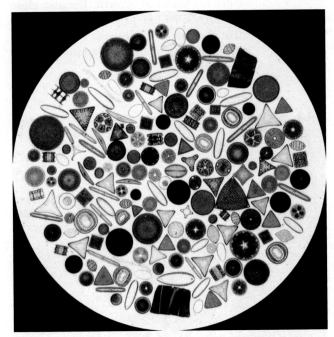

Figure 5-1. Diatoms as they appear when viewed with a compound light microscope. (Courtesy of Wipeter and Wikipedia.)

Volvox is a multicellular alga (sometimes referred to as a colonial alga or colony), consisting of as many as 60,000 interconnected, biflagellated cells, arranged to form a hollow sphere. The flagella beat in a coordinated manner, causing the *Volvox* colony to move through the water in a rolling motion. Sometimes, daughter colonies can be seen within a *Volvox* colony.

Euglena is a rather interesting alga, in that it possesses features possessed by both algae and protozoa. Like algae, *Euglena* contains chloroplasts, is photosynthetic, and stores energy in the form of starch. Protozoan features include the presence of a primitive mouth (called a *cytostome*) and the absence of a cell wall (hence, no cellulose). *Euglena* possesses a photosensing organelle called a stigma and a single flagellum. With its stigma, it can sense light; with its flagellum, it can swim into the light. When there is no light, *Euglena* can continue to obtain nutrients by ingesting food through its cytostome. Although it has no cell wall, *Euglena* does possess a pellicle, which serves the same function as a cell wall—protection.

Algae are easy to find. They include large seaweeds of various colors, brown kelp (up to 10 m in length) found along ocean shores, the green scum floating on

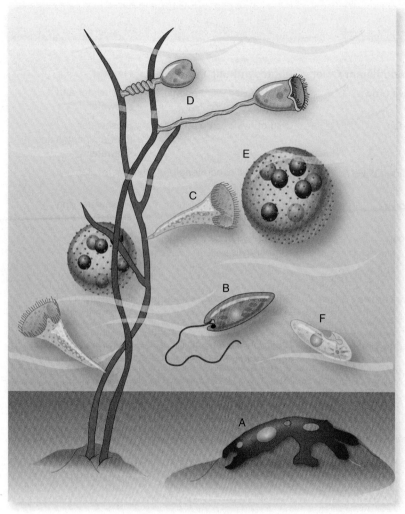

Figure 5-2. Common pond water algae and protozoa. A. *Amoeba* sp. **B.** *Euglena* sp. **C.** *Stentor* sp. **D.** *Vorticella* sp., in extended and contracted positions. **E.** *Volvox* sp. **F.** *Paramecium* sp. **(B)** and **(E)** are algae. **(A)**, **(C)**, **(D)**, and **(F)** are protozoa.

ponds, and the slippery green material on wet rocks (Fig. 5-3). Algae can also be found in the hot waters of thermal features at Yellowstone National Park (Fig. 5-4).

There are also many microscopic forms of algae in pond water that differ from the colorless, nonphotosynthetic protozoa in that they are pigmented and photosynthetic. Some algae (e.g., *Chlamydomonas*, *Euglena*, and *Volvox*) have characteristics (e.g., cytostome, pellicle, and flagella) that cause them to be classified as protozoa by some taxonomists. (Although there is some disagreement among taxonomists as to where *Chlamydomonas*, *Volvox*, and *Euglena* should be classified, they are referred to as algae in this book, primarily because they are photosynthetic. In this book, photosynthetic protists are considered to be algae, and nonphotosynthetic protists are considered to be protozoa.)

> In this book, photosynthetic protists are considered to be algae, and nonphotosynthetic protists are considered to be protozoa.

Algae are an important source of food, iodine and other minerals, fertilizers, emulsifiers for pudding, and stabilizers for ice cream and salad dressings; they are also used as a gelling agent for jams and nutrient media for bacterial growth. Because algae are nearly 50% oil, scientists are studying them as a source of biofuels. The agar used as a solidifying agent in laboratory culture

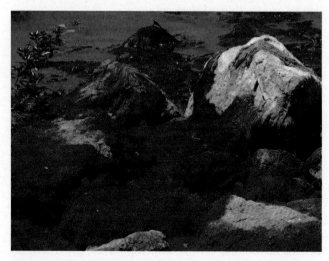

Figure 5-3. Green algae growing on rocks at the edge of a freshwater pond in Texas. (Courtesy of Biomed Ed, Round Rock, TX.)

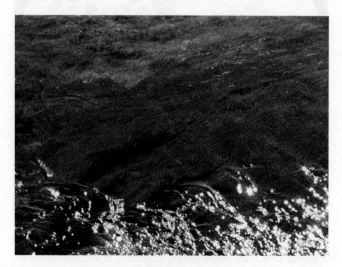

Figure 5-4. Green algae in hot water flowing from a thermal feature at Yellowstone National Park, WY. (Courtesy of Biomed Ed, Round Rock, TX.)

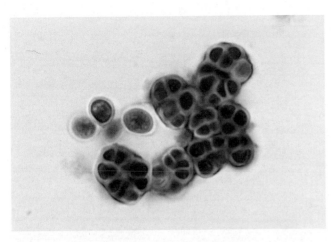

Figure 5-5. Microscopic appearance of *Prototheca* cells from a stained tissue sample. (Courtesy of the CDC.)

media is a complex polysaccharide derived from a red marine alga. On the down side, damage to water systems is frequently caused by algae clogging filters and pipes if many nutrients are present.

Medical Significance

One genus of algae (*Prototheca*) is a very rare cause of human infections (causing a disease known as protothecosis). *Prototheca* lives in soil and can enter wounds, especially those located on the feet (Fig. 5-5). It produces a small subcutaneous lesion that can progress to a crusty, warty-looking lesion. If the organism enters the lymphatic system, it may cause a debilitating, sometimes fatal infection, especially in immunosuppressed individuals. Algae in several other genera secrete substances (*phycotoxins*) that are poisonous to humans, fish, and other animals. For additional information on these toxins, see Appendix 1 on thePoint "Microbial Intoxications."

> Algae are only a very rare cause of human infections. Protothecosis is an example of a human algal infection.

Protozoa

Characteristics

Protozoa (sing., *protozoan*) are eukaryotic organisms that, together with algae, are classified in the second kingdom (Protista) of the Five-Kingdom System of Classification. As previously stated, not all taxonomists agree that algae and protozoa should be combined in the same kingdom. The study of protozoa is called protozoology, and a person who studies protozoa is called a protozoologist.

Most protozoa are unicellular (single-celled), ranging in length from 3 to 2,000 μm. Most of them

> Most protozoa are single-celled free-living microorganisms.

are free-living organisms, found in soil and water (Fig. 5-2). Protozoal cells are more animal-like than plantlike. All protozoal cells possess a variety of eukaryotic structures and organelles, including cell membranes, nuclei, endoplasmic reticulum, mitochondria, Golgi bodies, lysosomes, centrioles, and food vacuoles. In addition, some protozoa possess pellicles, cytostomes, contractile vacuoles, pseudopodia, cilia, and flagella. Protozoa have no chlorophyll and, therefore, cannot make their own food by photosynthesis. Some ingest whole algae, yeasts, bacteria, and smaller protozoans as their source of nutrients; others live on dead and decaying organic matter.

Protozoa do not have cell walls, but some, including some flagellates and some ciliates, possess a pellicle, which serves the same purpose as a cell wall—protection. Some flagellates and some ciliates ingest food through a primitive mouth or opening, called a cytostome. *Paramecium* spp. (common pond water ciliates) possess both a pellicle and a cytostome. Some pond water protozoa (such as amebae and *Paramecium*) contain an organelle called a *contractile vacuole*, which pumps water out of the cell. *Vorticella* spp. (pond water ciliates) have a contractile stalk (Fig. 5-2). Within the stalk is a primitive muscle fiber called a myoneme.

> *Paramecium* and *Vorticella* spp. are examples of free-living pond protozoa.

A typical protozoan life cycle consists of two stages: the trophozoite stage and the cyst stage. The **trophozoite** is the motile, feeding, dividing stage in a protozoan's life cycle, whereas the *cyst* is the nonmotile, dormant, survival stage. In some ways (e.g., the presence of a thick outer wall), cysts are like bacterial spores.

> A typical protozoan life cycle consists of two stages: a motile trophozoite stage and a nonmotile cyst stage.

Some protozoa are parasites. Parasitic protozoa break down and absorb nutrients from the body of the host in which they live. Many parasitic protozoa are pathogens, such as those that cause malaria, giardiasis, African sleeping sickness, and amebic dysentery (see Chapter 21). Other protozoa coexist with the host animal in a type of mutualistic symbiotic relationship—a relationship in which both organisms benefit. A typical example of such a symbiotic relationship is the termite and its intestinal protozoa. The protozoa digest the wood eaten by the termite, enabling both organisms to absorb the nutrients necessary for life. Without the intestinal protozoa, the termite would be unable to digest the wood that it eats and would starve to death. Symbiotic relationships are discussed in greater detail in Chapter 10.

> Malaria, giardiasis, African sleeping sickness, and amebic dysentery are examples of human diseases caused by parasitic protozoa.

Classification and Medical Significance

In some classification schemes, protozoa are divided into groups (variously referred to as phyla, subphyla, or classes) according to their method of locomotion (Table 5-3).

> Protozoa are sometimes classified taxonomically by their mode of locomotion. Some move by pseudopodia, others by flagella, others by cilia, and some are nonmotile.

Amebae (amebas) move by means of cytoplasmic extensions called **pseudopodia** (sing., *pseudopodium*; false feet) (Fig. 5-6). An **ameba** (pl., *amebae*) first extends a pseudopodium in the direction it intends to move, and then the rest of the cell slowly flows into it; this process is called ameboid movement. An ameba ingests a food particle (e.g., a yeast or bacterial cell) by surrounding the particle with pseudopodia, which then fuse together; this process is known as phagocytosis. The ingested particle, surrounded by a membrane, is referred to as a food vacuole (or phagosome). Digestive enzymes, released from lysosomes, then digest or break down the food into nutri-

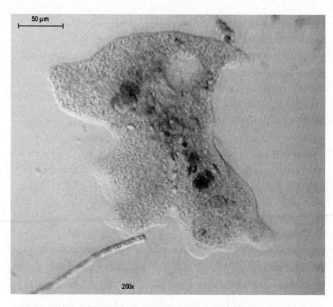

Figure 5-6. **A pond water ameba.** (Courtesy of Dr. Ralf Wagner and Wikidoc.)

ents. Some of the white blood cells in our bodies ingest and digest materials in the same manner as amebae. (Phagocytosis by white blood cells is discussed further in Chapter 15.) When fluids are ingested in a similar manner, the process is known as *pinocytosis*. One medically important ameba is *Entamoeba histolytica*, which causes amebic dysentery (amebiasis) and extraintestinal (meaning away from the intestine) amebic abscesses. Other amebae of medical significance, described in Chapter 21, include *Naegleria fowleri* (the causative agent of primary amebic meningoencephalitis) and *Acanthamoeba* spp. (which cause eye infections).

> Amebae (amebas), such as *Acanthamoeba*, *Entamoeba*, and *Naegleria spp.* move by means of cytoplasmic extensions called pseudopodia (false feet).

Ciliates (sing., *ciliate*) move about by means of large numbers of hairlike cilia on their surfaces. Cilia exhibit an oarlike motion. Ciliates are the most complex of all protozoa. A pathogenic ciliate, *Balantidium coli*, causes dysentery in underdeveloped countries (Fig. 5-7). It is usually transmitted to humans from drinking water that has been contaminated by swine feces. *B. coli* is the only ciliated protozoan that causes disease in humans. Examples of pond water ciliates are *Blepharisma*, *Didinium*, *Euplotes*, *Paramecium*, *Stentor*, and *Vorticella* spp., some of which are shown in Figure 5-2.

> Ciliates, such as *Balantidium*, *Paramecium*, *Stentor*, and *Vorticella* spp., move about by means of large numbers of hairlike cilia on their surfaces.

Flagellated protozoa or **flagellates** (sing., *flagellate*) move by means of whiplike flagella. A basal body (also called a kinetosome or kinetoplast) anchors each flagellum

Table 5-3 Characteristics of Major Protozoa

Category	Means of Movement	Method of Asexual Reproduction	Method of Sexual Reproduction	Representatives
Ciliates	Cilia	Transverse fission	Conjugation	*B. coli, Paramecium, Stentor, Tetrahymena, Vorticella*
Amebae (amebas)	Pseudopodia (false feet)	Binary fission	When present, involves flagellated sex cells	*Amoeba, Naegleria, E. histolytica*
Flagellates	Flagella	Binary fission	None	*Chlamydomonas, G. lamblia, Trichomonas, Trypanosoma*
Sporozoa	Generally nonmotile except for certain sex cells	Multiple fission	Involves flagellated sex cells	*Plasmodium, T. gondii, Cryptosporidium*

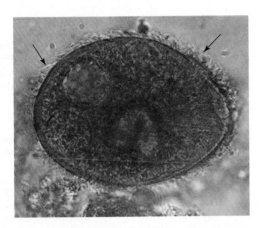

Figure 5-7. Photomicrograph of *Balantidium coli*, the only ciliated protozoan that causes human disease. *B. coli* causes a diarrheal disease called balantidiasis. Note the numerous short cilia (*arrows*) around the periphery of the cell. (Courtesy of the Oregon Public Health Laboratory and the Division of Parasitic Diseases, CDC.)

within the cytoplasm. Flagella exhibit a wavelike motion. Some flagellates are pathogenic. For example, *Trypanosoma brucei* subspecies *gambiense*, transmitted by the tsetse fly, causes African sleeping sickness in humans; *Trypanosoma cruzi* causes American trypanosomiasis (Chagas disease); *Trichomonas vaginalis* causes persistent sexually transmitted infections (trichomoniasis) of the male and female genital tracts; and *Giardia lamblia* (also known as *Giardia intestinalis*) causes a persistent diarrheal disease (giardiasis; Fig. 5-8).

> Flagellated protozoa (flagellates), such as Trypanosoma, Trichomonas, and *Giardia* spp., move by means of whiplike flagella.

Nonmotile protozoa—protozoa lacking pseudopodia, flagella, or cilia—are classified together in a category called **sporozoa**. The most important sporozoan pathogens are the *Plasmodium* spp. that cause malaria in many areas of the world. One of these species, *Plasmodium vivax*, causes a few cases of malaria annually in the United States. Malarial parasites are transmitted by female *Anopheles* mosquitoes, which become infected when they take a blood meal from a person with malaria. Another sporozoan, *Cryptosporidium parvum*, causes severe diarrheal disease (cryptosporidiosis) in immunosuppressed patients, especially those with acquired immunodeficiency syndrome (AIDS). A 1993 epidemic in Milwaukee, Wisconsin, caused by *Cryptosporidium* oocysts in drinking water, resulted in more than 400,000 cases of cryptosporidiosis, including some fatal cases. Other pathogenic sporozoans include *Babesia* spp. (the cause of babesiosis), *Cyclospora cayetanensis* (the cause of a diarrheal disease called cyclosporiasis), and *Toxoplasma gondii* (the cause of toxoplasmosis). Pathogenic protozoa are described in Chapter 21.

> *Babesia, Cryptosporidium, Cyclospora, Plasmodium,* and *Toxoplasma* spp. are examples of sporozoan protozoa that cause human infections. Sporozoan protozoa are nonmotile.

Fungi

Characteristics

In the Five-Kingdom System of Classification (described in Chapter 3), **fungi** (sing., *fungus*) are in a kingdom all by themselves—the Kingdom Fungi. The study of fungi is called mycology, and a person who studies fungi is called a mycologist.

> The study of fungi is called mycology.

Fungi are found almost everywhere on Earth, some (the saprophytic fungi) living on organic matter in water and soil, and others (the parasitic fungi) living on and within animals and plants. Some are harmful, whereas others are beneficial. Fungi also live on many unlikely materials, causing deterioration of leather and plastics and spoilage of jams, pickles, and many other foods. Beneficial fungi are important in the production of cheeses, beer, wine, and other foods, as well as certain drugs (e.g., the immunosuppressant drug cyclosporine) and antibiotics (e.g., penicillin).

Fungi are a diverse group of eukaryotic organisms that include yeasts, moulds, and mushrooms. As saprophytes, their main source of food is dead and decaying organic matter. Fungi are the "garbage disposers" of nature—the "vultures" of the microbial world. By secreting digestive enzymes into dead plant and animal matter, they decompose this material into absorbable nutrients for themselves and other living organisms; thus, they are the original "recyclers." Imagine living in a world without saprophytes, stumbling through endless piles of dead plants and animals and animal waste products. Not a pleasant thought!

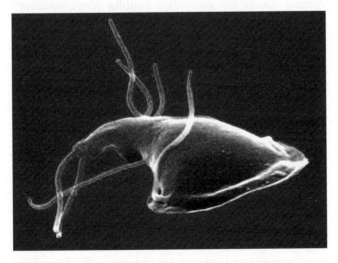

Figure 5-8. A digitally colorized scanning electron micrograph of *G. lamblia*, a flagellated protozoan that causes a human diarrheal disease known as giardiasis. (Courtesy of Dr. Stan Erlandsen, Dr. Dennis Feely, and the CDC.)

Fungi are sometimes incorrectly referred to as plants. They are not plants. One way that fungi differ from plants and algae is that they are not photosynthetic; they have no chlorophyll or other photosynthetic pigments. The cell walls of algal and plant cells contain cellulose (a polysaccharide), but fungal cell walls do not. Fungal cell walls do contain a polysaccharide called chitin, which is not found in the cell walls of any other microorganisms. Chitin is also found in the exoskeletons of arthropods.

> Neither algae nor fungi are plants. Algae are photosynthetic, but fungi are not.

Although many fungi are unicellular (e.g., yeasts), others grow as filaments called **hyphae** (sing., *hypha*), which intertwine to form a mass called a **mycelium** (pl., *mycelia*) or thallus; thus, they are quite different from bacteria, which are always unicellular. Also remember that bacteria are prokaryotic, whereas fungi are eukaryotic. Some fungi have *septate hyphae* (meaning that the cytoplasm within the hypha is divided into cells by cross-walls or septa), whereas others have *aseptate hyphae* (the cytoplasm within the hypha is not divided into cells; no septa). Aseptate hyphae contain multinucleated cytoplasm (described as being coenocytic). Learning whether the fungus possesses septate or aseptate hyphae is an important "clue" when attempting to identify a fungus that has been isolated from a clinical specimen (Fig. 5-9).

> Yeasts are unicellular, whereas moulds are multicellular.

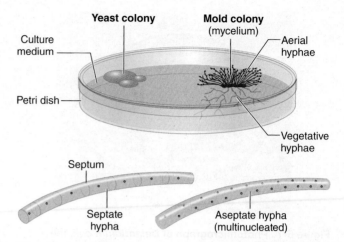

Figure 5-9. Fungal colonies and terms relating to hyphae.

Reproduction

Depending on the particular species, fungal cells can reproduce by budding, hyphal extension, or the formation of spores. There are two general categories of fungal spores: sexual spores and asexual spores.

> One of the ways in which fungi reproduce is spore production. The two general types of fungal spores are sexual and asexual spores.

Sexual spores are produced by the fusion of two gametes (thus, by the fusion of two nuclei). Sexual spores have a variety of names (e.g., ascospores, basidiospores, zygospores), depending on the exact manner in which they are formed. Fungi are classified taxonomically in accordance with the type of sexual spore that they produce or the type of structure on which the spores are produced (Fig. 5-10). Asexual spores are formed in many different ways, but not by the fusion of gametes (Fig. 5-11).

> Asexual fungal spores are known as conidia.

Asexual spores are also called **conidia** (sing., *conidium*). Some species of fungi produce both asexual and sexual spores. Fungal spores are very resistant structures that are carried great distances by wind. They are resistant to heat, cold, acids, bases, and other chemicals. Many people are allergic to fungal spores.

Classification

The taxonomic classification of fungi changes periodically. One current classification divides the Kingdom Fungi into five phyla. Classification of fungi into these phyla is based primarily on their mode of sexual reproduction. The two phyla known as "lower fungi" are the Zygomycotina (or Zygomycota) and the Chytridiomycotina (or Chytridiomycota). Zygomycotina include the common bread moulds and other fungi that cause food spoilage. Chytridiomycotina, which are not considered to be true fungi by some taxonomists, live in water ("water moulds") and soil. The two phyla known as "higher fungi" are the

STUDY AID

Decomposer versus Saprophyte

The term **decomposer** relates to what an organism "does for a living," so to speak—decomposers break materials down. The term **saprophyte** (or saprobe) relates to how an organism obtains nutrients; saprophytes absorb nutrients from dead and decaying organic matter. Sometimes the terms decomposer and saprophyte are used to describe the same organism. For example, all saprophytes are decomposers—they decompose organic materials, such as corpses, dead plants, and feces. However, not all decomposers are saprophytes. Some decomposers decompose materials such as minerals, rocks, inorganic industrial wastes, rubber, plastic, and textiles. Also note the difference between a saprophyte and a parasite. A parasite obtains nutrients from living organisms, whereas a saprophyte obtains nutrients from dead ones.

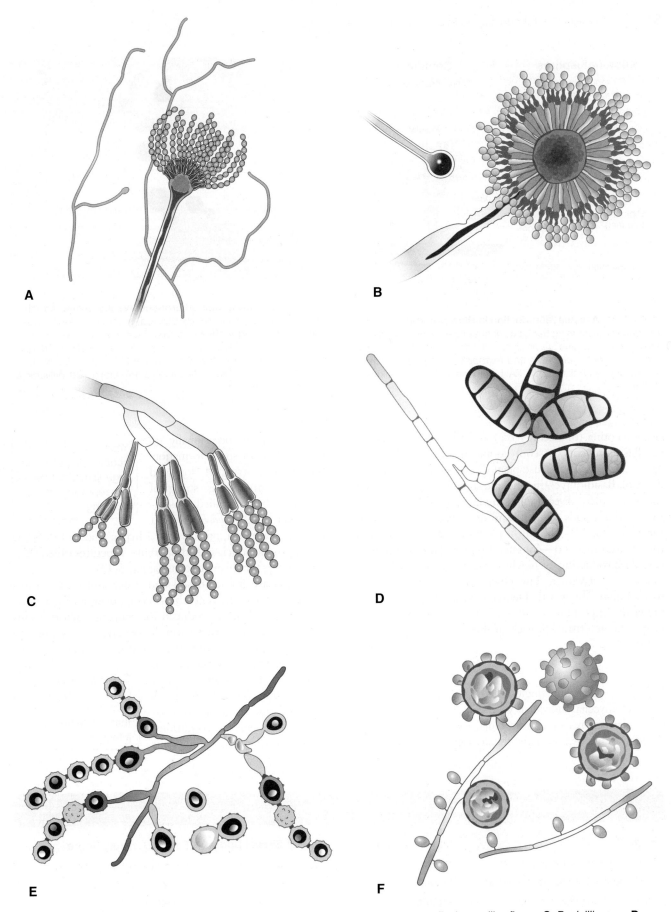

Figure 5-10. Microscopic appearance of various fungi. A. *Aspergillus fumigatus*. **B.** *Aspergillus flavus*. **C.** *Penicillium* sp. **D.** *Curvularia* sp. **E.** *Scopulariopsis* sp. **F.** *H. capsulatum*. (Redrawn from Winn WC Jr, et al. *Koneman's Color Atlas and Textbook of Diagnostic Microbiology*. 6th ed. Philadelphia, PA: Lippincott Williams & Wilkins; 2006.)

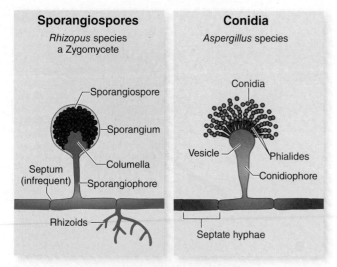

Figure 5-11. Asexual reproduction in *Rhizopus* and *Aspergillus* moulds. Illustrating the types of structures within and upon which asexual spores are produced. (Redrawn from Winn WC Jr, et al. *Koneman's Color Atlas and Textbook of Diagnostic Microbiology*. 6th ed. Philadelphia, PA: Lippincott Williams & Wilkins; 2006.)

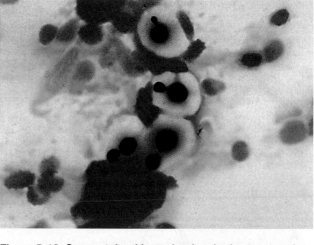

Figure 5-12. Gram-stained bronchoalveolar lavage specimen containing four darkly stained, narrow-necked, budding yeasts, suggestive of a *Cryptococcus* species. The negatively stained halos surrounding the yeast cells are dense polysaccharide capsules. (From Marler LM, Siders JA, Allen SD. *Direct Smear Atlas*. Philadelphia, PA: Lippincott Williams & Wilkins; 2001.)

Ascomycotina (or Ascomycota) and the Basidiomycotina (or Basidiomycota). Ascomycotina include certain yeasts and some fungi that cause plant diseases (e.g., Dutch Elm disease). Basidiomycotina include some yeasts, some fungi that cause plant diseases, and the large "fleshy fungi" that live in the woods (e.g., mushrooms, toadstools, bracket fungi, puffballs). The fifth phylum—Deuteromycotina (or Deuteromycota)—contains fungi having no mode of sexual reproduction, or in which the mode of sexual reproduction is not known. This phylum is sometimes referred to as Fungi Imperfecti. Deuteromycetes include certain medically important moulds such as *Aspergillus* and *Penicillium*. Characteristics of each of these phyla are shown in Table 5-4.

Yeasts

Yeasts are eukaryotic single-celled (unicellular) organisms that lack mycelia. Individual yeast cells, sometimes referred to as blastospores or blastoconidia, can be observed only through a microscope. They usually reproduce by budding

(Fig. 5-12), but occasionally do so by a type of spore formation. Sometimes a string of elongated buds is formed; this string of elongated buds is called a **pseudohypha** (pl., *pseudohyphae*). It resembles a hypha, but it is *not* a hypha (Fig. 5-13). Some yeasts produce thick-walled, sporelike structures called chlamydospores (or chlamydoconidia; Fig. 5-13).

> Yeasts are microscopic, single-celled organisms that usually reproduce by budding.

Yeasts are found in soil and water and on the skins of many fruits and vegetables. Wine, beer, and alcoholic beverages had been produced for centuries before Louis Pasteur discovered that naturally occurring yeasts on the skin of grapes and other fruits and grains were responsible for these fermentation processes. The common yeast *Saccharomyces cerevisiae* ("baker's yeast") ferments sugar to alcohol under anaerobic conditions. Under aerobic conditions, this

> *C. albicans* and *C. neoformans* are examples of yeasts that cause human infections.

Table 5-4	Selected Characteristics of the Phyla of Fungi		
Phylum	**Type of Hyphae**	**Type of Sexual Spore**	**Type of Asexual Spore**
Zygomycotina (Zygomycota)	Aseptate	Zygospore	Nonmotile sporangiospores
Chytridiomycotina (Chytridiomycota)	Aseptate	Oospore	Motile zoospores
Ascomycotina (Ascomycota)	Septate	Ascospore	Conidiospores
Basidiomycotina (Basidiomycota)	Septate	Basidiospore	Rare
Deuteromycotina (Deuteromycota)	Septate	None observed	Conidiospores

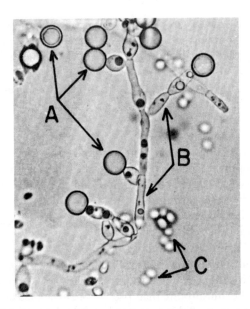

Figure 5-13. Microscopic examination of a culture of *C. albicans*. Seen here are **(A)** chlamydospores, **(B)** pseudohyphae (elongated yeast cells, linked end to end), and **(C)** budding yeast cells (blastospores). (From Davis BD, et al. *Microbiology*. 4th ed. Philadelphia, PA: Harper & Row; 1987.)

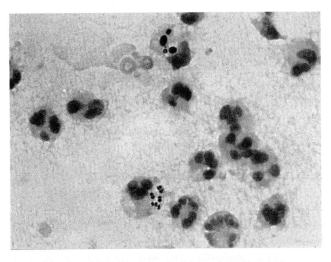

Figure 5-15. Gram-stained wound aspirate, illustrating the size differences between yeasts, bacteria, and white blood cells. Included in this photomicrograph are numerous white blood cells (red objects), two blue-stained budding yeast cells (top, center), and several Gram-positive cocci (small blue spheres near the bottom). The yeast and bacterial cells have been phagocytized by white blood cells. (From Marler LM, Siders JA, Allen SD. *Direct Smear Atlas*. Philadelphia, PA: Lippincott Williams & Wilkins; 2001.)

yeast breaks down simple sugars to carbon dioxide and water; for this reason, it has long been used as a leavening agent in bread production. Yeasts are also a good source of nutrients for humans because they produce many vitamins and proteins. Some yeasts (e.g., *Candida albicans* and *Cryptococcus neoformans*) are human pathogens. *C. albicans* is the yeast most frequently isolated from human clinical specimens, and is also the fungus most frequently isolated from human clinical specimens.

In the laboratory, yeasts produce colonies that are quite similar in appearance to bacterial colonies (Figs. 5-9 and 5-14). To distinguish between a yeast colony and a bacterial colony, a wet mount can be performed. A small portion of the colony is mixed with a drop of water or saline on a microscope slide, a coverslip is added, and the

preparation is examined under the microscope. Alternatively, the preparation can be stained using the Gram staining procedure. Yeasts are usually larger than bacteria (ranging from 3 to 8 µm in diameter) and are usually oval-shaped; some may be observed in the process of budding (Fig. 5-15). Bacteria do not produce buds.

Moulds

Although this category of fungi is frequently spelled "molds," mycologists prefer to use "moulds." Moulds are the fungi often seen in water and soil and on food (Fig. 5-16). They grow in the form of cytoplasmic filaments or hyphae that make up the mycelium of the

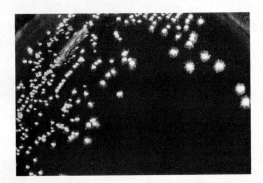

Figure 5-14. Colonies of the yeast, *C. albicans*, on a blood agar plate. Upon close examination, one can observe the foot-like extensions from the margins of the colonies, which are typical of this species. (Winn WC Jr, et al. *Koneman's Color Atlas and Textbook of Diagnostic Microbiology*. 6th ed. Philadelphia, PA: Lippincott Williams & Wilkins; 2006.)

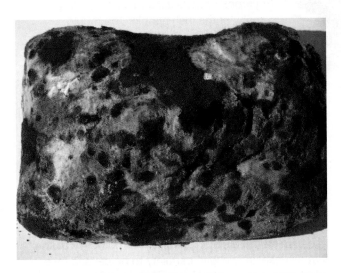

Figure 5-16. A variety of moulds growing on bread. (Courtesy of Biomed Ed, Round Rock, TX.)

mould. Some of the hyphae (called *aerial hyphae*) extend above the surface of whatever the mould is growing on, and some (called *vegetative hyphae*) are beneath the surface (Fig. 5-9). Reproduction is by spore formation, either sexually or asexually, on the aerial hyphae; for this reason, aerial hyphae are sometimes referred to as reproductive hyphae. Various species of moulds are found in each of the classes of fungi except Basidiomycotina. An interesting mould in class Chytridiomycotina is *Phytophthora infestans*, the potato blight mould that caused a famine in Ireland in the mid-19th century (see the following Historical Note).

Moulds have great commercial importance. For example, within the Ascomycotina are found many antibiotic-producing moulds, such as *Penicillium* and *Acremonium*. Penicillin, the first antibiotic to be discovered by a scientist, was actually discovered by accident (discussed in Chapter 9).

> Many of the commonly used antibiotics are produced by moulds.

Many additional antibiotics were later developed by culturing soil samples in laboratories and isolating any moulds that inhibited growth of bacteria. Today, to increase their spectrum of activity, antibiotics can be chemically altered in pharmaceutical company laboratories, as has been done with the various semisynthetic penicillins (e.g., ampicillin, amoxicillin, and carbenicillin).

Some moulds are also used to produce large quantities of enzymes (such as amylase, which converts starch to glucose), citric acid, and other organic acids that are used commercially. The flavor of cheeses such as bleu cheese, Roquefort, camembert, and limburger is the result of moulds that grow in them.

Fleshy Fungi

The large fungi that are encountered in forests, such as mushrooms, toadstools, puffballs, and bracket fungi, are collectively referred to as fleshy fungi (Fig. 5-17). Obviously, they are not microorganisms. Mushrooms are a class of true fungi that consist of a network of filaments or strands (the mycelium) that grow in the soil or in a rotting log, and a fruiting body (the mushroom that rises above the ground) that forms and releases spores. Each spore, much like the seed of a plant, germinates into a new organism. Many mushrooms are delicious to eat, but others, including some that resemble edible fungi, are extremely toxic and may cause permanent liver and brain damage or death if ingested. (thePoint contains information about the largest living organism—a type of mushroom.)

> Mushrooms, toadstools, puffballs, and bracket fungi (collectively referred to as fleshy fungi) are examples of fungi that are not microorganisms.

Medical Significance

A variety of fungi (including yeasts, moulds, and some fleshy fungi) are of medical, veterinary, and agricultural importance because of the diseases they cause in humans, animals, and plants. Many diseases of crop plants, grains, corn, and potatoes are caused by moulds. Some

> A variety of yeasts and moulds cause human infections (known as mycoses). Some moulds and fleshy fungi produce mycotoxins, which can cause human diseases called microbial intoxications.

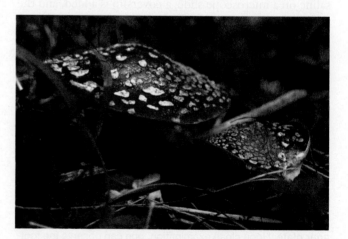

Figure 5-17. Fleshy fungi growing on the forest floor. The toxins produced by some fleshy fungi, such as the *Amanita* species shown here, can cause human disease. (Courtesy of Biomed Ed, Round Rock, TX.)

of these plant diseases are referred to as blights and rusts. Not only do these fungi destroy crops, but some produce toxins (*mycotoxins*) that cause disease in humans and animals (discussed in Appendix 1 on thePoint: "Microbial Intoxications"). Moulds and yeasts also cause a variety of infectious diseases of humans and animals—collectively referred to as *mycoses* (discussed later and in Chapter 20). Considering the large number of fungal species, very few are pathogenic for humans.

Fungal Infections of Humans

Fungal infections are known as **mycoses** (sing., *mycosis*), and are categorized as superficial, cutaneous, subcutaneous, or systemic mycoses. In some cases the infection may progress through all these stages. Representative mycoses are listed in Table 5-5.

Superficial and Cutaneous Mycoses. Superficial mycoses are fungal infections of the outermost areas of the human body: hair, fingernails, toenails, and the dead, outermost layers of the skin (the epidermis). Cutaneous mycoses are fungal infections of the living layers of skin (the dermis). A group of moulds, collectively referred to as dermatophytes, cause tinea infections, which are often referred to as "ringworm" infections. (Please note that ringworm infections have absolutely nothing to do with worms.) Tinea infections are named in accordance with the part of the anatomy that is infected; examples include tinea pedis (athlete's foot), tinea unguium (fingernails and toenails),

> The moulds that cause tinea (ringworm) infections are collectively referred to as dermatophytes.

tinea capitis (scalp), tinea barbae (face and neck), tinea corporis (trunk of the body), and tinea cruris (groin area).

C. albicans is an opportunistic yeast that lives harmlessly on the skin and mucous membranes of the mouth, gastrointestinal tract, and genitourinary tract. However, when conditions cause a reduction in the number of indigenous bacteria at these anatomic locations, *C. albicans* flourishes, leading to yeast infections of the mouth (thrush), skin, and vagina (yeast vaginitis). This type of local infection may become a focal site from which the organisms invade the bloodstream to become a generalized or systemic infection in many internal areas of the body.

Subcutaneous and Systemic Mycoses. Subcutaneous and systemic mycoses are more severe types of mycoses. Subcutaneous mycoses are fungal infections of the dermis and underlying tissues. These conditions can be quite grotesque in appearance. An example is Madura foot (a type of eukaryotic mycetoma), in which the patient's foot becomes covered with large, unsightly, fungus-containing bumps (see Figure 20-3 in Chapter 20).

> Subcutaneous and systemic mycoses are the more severe types of mycoses.

Systemic or generalized mycoses are fungal infections of internal organs of the body, sometimes affecting two or more different organ systems simultaneously (e.g., simultaneous infection of the respiratory system and the bloodstream, or simultaneous infection of the respiratory tract and the central nervous system).

Spores of some pathogenic fungi may be inhaled with dust from contaminated soil or dried bird and bat feces (guano), or they may enter through wounds of the hands

Table 5-5 Selected Fungal Diseases of Humans

Category	Genus/Species	Diseases
Yeasts	*C. albicans*	Thrush; yeast vaginitis, nail infections, systemic infection
	C. neoformans	Cryptococcosis (lung infection, meningitis, etc.)
Moulds	*Aspergillus* spp.	Aspergillosis (lung infection, systemic infection)
	Mucor and *Rhizopus* spp. and other species of bread moulds	Mucormycosis or zygomycosis (lung infection, systemic infection)
	Various dermatophytes	Tinea ("ringworm") infections
Dimorphic fungi	*B. dermatitidis*	Blastomycosis (primarily a disease of lungs and skin)
	C. immitis	Coccidioidomycosis (lung infection, systemic infection)
	H. capsulatum	Histoplasmosis (lung infection, systemic infection)
	S. schenckii	Sporotrichosis (a skin disease)
Other	*Pneumocystis jiroveci*	*Pneumocystis* pneumonia (PCP)

and feet. If the spores are inhaled into the lungs, they may germinate there to cause a respiratory infection similar to tuberculosis. Examples of deep-seated pulmonary infections are blastomycosis, coccidioidomycosis, cryptococcosis, and histoplasmosis. In each case, the pathogens may invade further to cause widespread systemic infections, especially in immunosuppressed individuals (see "Sick Building Syndrome" [Black Mould in Buildings] on thePoint).

Did you know that common bread moulds can cause human disease—even death? Inhalation of spores of bread moulds like *Rhizopus* and *Mucor* spp. by an immunosuppressed patient can lead to a respiratory disease called zygomycosis or mucormycosis. The mould can then become disseminated throughout the patient's body and can lead to death. *Rhizopus, Mucor,* and other bread moulds are primitive moulds with aseptate hyphae. As previously mentioned, the cytoplasm of aseptate hyphae is not divided into individual cells by cross-walls (septa).

To diagnose mycoses, clinical specimens are submitted to the mycology section of the clinical microbiology laboratory (discussed in Chapter 13). When isolated from clinical specimens, yeasts are identified (speciated) by inoculating them into a series of biochemical tests. In this way, the laboratory technologist can determine which substrates (usually carbohydrates) the yeast is able to use as nutrients; this depends on what enzymes the yeast possesses. Minisystems (miniaturized biochemical test systems) are commercially available for the identification of clinically important yeasts.

> In the mycology laboratory, yeasts are identified (speciated) by determining which substrates they are able to use as nutrients.

Biochemical tests are rarely used, however, for identification of moulds isolated from clinical specimens. Rather, moulds are identified by a combination of macroscopic and microscopic observations and the speed at which they grow. Macroscopic observations include the color, texture, and topography of the mould colony (mycelium). Microscopic examination of the mould reveals the types of structures on which or within which spores are produced (Fig. 5-10); the method of spore production varies from one species of mould to another. Immunodiagnostic procedures, including skin tests, are also available for diagnosing certain types of mycoses.

> In the mycology laboratory, moulds are identified by a combination of macroscopic and microscopic observations and the speed at which they grow.

Mycoses are most effectively treated with antifungal agents like nystatin, amphotericin B, or 5-fluorocytosine (discussed in Chapter 9). Because these chemotherapeutic agents may be toxic to humans, they are prescribed with due consideration and caution.

Dimorphic Fungi. A few fungi, including some human pathogens, can live either as yeasts or as moulds, depending on growth conditions. This phenomenon is called *dimorphism*, and the organisms are referred to as *dimorphic fungi* (Fig. 5-18). When grown in vitro at body temperature (37°C), dimorphic fungi exist as unicellular yeasts and produce yeast colonies. Within the human body (in vivo), dimorphic fungi exist as yeasts. However, when grown in vitro at room temperature (25°C), dimorphic fungi exist as moulds, producing mould colonies (mycelia). Dimorphic fungi that cause human diseases include *Histoplasma capsulatum* (which causes histoplasmosis), *Sporothrix schenckii* (which causes sporotrichosis), *Coccidioides immitis* (which causes coccidioidomycosis), and *Blastomyces dermatitidis* (which causes blastomycosis).

> Dimorphic fungi can live either as yeasts or as moulds, depending on growth conditions.

Lichens

Nearly everyone has seen lichens, usually while hiking in the woods.[c] They appear as colored, often circular patches on tree trunks and rocks. A **lichen** is actually a combination of two organisms—an alga (or a cyanobacterium) and a fungus—living together in such a close relationship that they appear to be one organism. Close relationships of this type are referred to as symbiotic relationships, and the partners in the relationship are referred to as symbionts. A lichen represents a particular type of symbiotic relationship known as mutualism—a relationship in which both parties benefit (discussed further in Chapter 10). The alga or cyanobacterium in a lichen is sometimes referred to as the photobiont (the photosynthetic partner in the relationship), and the fungus is referred to as the mycobiont. There are about 20,000 different species of lichens. Lichens may be gray, brown, black, orange, various shades of green, and other colors, depending on the specific combination of alga and fungus. Foliose lichens are leaflike, whereas crustose

> A lichen is a combination of two organisms: an alga (or a cyanobacterium) and a fungus.

---

[c]Lichens are sometimes misidentified as mosses (e.g., lichen-covered rocks are frequently referred to as "moss-covered" rocks). Mosses are plants, whereas lichens are not.

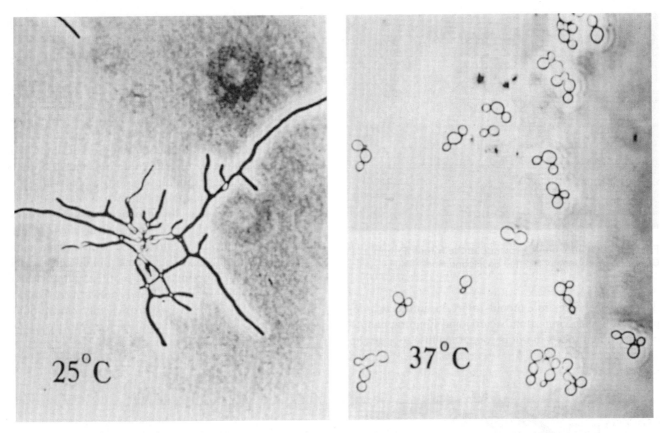

Figure 5-18. Dimorphism. Photomicrographs illustrating the dimorphic fungus, *H. capsulatum*, being grown at 25°C (left photo) and at 37°C (right photo). (From Schaeter M, et al., eds. *Mechanisms of Microbial Disease*. 3rd ed. Philadelphia, PA: Lippincott Williams & Wilkins; 1999.)

lichens appear as a crust on the rock or tree trunk surface (Fig. 5-19). Other lichens may be shrubby (fruticose lichens) or gelatinous. Lichens are classified as protists. They are not associated with human disease, but some substances produced by lichens have been shown to have antibacterial properties.

Slime Moulds

Slime moulds, which are found in soil and on rotting logs, have both fungal and protozoal characteristics and very interesting life cycles (Fig. 5-20). Some slime moulds

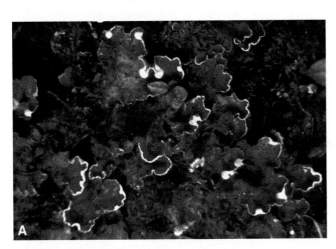

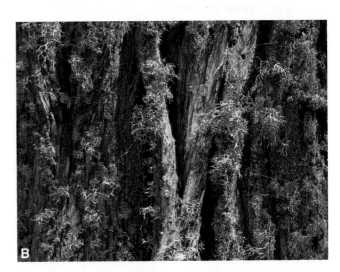

Figure 5-19. Examples of lichens. A. A foliose lichen in Colorado. **B.** Staghorn lichens growing on trees in Yosemite National Park, CA. (Courtesy of Biomed Ed, Round Rock, TX.)

Figure 5-20. Slime mould growing on the forest floor in Colorado. (Courtesy of Biomed Ed, Round Rock, TX.)

(known as cellular slime moulds) start out in life as independent amebae, ingesting bacteria and fungi by phagocytosis. When they run out of food, they fuse together to form a motile, multicellular form known as a slug, which is only about 0.5 mm long. The slug then becomes a fruiting body, consisting of a stalk and a spore cap. Spores produced within the spore cap become disseminated, and from each spore emerges an ameba (Fig. 5-21). Cellular slime moulds represent cell differentiation at the lowest level, and scientists are studying them in an attempt to determine how some of the cells in the slug know that they are to become part of the stalk, how others know that they are to become part of the spore cap, and still others know that they are to differentiate into spores within the spore cap. Other slime moulds, known as plasmodial (or acellular) slime moulds, also produce stalks and spores, but their life cycles differ somewhat from those of cellular slime moulds. In the life cycle of a plasmodial slime mould, haploid cells fuse to become diploid cells, which develop into very large masses of motile, multinucleated protoplasm, each such mass being known as a plasmodium (Fig. 5-21). Some taxonomists classify slime moulds as fungi, whereas others classify them as protists. They are not known to cause human disease.

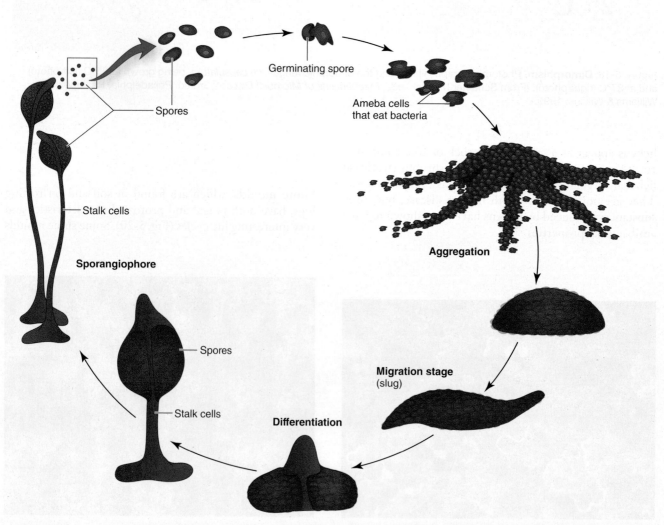

Figure 5-21. Life cycle of a slime mould. See text for details. (Courtesy of Mary Wu, Rich Kessin, Columbia University, and the National Science Foundation.)

ON thePoint

- Terms Introduced in This Chapter
- Review of Key Points
- A Closer Look: Sick Building Syndrome (Black Mould in Buildings)
- A Closer Look: the Largest Living Organism
- Increase Your Knowledge
- Critical Thinking
- Additional Self-Assessment Exercises

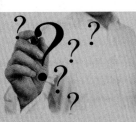

Self-Assessment Exercises

After studying this chapter, answer the following multiple-choice questions.

1. Which of the following statements about algae and fungi is (are) true?
   a. Algae are photosynthetic, whereas fungi are not
   b. Algal cell walls contain cellulose, whereas fungal cell walls do not
   c. Fungal cell walls contain chitin, whereas algal cell walls do not
   d. All of the above

2. All of the following are algae except:
   a. desmids
   b. diatoms
   c. dinoflagellates
   d. sporozoa

3. All of the following are fungi except:
   a. moulds
   b. *Paramecium*
   c. *Penicillium*
   d. yeasts

4. A protozoan may possess any of the following except:
   a. cilia
   b. flagella
   c. hyphae
   d. pseudopodia

5. Which one of the following terms is not associated with fungi?
   a. conidia
   b. hyphae
   c. mycelium
   d. pellicle

6. All of the following terms can be used to describe hyphae except:
   a. aerial and reproductive
   b. septate and aseptate
   c. sexual and asexual
   d. vegetative

7. A lichen usually represents a symbiotic relationship between which of the following pairs?
   a. a fungus and an ameba
   b. a yeast and an ameba
   c. an alga and a cyanobacterium
   d. an alga and a fungus

8. A stigma is a:
   a. light-sensing organelle
   b. primitive mouth
   c. thickened membrane
   d. type of plastid

9. If a dimorphic fungus is causing a respiratory infection, which of the following might be seen in a sputum specimen from that patient?
   a. amebae
   b. conidia
   c. hyphae
   d. yeasts

10. Which one of the following is not a fungus?
    a. *Aspergillus*
    b. *Candida*
    c. *Penicillium*
    d. *Prototheca*

6

The Biochemical Basis of Life

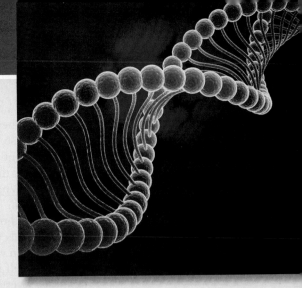

Artist rendering of a deoxyribonucleic acid (DNA) molecule.

 CHAPTER OUTLINE

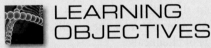 LEARNING OBJECTIVES

After studying this chapter, you should be able to:

- Name the four main categories of biochemical molecules discussed in this chapter
- State the major differences between trioses, tetroses, pentoses, hexoses, and heptoses
- Describe each of the following: monosaccharides, disaccharides, and polysaccharides, and cite two examples of each
- Compare and contrast a dehydration synthesis reaction and a hydrolysis reaction, and cite an example of each
- Differentiate between covalent, glycosidic, and peptide bonds
- Discuss the roles of enzymes in metabolism
- Define the following terms: apoenzyme, cofactor, coenzyme, holoenzyme, and substrate
- Cite three important differences between the structures of DNA and RNA
- State the major differences between DNA nucleotides and RNA nucleotides
- Define what is meant by "the Central Dogma"
- Describe the processes of DNA replication, transcription, and translation

Introduction

Some students are surprised to learn that they must study chemistry as part of a microbiology course. The reason why chemistry is an important component of a micro-

> Cells can be thought of as "bags" of chemicals. Even the bags themselves are composed of chemicals.

biology course is the answer to the question, "What exactly is a microorganism?" A cellular microbe can be thought of as a "bag" of chemicals that interact with each other in various ways. Even the bag itself is composed of chemicals. Everything a mi-

croorganism is and does relates to chemistry. The various ways microorganisms function and survive in their environment depend on their chemical makeup. The same things are true about the cells that make up any living organisms—including human beings; these cells, too, can be thought of as bags of chemicals.

To understand microbial cells and how they function, one must have a basic knowledge of the chemistry of atoms, molecules, and compounds. Appendix 3 on thePoint ("Basic Chemistry Concepts") contains such information. Students having little or no background in chemistry should study the material in Appendix 3 before attempting to learn the material in this chapter. Appendix 3 can also serve as a review for students who have already studied basic chemistry, either in a biology course or in an introductory chemistry course. Your instructor will inform you as to whether the material in Appendix 3 is "testable."

Even the most simple prokaryotic cells consist of very large molecules (*macromolecules*), such as deoxyribonucleic acid (DNA), ribonucleic acid (RNA), proteins, lipids, and polysaccharides, as well as many combinations of these macromolecules that combine to make up structures such as capsules, cell walls, cell membranes, and flagella. These macromolecules can be broken down into smaller units

> Cells contain many large biological molecules, known as macromolecules. Macromolecules include DNA, RNA, proteins, lipids, and polysaccharides.

or "building blocks," such as monosaccharides (simple sugars), fatty acids, amino acids, and nucleotides. The macromolecules and building blocks found in cells are collectively referred to as *biological molecules.* The building blocks can be broken down into even smaller molecules such as water, carbon dioxide, ammonia, sulfides, and

phosphates, which in turn can be broken down into atoms of carbon (C), hydrogen (H), oxygen (O), nitrogen (N), sulfur (S), phosphorus (P), etc.

Organic chemistry is the study of compounds that contain carbon; **inorganic chemistry** involves all other chemical reactions; **biochemistry** is the chemistry of living cells. Basic inorganic chemistry is introduced in Appendix 3 on thePoint ("Basic Chemistry Concepts");

organic chemistry and biochemistry are discussed in this chapter.

Only when all these molecules and compounds are in place and working together properly can the cell function like a well-managed factory. As in industry, a cell must have the appropriate machinery, regulatory molecules (enzymes) to control its activities, fuel (nutrients or light) to provide energy, and raw materials (nutrients) for manufacturing essential end products.

Everything that a microorganism is and does involves biochemistry. Biochemicals make up the structure of a microorganism, and a multitude of biochemical reactions take place within the microorganism. What is true for cellular microbes is also true for every other living organism. The characteristics that distinguish living organisms from inanimate objects—(a) their complex and highly organized structure; (b) their ability

> Everything that a cell is and does involves biochemistry.

to extract, transform, and use energy from their environment; and (c) their capacity for precise self-replication and self-assembly—all result from the nature, function, and interaction of biomolecules. Because biochemistry is a branch of organic chemistry, a brief introduction to organic chemistry will be presented first.

Organic Chemistry

Organic compounds are compounds that contain carbon, and organic chemistry is that branch of the science of chemistry that specializes in the study of organic compounds. The term *organic* is somewhat misleading, as it implies that all these compounds are produced by or are in some way related to liv-

ing organisms. This is not true. Although some organic compounds are associated with living organisms, many are not. A typical *Escherichia coli* cell contains more than 6,000 different kinds of organic compounds, including about 3,000 different proteins and approximately

> Organic compounds are compounds that contain carbon. Although many organic compounds are produced by or related to living organisms, some are not.

the same number of different molecules of nucleic acid. Proteins make up about 15% of the total weight of an *E. coli* cell, whereas nucleic acids, polysaccharides, and lipids make up about 7%, 3%, and 2%, respectively.

Organic chemistry is a broad and important branch of chemistry, involving the chemistry of fossil fuels (petroleum and coal), dyes, drugs, paper, ink, paints, plastics, gasoline, rubber tires, food, and clothing. The number of compounds that contain carbon far exceeds the number of compounds that do not contain carbon. Some carbon-containing compounds are very large and complex, some containing thousands of atoms.

Carbon Bonds

In our current understanding of life, carbon is the primary requisite for all living systems. The element carbon exists in three forms or allotropes: amorphous carbon, graphite, and diamond.

1. **Amorphous carbon** is also known as lampblack, gas black, channel black, and carbon black. It is the black soot that forms when a material containing carbon is burned with insufficient oxygen for it to burn completely. It is used to make inks, paints, rubber products, and the cores of dry cell batteries.
2. **Graphite** is one of the softest materials known. It is primarily used as a lubricant, although in a form called coke, is used in the production of steel. The black material in "lead" pencils is actually graphite.
3. **Diamond** is one of the hardest substances known. Naturally occurring diamonds are used for jewelry, whereas artificially produced diamonds are used to make diamond-tipped saw blades.

These three forms of carbon have dramatically different physical properties, making it difficult to believe that they are truly the same element. Carbon atoms have a valence of 4, meaning that a carbon atom can bond to four other atoms. For convenience, the carbon atom is illustrated in this text with the symbol C and four bonds.

The uniqueness of carbon lies in the ability of its atoms to bond to each other to form a multitude of compounds. The variety of carbon compounds increases still more when atoms of other elements also attach in different ways to the carbon atom.

There are three ways in which carbon atoms can bond to each other: **single bond**, **double bond**, and **triple bond**. In the following illustrations, each line between the carbon atoms represents a pair of shared electrons (known as a *covalent bond*). In a carbon–carbon single bond, the two carbon atoms share one pair of electrons; in a carbon–carbon double bond, two pairs of electrons; and in a carbon–carbon triple bond, three pairs of electrons. Covalent bonds are typical of the compounds of carbon and are the bonds of primary importance in organic chemistry. Organic chemistry is sometimes defined as the chemistry of carbon and its covalent bonds.

> Organic chemistry is sometimes defined as the chemistry of carbon and its covalent bonds.

Single bond   Double bond   Triple bond

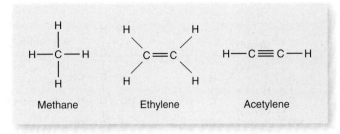

Figure 6-1. Simple hydrocarbons.

When atoms of other elements attach to available bonds of carbon atoms, compounds are formed. For example, if only hydrogen atoms are bonded to the available bonds, compounds called hydrocarbons are formed. In other words, a **hydrocarbon** is an organic molecule that contains only carbon and hydrogen atoms. Just a few of the many hydrocarbon compounds are shown in Figure 6-1.

> Hydrocarbons are organic compounds that contain only carbon and hydrogen.

When more than two carbons are linked together, longer molecules are formed. A series of many carbon atoms bonded together is referred to as a *chain*. Long-chain carbon compounds are usually liquids or solids, whereas short-chain carbon compounds, such as the hydrocarbons shown in Figure 6-1, are gases.

Cyclic Compounds

Carbon atoms may link to carbon atoms to close the chain, forming *rings* or *cyclic compounds*. An example is benzene, which has six carbons and six hydrogens, as shown in Figure 6-2. Although benzene contains six carbon atoms, other ring structures contain fewer or more carbon atoms, and some compounds contain fused rings (e.g., double- or triple-ringed compounds).

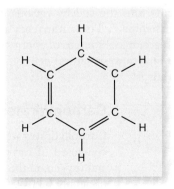

Figure 6-2. The benzene ring.

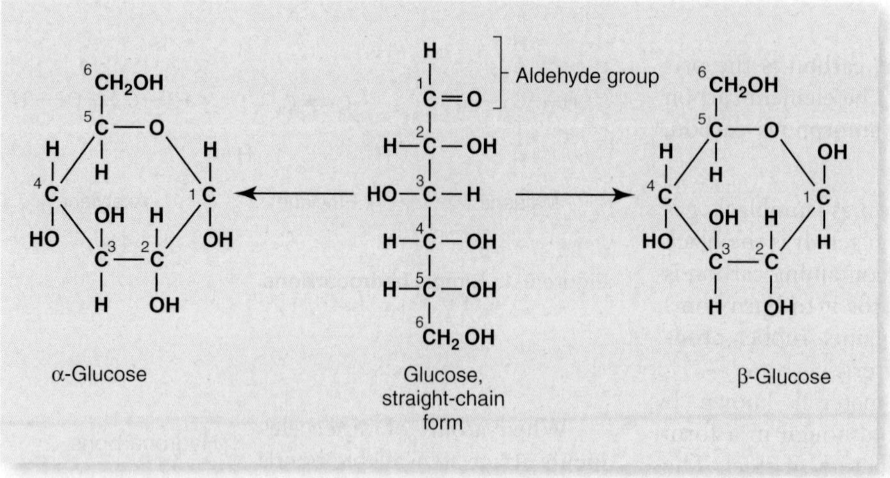

Figure 6-3. Forms of glucose. All three forms may exist in equilibrium in solution.

Biochemistry

Biochemistry is the study of biology at the molecular level and can thus be thought of as the chemistry of life or the chemistry of living organisms. Biochemistry is a branch of not only biology, but also organic chemistry. Biochemistry involves the study of the biomolecules that are present within living organisms. These biomolecules are usually large molecules (called *macromolecules*) and include carbohydrates, lipids, proteins, and nucleic acids. Other examples of biomolecules are vitamins, enzymes, hormones, and energy-carrying molecules, such as adenosine triphosphate (ATP).

Humans obtain their nutrients from the foods they eat. The carbohydrates, fats, nucleic acids, and proteins contained in these foods are digested, and their components are absorbed into the blood and carried to every cell in the body. Within cells, these components are then broken down and rearranged. In this way, the compounds necessary for cell structure and function are synthesized. Microorganisms also absorb their essential nutrients into the cell by various means, to be described in Chapter 7. These nutrients are then used in metabolic reactions as sources of energy and as building blocks for enzymes, structural macromolecules, and genetic materials.

> Biochemistry involves the study of biomolecules, and can be thought of as both a branch of chemistry and a branch of biology.

> Carbohydrates are biomolecules that are composed of carbon, hydrogen, and oxygen in the ratio of 1:2:1.

Carbohydrates

Carbohydrates are biomolecules composed of carbon, hydrogen, and oxygen, in the ratio of 1:2:1, or simply CH_2O. Glucose, fructose, sucrose, lactose, maltose, starch, cellulose, and glycogen are all examples of carbohydrates.

Monosaccharides

The simplest carbohydrates are sugars, and the smallest sugars (or simple sugars) are called **monosaccharides** (Greek *mono* meaning "one"; *sakcharon* meaning "sugar"). The "one" refers to the number of rings; in other words, monosaccharides are sugars composed of only one ring. The most important monosaccharide in nature is **glucose** ($C_6H_{12}O_6$), which may occur as a chain or in alpha or beta ring configurations, as shown in Figure 6-3. Monosaccharides may contain from three to nine carbon atoms (Table 6-1), although most of them contain five or six. A three-carbon monosaccharide is called a **triose**; one containing four carbons is called a **tetrose**; five, a **pentose**; six, a **hexose**; seven, a **heptose**; eight, an **octose**; and nine, a **nonose**. Ribose and deoxyribose are pentoses that are found in RNA and DNA, respectively. Glucose (also called *dextrose*) is a hexose. Octoses and nonoses are quite rare.

Glucose, the main source of energy for body cells, is found in most sweet fruits and in blood. The glucose that is carried in the blood to the cells is oxidized to produce the energy-carrying molecule ATP, with its high-energy phosphate bonds. ATP molecules are the main source of

> The simplest carbohydrates are simple sugars or monosaccharides. Trioses, pentoses, and hexoses are examples of monosaccharides.

Table 6-1	Monosaccharides	
Number of Carbon Atoms	**General Name**	**Examples**
3	Triose	Glyceraldehyde (glycerose), dihydroxyacetone
4	Tetrose	Erythrose
5	Pentose	Ribose, deoxyribose, arabinose, xylose, ribulose
6	Hexose	Glucose, fructose, galactose, mannose
7	Heptose	Sedoheptulose, mannoheptulose
8	Octose	Octoses have been synthetically prepared; they do not occur in nature
9	Nonose	Neuraminic acid

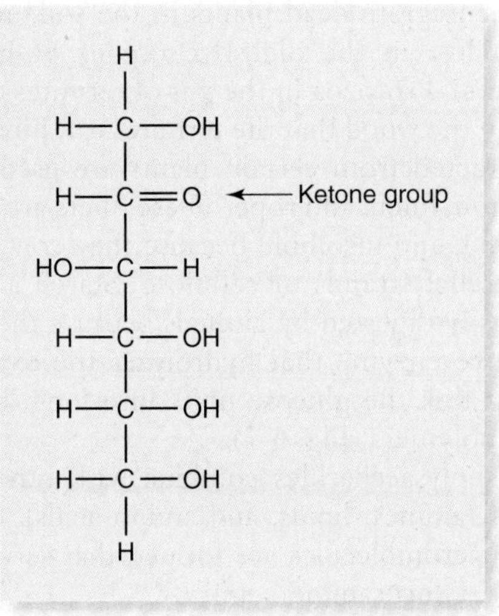

Figure 6-4. Fructose in straight-chain form. Fructose may also exist in the ring form shown in Figure 6-5.

the energy that is used to drive most metabolic reactions (Chapter 7). Galactose and fructose are other examples of hexoses. Fructose (Fig. 6-4), the sweetest of the monosaccharides, is found in fruits and honey.

Disaccharides

Disaccharides (*di* meaning "two") are double-ringed sugars that result from the combination of two monosaccharides. The synthesis of a disaccharide from two monosaccharides by removal of a water molecule is called a **dehydration synthesis reaction** (Fig. 6-5). The bond holding the two monosaccharides together is called a **glycosidic bond**; it is a type of covalent bond. Glucose is the major constituent of disaccharides. Sucrose (table sugar) is a sweet disaccharide made by joining together a glucose molecule and a fructose molecule. Sucrose comes from sugar cane, sugar beets, and maple sugar. Lactose (milk sugar) and maltose (malt sugar) are also disaccharides. Lactose is made by joining together a molecule of glucose and a molecule of galactose. People who lack the digestive enzyme lactase, needed to split lactose into its monosaccharide

> Sucrose, lactose, and maltose are examples of disaccharides.

components, are said to be lactose intolerant. Maltose is made by combining two molecules of glucose.

Disaccharides react with water in a process called a **hydrolysis reaction**, which causes them to break down into two monosaccharides:

$$\text{disaccharide} + H_2O \rightarrow \text{two monosaccharides}$$
$$\text{sucrose} + H_2O \rightarrow \text{glucose} + \text{fructose}$$
$$\text{lactose} + H_2O \rightarrow \text{glucose} + \text{galactose}$$
$$\text{maltose} + H_2O \rightarrow \text{glucose} + \text{glucose}$$

Peptidoglycan (mentioned in Chapter 3) is a complex macromolecular network found in the cell walls of all members of the domain *Bacteria*. Peptidoglycan consists of a repeating disaccharide, attached by polypeptides (proteins) to form a lattice that surrounds and protects the entire bacterial cell. Several antibiotics (including penicillin) prevent the final cross-linking of the rows of disaccharides, thus weakening the cell wall and leading to lysis (bursting) of the bacterial cell. Although most members of the domain *Archaea* have cell walls, their cell walls do not contain peptidoglycan.

> Bacterial cell walls contain peptidoglycan, a complex macromolecule consisting of a repeating disaccharide, attached by proteins.

Carbohydrates composed of three monosaccharides are called **trisaccharides**; those composed of four are called **tetrasaccharides**; those composed of five are called **pentasaccharides**; and so on, until one comes to polysaccharides.

Polysaccharides

The definition of a **polysaccharide** varies from one reference book to another, with some stating that a polysaccharide consists of more than 6 monosaccharides, others stating more than 8, and others stating more than 10. Poly means "many," and in reality, most polysaccharides contain many monosaccharides—up to hundreds or even thousands of monosaccharides. Thus, in this book, polysaccharides

> Polysaccharides can be defined as carbohydrates that contain many monosaccharides.

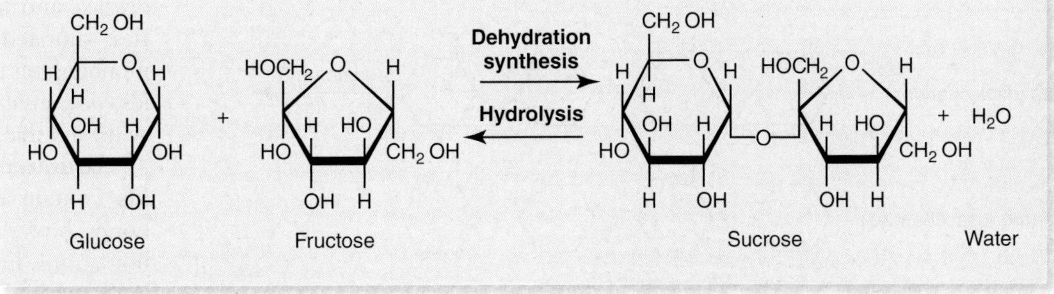

Figure 6-5. The dehydration synthesis and hydrolysis of sucrose.

Polysaccharides, such as glycogen, starch, and cellulose, are examples of polymers—molecules consisting of many similar subunits. In the case of polysaccharides, the repeating subunits are monosaccharides.

are defined as carbohydrate polymers containing many monosaccharides.

Examples include starch and glycogen, which are composed of hundreds of repetitive glucose units held together by different types of covalent bonds, known as glycosidic bonds (or glycosidic linkages). Glucose is the major constituent of polysaccharides. Polysaccharides are examples of **polymers**—molecules consisting of many similar subunits. Some of these molecules are so large that they are insoluble in water. In the presence of the proper enzymes or acids, polysaccharides may be hydrolyzed or broken down into disaccharides, and then finally into monosaccharides (Fig. 6-6).

Polysaccharides serve two main functions. One is to store energy that can be used when the external food supply is low. The common storage molecule in animals is **glycogen**, which is found in the liver and in muscles. In plants, glucose is stored as **starch** and is found in potatoes and other vegetables and seeds. Some algae store starch, whereas bacteria contain glycogen granules as a reserve nutrient supply. The other function of polysaccharides is to provide a "tough" molecule for structural support and protection. Many bacteria produce polysaccharide capsules, which protect them from being phagocytized (eaten) by white blood cells.

Cellulose is another example of a polysaccharide. Plant and algal cells have cellulose cell walls to provide support and shape as well as protection against the environment. Cellulose is insoluble in water and indigestible for humans and most animals. Some protozoa, fungi, and bacteria have enzymes that will break the β-glycosidic bonds linking the glucose units in cellulose. Some of these microorganisms (saprophytes) are

able to disintegrate dead plants in the soil, and others (parasites) live in the digestive organs of herbivores (plant eaters). Protozoa in the gut of termites digest the cellulose in the wood that the termites eat. Fibers of cellulose extracted from certain plants are used to make paper, cotton, linen, and rope. These fibers are relatively rigid, strong, and insoluble because they consist of 100 to 200 parallel strands of cellulose. Starch and glycogen are easily digested by animals because they possess the digestive enzyme that hydrolyzes the α-glycosidic bonds that link the glucose units into long, helical, or branched polymers (Fig. 6-7).

When polysaccharides combine with other chemical groups (amines, lipids, and amino acids), extremely complex macromolecules are formed that serve specific purposes. Glucosamine and galactosamine (amine derivatives of glucose and galactose, respectively) are important constituents of the supporting polysaccharides in connective tissue fibers, cartilage, and chitin. Chitin is the main component of the hard outer covering of insects, spiders, and crabs, and is also found in the cell walls of fungi. The main portion of the rigid cell wall of bacteria consists of amino sugars and short polypeptide chains that combine to form the peptidoglycan layer.

Bacterial cell walls contain peptidoglycan, algal cell walls contain cellulose, and fungal cell walls contain chitin. Peptidoglycan, cellulose, and chitin are examples of polysaccharides.

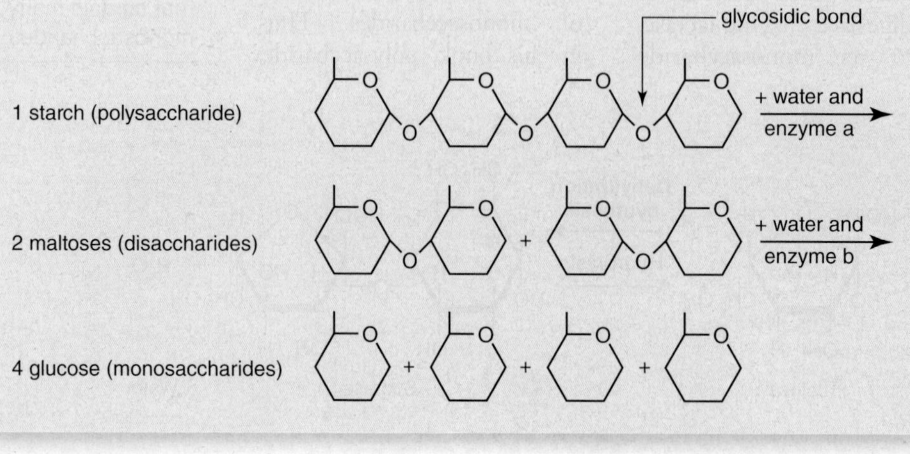

Lipids

Lipids constitute an important class of biomolecules. Most lipids are insoluble in water but soluble in fat solvents, such as ether, chloroform, and benzene. Lipids are essential constituents of almost all living cells.

Fatty Acids

Fatty acids can be thought of as the building blocks of lipids. Fatty acids are long-chain carboxylic acids that are insoluble in water. Fatty acids can be divided into four categories: saturated fatty acids, monounsaturated fatty acids, polyunsaturated fatty acids, and trans fats.

Saturated fatty acids contain only single bonds between the carbon atoms. Fats containing saturated fatty acids are usually solids at room

Figure 6-6. Steps in the hydrolysis of starch.

- 1 starch (polysaccharide)

- glycosidic bond

+ water and enzyme a

- 2 maltoses (disaccharides)

+ water and enzyme b

- 4 glucose (monosaccharides)

temperature. **Monounsaturated fatty acids** (such as those found in butter, olives, and peanuts) have one double bond in the carbon chain. **Polyunsaturated fatty acids** (such as those found in soybeans, safflowers, sunflowers, and corn) contain two or more double bonds. **Trans fats** are manufactured by the artificial addition of hydrogen atoms to unsaturated fats; the process is known as hydrogenation. Most fats containing unsaturated fatty acids are

> Monosaccharides are the building blocks of carbohydrates, whereas fatty acids are the building blocks of lipids.

liquids at room temperature, but trans fats are solid or semisolid fats, which are often incorporated into food products.

The terms saturated, monounsaturated, polyunsaturated fatty acids, and trans fats are often heard in discussions about human diet. Dieticians tell us that an increased intake of saturated and trans fats may increase the risk of coronary heart disease, whereas an increased intake of mono- and polyunsaturated fats may decrease that risk. Trans fats should be avoided because of their harmful effects on cholesterol levels and their link to heart disease.

Certain fatty acids, called **essential fatty acids**, cannot be synthesized in the human body and, thus, must be provided in the diet. Omega-3 fatty acid is an example of an essential fatty acid.

For purposes of discussion, lipids can be classified into the following categories (Fig. 6-8):

> Waxes, fats, oils, phospholipids, glycolipids, steroids, prostaglandins, and leukotrienes are all examples of lipids.

- Waxes
- Fats and oils
- Phospholipids
- Glycolipids
- Steroids
- Prostaglandins and leukotrienes

Waxes

A **wax** consists of a saturated fatty acid and a long-chain alcohol. Wax coatings on the fruits, leaves, and stems of

> Waxes in the cell walls of *Mycobacterium tuberculosis* (the causative agent of tuberculosis) protect phagocytized *M. tuberculosis* cells from being digested.

plants help to prevent loss of water and damage from pests. Waxes on the skin, fur, and feathers of animals and birds provide a waterproof coating. Lanolin, a mixture of waxes obtained from wool, is used in hand and body lotions to aid in retention of water, thus softening the skin. The waxes that are present in the cell walls of *Mycobacterium tuberculosis* (the causative agent of tuberculosis) are responsible for several interesting characteristics of this bacterium. For

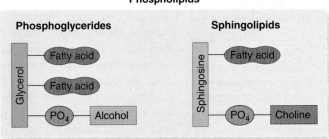

Figure 6-7. The difference between cellulose and starch.

example, should an *M. tuberculosis* cell be phagocytized by a phagocytic white blood cell (a phagocyte), the waxes protect the cell from being digested. This enables the bacterial cell to survive and multiply within the phagocyte. Also, the waxes in the cell walls of *M. tuberculosis* make the organism difficult to stain, and, once stained, the waxes make it difficult to remove the stain from the cell. In the acid-fast staining procedure, for example, it is necessary to heat the carbolfuchsin dye to drive it into the cell. Once the cell has been stained, the waxes prevent decolorization of the cell when a mixture of acid and alcohol is applied. Because the cell does not

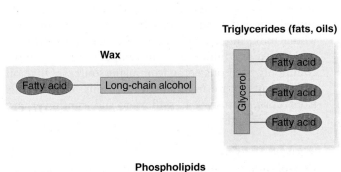
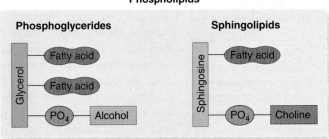
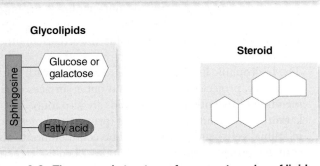

Figure 6-8. The general structure of some categories of lipids.

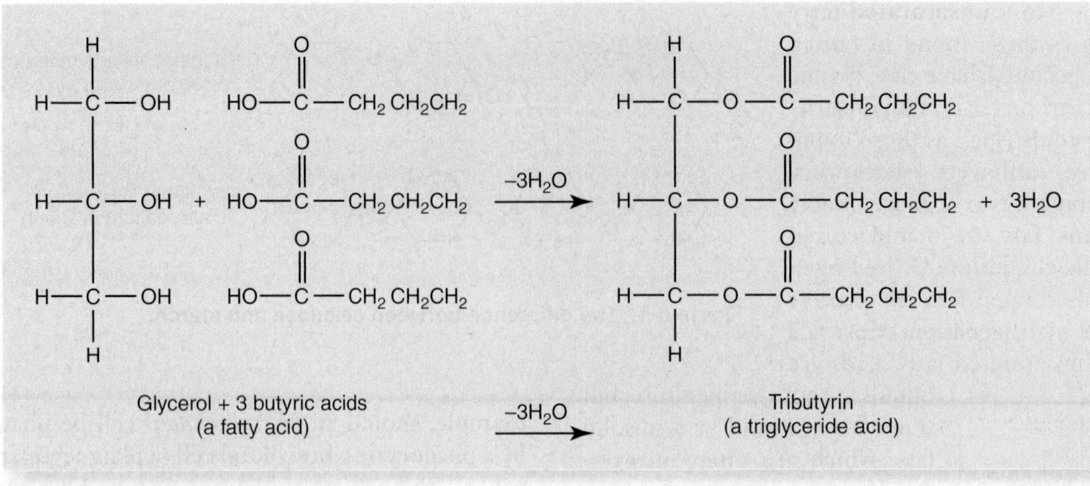

Glycerol + 3 butyric acids
(a fatty acid)

$-3H_2O$ →

Tributyrin
(a triglyceride acid)

Figure 6-9. The synthesis of a fat.

decolorize in the presence of acid, the organism is described as being acid-fast.

Fats and Oils

Fats and **oils** are the most common types of lipids. Fats and oils are also known as **triglycerides**, because they are composed of glycerol (a three-carbon alcohol) and three fatty acids (Fig. 6-9). Fats are triglycerides that are solid at room temperature. Most fats come from animal sources; examples include the fats found in meat, whole milk, butter, and cheese. Most oils are triglycerides that are liquid at room temperature. The most commonly used oils come from plant sources. Olive oil and peanut oil are monounsaturated oils, whereas oils from corn, cottonseed, safflower, and sunflower are polyunsaturated.

Phospholipids

Phospholipids contain glycerol, fatty acids, a phosphate group, and an alcohol. There are two types: *glycerophospholipids* (also called *phosphoglycerides*) and *sphingolipids*. Glycerophospholipids are the most abundant lipids in cell membranes. The basic structure of a cell membrane is a lipid bilayer, consisting of two rows of phospholipids, arranged tail-to-tail (Fig. 6-10). The hydrophobic tails, lacking an affinity for water molecules, point toward each other, enabling them to get as far away from water as possible. The hydrophilic heads, being able to associate with water molecules, project to the inner and outer surfaces of the membrane. Two other types of lipids are also found in eukaryotic cell membranes: steroids (primarily cholesterol, in animal cells) and glycolipids. The cell membrane also contains proteins, which have been described as "icebergs floating in a sea of lipids."

> Cell membranes consist of a lipid bilayer, composed of two rows of phospholipids, arranged tail-to-tail.

In addition to phospholipids, the outer membrane of Gram-negative bacterial cell walls contains lipoproteins and lipopolysaccharide (LPS). As the name implies, LPS consists of a lipid portion and a polysaccharide portion. The lipid portion is called lipid-A or endotoxin. When endotoxin is present in the human bloodstream, it can cause very serious physiologic conditions (e.g., fever and septic shock). The cell walls of Gram-positive bacteria do not contain LPS.

> When present in the human bloodstream, lipids found in the cell walls of Gram-negative bacteria can cause serious physiologic conditions, such as fever and shock.

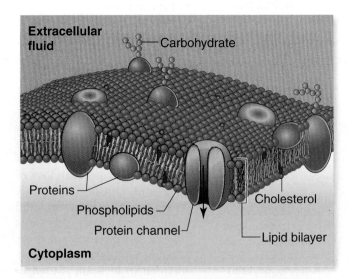

Figure 6-10. The lipid bilayer structure of cell membranes, showing the hydrophilic heads and hydrophobic tails of phospholipid molecules (blue). Cell membranes also contain protein molecules (pink), which have been described as resembling icebergs floating in a sea of lipids. (Redrawn from Cohen BJ. *Memmler's The Human Body in Health and Disease.* 11th ed. Philadelphia, PA: Lippincott Williams & Wilkins; 2009.)

Lecithins and cephalins are glycerophospholipids that are found in brain and nerve tissues as well as in egg yolks, wheat germ, and yeast.

Sphingolipids are phospholipids that contain an 18-carbon alcohol called sphingosine rather than glycerol. Sphingolipids are found in brain and nerve tissues. One of the most abundant sphingolipids is sphingomyelin, which makes up the white matter of the myelin sheath that coats nerve cells.

Glycolipids

Glycolipids are abundant in the brain and in the myelin sheaths of nerves. Some glycolipids contain glycerol plus two fatty acids and a monosaccharide. Cerebrosides and gangliosides are examples of glycolipids; both are found in the human nervous system. A person's blood group (A, B, AB, or O) is determined by the particular glycolipids that are present on the surface of that person's red blood cells (Chapter 16).

Steroids

Steroids are rather complex, four-ringed structures. Steroids include cholesterol, bile salts, fat-soluble vitamins, and steroid hormones. Cholesterol is a component of cell membranes, myelin sheath, and brain and nerve tissue. Bile salts are synthesized in the liver from cholesterol and stored in the gallbladder. The fat-soluble vitamins are vitamins A, D, E, and K.[a] Steroid hormones include male sex hormones (testosterone and androsterone) and female sex hormones (estrogens such as estradiol and progesterone). The adrenal corticosteroids (aldosterone and cortisone) are steroid hormones produced by the adrenal glands, one of which is located at the top of each kidney.

Prostaglandins and Leukotrienes

Prostaglandins and **leukotrienes** are derived from a fatty acid called *arachidonic acid*. Both have a wide variety of effects on body chemistry. They act as mediators of hormones, lower or raise blood pressure, cause inflammation, and induce fever. Leukotrienes are produced in leukocytes (for which they are named), but also occur in other tissues. Leukotrienes can produce long-lasting muscle contractions, especially in the lungs, where they cause asthma-like attacks.

> The complete collection of proteins within a given cell is known as that cell's proteome. Studies performed to explore the structure and activities of proteins are called **proteomics**.

Proteins

Proteins are among the most essential chemicals in all living cells, referred to by some scientists as "the substance of life." The complete collection of proteins within a given cell is known as that cell's **proteome**. The study of the structure and activities of proteins is called **proteomics**. Some proteins are the structural components of membranes, cells, and tissues, whereas others are enzymes and hormones that chemically control the metabolic balance within both the cell and the entire organism. All proteins are polymers of amino acids; however, they vary widely in the number of amino acids present and in the sequence of amino acids as well as their size, configuration, and functions. Proteins contain carbon, hydrogen, oxygen, nitrogen, and sometimes sulfur.

> Proteins contain carbon, hydrogen, oxygen, nitrogen, and sometimes sulfur.

Amino Acid Structure

A total of 23 different *amino acids* have been found in proteins—20 primary or naturally occurring amino acids plus 3 secondary amino acids (derived from primary amino acids). Each amino acid is composed of carbon, hydrogen, oxygen, and nitrogen; three of the amino acids also have sulfur atoms in the molecule. Humans can synthesize certain amino acids, but not others. Those that cannot be synthesized (called **essential amino acids**) must be ingested as part of our diets. The term *essential amino acids* is somewhat misleading, however, in view of the fact that *all* of the amino acids are necessary for protein synthesis. Because we cannot manufacture the essential amino acids, it is *essential* that they be included in our diets.

> Proteins are polymers that are composed of amino acids (i.e., amino acids are the building blocks of proteins).

The general formula for amino acids is shown in Figure 6-11. In this figure, the "R" group represents any of the 23 groups that may be substituted into that position to build the various amino acids. For instance, "H" in place of the "R" represents the amino acid glycine, and "CH$_3$" in that position results in the structural formula for the amino acid alanine.

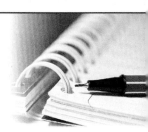

STUDY AID

Proteins

Proteins can be thought of as "strings of beads." The beads are amino acids. Proteins may contain as few as two amino acids to as many as 5,000 or more. The sequence of amino acids is referred to as the primary structure of a protein.

---

[a]Water-soluble vitamins (the eight B vitamins and vitamin C) dissolve easily in water, and are readily excreted from the body. Fat-soluble vitamins (A, D, E, K) are absorbed through the intestinal tract with the help of lipids, and are more likely to accumulate in the body than are water-soluble vitamins.

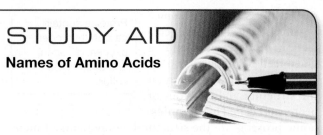

STUDY AID

Names of Amino Acids

Alanine	Glutamic acid	Isoleucine	Serine
(1°)	(1°)	(1°, E)	(1°)
Arginine	Glutamine	Leucine	Threonine
(1°, E*)	(1°)	(1°, E)	(1°, E)
Asparagine	Glycine	Lysine	Tryptophan
(1°)	(1°)	(1°, E)	(1°, E)
Aspartic	Histidine	Methionine	Tyrosine acid
(1°)	(1°, E*)	(1°, E)	(1°)
Cysteine	Hydroxylysine	Phenylalanine	Valine
(1°)	(2°)	(1°, E)	(1°, E)
Cystine	Hydroxyproline	Proline	
(2°)	(2°)	(1°)	

Key: 1°, a primary amino acid; 2°, a secondary amino acid; E, an essential amino acid; E*, additional essential amino acid in infants.

The thousands of different proteins in the human body are composed of a great variety of amino acids in various quantities and arrangements. The number of proteins that can be synthesized is virtually unlimited. Proteins are not limited by the number of different amino acids, just as the number of words in a written language is not limited by the number of letters in the alphabet. The actual number of proteins produced by an organism and the amino acid sequence of those proteins are determined by the particular genes present on the organism's chromosome(s).

Protein Structure

When water is removed, by dehydration synthesis, amino acids become linked together by a covalent bond, referred to as a **peptide bond** (as shown in Fig. 6-12). A **dipeptide** is formed by bonding two amino acids, whereas the bonding of three amino acids forms a **tripeptide**. A chain (polymer) consisting of more than three amino acids is referred to as a **polypeptide**. Polypeptides are said to have *primary protein structure*—a linear sequence of amino acids in a chain (Fig. 6-13).

> The monosaccharides in carbohydrates are joined together by glycosidic bonds. The amino acids in proteins are joined together by peptide bonds. Glycosidic bonds and peptide bonds are examples of covalent bonds.

Most polypeptide chains naturally twist into helices or sheets as a result of the charged side chains protruding from the carbon–nitrogen backbone of the molecule. This helical or sheetlike configuration is referred to as *secondary protein structure* and is found in fibrous proteins. Fibrous proteins are long, threadlike molecules that are insoluble in water. They make up keratin (found in hair, nails, wool, horns, feathers), collagen (in tendons), myosin (in muscles), and the microtubules and microfilaments of cells.

Because a long coil can become entwined by folding back on itself, a polypeptide helix may become globular (Fig. 6-13). In some areas, the helix is retained, but other areas curve randomly. This globular, *tertiary protein structure* is stabilized by not only hydrogen bonding but also disulfide bond cross-links between two sulfur groups (S–S). This three-dimensional configuration is characteristic of enzymes, which work by fitting on and into specific molecules (see the next section). Other examples of globular proteins include many hormones (e.g., insulin), albumin in eggs, and hemoglobin

Figure 6-11. The basic structure of an amino acid.

Figure 6-12. The formation of a dipeptide. R indicates any amino acid side chain.

Amino acid₁ + Amino acid₂ → Dipeptide

Peptide bond

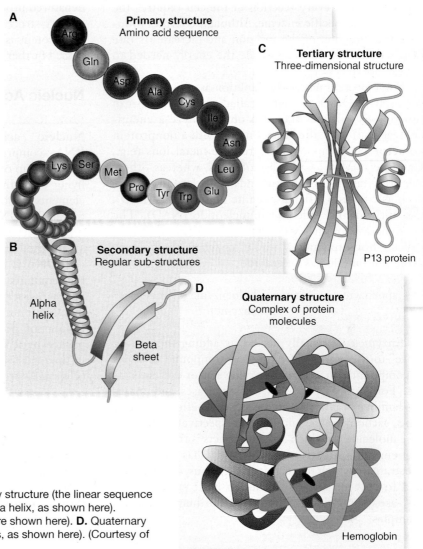

Figure 6-13. ▶ **Protein structure. A.** Primary structure (the linear sequence of amino acids). **B.** Secondary structure (e.g., a helix, as shown here). **C.** Tertiary structure (e.g., the globular structure shown here). **D.** Quaternary structure (e.g., four globular protein molecules, as shown here). (Courtesy of LadyofHats and Wikipedia.)

and fibrinogen in blood. Globular proteins are soluble in water.

When two or more polypeptide chains are bonded together by hydrogen and disulfide bonds, the resulting three-dimensional structure is referred to as *quaternary protein structure* (Fig. 6-13). For instance, hemoglobin consists of four globular myoglobins. The size, shape, and configuration of a protein are specific for the function it must perform. If the amino acid sequence and, thus, the configuration of hemoglobin in red blood cells are not perfect, the red blood cells may become distorted and assume a sickle shape (as in sickle cell anemia). In this state, they are unable to carry the oxygen that is necessary for cellular metabolism. Myoglobin, the oxygen-binding protein found in skeletal muscles, was the first protein to have its primary, secondary, and tertiary structure defined by scientists.

Should the secondary, tertiary, or quarternary structure of a protein be disrupted—for example, by heat, ultraviolet light, strong acids or alkalis, or enzymatic action—the protein molecule may lose its structural and functional characteristics. This process is known as denaturation, and the protein is said to be denatured.

Enzymes

Enzymes are protein molecules[b] produced by living cells as "instructed" by genes on the chromosomes. Enzymes are referred to as **biological catalysts**—biologic molecules that **catalyze** metabolic reactions. A **catalyst** is defined as an agent that speeds up a chemical reaction without being consumed in the process. In some cases, a particular metabolic reaction will not occur at all in the absence of an enzyme

> Enzymes are proteins that function as biological catalysts, meaning that they catalyze (speed up) metabolic reactions.

[b]Certain RNA molecules, called ribozymes, have been shown to have enzymatic activity. However, because most enzymes are proteins, enzymes are discussed in this book as if all of them were proteins.

catalyst. Almost every reaction in the cell requires the presence of a specific enzyme. Although enzymes influence the direction of the reaction and increase its rate of reaction, they do not provide the energy needed to activate the reaction.

Some protein molecules function as enzymes all by themselves. Other proteins (called **apoenzymes**) can function as enzymes (i.e., can only catalyze a chemical reaction) only after they link up with a nonprotein **cofactor**. Some apoenzymes require metal ions (e.g., Ca^{2+}, Fe^{2+}, Mg^{2+}, Cu^{2+}) as cofactors, whereas others require vitamin-type compounds (called **coenzymes**), such as vitamin C, flavin-adenine dinucleotide (FAD), and nicotinamide-adenine dinucleotide (NAD). The combination of the apoenzyme plus the cofactor is called a **holoenzyme** (a "whole" enzyme); the holoenzyme can function as an enzyme.

apoenzyme + cofactor = holoenzyme (a functional enzyme)

Enzymes are usually named by adding the ending "-ase" to the word, indicating the compound or types of compounds on which an enzyme acts or exerts its effect. For example, proteases, carbohydrases, and lipases are families of enzymes that exert their effects on proteins, carbohydrates, and lipids, respectively. The specific molecule on which an enzyme acts is referred to as that enzyme's **substrate**. Each enzyme has a particular substrate on which it exerts its effect; thus, enzymes are said to be very specific. Although most enzymes end in "-ase," some do not; lysozyme and hemolysins are examples.

Some toxins and other poisonous substances cause damage to the human body by interfering with the action of certain necessary enzymes. For example, cyanide poison binds to the iron and copper ions in the cytochrome systems of the mitochondria of eukaryotic cells. As a result, the cells cannot use oxygen to synthesize ATP, which is essential for energy production, and they soon die.

Proteins, including enzymes, may be denatured (structurally altered) by heat or certain chemicals. In a denatured protein, the bonds that hold the molecule in a tertiary structure are broken. With these bonds broken, the protein is no longer functional. Enzymes are discussed further in Chapter 7.

Nucleic Acids

Function

Nucleic acids—DNA and RNA—comprise the fourth major group of biomolecules in living cells. In addition to the elements carbon (C), hydrogen (H), oxygen (O), and nitrogen (N), DNA and RNA also contain phosphorus (P).

> Nucleic acids contain C, H, O, N, and P.

Nucleic acids play extremely important roles in a cell; they are critical to the proper functioning of a cell. DNA is the "hereditary molecule"—the molecule that contains the genes and genetic code. DNA makes up the major portion of chromosomes. The information in DNA must flow to the rest of the cell for the cell to function properly; this flow of information is accomplished by RNA molecules. RNA molecules participate in the conversion of the genetic code into proteins and other gene products.

Structure

The building blocks of nucleic acid polymers are called **nucleotides**. These are more complex monomers (single molecular units that can be repeated to form a polymer) than amino acids, which are the building blocks of proteins. Nucleotides consist of three subunits: a nitrogen-containing (nitrogenous) base, a five-carbon sugar (pentose), and a phosphate group, joined together, as shown in Figure 6-14.

> The building blocks of nucleic acids are called nucleotides, each of which contains three components: a nitrogenous base, a pentose, and a phosphate group.

The building blocks of DNA are called **DNA nucleotides**; they contain a nitrogenous base, deoxyribose (a pentose), and a phosphate group. The building blocks of RNA are called **RNA nucleotides**; they contain a nitrogenous base, ribose (a pentose), and a phosphate group.

> The building blocks of DNA are called DNA nucleotides, whereas the building blocks of RNA are called RNA nucleotides.

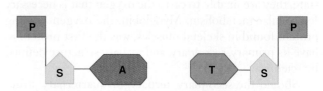

Figure 6-14. Two nucleotides, each consisting of a nitrogenous base (A or T), a five-carbon sugar (S), and a phosphate group (P).

As previously stated, there are two kinds of nucleic acids in cells: DNA and RNA. DNA contains deoxyribose as its pentose, whereas RNA contains ribose as its pentose. There are three types of RNA, which are named for the function they serve: *messenger RNA* (mRNA), *ribosomal RNA* (rRNA), and *transfer RNA* (tRNA).

> The three types of RNA in a cell are mRNA, rRNA, and tRNA.

The five nitrogenous bases in nucleic acids are adenine (A), guanine (G), thymine (T), cytosine (C), and uracil (U). Thymine is found in DNA, but not in RNA. Uracil is found in RNA, but not in DNA. The other three bases (A, G, C) are present in both DNA and RNA. Both A and G are **purines** (double-ring structures), whereas T, C, and U are pyrimidines (single-ring structures; Fig. 6-15).

> The nitrogenous bases adenine, guanine, and cytosine are found in both DNA and RNA. However, thymine is found only in DNA, and uracil is found only in RNA.

The nucleotides join together (via covalent bonds) between their sugar and phosphate groups to form very long polymers—100,000 or more monomers long—as shown in Figure 6-16.

DNA Structure

For a double-stranded DNA molecule to form, the nitrogenous bases on the two separate strands must bond together.

STUDY AID

Nucleotides

Three Parts to Every Nucleotide	Four DNA Nucleotides (Deoxyribonucleotides)	Four RNA Nucleotides (Ribonucleotides)
1. Nitrogenous base	Adenine (a purine)	Adenine (a purine)
	Guanine (a purine)	Guanine (a purine)
	Cytosine (a pyrimidine)	Cytosine (a pyrimidine)
	Thymine (a pyrimidine)	Uracil (a pyrimidine)
2. Pentose	Deoxyribose	Ribose
3. Phosphate group	Phosphate group	Phosphate group

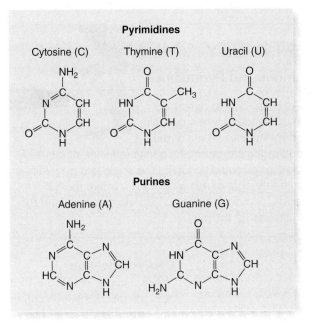

Figure 6-15. The pyrimidines and purines found in DNA and RNA. Note that pyrimidines are single-ring structures, whereas purines are double-ring structures.

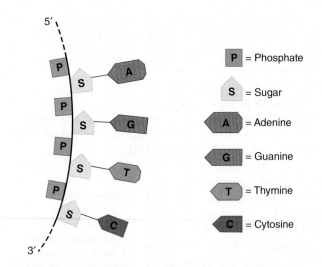

Figure 6-16. One small section of a nucleic acid polymer.

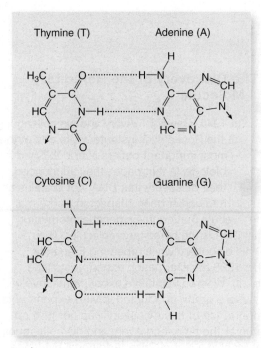

Figure 6-17. Base pairs that occur in double-stranded DNA molecules. Note that A and T are connected by two hydrogen bonds, whereas G and C are connected by three hydrogen bonds. The arrows represent the points at which the bases are bonded to deoxyribose molecules.

> Within a double-stranded DNA molecule, A in one strand always bonds with T in the complementary strand, and G in one strand always bonds with C in the complementary strand. A–T and G–C are known as base pairs.

Because of the size and bonding attraction between the two strands, A (a purine) always bonds with T (a pyrimidine) via two hydrogen bonds, and G (a purine) always bonds with C (a pyrimidine) via three hydrogen bonds (Fig. 6-17). (A–T and G–C are known as "base pairs.") The bonding forces of the double-stranded polymer cause it to assume the shape of a double α-helix, which is similar to a right-handed spiral staircase (Fig. 6-18).

occurs by separation of the DNA strands and the building of complementary strands by the addition of the correct DNA nucleotides, as illustrated in Figure 6-19. The point on the molecule where DNA replication starts is called the *replication fork*. The most important enzyme required for DNA replication is **DNA polymerase** (also known as DNA-dependent DNA polymerase). Other enzymes are also required, including DNA helicase and DNA topoisomerase (which initiate the separation of the two strands of the DNA molecule), primase (which synthesizes a short RNA primer), and DNA ligase (which connects fragments of newly synthesized DNA).

STUDY AID

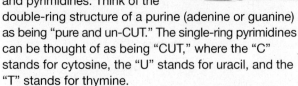

Purines and Pyrimidines

Here is one way to remember the difference between purines and pyrimidines. Think of the double-ring structure of a purine (adenine or guanine) as being "pure and un-CUT." The single-ring pyrimidines can be thought of as being "CUT," where the "C" stands for cytosine, the "U" stands for uracil, and the "T" stands for thymine.

DNA Replication

When a cell is preparing to divide, all the DNA molecules in the chromosomes of that cell must duplicate, thereby ensuring that the same genetic information is passed on to both daughter cells. This process is called **DNA replication**. It

> The most important enzyme taking part in DNA replication is DNA polymerase (also known as DNA-dependent DNA polymerase).

HISTORICAL NOTE

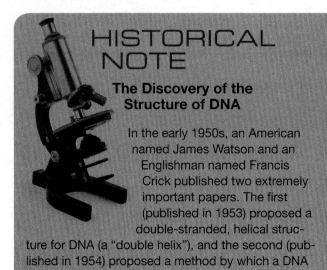

The Discovery of the Structure of DNA

In the early 1950s, an American named James Watson and an Englishman named Francis Crick published two extremely important papers. The first (published in 1953) proposed a double-stranded, helical structure for DNA (a "double helix"), and the second (published in 1954) proposed a method by which a DNA molecule could copy (replicate) itself exactly, so that identical genetic information could be passed on to each daughter cell. The idea for the double-helical structure was based on an x-ray diffraction photograph of crystallized DNA that Watson had seen in the London laboratory of Maurice Wilkins. The now famous photograph had been produced by Rosalind Franklin, an x-ray crystallographer. Watson, Crick, and Wilkins received a Nobel Prize in Chemistry in 1962 for their contributions to our understanding of DNA. Franklin did not share the prize because she had died before 1962; the Nobel Prize is not awarded posthumously.

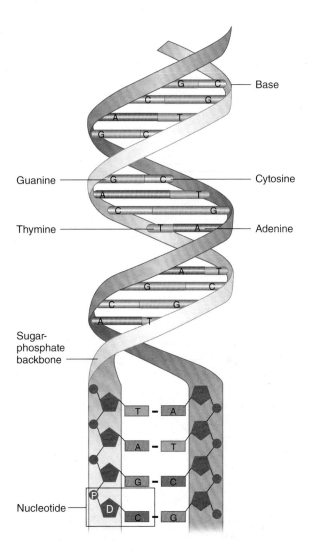

Figure 6-18. Double-stranded DNA molecule, also referred to as a double helix.

STUDY AID

Major Differences Between DNA and RNA

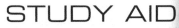

DNA is double-stranded, whereas RNA is single-stranded.
DNA contains deoxyribose, whereas RNA contains ribose.
DNA contains thymine, whereas RNA contains uracil.

STUDY AID

DNA Replication

Francis Crick provided this method of visualizing what happens during DNA replication. First, remember that DNA is a double-stranded molecule. Think of it as a hand within a glove. When the hand is removed from the glove, a new glove is formed around the hand. Simultaneously, a new hand is formed within the glove. What you end up with are two gloved hands, each of which is identical to the original gloved hand.

The duplicated DNA of the chromosomes can then be separated during cell division, so that each daughter cell contains the same number of chromosomes, the same genes, and the same amount of DNA as in the parent cell (except during meiosis, the reduction division by which ova and sperm cells—haploid cells—are produced in eukaryotes). There are subtle differences between DNA replication in prokaryotes and eukaryotes; these differences are beyond the scope of this book.

Gene Expression

As you learned in Chapter 3, a gene is a particular segment of a DNA molecule or chromosome. A gene contains the instructions (the "recipe" or "blueprint") that will enable a cell to make what is known as a *gene product* (in some cases, more than one gene product). The **genetic code** contains four "letters" (the letters that stand for the four nitrogenous bases found in DNA): "A" for adenine, "G" for guanine, "C" for cytosine, and "T" for thymine. It is the sequence of these four bases that spell out the instructions for a particular gene product.

> The genetic code consists of four letters: A, T, G, and C.

Although most genes code for proteins (meaning that each gene contains the instructions for the production of a particular protein), some code for rRNA and tRNA molecules. However, because the vast majority of gene

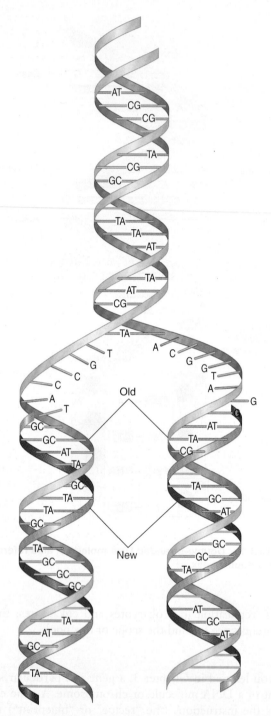

Figure 6-19. DNA replication. See text for details. (An animated version of this figure can be found on thePoint.)

products are proteins, gene products are discussed in this chapter as if all of them are proteins.

The Central Dogma. It was Francis Crick who, in 1957, proposed what is referred to as the **Central Dogma** to explain the flow of genetic information within a cell:

$$DNA \rightarrow mRNA \rightarrow protein$$

The Central Dogma (also known as the "one gene–one protein hypothesis") states the following:

1. The genetic information contained in one gene of a DNA molecule is used to make one molecule of mRNA by a process known as transcription.
2. The genetic information in that mRNA molecule is then used to make one protein by a process known as translation.[c]

STUDY AID

The Central Dogma

The term "dogma" usually refers to a basic or fundamental doctrinal point in religion or philosophy. Francis Crick's use of the term "Central Dogma" refers to the most fundamental process of molecular biology—the flow of genetic information within a cell. Although originally referred to as the one gene–one protein hypothesis, it is now known that a particular gene may code for one or more proteins.

When the information in a gene has been used by the cell to make a gene product, the gene that codes for that particular gene product is said to have been *expressed*. All the genes on the chromosome are not being expressed at any one time. That would be a terrible waste of energy! For example, it would not be logical for a cell to produce a particular enzyme if that enzyme was not actually needed. Genes that are expressed at all times are called **constitutive genes**. Those that are expressed only when the gene products are needed are called **inducible genes**.

> Genes that are expressed at all times are called constitutive genes, whereas those that are expressed only when the gene products are needed are called inducible genes.

Transcription. When a cell is stimulated (by need) to produce a particular protein, the DNA of the appropriate gene is activated to unwind temporarily from its helical configuration. This unwinding exposes the bases, which then attract the bases of free RNA nucleotides, and an mRNA molecule begins to be assembled alongside one of the strands of the unwound DNA. Thus, one of the DNA strands has served as a template, or pattern (referred to as the *DNA template*), and has coded for a complementary

---

[c]At the time the Central Dogma was proposed, it was thought that a particular gene codes for only one protein. It is now known that a gene may code for more than one protein, depending on several factors (including the manner in which the gene is transcribed and whether or not the final gene product is cut into several proteins).

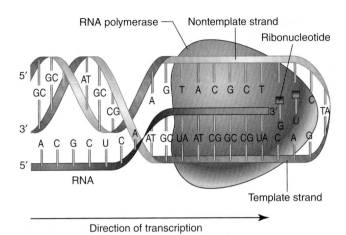

Figure 6-20. **Transcription.**

> The process by which the information in a single gene is used to make an mRNA molecule is known as transcription.

mirror image of its structure in the mRNA molecule. On the growing mRNA molecule, an A will be introduced opposite a T on the DNA molecule, a G opposite a C, a C opposite a G, and a U opposite an A (see the following Study Aid). Remember that there is no T in RNA molecules. This process is called **transcription** because the genetic code from the DNA molecule is transcribed to produce an mRNA molecule (Fig. 6-20). After the mRNA has been synthesized over the length of the gene, it is released from the DNA strand to carry the message to the cytoplasm and direct the synthesis of a particular protein.

let the RNA polymerase know where to start and stop the transcription process (i.e., the traffic signals are the starting and stopping points for each gene). Each mRNA molecule contains the same genetic information that was contained in the gene on the DNA template. Note, however, that the genetic code in the mRNA molecule is made up of RNA nucleotides, whereas the genetic code in the DNA template is made up of DNA nucleotides. The information in the mRNA molecule will then be used to synthesize one or more proteins.

> The primary enzyme involved in transcription is called RNA polymerase (also known as DNA-dependent RNA polymerase).

In eukaryotes, transcription occurs within the nucleus. The newly formed mRNA molecules then travel through the pores of the nuclear membrane, out into the cytoplasm, where they take up positions on the protein "assembly line." Ribosomes, which are composed of proteins and rRNA, attract the mRNA molecules. In eukaryotic cells, ribosomes are usually attached to endoplasmic reticulum membranes, creating what is called rough endoplasmic reticulum (RER).

In prokaryotes, transcription occurs in the cytoplasm. Ribosomes attach to the mRNA molecules as they are being transcribed at the DNA; thus, transcription and translation (protein synthesis) may occur simultaneously.

Translation (Protein Synthesis). The base sequence of the mRNA molecule is read or interpreted in groups of three bases, called *codons*. The sequence of a codon's three bases is the code that determines which amino acid is inserted in that position in the protein being synthesized. Also located on the mRNA molecule are various codons that act as start and stop signals.

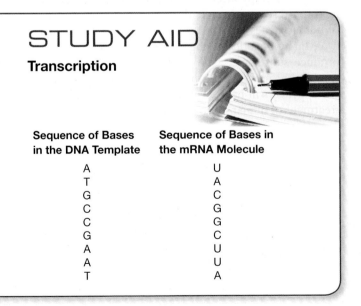

STUDY AID
Transcription

Sequence of Bases in the DNA Template	Sequence of Bases in the mRNA Molecule
A	U
T	A
G	C
C	G
C	G
G	C
A	U
A	U
T	A

The primary enzyme involved in transcription is called **RNA polymerase** (also known as DNA-dependent RNA polymerase). Located along the DNA template are various nucleotide sequences known as "traffic signals" that

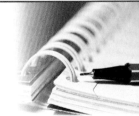

STUDY AID
Where Various Processes Occur

	Prokaryotic Cells	Eukaryotic Cells
DNA replication	In the cytoplasm	In the nucleus
Transcription	In the cytoplasm	In the nucleus
Translation	In the cytoplasm	In the cytoplasm

Before they can be used to build a protein molecule, amino acids must first be "activated." Each amino acid is activated by attaching to an appropriate tRNA molecule, which then carries (transfers) the amino acid from the cytoplasmic matrix to the site of protein assembly. The enzyme responsible for attaching amino acids to their corresponding tRNA molecules is amino acyl-tRNA synthetase.

The three-base sequence of the codon determines which tRNA brings its specific amino acid to the ribosome, because the tRNA molecule contains an **antico-don**: a three-base sequence that is complementary to, or attracted to, the codon of the mRNA. For example, the tRNA with the anticodon base sequence UUU carries the amino acid lysine to the mRNA codon AAA. Similarly, the mRNA codon CCG codes for the tRNA anticodon GGC, which carries the amino acid proline. The following chart illustrates the sequence of three bases (GGC) in the DNA template that codes for a particular codon (CCG) in mRNA, which, in turn, attracts a particular anticodon (GGC) on the tRNA carrying a specific amino acid (proline).

> Codons are located on mRNA molecules, whereas anticodons are located on tRNA molecules.

DNA Template	mRNA (Codon)	tRNA (Anticodon)	Amino Acid
G	C	G	
G	C	G	Proline
C	G	C	

The process of translating the message carried by the mRNA, whereby particular tRNAs bring amino acids to be bound together in the proper sequence to make a specific protein, is called **translation** (summarized in Fig. 6-21). In this context, translation and protein synthesis are synonyms. It should be noted that a eukaryotic cell is constantly producing mRNAs in its nucleus, which direct the synthesis of all the proteins, including metabolic enzymes necessary for the normal functions of that specific type of cell. Also, mRNA and tRNA are short-lived nucleic acids that may be reused many times and then destroyed and resynthesized. The rRNA molecules are made in the dense portion of the nucleus called the nucleolus. Ribosomes last longer in the cell than do mRNA molecules.

> The process by which the genetic information within an mRNA molecule is used to make a specific protein is called translation. Translation occurs at a ribosome.

As tRNA molecules attach to mRNA while it is sliding over the ribosome, they bring the correct activated amino acids into contact with each other so that peptide bonds are formed and a polypeptide is synthesized. Recent evidence suggests a role for rRNA (a structural component of the ribosome) in the formation of the peptide bonds. As the polypeptide grows and becomes a protein, it folds into the unique shape determined by the amino acid sequence. This characteristic shape allows the protein to perform its specific function. If one of the bases of a DNA gene is incorrect or out of sequence (known as a *mutation*), the amino acid sequence of the gene product will be incorrect and the altered protein configuration may not allow the protein to function properly. For example, some diabetics may not produce a functional insulin molecule because a mutation in one of their chromosomes caused a rearrangement of the bases in the gene that codes for insulin. Such errors are the basis for most genetic and inherited diseases, such as phenylketonuria (PKU), sickle cell anemia, cerebral palsy, cystic fibrosis, cleft lip, clubfoot, extra fingers, albinism, and many other birth defects. Likewise, nonpathogenic microbes may mutate to become pathogens, and pathogens may lose the ability to cause disease by mutation. Mutations are discussed further in Chapter 7.

The relatively new sciences of genetic engineering and gene therapy attempt to repair the genetic damage in some diseases. As yet, the morality of manipulation of human genes has not been resolved by society. However, many genetically engineered microbes are able to produce substances, such as human insulin, interferon, growth hormones, new pharmaceutical agents, and vaccines, which will have a substantial effect on the medical treatment of humans (see Chapter 7).

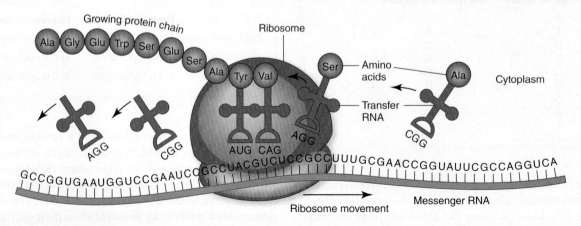

Figure 6-21. Translation (protein synthesis). See text for details. (An animated version of this figure can be found on thePoint.)

ON thePoint

- Terms Introduced in This Chapter
- Review of Key Points
- Increase Your Knowledge
- Critical Thinking
- Additional Self-Assessment Exercises

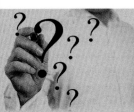

Self-Assessment Exercises

After studying this chapter, answer the following multiple-choice questions.

1. Which one of the following are the building blocks of proteins?
   a. amino acids
   b. monosaccharides
   c. nucleotides
   d. peptides

2. Glucose, sucrose, and cellulose are examples of:
   a. carbohydrates
   b. disaccharides
   c. monosaccharides
   d. polysaccharides

3. Which of the following nitrogenous bases is *not* found in an RNA molecule?
   a. adenine
   b. guanine
   c. thymine
   d. uracil

4. Which of the following are purines?
   a. adenine and guanine
   b. adenine and thymine
   c. guanine and uracil
   d. guanine and cytosine

5. Which one of the following is *not* found at the site of protein synthesis?
   a. DNA
   b. mRNA
   c. rRNA
   d. tRNA

6. Which of the following statements about DNA is (are) true?
   a. DNA contains thymine but not uracil
   b. DNA molecules contain deoxyribose
   c. In a double-stranded DNA molecule, adenine on one strand will be connected to thymine on the complementary strand by two hydrogen bonds
   d. All of the above statements are true

7. The amino acids in a polypeptide chain are connected by:
   a. covalent bonds
   b. glycosidic bonds
   c. peptide bonds
   d. both a and c

8. Which of the following statements about nucleotides is (are) true?
   a. A nucleotide contains a nitrogenous base
   b. A nucleotide contains a pentose
   c. A nucleotide contains a phosphate group
   d. All of the above statements are true

9. A heptose contains how many carbon atoms?
   a. 4
   b. 5
   c. 6
   d. 7

10. Virtually all enzymes are:
    a. carbohydrates
    b. nucleic acids
    c. proteins
    d. substrates

7

Microbial Physiology and Genetics

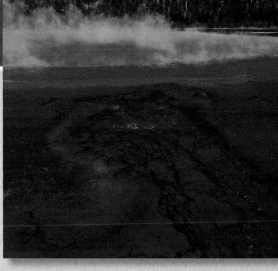

Colorful, thermophilic, photosynthetic cyanobacteria living in a thermal feature at Yellowstone National Park, Wyoming.

CHAPTER OUTLINE

LEARNING OBJECTIVES

After studying this chapter, you should be able to:

- Define phototroph, chemotroph, autotroph, heterotroph, photoautotroph, chemoheterotroph, endoenzyme, exoenzyme, plasmid, R-factor, "superbug," mutation, mutant, and mutagen
- Discuss the relationships among apoenzymes, coenzymes, and holoenzymes
- Differentiate between catabolism and anabolism
- Explain the role of adenosine triphosphate (ATP) molecules in metabolism
- Briefly describe each of the following: biochemical pathway, aerobic respiration, glycolysis, the Krebs cycle, the electron transport chain, oxidation–reduction reactions, and photosynthesis
- Explain the differences between beneficial, harmful, and silent mutations
- Briefly describe each of the following ways in which bacteria acquire genetic information: lysogenic conversion, transduction, transformation, and conjugation

---

Microbial Physiology

Introduction

Physiology is the study of the vital life processes of organisms, especially how these processes normally function in living organisms. *Microbial physiology* concerns the vital life processes of microorganisms. Microorganisms, especially bacteria, are ideally suited for use in studies of the basic metabolic reactions that occur within cells. Bacteria are inexpensive to maintain in the laboratory, take up little space, and reproduce quickly. Their morphology, nutritional needs, and metabolic reactions are easily observable. Of special importance is the fact that species of bacteria can be found that represent each of the nutritional types of organisms on Earth. Scientists can learn a great deal about cells—including human cells—by studying the nutritional needs of bacteria; their metabolic pathways; and why they live, grow, multiply, or die under certain conditions.

> Microbial physiology is the study of the life processes of microorganisms.

Each tiny single-celled bacterium strives to produce more cells like itself, and, as long as water and an adequate nutrient supply are available, it often does so at an alarming rate. Under favorable conditions, in 24 hours, the offspring (progeny) of a single *Escherichia coli* cell would outnumber the entire human population on Earth! Because some bacteria, fungi, and viruses produce generation after generation so rapidly, they have been used extensively in genetic studies. In fact, most of today's genetic knowledge was and still is being obtained by studying these microbes.

Microbial Nutritional Requirements

Studies of bacterial nutrition and other aspects of microbial physiology enable scientists to understand the vital chemical processes that occur within every living cell, including those of the human body. All living protoplasm contains six major chemical elements: carbon, hydrogen, oxygen, nitrogen, phosphorus, and sulfur. Other elements, usually required in lesser amounts, include sodium, potassium, chlorine, magnesium, calcium, iron, iodine, and some trace elements. Combinations of all these elements make up the vital macromolecules of life, including carbohydrates, lipids, proteins, and nucleic acids.

To build necessary cellular materials, every organism requires a source (or sources) of energy, a source (or sources) of carbon, and additional nutrients. Those materials that organisms are unable to synthesize, but are required for the building of macromolecules and sustaining life, are termed *essential nutrients*. Essential nutrients (e.g., essential amino acids and essential fatty acids) must be continually supplied to an organism for it to survive. Essential nutrients vary from species to species.

> All organisms require a source of energy, a source of carbon, and additional nutrients.

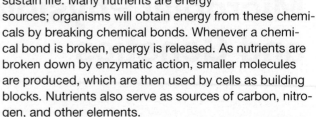

Categorizing Microorganisms According to Their Energy and Carbon Sources

Since the beginning of life on Earth, microorganisms have been evolving, some in different directions than others. Today, there are microbes representing each of the four major nutritional categories (photoautotrophs, photoheterotrophs, chemoautotrophs, and chemoheterotrophs; these terms are defined later in this chapter). Various terms are used to indicate an organism's energy source and carbon source. As you will see, these terms can be used in combination (Table 7-1).

Terms Relating to an Organism's Energy Source

The terms phototroph and chemotroph pertain to what an organism uses as an energy source. **Phototrophs** use light as an energy source. The process by which organisms convert light energy into chemical energy is called *photosynthesis*. **Chemotrophs** use either inorganic or organic chemicals as an energy source. Chemotrophs can be subdivided into two categories: chemolithotrophs and chemoorganotrophs. **Chemolithotrophs** (or simply lithotrophs) are organisms that use inorganic chemicals as an energy source. **Chemoorganotrophs** (or simply organotrophs) are organisms that use organic chemicals as an energy source.

> Phototrophs use light as an energy source, whereas chemotrophs use chemicals as a source of energy.

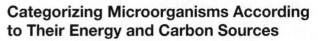

Terms Relating to an Organism's Carbon Source

The terms autotroph and heterotroph pertain to what an organism uses as a carbon source. **Autotrophs** use carbon dioxide (CO_2) as their sole source of carbon. Photosynthetic organisms such as plants, algae, and cyanobacteria are examples of autotrophs. **Heterotrophs** are organisms

Table 7-1	Terms Relating to Energy and Carbon Sources	
Terms Relating to Energy Source	**Terms Relating to Carbon Source**	
	Autotrophs (organisms that use CO_2 as a carbon source)	**Heterotrophs** (organisms that use organic compounds other than CO_2 as a carbon source)
Phototrophs (organisms that use light as an energy source)	**Photoautotrophs** (e.g., algae, plants, some photosynthetic bacteria including cyanobacteria)	**Photoheterotrophs** (e.g., some photosynthetic bacteria)
Chemotrophs[a] (organisms that use chemicals as an energy source)	**Chemoautotrophs** (e.g., some bacteria)	**Chemoheterotrophs** (e.g., protozoa, fungi, animals, most bacteria)

[a]Chemotrophs can be divided into two categories: (1) chemolithotrophs (or simply lithotrophs) are organisms that use inorganic chemicals as an energy source and (2) chemoorganotrophs (or simply organotrophs) are organisms that use organic chemicals as an energy source.

> Autotrophs use carbon dioxide as their sole source of carbon, whereas heterotrophs use other carbon-containing compounds as their carbon source.

that use organic compounds other than CO_2 as their carbon source. (Recall that all organic compounds contain carbon.) Humans, animals, fungi, and protozoa are examples of heterotrophs. Both saprophytic fungi, which live on dead and decaying organic matter, and parasitic fungi are heterotrophs. Most bacteria are also heterotrophs.

The terms relating to energy source can be combined with the terms relating to carbon source, yielding terms that indicate *both* an organism's energy source and carbon source. For example, **photoautotrophs** are organisms (such as plants, algae, cyanobacteria, and purple and green sulfur bacteria) that use light as an energy source and CO_2 as a carbon source. **Photoheterotrophs**, such as purple nonsulfur and green nonsulfur bacteria, use light as an energy source and organic compounds other than CO_2 as a carbon source. **Chemoautotrophs** (such as nitrifying, hydrogen, iron, and sulfur bacteria) use chemicals as an energy source and CO_2 as a carbon source. **Chemoheterotrophs** use chemicals as an energy source and organic compounds other than CO_2 as a carbon source. All animals, all protozoa, all fungi, and most bacteria are chemoheterotrophs. All medically important bacteria are chemoheterotrophs.

Ecology is the study of the interactions between organisms and the world around them. The term *ecosystem* refers to the interactions between living organisms and their nonliving environment. Interrelationships among the different nutritional types are of prime importance in the functioning of the ecosystem. Phototrophs (like algae and plants) are the producers of food and oxygen for chemoheterotrophs (such as animals). Dead plants and animals would clutter the earth if chemoheterotrophic, saprophytic decomposers (certain fungi and bacteria) did not break down the dead organic matter into

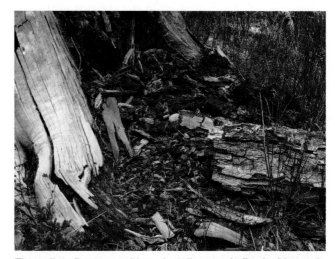

Figure 7-1. Decomposition of a fallen tree in Rocky Mountain National Park, CO. (Courtesy of Biomed Ed, Round Rock, TX.)

small inorganic and organic compounds (carbon dioxide, nitrates, phosphates) in soil, water, and air—compounds that are then used and recycled by chemotrophs (Fig. 7-1). Photoautotrophs contribute energy to the ecosystem by trapping energy from the sun and using it to build organic compounds (carbohydrates, lipids, proteins, and nucleic acids) from inorganic materials in the soil, water, and air. In oxygenic photosynthesis (described later), oxygen is released for use by aerobic organisms, such as animals and humans.

Metabolic Enzymes

The term *metabolism* refers to all the chemical reactions that occur within any cell. These chemical reactions are referred to as *metabolic reactions*. The metabolic processes that occur in microbes are similar to those that occur in cells of the human body. Metabolic reactions are enhanced and regulated by enzymes, known as *metabolic enzymes*. A cell can only perform a certain metabolic reaction if it possesses the appropriate metabolic enzyme, and it can only possess that enzyme if the genome of the cell contains the gene that codes for production of that enzyme.

> Metabolism refers to all of the chemical reactions (metabolic reactions) that occur within a living cell.

Biologic Catalysts (Enzymes)

As you learned in Chapter 6, enzymes are known as *biologic catalysts*. Enzymes are proteins that catalyze (speed up or accelerate) the rate of biochemical reactions. In some cases, the reaction will not occur at all in the absence of the enzyme. Thus, a complete definition of a biologic catalyst would be a protein that either causes a particular chemical reaction to occur or accelerates it.

> Enzymes are proteins that catalyze (accelerate) biochemical reactions.

Recall that enzymes are very specific. A particular enzyme can catalyze only one particular chemical reaction. In most cases, a particular enzyme can exert its effect or act on only one particular substance—known as the *substrate* for that enzyme. The unique three-dimensional shape of the enzyme enables it to fit the combining site of the substrate, much like a key fits into a lock (Fig. 7-2).

> The substance upon which an enzyme acts is known as that enzyme's substrate.

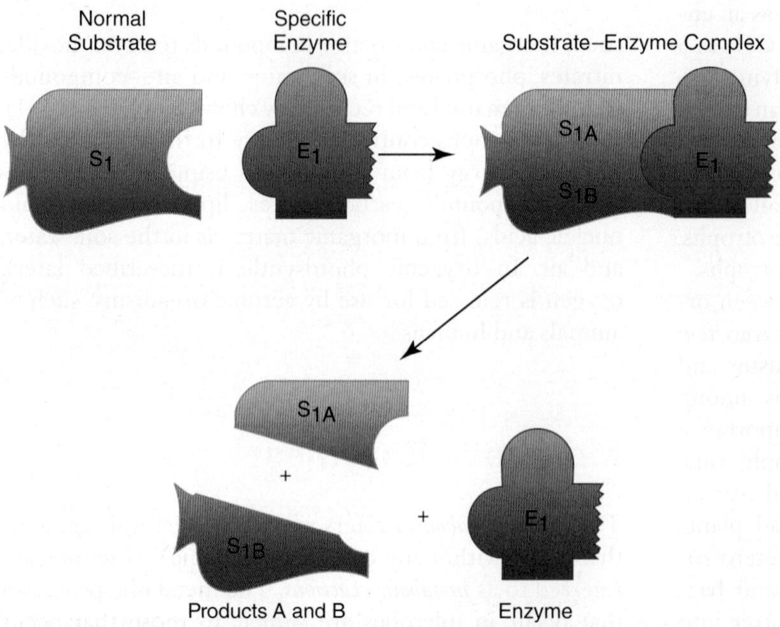

An enzyme does not become altered during the chemical reaction that it catalyzes. At the conclusion of the reaction, the enzyme is unchanged and is available to drive that reaction over and over. The enzyme moves from substrate molecule to substrate molecule at a rate of several hundred each second, producing a supply of the end product for as long as this particular end product is needed by the cell. However, enzymes do not last indefinitely; they finally degenerate and lose their activity. Therefore, the cell must synthesize and replace these important proteins. Because there are thousands of metabolic reactions continually occurring in the cell, there are thousands of enzymes available to control and direct the essential metabolic pathways. At any particular time, all the required enzymes need not be present; this situation is controlled by genes on the chromosomes and the needs of the cell, which are determined by the internal and external environments. For example, if no lactose is present in the organism's external environment, the organism does not need the enzyme required to break down lactose.

Enzymes produced within a cell that remain within the cell—to catalyze reactions within the cell—are called *endoenzymes*. The digestive enzymes within phagocytes are good examples of endoenzymes; they are used to digest materials that the phagocytes have ingested. Enzymes produced within a cell that are then released from the cell—to catalyze extracellular reactions—are called *exoenzymes*. Examples of exoenzymes are cellulase and pectinase, which are secreted by saprophytic fungi to digest cellulose and pectin in the external environment (e.g., in rotting leaves on the forest floor). Cellulose and pectin molecules are too large to be absorbed into fungal cells. The exoenzymes cellulase and pectinase break down these large molecules into smaller molecules, which can then be absorbed into the cells.

> Endoenzymes remain within the cell that produced them, whereas exoenzymes leave the cell to catalyze reactions outside of the cell.

Hydrolases and polymerases are additional examples of metabolic enzymes. Hydrolases break down macromolecules by the addition of water, in a process called *hydrolysis* or a *hydrolysis reaction*. These hydrolytic processes enable saprophytes to break apart such complex materials as leather, wax, cork, wood, rubber, hair, and some plastics. Some of the enzymes involved in the formation of large polymers such as DNA and RNA are called *polymerases*. As was discussed in Chapter 6, DNA polymerase is active each time the DNA of a cell is replicated, and RNA polymerase is required for the synthesis of messenger RNA (mRNA) molecules.

As discussed in Chapter 6, some proteins (called *apoenzymes*) cannot, on their own,

Figure 7-2. **Action of a specific enzyme (E) breaking down a substrate (S) molecule.**

Normal Substrate — S_1

Specific Enzyme — E_1

Substrate–Enzyme Complex — S_{1A} S_{1B} E_1

S_{1A} + S_{1B} + E_1

Products A and B   Enzyme

catalyze a chemical reaction. An apoenzyme must link up with a cofactor to catalyze a chemical reaction. Cofactors are either mineral ions (e.g., magnesium, calcium, or iron cations) or coenzymes. Coenzymes are small organic, vitamin-type molecules such as flavin adenine dinucleotide (FAD) and nicotinamide adenine dinucleotide (NAD). These particular coenzymes participate in the Krebs cycle, which is discussed later in this chapter. Like enzymes, coenzymes do not have to be present in large amounts because they are not altered during the chemical reaction that they catalyze; thus, they are available for use over and over. However, a lack of certain vitamins from which the coenzymes are synthesized will halt all reactions involving that particular coenzyme.

> To catalyze a reaction, an apoenzyme must first link up with a cofactor (either a mineral ion or a coenzyme).

Factors That Affect the Efficiency of Enzymes

Many factors affect the efficiency or effectiveness of enzymes. Certain physical or chemical changes can diminish or completely stop enzyme activity, because enzymes function properly only under optimum conditions. Optimum conditions for enzyme activity include a relatively limited range of pH and temperature as well as the appropriate concentration of enzyme and substrate. Extremes in heat and acidity can denature (or alter) enzymes by breaking the bonds responsible for their three-dimensional shape, resulting in the loss of enzymatic activity.

An enzyme will function at peak efficiency over a particular pH range. If the pH is too high or too low, the enzyme will not function at peak efficiency, and the reaction that the enzyme catalyzes will not proceed at its maximum rate. Likewise, an enzyme will function at peak efficiency over a particular temperature range. If the temperature is too high or too low, the enzyme will not function at peak efficiency, and the reaction that the enzyme catalyzes will not proceed at its maximum rate.

This explains why a particular bacterium grows best at a certain temperature and pH; these are the optimal conditions for the enzymes possessed by that bacterium. The optimal pH and temperature for growth vary from one species to another.

Substrate concentration is another factor that influences the efficiency of an enzyme. If the substrate concentration is too high or too low, the enzyme will not function at peak efficiency, and the reaction that the enzyme catalyzes will not proceed at its maximum rate.

Although certain mineral ions (e.g., calcium, magnesium, and iron) enhance the activity

> Enzyme efficiency is influenced by various factors, including pH, temperature, and the concentration of the substrate.

of enzymes by serving as cofactors, other heavy metal ions (e.g., lead, zinc, mercury, and arsenic) usually act as poisons to the cell. These toxic ions inhibit enzyme activity by replacing the cofactors at the combining site of the enzyme, thus inhibiting normal metabolic processes. Some disinfectants containing mineral ions are effective in inhibiting the growth of bacteria in this manner.

Sometimes, a molecule that is similar in structure to the substrate can be used as an inhibitor to deliberately interfere with a particular metabolic pathway. The enzyme binds to the molecule having a similar structure to the substrate, thus tying the enzyme up, so that it cannot attach to the substrate and cannot catalyze the chemical reaction. If that reaction is essential for the life of the cell, the cell will stop growing and may die. For example, a chemotherapeutic agent, such as a sulfonamide drug, can bind to certain bacterial enzymes, blocking attachment of the enzymes to their substrates and preventing essential metabolites from being formed. This could lead to the death of the bacteria.

Metabolism

As previously mentioned, the term metabolism refers to all the chemical reactions occurring within a cell. The reactions are referred to as metabolic reactions. A *metabolite* is any molecule that is a nutrient, an intermediary product, or an end product in a metabolic reaction. Within a cell, many metabolic reactions proceed simultaneously, breaking down some compounds and synthesizing (building) others. Most metabolic reactions fall into two categories: catabolism and anabolism (Fig. 7-3).

The term *catabolism* refers to all the catabolic reactions that are occurring in a cell. *Catabolic reactions*, which are described in greater detail in a subsequent section, involve the breaking down of larger molecules into smaller molecules, requiring the breaking of bonds. **Any time that chemical bonds are broken, energy is released. Catabolic reactions are a cell's major source of energy**. Catabolic reactions in bacteria are quite diverse, because energy sources range from inorganic compounds (e.g., sulfide, ferrous ion, hydrogen) to organic compounds (e.g., carbohydrates, lipids, amino acids).

> Catabolic reactions involve the breaking of chemical bonds and the release of energy.

Anabolism refers to all the anabolic reactions that are occurring in a cell. *Anabolic reactions*, which are described in greater detail in a subsequent section, involve the assembly of smaller molecules into larger molecules, requiring the formation of bonds. **Energy is required for bond formation. Once formed, the bonds**

> Anabolic reactions involve the formation of bonds, which requires energy.

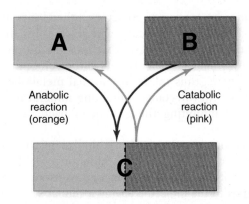

Figure 7-3. Anabolic and catabolic reactions. An anabolic reaction joins smaller molecules **(A, B)** together to produce a larger molecule **(C)**. A catabolic reaction breaks a larger molecule (C) down into smaller molecules (A, B).

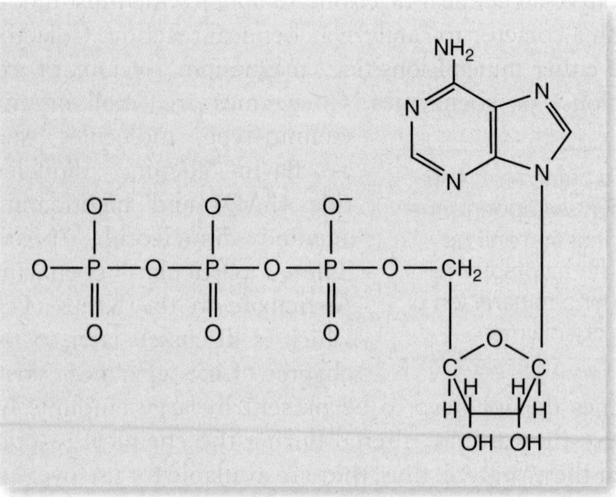

represent stored energy. Anabolic reactions tend to be quite similar for all types of cells; the pathways for the biosynthesis of macromolecules do not differ much among organisms. Table 7-2 illustrates the key differences between catabolism and anabolism.

The energy that is released during catabolic reactions is used to drive anabolic reactions. A kind of energy balancing act occurs within a cell, with some metabolic reactions releasing energy and other metabolic reactions requiring energy. The energy required by a cell may be

> ATP molecules are the major energy-storing or energy-carrying molecules within a cell.

trapped from the rays of the sun (as in photosynthesis), or it may be produced by certain catabolic reactions. Then the energy can be temporarily stored within high-energy bonds in special molecules, usually ATP molecules (Fig. 7-4). Although ATP molecules are not the only high-energy compounds found within a cell, they are

Figure 7-4. Adenosine triphosphate (ATP) molecule. As the name implies, ATP molecules contain three phosphate groups.

the most important ones. ATP molecules are the major energy-storing or energy-carrying molecules within a cell.

ATP molecules are found in all cells because they are used to transfer energy from energy-yielding molecules, such as glucose, to an energy-requiring reaction. Thus, ATP is a temporary, intermediate molecule. If ATP is not used shortly after it is formed, it is soon hydrolyzed to adenosine diphosphate (ADP), a more stable molecule; the hydrolysis of ATP is an example of a catabolic reaction. If a cell runs out of ATP molecules, ADP molecules can be used as an emergency energy source by the removal of another phosphate group to produce adenosine monophosphate (AMP); the hydrolysis of ADP is also a catabolic reaction. Figure 7-5 illustrates the interrelationships between ATP, ADP, and AMP molecules.

In addition to the energy required for metabolic pathways, energy is also required by the organism for growth, reproduction, sporulation, movement, and the active transport of substances across membranes. Some organisms (e.g., certain planktonic dinoflagellates) even use energy for bioluminescence. They cause a glowing that can sometimes be seen at the surface of an ocean, in a ship's wake, or as waves break on a beach. The value of bioluminescence to these organisms is unclear.

Chemical reactions are essentially energy transformation processes during which the energy that is stored in chemical bonds is transferred to produce new chemical bonds. The cellular mechanisms that release small amounts of energy as the cell needs it usually involve a sequence of catabolic and anabolic reactions.

Catabolism

As previously stated, the term catabolism refers to all the catabolic reactions that occur within a cell. **The key thing about catabolic reactions is that they release**

Table 7-2	Differences between Catabolism and Anabolism	
Catabolism	**Anabolism**
All the catabolic reactions in a cell	All the anabolic reactions in a cell
Catabolic reactions release energy	Anabolic reactions require energy
Catabolic reactions involve the breaking of bonds; whenever chemical bonds are broken, energy is released	Anabolic reactions involve the creation of bonds; it takes energy to create chemical bonds
Larger molecules are broken down into smaller molecules (sometimes referred to as degradative reactions)	Smaller molecules are bonded together to create larger molecules (sometimes referred to as biosynthetic reactions)

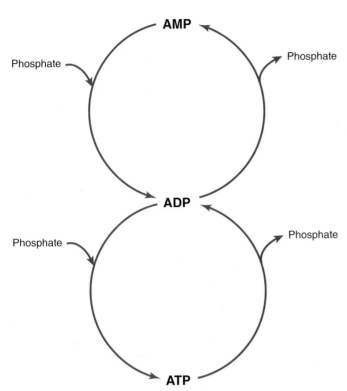

Figure 7-5. **Interrelationships between ATP, ADP, and AMP molecules.**

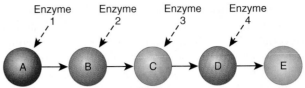

Figure 7-6. **A biochemical pathway.** There are four steps in this hypothetical biochemical pathway, in which compound A is ultimately converted to compound E. Compound A is first converted to compound B, which in turn is converted to compound C, which in turn is converted to compound D, which in turn is converted to compound E. Compound A is referred to as the starting material; compounds B, C, and D are referred to as intermediate (or intermediary) products; and compound E is referred to as the end product. A total of four enzymes are required in this pathway. The substrate for enzyme 1 is compound A; the substrate for enzyme 2 is compound B, and so on.

energy. Catabolic reactions are a cell's major source of energy. Catabolic reactions involve the breaking of chemical bonds. Any time chemical bonds are broken, energy is released. The energy produced by catabolic reactions can be used to wiggle flagella and actively transport substances through membranes, but most of the energy produced by catabolic reactions is used to drive anabolic reactions. Unfortunately, some of the energy is lost as heat. Catabolic reactions are often referred to as *degradative reactions*; they degrade larger molecules down into smaller molecules. For example, breaking down a disaccharide into its two original monosaccharides—a hydrolysis reaction—is an example of a catabolic reaction.

> Catabolic reactions release energy because chemical bonds are broken.

Biochemical Pathways

A biochemical pathway is a series of linked biochemical reactions that occur in a stepwise manner, leading from a starting material to an end product (Fig. 7-6).

Glucose is the favorite "food" or nutrient of cells, including microorganisms. **Nutrients should be thought of as energy sources, and**

> Nutrients should be thought of as energy sources, and chemical bonds should be thought of as stored energy.

chemical bonds should be thought of as stored energy. Whenever the chemical bonds within the nutrients are broken, energy is released.

There are many chemical processes by which glucose is catabolized within cells. Two common processes are the biochemical pathways known as aerobic respiration and fermentation reactions, which will be discussed in this chapter. Additional pathways for catabolizing glucose, such as the Entner–Doudoroff pathway, the pentose phosphate pathway, and anaerobic respiration, will not be described because they are beyond the scope of this book.

Aerobic Respiration of Glucose

The complete catabolism of glucose by the process known as aerobic respiration (or cellular respiration) occurs in three phases, each of which is a biochemical pathway: (a) glycolysis, (b) the Krebs cycle, and (c) the electron transport chain. Although the first phase—glycolysis—is an anaerobic process, the other two phases require aerobic conditions; hence the name *aerobic* respiration.

> Aerobic respiration involves (a) glycolysis, (b) the Krebs cycle, and (c) the electron transport chain.

STUDY AID

A Biochemical Pathway

Think of a biochemical pathway as a journey by car. To drive from city A to city E, you must pass through cities B, C, and D. City A is the starting point. City E is the destination or end point. Cities B, C, and D are intermediate points along the journey.

Glycolysis. Glycolysis, also known as the *glycolytic pathway*, the Embden–Meyerhof pathway, and the Embden–Meyerhof–Parnas pathway, is a nine-step biochemical pathway, involving nine separate biochemical reactions, each of which requires a specific enzyme (Fig. 7-7).

In glycolysis, a six-carbon molecule of glucose is ultimately broken down into two three-carbon molecules of pyruvic acid (also called *pyruvate*). Glycolysis can take place in either the presence or the absence of oxygen; oxygen does not participate in this phase of aerobic respiration. Glycolysis produces very little energy—a net yield

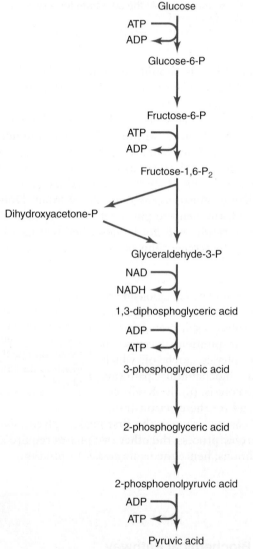

Figure 7-7. Glycolysis. Each of the compounds from glucose to fructose-1,6-P_2 contains six-carbon atoms. Fructose-1,6-P_2 is broken into two three-carbon compounds: dihydroxyacetone-P and glyceraldehyde-3-P, each of which is ultimately transformed into a molecule of pyruvic acid. Thus, in glycolysis, one six-carbon molecule of glucose is converted to two three-carbon molecules of pyruvic acid. (See text for additional details.) (From Volk WA, et al. *Essentials of Medical Microbiology.* 5th ed. Philadelphia, PA: Lippincott-Raven, 1996.)

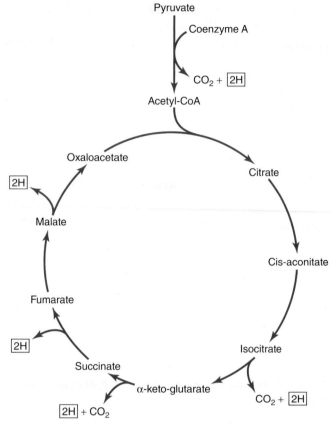

Figure 7-8. The Krebs cycle. See text for details. (From Volk WA, et al. *Essentials of Medical Microbiology.* 5th ed. Philadelphia, PA: Lippincott-Raven; 1996.)

of only two molecules of ATP. Glycolysis takes place in the cytoplasm of both prokaryotic and eukaryotic cells.

Krebs Cycle. The pyruvic acid molecules produced during glycolysis are converted into acetyl-coenzyme A (acetyl-CoA) molecules, which then enter the Krebs cycle (Fig. 7-8).

The Krebs cycle is a biochemical pathway consisting of eight separate reactions, each of which is controlled by a different enzyme. In the first step of the Krebs cycle, acetyl-CoA combines with oxaloacetate to produce citric acid (a tricarboxylic acid [TCA]); hence, the other names for the Krebs cycle—the citric acid cycle, the tricarboxylic acid cycle, and the TCA cycle. It is referred to as a cycle because at the end of the eight reactions, the biochemical pathway ends up back at its starting point—oxaloacetate. Only two ATP molecules are produced during the Krebs cycle, but several products (e.g., NADH, FADH$_2$, and hydrogen ions) that are formed during the Krebs cycle enter the electron transport chain. (NADH is the reduced form of NAD, and FADH$_2$ is the reduced form of FAD.[a] In eukaryotic cells, the Krebs cycle and the electron transport chain

---

[a]NAD and FAD were mentioned earlier in this chapter.

are located within mitochondria. (Recall from Chapter 3 that mitochondria are referred to as "energy factories" or "power houses.") In prokaryotic cells, both the Krebs cycle and the electron transport chain occur at the inner surface of the cell membrane.

Electron Transport Chain. As previously mentioned, certain of the products produced during the Krebs cycle enter the *electron transport chain* (also called the electron transport system or respiratory chain). The electron transport chain consists of a series of oxidation–reduction reactions (described in a subsequent section), whereby energy released as electrons is transferred from one compound to another. These compounds include flavoproteins, quinones, nonheme iron proteins, and cytochromes. Oxygen is at the end of the chain; it is referred to as the final or terminal electron acceptor.

Many different enzymes are involved in the electron transport chain, including cytochrome oxidase (also called cytochrome *c*, or merely oxidase), the enzyme responsible for transferring electrons to oxygen, the final electron acceptor. In the clinical microbiology laboratory, the oxidase test is useful in the identification (speciation) of a Gram-negative bacillus that has been isolated from a clinical specimen. Whether or not the organism possesses oxidase is an important clue to the organism's identity.

During the electron transport chain, a large number of ATP molecules are produced by a process known as oxidative phosphorylation—oxidation referring to a loss of electrons and phosphorylation referring to the conversion of ADP molecules to ATP molecules. The net yield of ATP molecules from the catabolism of one glucose molecule by aerobic respiration is 38 in prokaryotic cells and 36 to 38 in eukaryotic cells (Table 7-3). That is a great deal of energy from one molecule of glucose! Aerobic respiration is a very efficient system. It produces 18 to

> The breakdown of glucose by aerobic respiration produces 38 ATP molecules in prokaryotic cells and 36 to 38 ATP molecules in eukaryotic cells.

19 times as much energy as does fermentation of glucose (discussed in a subsequent section).

The chemical equation representing aerobic respiration is:

$$C_6H_{12}O_6 + 6\,O_2 + 38\,ADP + 38\,\circledP \rightarrow 6\,H_2O + 6\,CO_2 + 38\,ATP$$

where $\circledP$ indicates an activated phosphate group.

The catabolism of glucose by aerobic respiration is just one of many ways in which cells can catabolize glucose molecules. How glucose is utilized by a cell depends on the individual organism, its available nutrient and energy resources, and the enzymes it is able to produce. Some bacteria degrade glucose to pyruvic acid by other metabolic pathways. Also, glycerol, fatty acids from lipids, and amino acids from protein digestion may enter the Krebs cycle to produce energy for the cell when necessary (i.e., when there are insufficient carbohydrates available).

Fermentation of Glucose

The first thing to note about *fermentation* reactions is that they do not involve oxygen; therefore, fermentations usually take place in anaerobic environments. The first step in the fermentation of glucose is glycolysis, which occurs exactly as previously described. Remember that glycolysis does not involve oxygen, and very little energy (two ATP molecules) is produced by glycolysis.

> Oxygen does not participate in fermentation reactions.

The next step in fermentation reactions is the conversion of pyruvic acid into an end product. The particular end product that is produced depends on the specific organism involved. The various end products of fermentation have many industrial applications. For example, certain yeasts (*Saccharomyces* spp.) and bacteria (*Zymomonas* spp.) convert pyruvic acid into ethyl alcohol (ethanol) and CO_2. Such yeasts are used to make wine, beer, other alcoholic beverages, and bread.

A group of Gram-positive bacteria, called *lactic acid bacteria*, convert pyruvic acid to lactic acid. These bacteria are used to make various food products, including cheeses, yogurt, pickles, and cured sausages. In human muscle cells, the lack of oxygen during extreme exertion results in pyruvic acid being converted to lactic acid. The presence of lactic acid in muscle tissue is the cause of soreness that develops in exhausted muscles. Some oral bacteria (e.g., various *Streptococcus* spp.) convert glucose into lactic acid, which then eats away the enamel on our teeth, leading to tooth decay. The presence of lactic acid bacteria in milk causes the souring of milk into curd and whey.

Some bacteria convert pyruvic acid into propionic acid. *Propionibacterium* spp. are used in the production of Swiss cheese. The propionic acid they produce gives the

Table 7-3	Recap of the Theoretical Maximum Yield of ATP Molecules Produced from One Molecule of Glucose by Aerobic Respiration	
	Prokaryotic Cells	**Eukaryotic Cells**
Glycolysis	2	2
Krebs cycle	2	2
Electron transport chain	34	32–34[a]
Total ATP molecules	38	36–38[a]

[a]Varies depending upon how many NADH molecules produced during glycolysis enter the mitochondria.

cheese its characteristic flavor, and the CO_2 that is produced creates the holes. Other end products of fermentation include acetic acid, acetone, butanol, butyric acid, isopropanol, and succinic acid.

Fermentation reactions produce very little energy (approximately two ATP molecules); therefore, they are very inefficient ways to catabolize glucose. Aerobes and facultative anaerobes are much more efficient in energy production than obligate anaerobes because they are able to catabolize glucose via aerobic respiration.

> The breakdown of glucose by fermentation produces only two ATP molecules.

Oxidation–Reduction (Redox) Reactions

Oxidation–reduction reactions are paired reactions in which electrons are transferred from one compound to another (Fig. 7-9). Whenever an atom, ion, or molecule loses one or more electrons (e–) in a reaction, the process is called *oxidation*, and the molecule is said to be *oxidized*. The electrons that are lost do not float about at random but, because they are very reactive, attach immediately to another molecule. The resulting gain of one or more electrons by a molecule is called *reduction*, and the molecule is said to be *reduced*. Within the cell, an oxidation reaction is always paired (or coupled) with a reduction reaction; thus the term oxidation–reduction or "redox" reactions. In a redox reaction, the electron donor is referred to as the reducing agent and the electron acceptor is referred to as the oxidizing agent. Thus, in Figure 7-9, compound A is the reducing agent and compound B is the oxidizing agent.

> Oxidation reactions involve the loss of an electron, whereas reduction reactions involve the gain of an electron.

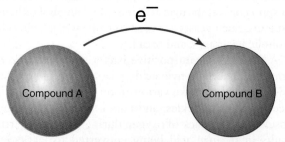

Figure 7-9. An oxidation–reduction reaction. In this illustration, an electron has been transferred from compound A to compound B. Two reactions have occurred simultaneously. Compound A has lost an electron (an oxidation reaction), and compound B has gained an electron (a reduction reaction). Oxidation is the loss of an electron. Reduction is the gain of an electron. Compound A has been oxidized, and compound B has been reduced. The term *reduction* relates to the fact that an electron has a negative charge. When compound B receives an electron, its electrical charge is reduced.

As stated earlier, the electron transport chain consists of a series of oxidation–reduction reactions, whereby energy released as electrons is transferred from one compound to another. Many biologic oxidations are referred to as *dehydrogenation reactions* because hydrogen ions (H^+) as well as electrons are removed. Concurrently, those hydrogen ions must be picked up in a reduction reaction. Many good illustrations are found in the aerobic respiration of glucose, in which the hydrogen ions released during the Krebs cycle enter the electron transport chain. (See "Why Anaerobes Die in the Presence of Oxygen" on thePoint.)

Anabolism

As previously stated, anabolism refers to all the *anabolic reactions* that are occurring in a cell. **Anabolic reactions require energy because chemical bonds are being formed.** It takes energy to create a chemical bond. **Most of the energy required for anabolic reactions is provided by the catabolic reactions that are occurring simultaneously in the cell.** Anabolic reactions are often referred to as biosynthetic reactions. Examples of anabolic reactions include creating a disaccharide from two monosaccharides by dehydration synthesis, the biosynthesis of polypeptides by linking amino acid molecules together, and the biosynthesis of nucleic acid molecules by linking nucleotides together.

> Anabolic reactions require energy because chemical bonds are being formed.

Biosynthesis of Organic Compounds

The biosynthesis of organic compounds requires energy and may occur through either photosynthesis (biosynthesis using light energy) or **chemosynthesis** (biosynthesis using chemical energy).

Photosynthesis. In photosynthesis, light energy is converted to chemical energy in the form of chemical bonds. Phototrophs that use CO_2 as their carbon source are called photoautotrophs; examples are algae, plants, cyanobacteria, and certain other photosynthetic bacteria. Phototrophs that use small organic molecules, such as acids and alcohols, to build organic molecules are called photoheterotrophs; some types of bacteria are photoheterotrophs.

The goal of photosynthetic processes is to trap the radiant energy of light and convert it into chemical bond energy in ATP molecules and carbohydrates, particularly glucose, which can then be converted into more ATP molecules at a later time through aerobic respiration. Bacteria that produce oxygen by photosynthesis are called *oxygenic photosynthetic bacteria*, and the process is known as *oxygenic photosynthesis*. The oxygenic photosynthesis reaction is

$$6\ CO_2 + 12\ H_2O \xrightarrow[\text{ATP}]{\text{light}} C_6H_{12}O_6 + 6\ O_2 + 6\ H_2O + ATP + \textcircled{P}$$

Note that this reaction is almost the reverse of the aerobic respiration reaction; it is nature's way of balancing substrates in the environment. In aerobic respiration, glucose and oxygen are ultimately converted into water and carbon dioxide. In oxygenic photosynthesis, water and carbon dioxide are converted into glucose and oxygen.

Photosynthetic reactions do not always produce oxygen. Purple sulfur bacteria and green sulfur bacteria (which are obligate anaerobic photoautotrophs) are referred to as *anoxygenic photosynthetic bacteria* because their photosynthetic processes do not produce oxygen (*anoxygenic photosynthesis*). These bacteria use sulfur, sulfur compounds (e.g., H_2S gas), or hydrogen gas to reduce CO_2, rather than H_2O.

Bacterial photosynthetic pigments use shorter wavelengths of light, which penetrate deep within a body of water or into mud where it appears to be dark. In the absence of light, some phototrophic organisms may survive anaerobically by the fermentation process alone. Other phototrophic bacteria also have a limited ability to use simple organic molecules in photosynthetic reactions; thus, they become photoheterotrophic organisms under certain conditions.

Chemosynthesis. The chemosynthetic process involves a chemical source of energy and raw materials for synthesis of the metabolites and macromolecules required for growth and function of the organisms. Chemotrophs that use CO_2 as their carbon source are called chemoautotrophs. Examples of chemoautotrophs are a few primitive types of bacteria. You will recall that some archaea are methanogens; they are chemoautotrophs also. Methanogens produce methane in the following manner:

$$4\ H_2 + CO_2 \rightarrow CH_4 + 2\ H_2O$$

Chemotrophs that use organic molecules other than CO_2 as their carbon source are called chemoheterotrophs. Most bacteria, as well as all protozoa, fungi, animals, and humans, are chemoheterotrophs.

Bacterial Genetics

It would be impossible to discuss the genetics of all types of microorganisms in a book of this size. (Recall that some microbes are prokaryotic and others are eukaryotic.) Therefore, the following discussion of bacterial genetics will serve as an introduction to the subject of microbial genetics.

Genetics—the study of heredity—involves many subtopics, some of which (e.g., DNA, genes, the genetic code, chromosomes, DNA replication, transcription, translation) have already been addressed in this book. The topics thus far discussed all relate to molecular genetics—genetics at the molecular level.

An organism's *genotype* (or *genome*) is its complete collection of genes, whereas an organism's *phenotype* is all the organism's physical traits, attributes, or characteristics. Phenotypic characteristics of humans include hair, eye, and skin color. Phenotypic characteristics of bacteria include the presence or absence of certain enzymes and such structures as capsules, flagella, and pili. An organism's phenotype is dictated by that organism's genotype. **Phenotype is the manifestation of genotype.** For example, an organism cannot produce a particular enzyme unless it possesses the gene that codes for that enzyme. It cannot produce flagella unless it possesses the genes necessary for flagella production.

> An organism's genotype (or genome) is its complete collection of genes, whereas an organism's phenotype is all the physical traits, attributes, or characteristics of the organism.

Most bacteria possess one chromosome, which usually consists of a long, continuous (circular), double-stranded DNA molecule, with no protein on the outside (as is found in eukaryotic chromosomes). A particular segment of the chromosome constitutes a gene. The chromosome can be thought of as a circular strand of genes, all linked together—somewhat like a string of beads. Genes are the fundamental units of heredity that carry the information needed for the special characteristics of each different species of bacteria. **Genes direct all functions of the cell, providing it with its own particular traits and individuality.**

As you learned in Chapter 6, the information in a gene is used by the cell to make an mRNA molecule (via the process known as transcription). Then, the information in the mRNA molecule is used to make a *gene product* (via the process known as translation). Most gene products are proteins, but ribosomal RNA (rRNA) and transfer RNA (tRNA) molecules are also coded for by genes and, therefore, represent other types of gene products. When the information in a gene has been used by the cell to make a gene product, the gene coding for that particular gene product is said to have been *expressed*. All the genes on the chromosome

> Constitutive genes are expressed at all times, whereas inducible genes are expressed only when needed.

are not being expressed at any given time. That would be a terrible waste of energy! For example, it would be pointless for a cell to produce a particular enzyme if that enzyme was not needed. Genes that are expressed at all times are called *constitutive genes*. Those that are expressed only when the gene products are needed are called *inducible genes*.

Because there is only one chromosome that replicates just before cell division, identical traits of a species are passed from the parent bacterium to the daughter cells after binary fission has occurred. DNA replication must precede binary fission to ensure that each daughter cell has exactly the same genetic composition as the parent cell.

Mutations

The DNA of any gene on the chromosome is subject to accidental alteration (e.g., the deletion of a base pair), which alters the gene product and perhaps also alters the trait that is controlled by that gene. If the change in the gene alters or eliminates a trait in such a way that the cell does not die or become incapable of division, the altered trait is transmitted to the daughter cells of each succeeding generation. A change in the characteristics of a cell caused by a change in the DNA molecule (genetic alteration) that is transmissible to the offspring is called a *mutation*. There are three categories of mutations: beneficial mutations, harmful (and sometimes lethal) mutations, and silent mutations.

Beneficial mutations, as the name implies, are of benefit to the organism. An example would be a mutation that enables the organism to survive in an environment where organisms without that mutation would die. Perhaps the mutation enables the organism to be resistant to a particular antibiotic.

An example of a *harmful mutation* would be a mutation that leads to the production of a nonfunctional enzyme. A nonfunctional enzyme is unable to catalyze the chemical reaction that it would normally catalyze if it were functional. If it happens to be an enzyme that catalyzes a metabolic reaction essential to the life of the cell, the cell will die. Thus, this is an example of a *lethal mutation*. Not all harmful mutations are lethal.

> Beneficial mutations are of benefit to an organism, whereas harmful mutations result in the production of nonfunctional enzymes. Some harmful mutations are lethal to the organism.

In all likelihood, most mutations are *silent mutations* (or neutral mutations), meaning that they have no effect on the cell. For example, if the mutation causes an incorrect amino acid to be placed near the center of a large, highly convoluted enzyme, composed of hundreds of amino acids, it is doubtful that the mutation would cause any change in the structure or function of that enzyme. If the mutation causes no change in function, it is considered silent.

Most likely, spontaneous mutations (random mutations that occur naturally) occur more or less constantly throughout a bacterial genome. However, some genes are more prone to spontaneous mutations than others. The rate at which spontaneous mutations occur is usually expressed in terms of the frequency at which a mutation will occur in a particular gene. This rate varies from one mutation every 10^4 (10,000) rounds of DNA replication to one mutation every 10^{12} (1 trillion) rounds of DNA replication. The average spontaneous mutation rate is about one mutation every 10^6 (1 million) rounds of DNA replication. In other words, the odds that a spontaneous mutation will occur in a particular gene are about one mutation per million cell divisions.

The mutation rate can be increased by exposing cells to physical or chemical agents that affect the chromosome. Such agents are called *mutagens*. In research laboratories, x-rays, ultraviolet light, and radioactive substances, as well as certain chemical agents, are used to increase the mutation rate of bacteria, thus causing more mutations to occur. The organism containing the mutation is called a *mutant*. Bacterial mutants are used in genetic and medical research and in the development of vaccines. The types of mutagenic changes

> Physical or chemical agents that cause an increased mutation rate are called mutagens.

frequently observed in bacteria involve cell shape, biochemical activities, nutritional needs, antigenic sites, colony characteristics, virulence, and drug resistance. Nonpathogenic "live" virus vaccines, such as the Sabin vaccine for polio, are examples of laboratory-induced mutations of pathogenic microbes.

In a test procedure called the *Ames test* (developed by Bruce Ames in the 1960s), a mutant strain of *Salmonella* is used to learn whether a particular chemical (e.g., a food additive or a chemical used in some type of cosmetic product) is a mutagen. If exposure to the chemical causes a reversal of the organism's mutation (known as a back mutation), then the chemical has been shown to be mutagenic. If the chemical is mutagenic, then it might also be carcinogenic (cancer-causing) and should be tested using laboratory animals or cell cultures. Many substances found to be mutagenic by the Ames test have been shown to be carcinogenic in laboratory animals. Substances that are carcinogenic in laboratory animals might also be carcinogenic in humans.

Ways in Which Bacteria Acquire New Genetic Information

There are at least four additional ways that the genetic composition of bacteria can be changed: lysogenic conversion, transduction, transformation, and conjugation. These are ways in which bacteria acquire new genetic information (i.e., acquire new genes). If the new genes

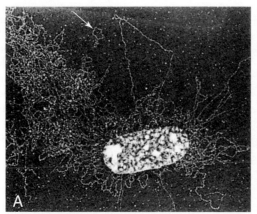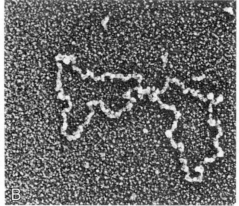

Figure 7-10. Plasmids. (A) Disrupted *E. coli* cell. The DNA has spilled out and a plasmid can be seen slightly to the left of top center (*arrow*). **(B)** Enlargement of a plasmid, which is about 1 μm from side to side. (From Volk WA, et al. *Essentials of Medical Microbiology*. 4th ed. Philadelphia, PA: JB Lippincott, 1991.)

remain in the cytoplasm of the cell, the DNA molecule on which they are located is called a *plasmid* (Fig. 7-10). Because they are not part of the chromosome, plasmids are referred to as extrachromosomal DNA. Many different types of plasmids have been discovered, and information about them all would fill many books. Some plasmids contain many genes, others only a few, but, in all cases, the cell is changed by the acquisition of these genes. Some plasmids replicate simultaneously with chromosomal DNA replication; others replicate independently at various other times. A plasmid that either can exist autonomously (by itself) or can integrate into the chromosome is referred to as an *episome*. Some plasmid genes can be expressed as extrachromosomal genes, but others must integrate into the chromosome before the genes become functional.

Lysogenic Conversion

As mentioned in Chapter 4, there are two categories of bacteriophages (phages): virulent phages and temperate phages. Virulent phages (which were described in Chapter 4) always cause the lytic cycle to occur, ending with the destruction (lysis) of the bacterial cell.

After *temperate phages* (also known as lysogenic phages) inject their DNA into the bacterial cell, the phage DNA integrates into (becomes part of) the bacterial chromosome but does not cause the lytic cycle to occur. This situation—in which the phage genome is present in the cell but is not causing the lytic cycle to occur—is known as *lysogeny*. During lysogeny, all that remains of the phage is its DNA; in this form, the phage is referred to as a *prophage*. The bacterial cell containing the prophage is referred to as a *lysogenic cell* or *lysogenic bacterium*. Each time a lysogenic cell undergoes binary fission, the phage DNA is replicated along with the bacterial DNA and is passed on to each of the daughter cells. Thus, the daughter cells are also lysogenic cells.

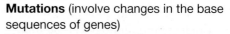
Although the prophage does not usually cause the lytic cycle to occur, certain events (e.g., exposure of the bacterial cell to ultraviolet light or certain chemicals) can trigger it to do so. While the prophage is integrated into the bacterial chromosome, the bacterial cell can produce gene products that are coded for by the prophage genes. The bacterial cell will exhibit new properties—a phenomenon known as *lysogenic conversion* (or *phage conversion*). In other words, the bacterial cell has been converted as a result of lysogeny and is now able to produce one or more gene products that it previously was unable to produce.

A medically related example of lysogenic conversion involves the disease diphtheria. Diphtheria is caused by

> A lysogenic bacterium is capable of producing one or more new gene products as a result of infection by a temperate bacteriophage.

a toxin—called diphtheria toxin—that is produced by a Gram-positive bacillus named *Corynebacterium diphtheriae*. Interestingly, the *C. diphtheriae* genome does not normally contain the gene that codes for diphtheria toxin. Only cells of *C. diphtheriae* that contain a prophage can produce diphtheria toxin, because it is actually a phage gene (called the tox gene) that codes for the toxin. Strains of *C. diphtheriae* capable of producing diphtheria toxin are called *toxigenic strains*, and those unable to produce the toxin are called *nontoxigenic strains*. A nontoxigenic *C. diphtheriae* cell can be converted to a toxigenic cell as a result of lysogeny. As previously mentioned, conversion as a result of lysogeny is referred to as lysogenic conversion. The phage that infects *C. diphtheriae*—the phage having the tox gene in its genome—is called a corynebacteriophage.

Other medically related examples of lysogenic conversion involve *Streptococcus pyogenes*, *Clostridium botulinum*, and *Vibrio cholerae*. Only strains of *S. pyogenes* that carry a prophage are capable of producing erythrogenic toxin—the toxin that causes scarlet fever. Only strains of *C. botulinum* that carry a prophage can produce botulinal toxin, and only strains of *V. cholerae* that carry a prophage can produce cholera toxin. Thus, without being infected by bacteriophages, these bacteria could not cause scarlet fever, botulism, and cholera, respectively. A recap of bacteriophage terminology can be found in Table 7-4.

Transduction

Transduction also involves bacteriophages. Transduction means "to carry across." Some bacterial genetic material may be carried across from one bacterial cell to another by a bacterial virus. This phenomenon may occur after infection of a bacterial cell by a temperate bacteriophage. The viral DNA combines with the bacterial chromosome, becoming a prophage. If a stimulating chemical, heat, or ultraviolet light activates the prophage, it begins to produce new viruses via the production of phage DNA and proteins. As the chromosome disintegrates, small pieces of bacterial DNA may remain attached to the maturing phage DNA. During the assembly of the virus particles, one or more bacterial genes may be incorporated into some of the mature bacteriophages. When all the phages are released by cell lysis, they proceed to infect other cells, some injecting bacterial genes as well as viral genes. Thus, bacterial genes that are attached to the phage DNA are carried to new cells by the virus. As explained on thePoint ("A Closer Look at Transduction"), there are two types of transduction: generalized transduction and specialized transduction. Generalized transduction is illustrated in Figure 7-11.

> Only small segments of DNA are transferred from cell to cell by transduction compared with the amount that can be transferred by transformation and conjugation.

Transformation

In *transformation*, a bacterial cell becomes genetically transformed after the uptake of DNA fragments ("naked DNA") from the environment (Fig. 7-12). Transformation experiments, performed by Oswald Avery and his colleagues, proved that DNA is indeed the genetic material (see the following Historical Note). In those experiments, a DNA extract from encapsulated, pathogenic *Streptococcus pneumoniae* bacteria (referred to as *S. pneumoniae* type 1) was added to a broth culture of

> In transformation, a bacterial cell becomes genetically transformed following uptake of DNA fragments ("naked DNA") from the environment.

Table 7-4	Recap of Bacteriophage Terminology
Term	**Meaning**
Bacteriophage (or phage)	A virus that infects bacteria
Lysogenic cell (or lysogenic bacterium)	A bacterial cell with bacteriophage DNA integrated into its chromosome
Lysogenic conversion	When a bacterial cell has acquired new phenotypic characteristics as a result of lysogeny
Lysogeny	When the bacteriophage DNA is integrated into the bacterial chromosome; the bacteriophage DNA replicates along with the chromosome
Lytic cycle	The sequence of events in the multiplication of a virulent bacteriophage; ends with lysis of the bacterial cell
Prophage	The name given to the bacteriophage when all that remains of it is its DNA, integrated into the bacterial chromosome
Temperate bacteriophage (or lysogenic bacteriophage)	A bacteriophage whose DNA integrates into the bacterial chromosome but does not immediately cause the lytic cycle to occur
Virulent bacteriophage	A bacteriophage that always causes the lytic cycle to occur

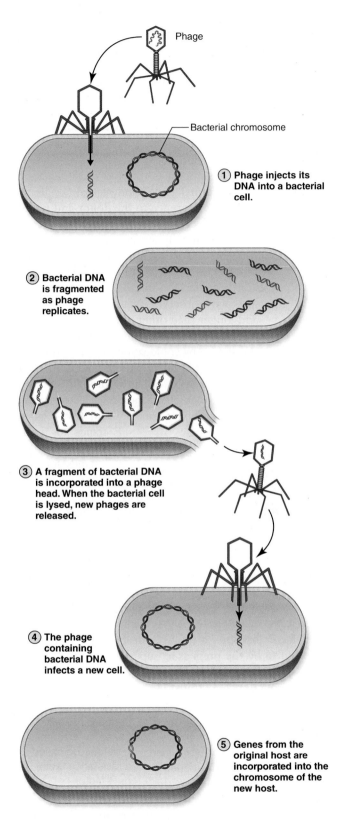

① **Phage injects its DNA into a bacterial cell.**

② **Bacterial DNA is fragmented as phage replicates.**

③ **A fragment of bacterial DNA is incorporated into a phage head. When the bacterial cell is lysed, new phages are released.**

④ **The phage containing bacterial DNA infects a new cell.**

⑤ **Genes from the original host are incorporated into the chromosome of the new host.**

Figure 7-11. Generalized transduction. (An animated version of this figure can be found on thePoint.)

nonencapsulated, nonpathogenic *S. pneumoniae* (referred to as *S. pneumoniae* type 2). Thus, at the beginning of the experiment, there were no live encapsulated bacteria in the culture. After incubation, however, live type 1

(encapsulated) bacteria were recovered from the culture. How was that possible? The only possible explanation was that some of the live type 2 bacteria must have taken up (absorbed) some of the type 1 DNA from the broth. Type 2 bacteria that absorbed pieces of type 1 DNA containing the gene(s) for capsule production were now able to produce capsules. In other words, type 2 (nonencapsulated) bacteria were converted to type 1 (encapsulated) bacteria as a result of the uptake of the genes that code for capsule production.

Transformation is probably not widespread in nature. In the laboratory, it has been demonstrated to occur in several genera of bacteria including *Bacillus*, *Escherichia*, *Haemophilus*, *Pseudomonas*, and *Neisseria*. Transformations have even been shown to occur between two different species (e.g., between *Staphylococcus* and *Streptococcus*). Extracellular pieces of DNA molecules can only penetrate the cell wall and cell membrane of certain bacteria. The ability to absorb naked DNA into the cell is referred to as *competence*, and bacteria capable of taking up naked DNA molecules are said to be *competent bacteria*.

Some competent bacterial cells have incorporated DNA fragments from certain animal viruses (e.g., cowpox), retaining the latent virus genes for long periods. This knowledge may have some importance in the study

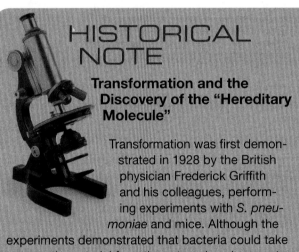

HISTORICAL NOTE

Transformation and the Discovery of the "Hereditary Molecule"

Transformation was first demonstrated in 1928 by the British physician Frederick Griffith and his colleagues, performing experiments with *S. pneumoniae* and mice. Although the experiments demonstrated that bacteria could take up genetic material from the external environment and, thus, be transformed, it was not known at that time what molecule actually contained the genetic information. It was not until 1944 that Oswald Avery, Colin MacLeod, and Maclyn McCarthy, who also experimented with *S. pneumoniae*, first demonstrated that DNA was the molecule that contained genetic information. Whereas Griffith's experiments were conducted in vivo, Avery's experiments were conducted in vitro. Experiments conducted in 1952 by Alfred Hershey and Martha Chase, using *E. coli* and bacteriophages, confirmed that DNA carried the genetic code.

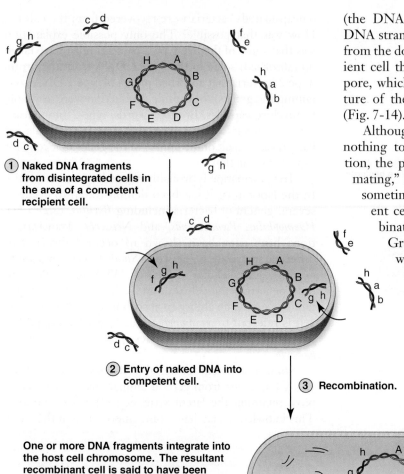

① **Naked DNA fragments from disintegrated cells in the area of a competent recipient cell.**

② **Entry of naked DNA into competent cell.**

③ **Recombination.**

One or more DNA fragments integrate into the host cell chromosome. The resultant recombinant cell is said to have been genetically transformed. It can now express the foreign genes it has received and pass them on to its progeny.

DNA that has not recombined is broken down by enzymes.

◀ **Figure 7-12. Transformation.** (An animated version of this figure can be found on thePoint.)

of viruses that remain latent in humans for many years before they finally cause disease, as may be the case in Parkinson disease. These human virus genes may hide in the bacteria of the indigenous microbiota until they are released to cause disease.

Conjugation

The transfer of genetic material by the process known as conjugation was discovered by Joshua Lederberg and Edward Tatum in 1946, while experimenting with *E. coli.* Conjugation involves a specialized type of pilus called a sex pilus (sometimes referred to as an F pilus or a conjugation bridge). A bacterial cell (called the donor cell or F^+ cell) possessing a sex pilus attaches to another bacterial cell (called the recipient cell or F^- cell) by means of the sex pilus (Fig. 7-13). Pilus retraction then brings the two cells into tight contact. Within the donor cell, an enzyme called relaxase nicks the double-stranded F plasmid DNA and guides one of the strands to a coupling protein

(the DNA pump). The single DNA strand is then transferred from the donor cell to the recipient cell through a conjugative pore, which forms at the juncture of the two bacterial cells (Fig. 7-14).[b]

Although conjugation has nothing to do with reproduction, the process is sometimes referred to as "bacterial mating," and the terms "male" and "female" cells are sometimes used in reference to the donor and recipient cells, respectively. This type of genetic recombination occurs mostly among species of enteric, Gram-negative bacilli, but has been reported within species of *Pseudomonas* and *Streptococcus* as well. In electron micrographs, microbiologists have observed that sex pili are thicker and longer than other pili.

Although many different genes may be transferred by conjugation, the ones most frequently noted include those coding for antibiotic resistance, colicin (a protein produced by *E. coli* that kills certain other bacteria), and fertility factors (F^+ and Hfr^+), where F stands for fertility and Hfr stands for high frequency of recombination. Check thePoint for "A Closer Look at Fertility Factors."

If a plasmid contains multiple genes for antibiotic resistance, the plasmid is referred to as a resistance factor or *R-factor*. A recipient cell that receives an R-factor becomes a multiply drug-resistant organism (referred to by the press as a "superbug"). Superbugs are discussed in detail in Chapter 9.

Transduction, transformation, and conjugation are excellent tools for mapping bacterial chromosomes and for studying bacterial and viral genetics. Although all these methods are frequently used in the laboratory, it is believed that they also occur in natural environments under certain circumstances.

> In conjugation, genetic material, usually in the form of a plasmid, is transferred through a conjugative pore from a donor cell to a recipient cell.

> A plasmid that contains multiple genes for antibiotic resistance is called a resistance factor or R-factor.

---

[b]For many years, it was assumed that the sex pilus was hollow, and that donor cell DNA was transferred to the recipient cell *through* the sex pilus. Recent evidence indicates that this is not the case.

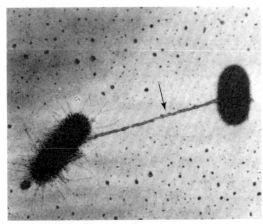

Figure 7-13. Conjugation in *E. coli*. The donor cell (the cell on the left, possessing numerous short pili) is connected to the recipient cell by a sex pilus (*arrow*). Contraction of the sex pilus will draw the recipient cell closer to the donor cell. (From Volk WA, et al. *Essentials of Medical Microbiology*. 5th ed. Philadelphia, PA: Lippincott-Raven, 1996.)

Genetic Engineering

An array of techniques has been developed to transfer eukaryotic genes, particularly human genes, into other easily cultured cells to facilitate the large-scale production of important gene products (proteins, in most cases). This process is known as *genetic engineering* or recombinant DNA technology (see Study Aid). Plasmids are frequently used as vectors or vehicles for inserting genes into cells. Bacteria, yeasts, human leukocytes, macrophages, and fibroblasts have been used as genetically engineered "manufacturing plants" for proteins such as human growth hormone (somatotropin), somatostatin (which inhibits the release of somatotropin), plasminogen-activating factor, insulin, and interferon. For example, the

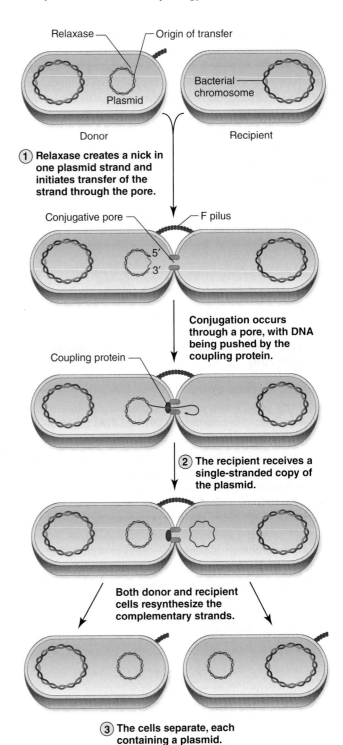

① **Relaxase creates a nick in one plasmid strand and initiates transfer of the strand through the pore.**

Conjugation occurs through a pore, with DNA being pushed by the coupling protein.

② **The recipient receives a single-stranded copy of the plasmid.**

Both donor and recipient cells resynthesize the complementary strands.

③ **The cells separate, each containing a plasmid.**

Figure 7-14. Conjugation. (See text for details.) Note that the donor cell does not lose its plasmid in the process. (Redrawn with permission from Sinauer Associates, Inc. An animated version of this figure can be found on thePoint.)

human gene that codes for insulin was inserted into *E. coli* cells, so that those cells and all of their progeny were able to produce human insulin. Somatostatin and insulin were first produced by recombinant DNA technology in 1978.

Many industrial and medical benefits may be derived from genetic engineering research. In agriculture, there is a potential for incorporating nitrogen-fixing capabilities into additional soil microorganisms; to make plants that are resistant to insects, as well as to bacterial and fungal diseases; and to increase the size and nutritional value of foods.

Genetically engineered microorganisms can also be used to clean up the environment (e.g., to get rid of toxic wastes). Consider this hypothetical example. A soil bacterium contains a gene that enables the organism to break oil down into harmless by-products, but, because the organism cannot survive in salt water, it cannot be used to clean up oil spills at sea. Remove the gene from the soil bacterium, and, using a plasmid vector, insert it into a marine bacterium. Now the marine bacterium has the ability to break down oil and, in large numbers, can be used to clean up oil spills at sea.

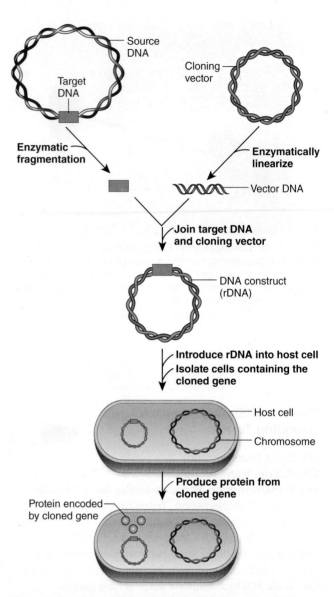

Figure 7-15. Recombinant DNA technology and genetic engineering. Plasmids are the most widely used vectors, but bacteriophages, artificial bacterial and yeast chromosomes, and disabled retroviruses have also been used.

STUDY AID

Recombinant DNA Technology vs. Genetic Engineering

Although these terms are frequently used interchangeably, there is a difference between them. **Recombinant DNA (rDNA) technology** can be thought of as the process by which rDNA is produced. This involves inserting a molecule or portion of a molecule of DNA into a different molecule or portion of a different molecule of DNA. The two molecules combine to form a single molecule, and the product is referred to as rDNA. **Genetic engineering** can be thought of as the process by which rDNA is used to modify an organism's genome—often to enable that organism to produce a particular gene product that it was previously unable to produce or to accomplish a task that it was previously unable to accomplish. Both processes—production of rDNA and genetic engineering—are illustrated in Figure 7-15.

In medicine, there is potential for making engineered antibodies, antibiotics, and drugs; for synthesizing important enzymes and hormones for treatment of inherited diseases; and for making vaccines. Such vaccines would contain only part of the pathogen (e.g., the capsid proteins of a virus) to which the person would form protective antibodies (see "Genetically Engineered Bacteria and Yeasts" on thePoint).

Gene Therapy

Gene therapy of human diseases involves the insertion of a normal gene into cells to correct a specific genetic or acquired disorder that is being caused by a defective gene. The first gene therapy trials were conducted in the United States in 1990. Viral delivery is currently the most common method for inserting genes into cells, in which specific viruses are selected to target the DNA of specific cells. For example, a virus capable of infecting liver cells would be used to insert a therapeutic gene or genes into the DNA of liver cells. Viruses currently being used or considered for use as vectors include adenoviruses, retroviruses, adeno-associated virus, and herpesviruses.

Certain genera of bacteria, including *Shigella*, *Salmonella*, *Listeria*, and others capable of entering mammalian cells are also being studied as possible vectors for use in gene therapy, cancer treatment, and vaccination. When these bacteria enter host cells (a process known as bactofection), they lyse and release their plasmids into the host cell cytoplasm. Plasmid genes can then enter the host cell nucleus and be expressed.

Since 1990, there have been hundreds of human gene therapy trials for many diseases. Nearly all have failed because of the difficulties of inserting a working gene into cells without causing harmful side effects. Nevertheless, scientists remain hopeful that genes will someday be regularly prescribed as "drugs" in the treatment of certain diseases (e.g., autoimmune diseases, sickle cell anemia, cancer, certain liver and lung diseases, cystic fibrosis, heart disease, hemoglobin defects, hemophilia, muscular dystrophy, and various immune deficiencies). In the future, synthetic vectors, rather than viruses or bacteria, may be used to insert genes into cells.

ON thePoint

- Terms Introduced in This Chapter
- Review of Key Points
- Why Anaerobes Die in the Presence of Oxygen
- A Closer Look at Transduction
- A Closer Look at Fertility Factors
- Genetically Engineered Bacteria and Yeasts
- Increase Your Knowledge
- Critical Thinking
- Additional Self-Assessment Exercises

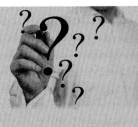

Self-Assessment Exercises

After studying this chapter, answer the following multiple-choice questions.

1. Which of the following characteristics do animals, fungi, and protozoa have in common?
   a. They obtain their carbon from carbon dioxide
   b. They obtain their carbon from inorganic compounds
   c. They obtain their energy and carbon atoms from chemicals
   d. They obtain their energy from light

2. Most ATP molecules are produced during which phase of aerobic respiration?
   a. electron transport chain
   b. fermentation
   c. glycolysis
   d. Krebs cycle

3. Which of the following processes does not involve bacteriophages?
   a. lysogenic conversion
   b. lytic cycle
   c. transduction
   d. transformation

4. In transduction, bacteria acquire new genetic information in the form of:
   a. bacterial genes
   b. naked DNA
   c. R-factors
   d. viral genes

5. The process whereby naked DNA is absorbed into a bacterial cell is known as:
   a. transcription
   b. transduction
   c. transformation
   d. translation

6. In lysogenic conversion, bacteria acquire new genetic information in the form of:
   a. bacterial genes
   b. naked DNA
   c. R-factors
   d. viral genes

7. Saprophytic fungi are able to digest organic molecules outside of the organism by means of:
   a. apoenzymes
   b. coenzymes
   c. endoenzymes
   d. exoenzymes

8. The process by which a nontoxigenic *C. diphtheriae* cell is changed into a toxigenic cell is called:
   a. conjugation
   b. lysogenic conversion
   c. transduction
   d. transformation

9. Which of the following does (do) not occur in anaerobes?
   a. anabolic reactions
   b. catabolic reactions
   c. electron transport chain
   d. fermentation reactions

10. Proteins that must link up with a cofactor to function as an enzyme are called:
    a. apoenzymes
    b. coenzymes
    c. endoenzymes
    d. holoenzymes

8

Controlling Microbial Growth In Vitro

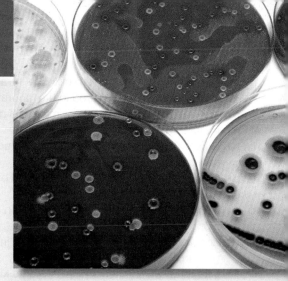

Bacterial colonies on various types of solid culture media.

CHAPTER OUTLINE

Introduction

Factors That Affect Microbial Growth

Availability of Nutrients
Moisture
Temperature
pH
Osmotic Pressure and Salinity
Barometric Pressure
Gaseous Atmosphere

Encouraging the Growth of Microbes In Vitro

Culturing Bacteria in the Laboratory
Bacterial Growth
Culture Media
Inoculation of Culture Media
Importance of Using "Aseptic Technique"
Incubation
Bacterial Population Counts
Bacterial Population Growth Curve
Culturing Viruses and Other Obligate Intracellular
  Pathogens in the Laboratory
Culturing Fungi in the Laboratory
Culturing Protozoa in the Laboratory

Inhibiting the Growth of Microbes In Vitro

Definition of Terms
Sterilization
Disinfection, Pasteurization, Disinfectants,
  Antiseptics, and Sanitization
Microbicidal Agents
Microbistatic Agents
Sepsis, Asepsis, Aseptic Technique, Antisepsis,
  and Antiseptic Technique
Sterile Technique

Using Physical Methods to Inhibit Microbial Growth
Heat
Cold
Desiccation
Radiation
Ultrasonic Waves
Filtration
Gaseous Atmosphere
Using Chemical Agents to Inhibit Microbial Growth
Disinfectants
Antiseptics
Controversies Relating to the Use of Antimicrobial
  Agents in Animal Feed and Household Products

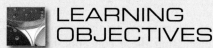

LEARNING OBJECTIVES

After studying this chapter, you should be able to:

• List several factors that affect the growth of microorganisms
• Describe the following types of microorganisms: psychrophilic, mesophilic, thermophilic, halophilic, haloduric, alkaliphilic, acidophilic, and piezophilic
• List three in vitro sites where microbial growth is encouraged
• Differentiate among enriched, selective, and differential media, and cite two examples of each
• Explain the importance of using "aseptic technique" in the microbiology laboratory
• Describe the three types of incubators that are used in the microbiology laboratory
• Draw a bacterial growth curve and label its four phases
• Cite two reasons why bacteria die during the death phase

- Name three ways in which obligate intracellular pathogens can be cultured in the laboratory
- List three in vitro sites where microbial growth must be inhibited
- Differentiate among sterilization, disinfection, and sanitization
- Differentiate between bactericidal and bacteriostatic agents
- Explain the processes of pasteurization and lyophilization
- List several physical methods used to inhibit the growth of microorganisms
- Cite three ways in which disinfectants kill microorganisms
- Identify several factors that can influence the effectiveness of disinfectants
- Explain briefly why the use of antibiotics in animal feed and household products is controversial

Introduction

In certain locations, such as within microbiology laboratories, the growth[a] of microbes is encouraged; in other words, scientists *want* them to grow. In other locations—such as on hospital wards, in intensive care units, in operating rooms, in kitchens, bathrooms, and restaurants—it is necessary or desirable to *inhibit* the growth of microbes. Both concepts, encouraging and inhibiting the in vitro growth of microbes, are discussed in this chapter. (Recall from Chapter 1 that, as used in this book, *in vitro* refers to events that occur outside the body, whereas *in vivo* refers to events that occur inside the body.) Before discussing these concepts, however, various factors that affect the growth of microbes are examined.

Factors That Affect Microbial Growth

Microbial growth is affected by many different environmental factors, including the availability of nutrients and moisture, temperature, pH, osmotic pressure, barometric pressure, and composition of the atmosphere. These environmental factors affect microorganisms in our daily lives and play important roles in the control of microorganisms in laboratory, industrial, and hospital settings. Whether scientists wish to encourage or inhibit the growth of microorganisms, they must first understand the fundamental needs of microbes.

Availability of Nutrients

As discussed in Chapter 7, all living organisms require nutrients—the various chemical compounds that organisms use to sustain life. Therefore, to survive in a particular environment, appropriate nutrients must be available. Many nutrients are energy sources; organisms will obtain energy from these chemicals by breaking chemical bonds. Nutrients also serve as sources of carbon, oxygen, hydrogen, nitrogen, phosphorus, and sulfur as well as other elements (e.g., sodium; potassium; chlorine; magnesium; calcium; and trace elements such as iron, iodine, and zinc) that are usually required in lesser amounts. About two dozen of the approximately 92 naturally occurring elements are essential to life.[b]

Moisture

On Earth, water is essential for life as we know it. Cells consist of anywhere between 70% and 95% water. All living organisms require water to carry out their normal metabolic processes, and most will die in environments containing too little moisture. There are certain microbial stages (e.g., bacterial endospores, protozoan cysts), however, that can survive the complete drying process (**desiccation**). The organisms contained within the spores and cysts are in a dormant or resting state; if they are placed in a moist, nutrient-rich environment, they will grow and reproduce normally.

> Water is essential for life, as we know it. Cells are composed of 70% to 95% water.

Temperature

Every microorganism has an optimum growth temperature—the temperature at which the organism grows best. Every microorganism also has a minimum growth temperature, below which it ceases to grow, and a maximum growth temperature, above which it dies. The temperature range (i.e., the range of temperatures from the minimum growth temperature to the maximum growth temperature) at which an organism grows can differ greatly from one microbe to another. To a large extent, the temperature and pH ranges over which an organism grows best are determined by the enzymes present within the organism. As discussed in Chapter 7, enzymes have optimum temperature and pH ranges at which they operate at peak efficiency. If an organism's enzymes are operating at peak efficiency, the organism will be metabolizing and growing at its maximum rate.

> Every microorganism has an optimal, a minimum, and a maximum growth temperature.

---

[a]The word "growth" is used in this chapter to mean proliferation or multiplication.

[b]Scientists continue to debate the actual number of naturally occurring elements, but most would agree that the number lies between 88 and 94.

Table 8-1 Temperatures at Which Various Organisms Can Be Found in Bodies of Water at Yellowstone National Park

Temperature	Organisms
163°F (73°C) or lower	Cyanobacteria
144°F (62°C) or lower	Fungi
140°F (60°C) or lower	Algae
133°F (56°C) or lower	Protozoa
122°F (50°C) or lower	Mosses, crustaceans, insects
80°F (27°C) or lower	Fish

Table 8-1 contains information regarding temperatures at which various organisms live in bodies of water at Yellowstone National Park.

Microorganisms that grow best at high temperatures are called **thermophiles** (meaning organisms that love heat). Thermophiles can be found in hot springs, compost pits, and silage as well as in and near hydrothermal vents at the bottom of the ocean (check thePoint for "A Closer Look at Hydrothermal Vents"). Thermophilic cyanobacteria, certain other types of bacteria, and algae cause many of the colors observed in the near-boiling hot springs found in Yellowstone National Park (Fig. 8-1). Organisms that favor temperatures above 100°C are referred to as hyperthermophiles (or extreme thermophiles). The highest temperature at which a bacterium has been found living is around 113°C; it was an archaeon named *Pyrolobus fumarii*.

> Thermophiles are organisms that "love" high temperatures.

Microbes that grow best at moderate temperatures are called **mesophiles**. This group includes most of the species that grow on plants and animals and in warm soil and water. Most pathogens and members of the indigenous microbiota are mesophilic, because they grow best at normal body temperature (37°C).

Psychrophiles prefer cold temperatures. They thrive in cold ocean water. At high altitudes, algae (often pink) can be seen living on snow. Biologists studying microbial life in the Antarctic have reported finding bacteria in a lake that has been iced over for at least 2,000 years.[c] These microbes thrive in an environment that is –13°C, has 20% salinity, and contains high concentrations of ammonia and sulfur.

Ironically, the optimum growth temperature of one group of psychrophiles (called **psychrotrophs**) is refrigerator temperature (4°C); perhaps you encountered some of these microbes (bread molds, for example) the last time you cleaned out your refrigerator. Microorganisms that prefer warmer temperatures, but can tolerate or endure very cold temperatures and can be preserved in the frozen state, are known as **psychroduric organisms**. Refer to Table 8-2 for the temperature ranges of psychrophilic, mesophilic, and thermophilic bacteria.

> Psychrophiles are organisms that "love" cold temperatures.

pH

The term "pH" refers to the hydrogen ion concentration of a solution and, thus, the acidity or alkalinity of the solution (see Appendix 3 on thePoint: "Basic Chemistry Concepts"). Most microorganisms prefer a neutral or slightly alkaline growth medium (pH 7.0–7.4), but *acidophilic* microbes (**acidophiles**), such as those that can live in the human stomach and in pickled foods, prefer a pH of 2 to 5. Fungi prefer acidic environments. Acidophiles thrive in highly acidic environments, such as those created by the production of sulfurous gases in hydrothermal vents and hot springs as well as in the debris produced from coal mining. **Alkaliphiles** prefer an alkaline environment (pH >8.5), such as that found inside the intestine (pH approximately 9), in soils laden with carbonate, and in so-called soda lakes. *Vibrio cholerae*—the bacterium that causes cholera—is the only human pathogen that grows well above pH 8.

> Acidophiles prefer acidic environments, whereas alkaliphiles prefer environments that are alkaline.

Osmotic Pressure and Salinity

Osmotic pressure is the pressure that is exerted on a cell membrane by solutions both inside and outside the cell. When cells are suspended in a solution, the

> Cells lose water and shrink when placed into a hypertonic solution.

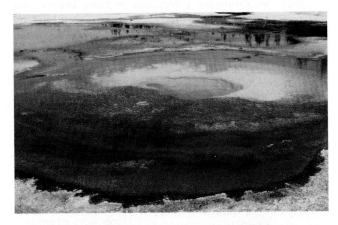

Figure 8-1. Colorful thermophiles living in a geothermal feature at Yellowstone National Park, WY. (Courtesy of Biomed Ed, Round Rock, TX.)

[c]www.pnas.org/cgi/doi/10.1073/pnas.1208607109

Table 8-2 Categories of Bacteria on the Basis of Growth Temperature

Category	Minimum Growth Temperature (°C)	Optimum Growth Temperature (°C)	Maximum Growth Temperature (°C)
Thermophiles	25	50–60	113
Mesophiles	10	20–40	45
Psychrophiles	−5	10–20	30

ideal situation is that the pressure inside the cell is equal to the pressure of the solution outside the cell. Substances dissolved in liquids are referred to as solutes. When the concentration of solutes in the environment outside of a cell is greater than the concentration of solutes inside the cell, the solution in which the cell is suspended is said to be **hypertonic**. In such a situation, whenever possible, water leaves the cell by osmosis in an attempt to equalize the two concentrations. **Osmosis** is defined as the movement of a solvent (e.g., water), through a permeable membrane, from a solution having a lower concentration of solute to a solution having a higher concentration of solute. If the cell is a human cell, such as a red blood cell (erythrocyte), the loss of water causes the cell to shrink; this shrinkage is called **crenation** and the cell is said to be **crenated** (Fig. 8-2). If the cell is a bacterial cell, having a rigid cell wall, the cell does not shrink. Instead, the cell membrane and cytoplasm shrink away from the cell wall. This condition, known as **plasmolysis**, inhibits bacterial cell growth and multiplication. Salts and sugars are added to certain foods as a way of preserving them. Bacteria that

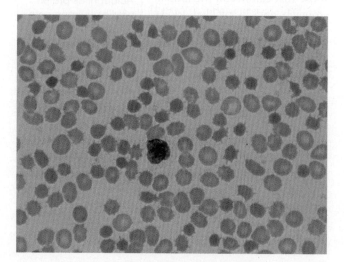

Figure 8-2. Stained peripheral blood smear showing numerous crenated red blood cells, which are also known as acanthocytes. The crenated red blood cells have developed a number of cell wall projections, thus giving the cells a spiked or "thorny" appearance. Acanthocytosis—the formation of acanthocytes—can be indicative of a number of hematologic disease processes. The larger purple-stained cell in the center of the photomicrograph is a white blood cell. (Courtesy of R. Zamel, R. Khan, RL Pollex, RA Hegele, and Wikimedia Commons.)

enter such hypertonic environments will die as a result of loss of water and desiccation.

When the concentration of solutes outside a cell is less than the concentration of solutes inside the cell, the solution in which the cell is suspended is said to be **hypotonic**. In such a situation, whenever possible, water enters the cell in an attempt to equalize the two concentrations. If the cell is a human cell, such as an erythrocyte, the increased water within the cell causes the cell to swell. If sufficient water enters, the cell will burst (lyse). In the case of erythrocytes, this bursting is called **hemolysis**. If a bacterial cell is placed in a hypotonic solution (such as distilled water), the cell may not burst (because of the rigid cell wall), but the fluid pressure within the cell increases greatly. This increased pressure occurs in cells having rigid cell walls such as plant cells and bacteria. If the pressure becomes so great that the cell ruptures, the escape of cytoplasm from the cell is referred to as **plasmoptysis**.

> Cells swell up, and sometimes burst, when placed into a hypotonic solution.

When the concentration of solutes outside a cell equals the concentration of solutes inside the cell, the solution is said to be **isotonic**. In an isotonic environment, excess water neither leaves nor enters the cell and, thus, no plasmolysis or plasmoptysis occurs; the cell has normal turgor (fullness). Refer to Figure 8-3 for a comparison of the effects of various solution concentrations on bacterial cells and red blood cells.

Sugar solutions for jellies and pickling brines (salt solutions) for meats preserve these foods by inhibiting the growth of most microorganisms. However, some types of molds and bacteria can survive and even grow in a salty environment.

Those microbes that actually prefer salty environments (such as the concentrated salt water found in the Great Salt Lake and solar salt evaporation ponds) are called **halophilic organisms**, *halo* referring to "salt" and *philic* meaning "to love." Microbes that live in the ocean, such as *V. cholerae* (mentioned earlier) and other *Vibrio* species, are halophilic. Organisms that do not prefer to live in salty environments but are capable of surviving there (such as *Staphylococcus aureus*) are referred to as **haloduric organisms**.

> Microorganisms that prefer salty environments are called halophiles.

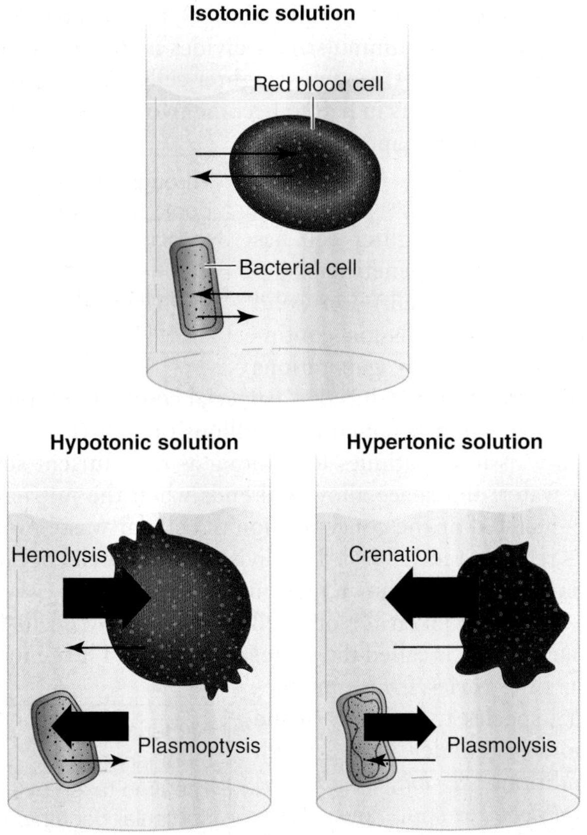

Isotonic solution

Red blood cell

Bacterial cell

Hypotonic solution

Hemolysis

Plasmoptysis

Hypertonic solution

Crenation

Plasmolysis

Figure 8-3. Effects of changes in osmotic pressure. No change in pressure occurs within the cell in an isotonic solution. Internal pressure is increased in a hypotonic solution, resulting in swelling of the cell. Internal pressure is decreased in a hypertonic solution, resulting in shrinking of the cell. (*Arrows* indicate the direction of water flow. The larger the arrow, the greater the amount of water flowing in that direction.)

Barometric Pressure

Most bacteria are not affected by minor changes in barometric pressure. Some thrive at normal atmospheric pressure (about 14.7 pounds per square inch [psi]). Others, known as **piezophiles**, thrive deep in the ocean and in oil wells, where the atmospheric pressure is very high. Some archaea, for example, are piezophiles, capable of living in the deepest parts of the ocean. Check thePoint for "A Closer Look at Barometric Pressure."

Gaseous Atmosphere

As discussed in Chapter 4, microorganisms vary with respect to the type of gaseous atmosphere that they require. For example, some microbes (obligate aerobes) prefer the same atmosphere that humans do (i.e., about 20%–21% oxygen and 78%–79% nitrogen, with all other atmospheric gases combined representing less than 1%). Although microaerophiles also require oxygen, they require reduced concentrations of oxygen (around 5%).

Obligate anaerobes are killed by the presence of oxygen. Thus, in nature, the types and concentrations of gases present in a particular environment determine which species of microbes are able to live there. To grow a particular microorganism in the laboratory, it is necessary to provide the atmosphere that it requires. For example, to obtain maximum growth in the laboratory, capnophiles require increased concentrations of carbon dioxide (usually from 5% to 10%).

STUDY AID

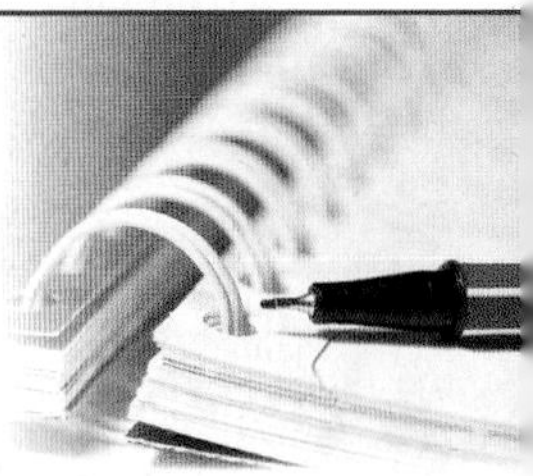

-Phile

The suffix *-phile* means to love something. For example, acidophiles are organisms that love acidic conditions; therefore, they live in acidic environments. Alkaliphiles live in alkaline environments. Halophiles live in salty environments. Piezophiles (formerly called barophiles) live in environments where there is high barometric pressure, such as at the bottom of the ocean. Thermophiles prefer hot temperatures. Mesophiles prefer moderate temperatures. Psychrophiles prefer cold temperatures. Microaerophiles live in environments containing reduced concentrations of oxygen (around 5% oxygen). Capnophiles grow best in environments rich in carbon dioxide.

Encouraging the Growth of Microbes In Vitro

There are many reasons why the growth of microbes is encouraged in microbiology laboratories. For example, technologists and technicians who work in clinical microbiology laboratories must be able to isolate microorganisms from clinical specimens and grow them on culture media so they can then gather information that will enable identification of any pathogens that are present. In microbiology research laboratories, scientists must culture microbes so that they can learn more about them, harvest antibiotics and other microbial products, test new antimicrobial agents, and produce vaccines. Microbes must also be cultured in genetic engineering laboratories and in the laboratories of certain food and beverage companies, as well as other industries.

Many different types of microbes can be cultured (grown) in vitro, including viruses, bacteria, fungi, and protozoa. In this chapter, emphasis is placed on culturing bacteria. Culturing other types of microbes will be mentioned only briefly.

Culturing Bacteria in the Laboratory

In many ways, modern microbiology laboratories resemble those of 50, 100, or even 150 years ago. Today's laboratories still use many of the same basic tools that were used in the past. For example, microbiologists still use compound light microscopes, Petri dishes containing solid culture media, tubes containing liquid culture media, Bunsen burners, wire inoculating loops, bottles of staining reagents, and incubators. However, a closer inspection will reveal many modern, commercially available products and instruments that would have been inconceivable in the days of Louis Pasteur and Robert Koch.

HISTORICAL NOTE

Culturing Bacteria in the Laboratory

The earliest successful attempts to culture microorganisms in a laboratory setting were made by Ferdinand Cohn (1872), Joseph Schroeter (1875), and Oscar Brefeld (1875). Robert Koch described his culture techniques in 1881. Initially, Koch used slices of boiled potatoes on which to culture bacteria, but he later developed both liquid and solid forms of artificial media. Gelatin was initially used as a solidifying agent in Koch's culture media, but in 1882, Fanny Hesse, the wife of Dr. Walther Hesse—one of Koch's assistants—suggested the use of agar. Frau Hesse (as she is most commonly called) had been using agar in her kitchen for many years as a solidifying agent in fruit and vegetable jellies. Another of Koch's assistants, Richard Julius Petri, invented glass Petri dishes in 1887 for use as containers for solid culture media and bacterial cultures. The Petri dishes in use today are virtually unchanged from the original design, except that most of today's laboratories use plastic, presterilized, disposable Petri dishes. In 1878, Joseph Lister became the first person to obtain a pure culture of a bacterium (*Streptococcus lactis*) in a liquid medium. As a result of their ability to obtain pure cultures of bacteria in their laboratories, Louis Pasteur and Robert Koch made significant contributions to the germ theory of disease.

Bacterial Growth

With respect to humans, the term *growth* refers to an increase in size; for example, going from a tiny newborn baby to a large adult. Although bacteria do increase in size before cell division, *bacterial growth* refers to an increase in the *number* of organisms rather than an increase in their size. Thus, with respect to bacteria, *growth* refers to

their proliferation or multiplication. When each bacterial cell reaches its optimum size, it divides by binary fission (bi meaning "two") into two daughter cells (i.e., each bacterium simply splits in half to become two identical cells). (Recall from Chapter 3 that DNA replication must occur before binary fission occurs, so that each daughter cell has exactly the same genetic makeup as the parent cell.) On solid medium, binary fission continues through many generations until a colony is produced. A bacterial colony is a mound or pile of bacteria containing millions of cells (Fig. 8-4). Binary fission continues for as long as the nutrient supply, water, and space allow and ends when the nutrients are depleted or the concentration of cellular waste products reaches a toxic level. The division of staphylococci by binary fission was shown in Figure 2-12.

> Throughout this book, the term *bacterial growth* refers to the proliferation or multiplication of bacteria.

The time taken for one cell to become two cells by binary fission is called the **generation time**. The generation time varies from one bacterial species to another. In the laboratory, under ideal growth conditions, *E. coli*, *V. cholerae*, *Staphylococcus* spp., and *Streptococcus* spp. all have a generation time of about 20 minutes, whereas some *Pseudomonas* and *Clostridium* spp. may divide every 10 minutes, and *Mycobacterium tuberculosis* may divide only every 18 to 24 hours. Bacteria with short generation times are referred to as rapid growers, whereas those with long generation times are referred to as slow growers.

> Bacteria multiply by binary fission. The time taken by a particular bacterial species to undergo binary fission is called that organism's generation time.

The growth of microorganisms in the body, in nature, or in the laboratory is greatly influenced by temperature,

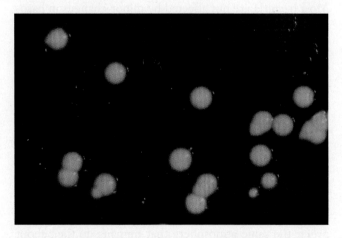

Figure 8-4. Bacterial colonies on the surface of a solid culture medium. These are colonies of *Klebsiella pneumoniae*, a fairly common cause of pneumonia and UTIs. The appearance (morphology) of bacterial colonies varies from species to species. (Courtesy of the CDC.)

pH, moisture content, available nutrients, and the characteristics of other organisms present. Therefore, the number of bacteria in nature fluctuates unpredictably because these factors vary with the seasons, rainfall, temperature, and time of day.

In the laboratory, however, a pure culture of a single species of bacteria can usually be maintained if the appropriate growth medium and environmental conditions are provided. The temperature, pH, and proper atmosphere are quite easily controlled to provide the optimum conditions for growth. Appropriate nutrients must be provided in the growth medium, including an appropriate energy and carbon source. Some bacteria, described as being *fastidious*, have complex nutritional requirements. Often, special mixtures of vitamins and amino acids must be added to the medium to culture these fastidious organisms. Some organisms will not grow at all on artificial culture media; these include obligate intracellular pathogens, such as viruses, rickettsias, and chlamydias. To propagate obligate intracellular pathogens in the laboratory, they must be inoculated into live animals, embryonated chicken eggs, or cell cultures. Other microorganisms that will not grow on artificial media include *Treponema pallidum* (the bacterium that causes syphilis) and *Mycobacterium leprae* (the bacterium that causes leprosy).

> Microorganisms that are difficult to grow in the laboratory are said to be fastidious.

Culture Media

The media (sing., medium) that are used in microbiology laboratories to culture bacteria are referred to as **artificial media** or **synthetic media**, because they do not occur naturally; rather, they are prepared in the laboratory. There are a number of ways of categorizing the media that are used to culture bacteria.

One way to classify culture media is based on whether the exact contents of the media are known. A **chemically defined medium** is one in which all the ingredients are known; this is because the medium was prepared in the laboratory by adding a certain number of grams of each of the components (e.g., carbohydrates, amino acids, salts). A **complex medium** is one in which the exact contents are not known. Complex media contain ground-up or digested extracts from animal organs (e.g., hearts, livers, brains), fish, yeasts, and plants, which provide the necessary nutrients, vitamins, and minerals.

Culture media can also be categorized as liquid or solid (Fig. 8-5). Liquid media (also known as broths) are contained in tubes and are thus often referred to as tubed media. Solid media are prepared by adding agar to liquid media and then pouring the media into tubes or Petri dishes, where the media solidifies. Bacteria are then grown on the surface of the agar-containing solid media. Agar is a complex polysaccharide that is obtained from a red marine alga; it is used as a solidifying agent, much like gelatin is used as a solidifying agent in the kitchen.

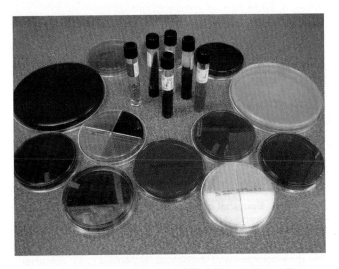

Figure 8-5. Examples of solid and liquid culture media used in a Clinical Microbiology Laboratory. (Courtesy of Dr. Robert Fader and Biomed Ed, Round Rock, TX.)

An **enriched medium** is a broth or solid medium containing a rich supply of special nutrients that promotes the growth of fastidious organisms. It is usually prepared by adding extra nutrients to a medium called nutrient agar. Blood agar (nutrient agar plus 5% sheep red blood cells) and chocolate agar (nutrient agar plus powdered hemoglobin) are examples of solid enriched media that are used routinely in the clinical bacteriology laboratory. Blood agar is bright red, whereas chocolate agar is brown (the color of chocolate). Although both of these media contain hemoglobin, chocolate agar is considered to be more enriched than blood agar because the hemoglobin is more readily accessible in chocolate agar. Chocolate agar is used to culture important, fastidious, bacterial pathogens, such as *Neisseria gonorrhoeae* and *Haemophilus influenzae*, which will not grow on blood agar.

> Blood agar and chocolate agar are examples of enriched media.

A **selective medium** has added inhibitors that discourage the growth of certain organisms without inhibiting growth of the organism being sought. For example, MacConkey agar inhibits growth of Gram-positive bacteria and thus is selective for Gram-negative bacteria. Phenylethyl alcohol (PEA) agar and colistin–nalidixic acid (CNA) agar inhibit growth of Gram-negative bacteria and are thus selective for Gram-positive bacteria. Thayer–Martin agar and Martin-Lewis agar (chocolate agars containing extra nutrients plus several antimicrobial agents) are selective for *N. gonorrhoeae*. Only salt-tolerant (haloduric) bacteria can grow on mannitol salt agar (MSA).

> A selective medium is used to discourage the growth of certain organisms without inhibiting growth of the organism being sought.

A **differential medium** permits the differentiation of organisms that grow on the medium. For example,

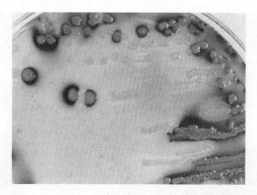

Figure 8-6. Bacterial colonies on MacConkey agar, which is a selective and differential medium. It is selective for Gram-negative bacteria, meaning that only Gram-negative bacteria will grow on this medium. Colonies of lactose fermenters (pink colonies) and nonlactose fermenters (clear colonies) can be seen. (From Winn WC Jr, et al. *Koneman's Color Atlas and Textbook of Diagnostic Microbiology*. 6th ed. Philadelphia, PA: Lippincott Williams & Wilkins; 2006.)

MacConkey agar is frequently used to differentiate among various Gram-negative bacilli that are isolated from fecal specimens. Gram-negative bacteria capable of fermenting lactose (an ingredient of MacConkey agar) produce pink colonies, whereas those that are unable to ferment lactose produce colorless colonies (Fig. 8-6). Thus, MacConkey agar differentiates between lactose-fermenting (LF) and nonlactose-fermenting (NLF) Gram-negative bacteria. MSA is used to screen for *S. aureus*; *S. aureus* not only will grow on MSA, but also turns the originally pink medium to yellow because of its ability to ferment mannitol (Fig. 8-7). In a sense, blood

> A differential medium allows one to readily differentiate among the various types of organisms that are growing on the medium.

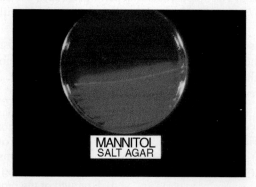

MANNITOL
SALT AGAR

Figure 8-7. MSA, a selective and differential medium, is used to screen for *Staphylococcus aureus*. Any bacteria capable of growing in a 7.5% sodium chloride concentration will grow on this medium, but *S. aureus* will turn the medium yellow because of its ability to ferment the mannitol in the medium. The organism growing on the upper section of the plate is unable to ferment mannitol, but the organism growing on the lower section is a mannitol fermenter. (From Koneman E, et al. *Color Atlas and Textbook of Diagnostic Microbiology*. 5th ed. Philadelphia, PA: Lippincott Williams & Wilkins; 1997.)

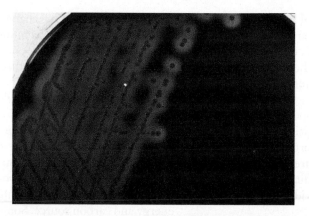

Figure 8-8. Colonies of β-hemolytic *Streptococcus pyogenes* on a blood agar plate. The clear zones (β-hemolysis) surrounding the colonies are caused by enzymes (hemolysins) that lyse the red blood cells in the agar. (Note: Information about the Greek alphabet can be found in Appendix D.) (From Winn WC Jr, et al. *Koneman's Color Atlas and Textbook of Diagnostic Microbiology*. 6th ed. Philadelphia, PA: Lippincott Williams & Wilkins; 2006.)

agar is also a differential medium because it is used to determine the type of hemolysis (alteration or destruction of red blood cells) that the bacterial isolate produces (Fig. 8-8).

The various categories of media (enriched, selective, and differential) are not mutually exclusive. For example, as just seen, blood agar is enriched and differential. MacConkey agar and MSA are selective and differential. PEA and CNA are enriched and selective: they are blood agars to which selective inhibitory substances have been added. Thayer–Martin and Martin-Lewis agars are highly enriched and highly selective.

Thioglycollate broth (THIO) is a very popular liquid medium for use in the bacteriology laboratory. THIO supports the growth of all categories of bacteria from obligate aerobes to obligate anaerobes. How is this possible? Within the tube of THIO there is a concentration gradient of dissolved oxygen. The concentration of oxygen decreases with depth. The concentration of oxygen in the broth at the top of the tube is about 20% to 21%. At the bottom of the tube, there is no oxygen in the broth. Organisms will grow only in that part of the broth where the oxygen concentration meets their needs (Fig. 8-9). For example, microaerophiles will grow where there is around 5% oxygen, and obligate anaerobes will grow only at the very bottom of the tube where there is no oxygen. Facultative anaerobes can grow anywhere in the tube. (Recall that facultative anaerobes can live in the presence or absence of oxygen.)

Inoculation of Culture Media

In clinical microbiology laboratories, culture media are routinely inoculated with clinical specimens (i.e., specimens that have been collected from patients suspected of having infectious diseases). **Inoculation** of a liquid medium involves adding a portion of the specimen to

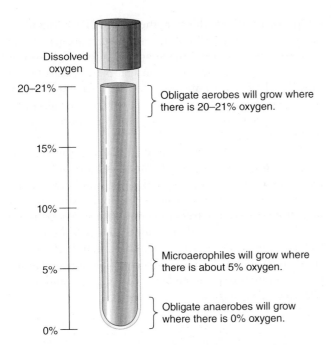

Dissolved oxygen

20–21% ⎱ Obligate aerobes will grow where there is 20–21% oxygen.

Microaerophiles will grow where there is about 5% oxygen.

Obligate anaerobes will grow where there is 0% oxygen.

Figure 8-9. Thioglycollate broth contains a concentration gradient of dissolved oxygen, ranging from 20% to 21% O_2 at the top of the tube to 0% O_2 at the bottom of the tube. A particular bacterium will grow only in that part of the broth containing the concentration of oxygen that it requires.

the medium. Inoculation of a solid or plated medium involves the use of a sterile inoculating loop to apply a portion of the specimen to the surface of the medium; a process commonly referred to as *streaking* (Fig. 8-10).

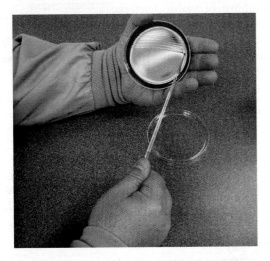

Figure 8-10. Laboratory professional demonstrating the proper method of inoculating the surface of an agar plate. The plate is held in the palm of one hand. The other hand is used to lightly drag the inoculating loop over the surface of the solid culture medium. The inoculating loop is held in much the same manner as a small camel-hair paint brush is held by an artist when applying paint to the surface of a canvas. This person would be wearing gloves if an actual specimen was being inoculated to the agar plate. (Additional information regarding the proper method of "streaking" can be found on thePoint.) (Courtesy of Dr. Robert Fader and Biomed Ed, Round Rock, TX.)

The proper method of inoculating plated media to obtain well-isolated colonies is described in Appendix 5 on thePoint: "Clinical Microbiology Laboratory Procedures."

Importance of Using "Aseptic Technique"

Individuals working in a microbiology laboratory must practice what is known as **aseptic technique** and must understand its importance. Aseptic technique is practiced to prevent (a) microbiology professionals from becoming infected, (b) contamination of their work environment, and (c) contamination of clinical specimens, cultures, and subcultures. For example, when inoculating plated media, it is important to keep the Petri dish lid in place at all times, except for the few seconds that it takes to inoculate the specimen to the surface of the culture medium. Every additional second that the lid is off provides an opportunity for airborne organisms (e.g., bacterial and fungal spores) to land on the surface of the medium, where they will then grow. Such unwanted organisms are referred to as **contaminants**, and the plate is said to be *contaminated*. Of equal importance is to maintain the sterility of the media before inoculation and to avoid touching the agar surface with fingertips or other nonsterile objects. Inoculating media within a biologic safety cabinet (BSC) minimizes the possibility of contamination and protects the laboratory worker from becoming infected with the organism(s) that he or she is working with. BSCs are further discussed in Appendix 4 on thePoint: "Responsibilities of the Clinical Microbiology Laboratory."

> Aseptic technique is practiced in the microbiology laboratory to prevent infection of individuals and contamination of the work environment, clinical specimens, and cultures.

Incubation

After media are inoculated, they must be incubated (i.e., they must be placed into a chamber [called an *incubator*] that contains the appropriate atmosphere and moisture level and is set to maintain the appropriate temperature). This is called **incubation**. To culture most human pathogens, the incubator is set at 35° to 37°C. Three types of incubators are used in a clinical microbiology laboratory:

> The three types of incubators used in the microbiology laboratory are CO_2 incubators, non-CO2 incubators, and anaerobic incubators.

1. A CO_2 (carbon dioxide) incubator is an incubator to which a cylinder of CO_2 is attached. CO_2 is periodically introduced into the incubator to maintain a CO_2 concentration of about 5% to 10%. Such an incubator is used to isolate capnophiles (organisms that grow best in atmospheres containing increased CO_2). It is important to keep in mind that a CO_2 incubator

contains oxygen (about 15% to 20%) in addition to CO_2. Thus, a CO_2 incubator is *not* an anaerobic incubator.

2. A non-CO_2 incubator is an incubator containing room air; thus, it contains about 20% to 21% oxygen.
3. An anaerobic incubator is an incubator containing an atmosphere devoid of oxygen.

Once a particular species of bacteria has been isolated from a clinical specimen, it can be separated from any other organisms that were present in the specimen and can be grown as a pure culture. The term *pure culture* refers to the fact that there is only one bacterial species present. The changes in a bacterial population over an extended period follow a definite predictable pattern that can be shown by plotting the population growth curve on a graph (discussed later in this chapter).

> A pure culture is a culture that contains only one species of organism.

Bacterial Population Counts

Microbiologists sometimes need to know how many bacteria are present in a particular liquid at any given time (e.g., to determine the degree of bacterial contamination in drinking water, milk, and other foods). The microbiologist may (a) determine the total number of bacterial cells in the liquid (the total number would include both viable and dead cells) or (b) determine the number of viable (living) cells.

Various types of instruments are available to determine the total number of cells (e.g., a spectrophotometer could be used). In a spectrophotometer, a beam of light is passed through the liquid. When no bacteria are present in the liquid, the liquid is clear, and a large amount of light passes through. As bacteria increase in number, the liquid becomes turbid (cloudy), and less light passes through. Turbidity increases (i.e., the solution becomes more cloudy) as the number of organisms increases; therefore, the amount of transmitted light decreases as the bacteria increase in number. Formulas are available to equate the amount of transmitted light to the concentration of organisms in the liquid, which is usually expressed as the number of organisms per milliliter (mL) of suspension.

The **viable plate count** is used to determine the number of viable bacteria in a liquid sample, such as milk, water, ground food diluted in water, or a broth culture. In this procedure, serial dilutions of the sample are prepared, and then 0.1-mL or 1-mL aliquots (portions) are inoculated onto plates of nutrient agar. After overnight incubation, the number of colonies is counted. (Usually, a plate containing 30 to 300 colonies is used.) To determine the concentration of bacteria in the original sample, the number of colonies must be multiplied by the dilution factor(s). For example, if 220 colonies were counted on an agar plate that had been inoculated with a 1.0-mL

sample of a 1:10,000 dilution, there were $220 \times 10,000 = 2,200,000$ bacteria/mL of the original material at the time the dilutions were made and cultured. If, however, 220 colonies were counted on an agar plate that had been inoculated with a 0.1-mL sample of a 1:10,000 dilution, there were $220 \times 10 \times 10,000 = 22,000,000$ bacteria/mL of the original material at the time the dilutions were made and cultured.

In the clinical microbiology laboratory, a viable cell count is an important part of a urine culture. (The technique is described in Chapter 13.) The number of viable bacteria per milliliter of a urine specimen is used as an indicator of a urinary tract infection (UTI). As explained in Chapter 13, high colony counts may also be caused by contamination of the urine specimen with indigenous microbiota during specimen collection or failure to refrigerate the specimen between collection and transport to the laboratory.

Bacterial Population Growth Curve

A **population growth curve** for any particular species of bacterium may be determined by growing a pure culture of the organism in a liquid medium at a constant temperature. Samples of the culture are collected at fixed intervals (e.g., every 30 minutes), and the number of viable organisms in each sample is determined. The data are then plotted on logarithmic graph paper. The graph in Figure 8-11 was obtained by plotting the logarithm (log_{10}) of the number of viable bacteria (on the vertical or *y*-axis) against the incubation time (on the horizontal or *x*-axis). (If you are not familiar with logarithms, use an Internet search engine or refer to a math book.)

> A bacterial population growth curve consists of four phases: a lag phase, a log phase, a stationary phase, and a death phase.

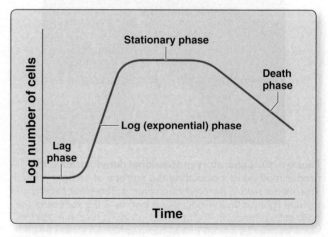

Figure 8-11. A population growth curve of living organisms. The logarithm of the number of bacteria per milliliter of medium is plotted against time. See text for details. (Redrawn from Harvey RA, et al. *Lippincott's Illustrated Reviews: Microbiology.* 3rd ed. Philadelphia, PA: Lippincott Williams & Wilkins; 2013.)

The growth curve consists of the following four phases:

1. The first phase of the growth curve is the **lag phase**, during which the bacteria absorb nutrients, synthesize enzymes, and prepare for cell division. The bacteria do not increase in number during the lag phase.

2. The second phase of the growth curve is the **logarithmic growth phase** (also known as the **log phase** or exponential growth phase). In the log phase, the bacteria multiply so rapidly that the number of organisms doubles with each generation time (i.e., the number of bacteria increases exponentially). Growth rate is the greatest during the log phase. The log phase is always brief, unless the rapidly dividing culture is maintained by constant addition of nutrients and frequent removal of waste products. When plotted on logarithmic graph paper, the log phase appears as a steeply sloped straight line.

3. As the nutrients in the liquid medium are used up and the concentration of toxic waste products from the metabolizing bacteria build up, the rate of division slows, such that the number of bacteria that are dividing equals the number that are dying. The result is the **stationary phase**. It is during this phase that the culture is at its greatest population density.

4. As overcrowding occurs, the concentration of toxic waste products continues to increase and the nutrient supply decreases. The microorganisms then die at a rapid rate; this is the **death phase** or **decline phase**. The culture may die completely, or a few microorganisms may continue to survive for months. If the bacterial species is a spore former, it will produce spores to survive beyond this phase. When cells are observed in old cultures of bacteria in the death phase, some of them look different from healthy organisms seen in the log phase. As a result of unfavorable conditions, morphologic changes in the cells may appear. Some cells undergo involution and assume various shapes, becoming long, filamentous rods or branching or globular forms that are difficult to identify. Some develop without a cell wall and are referred to as protoplasts, spheroplasts, or L-phase variants (L-forms). When these involuted forms are inoculated into a fresh nutrient medium, they usually revert to the original shape of the healthy bacteria.

Many industrial and research procedures depend on the maintenance of an essential species of microorganism. These are continuously cultured in a controlled environment called a *chemostat* (Fig. 8-12), which regulates the supply of nutrients and the removal of waste products and excess microorganisms. Chemostats are used in industries where yeast is grown to produce beer and wine, where fungi and bacteria are cultivated to produce antibiotics, where *E. coli* cells are grown for genetic research, and in any other process needing a constant source of microorganisms.

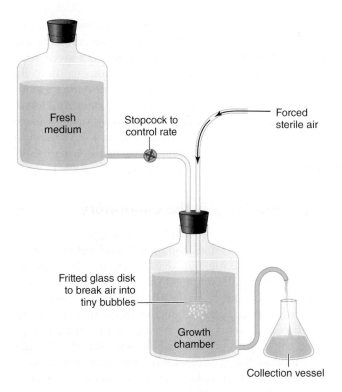

Figure 8-12. Chemostat used for continuous cultures. Rates of growth can be controlled either by controlling the rate at which new medium enters the growth chamber or by limiting a required growth factor in the medium.

Culturing Viruses and Other Obligate Intracellular Pathogens in the Laboratory

Recall from Chapter 4 that obligate intracellular pathogens are microbes that can survive and multiply only within living cells (called host cells). Obligate intracellular pathogens include viruses and two groups of Gram-negative bacteria—rickettsias and chlamydias. Because obligate intracellular pathogens will not grow on artificial (synthetic) media, they present a challenge to laboratorians when large numbers of the organisms are required for diagnostic or research purposes (e.g., development of vaccines and new drugs). To grow such organisms in the laboratory, they must be inoculated into embryonated chicken eggs, laboratory animals, or cell cultures.

> Obligate intracellular pathogens can be propagated in the laboratory using embryonated chicken eggs, laboratory animals, or cell cultures.

In the virology laboratory, cell cultures are primarily used for the propagation of viruses. Because a given virus can only attach to and infect cells that bear appropriate cell surface receptors, it is necessary to maintain several different types of cell lines in the virology laboratory. Examples of cell lines are kidney cells from monkeys, rabbits, or humans, human and mink lung cells, and various cancer cell lines. After appropriate cells are inoculated with a clinical specimen suspected of containing a specific type of virus, the cells are incubated for several days, and then examined microscopically. If present, a given virus will cause specific morphologic alterations to the cells. These changes are called cytopathic effect (CPE). Examples of CPE include rounding, swelling, and shrinking of cells, or cells may become granular, glassy, vacuolated, or fused (illustrated in Fig. 13-20 in Chapter 13). Viruses can then be identified, based upon the particular type of CPE that they cause in a specific cell line.

Culturing Fungi in the Laboratory

Fungi (including yeasts, molds, and dimorphic fungi) will grow on and in various solid and liquid culture media. There is no one medium that is best for all medically important fungi. Examples of solid culture media used to grow fungi include brain–heart infusion (BHI) agar, BHI agar with blood, and Sabouraud dextrose agar (SDA). Antibacterial agents are often added to the media to suppress the growth of bacteria. The low pH of SDA (pH 5.6) inhibits the growth of most bacteria; thus, SDA is selective for fungi. Laboratory personnel must exercise caution when culturing fungi, because the spores of certain fungi are highly infectious. Because of the potential danger, a Class II BSC must be used.

Culturing Protozoa in the Laboratory

Most clinical microbiology laboratories do not culture protozoa, but techniques are available for culturing protozoa in reference and research laboratories. Examples of protozoa that can be cultured in vitro are amebae (e.g., *Acanthamoeba* spp., *Balamuthia* spp., *Entamoeba histolytica, Naegleria fowleri), Giardia lamblia, Leishmania* spp., *Toxoplasma gondii, Trichomonas vaginalis,* and *Trypanosoma cruzi.* Of these protozoa, it is of greatest importance to culture *Acanthamoeba, Balamuthia,* and *N. fowleri* in a clinical microbiology laboratory. These amebae can cause serious (often fatal) infections of the central nervous system—infections that are difficult to diagnose by other methods. Parasitic protozoa are further discussed in Chapter 21.

Inhibiting the Growth of Microbes In Vitro

In certain environments, it is necessary or desirable to inhibit the growth of microbes. In hospitals, nursing homes, and other healthcare institutions, for example, it is necessary to inhibit the growth of pathogens so that they will not infect patients, staff members, or visitors. Other environments in which it is necessary or desirable to inhibit microbial growth include food and beverage processing plants, restaurants, kitchens, and bathrooms.

Definition of Terms

Before discussing the various methods used to destroy or inhibit the growth of microbes, a number of terms should be understood as they apply to microbiology.

Sterilization

Sterilization involves the destruction or elimination of *all* microbes, including cells, spores, and viruses. When something is *sterile*, it is devoid of microbial life. In healthcare facilities, sterilization of objects can be accomplished by physical or chemical methods. Dry heat, autoclaving (steam under pressure), ethylene oxide gas, and various liquid chemicals (such as formaldehyde) are the principal sterilizing agents in healthcare facilities. In some situations, certain types of radiation (e.g., ultraviolet light and gamma rays) are also used. These techniques are discussed later in this chapter.

> Sterilization involves the destruction or elimination of all microbes.

Disinfection, Pasteurization, Disinfectants, Antiseptics, and Sanitization

Disinfection describes the elimination of most or all pathogens (except bacterial spores) from nonliving objects. In healthcare settings, objects usually are disinfected by liquid chemicals or wet pasteurization. The heating process developed by Pasteur to kill microbes in wine—*pasteurization*—is a method of disinfecting liquids. Pasteurization is used today to eliminate pathogens from milk and most other beverages. It should be remembered that pasteurization is not a sterilization procedure, because not all microbes are destroyed.

> Disinfection involves the elimination of most or all pathogens (except bacterial spores) from nonliving objects.

Chemicals used to disinfect inanimate objects, such as bedside equipment and operating rooms, are called **disinfectants**. Disinfectants do not kill spores (i.e., they are not sporicidal). Because they are strong chemical substances, disinfectants cannot be used on living tissue. **Antiseptics** are solutions used to disinfect skin and other living tissues. **Sanitization** is the reduction of microbial populations to levels considered safe by public health standards, such as those applied to restaurants.

Microbicidal Agents

The suffix *-cide* or *-cidal* refers to "killing," as in the words homicide, suicide, and genocide. General terms like **germicidal agents** (*germicides*), **biocidal agents** (*biocides*), and **microbicidal agents** (*microbicides*) are disinfectants or antiseptics that kill microbes. **Bactericidal agents**

> Agents having the suffix "-cidal" kill organisms, whereas agents having the suffix "-static" merely inhibit their growth and reproduction.

(*bactericides*) specifically kill bacteria, but not necessarily bacterial endospores. Because spore coats are thick and resistant to the effects of many disinfectants, **sporicidal agents** are required to kill bacterial endospores. **Fungicidal agents** (*fungicides*) kill fungi, including fungal spores. **Algicidal agents** (*algicides*) are used to kill algae in swimming pools and hot tubs. **Viricidal agents** (or *viricidal agents*) destroy viruses. **Pseudomonicidal agents** kill *Pseudomonas* species, and **tuberculocidal agents** kill *M. tuberculosis*.

Microbistatic Agents

A **microbistatic agent** is a drug or chemical that inhibits reproduction of microorganisms, but does not necessarily kill them. A **bacteriostatic agent** is one that specifically inhibits the metabolism and reproduction of bacteria. Some of the drugs used to treat bacterial diseases are bacteriostatic, whereas others are bactericidal. Freeze-drying (lyophilization) and rapid freezing (using liquid nitrogen) are microbistatic techniques that are used to preserve microbes for future use or study.

Lyophilization is a process that combines dehydration (drying) and freezing. Lyophilized materials are frozen in a vacuum; the container is then sealed to maintain the inactive state. This freeze-drying method is widely used in industry to preserve foods, antibiotics, antisera, microorganisms, and other biologic materials. It should be remembered that lyophilization cannot be used to kill microorganisms, but, rather, is used to prevent them from reproducing and to store them for future use.

> Lyophilization is a good method of preserving microorganisms for future use.

Sepsis, Asepsis, Aseptic Technique, Antisepsis, and Antiseptic Technique

Sepsis refers to the presence of pathogens in blood or tissues, whereas **asepsis** means the absence of pathogens. The two general categories of aseptic technique—medical and surgical asepsis—are described in detail in Chapter 12. Various techniques, collectively referred to as **aseptic techniques**, are used to eliminate and exclude pathogens. Earlier in this chapter, you learned of the importance of using aseptic technique in the microbiology laboratory when inoculating culture media. In other areas of the hospital, aseptic techniques include hand hygiene[d]; the use of sterile gloves, masks, and gowns; sterilization of surgical instruments and other equipment; and the use of disinfectants and antiseptics. **Antisepsis** is the prevention of infection. **Antiseptic technique**, developed by Joseph Lister in 1867, refers to the use of

antiseptics. Antiseptic technique is a type of aseptic technique. Lister used dilute carbolic acid (phenol) to cleanse surgical wounds and equipment and a carbolic acid aerosol to prevent harmful microorganisms from entering the surgical field or contaminating the patient.

Sterile Technique

Sterile technique is practiced when it is necessary to exclude *all* microorganisms from a particular area, so that the area will be sterile. In Chapter 12, you will learn how sterile technique is used in areas of the hospital such as the operating room.

Using Physical Methods to Inhibit Microbial Growth

The methods used to destroy or inhibit microbial life are either physical or chemical, and sometimes both types are used. Physical methods commonly used in hospitals, clinics, and laboratories to destroy or control pathogens include heat, the combination of heat and pressure, desiccation, radiation, sonic disruption, and filtration. Each of these methods will now be briefly discussed.

Heat

Heat is the most practical, efficient, and inexpensive method of sterilization of those inanimate objects and materials that can withstand high temperatures. Because of these advantages, it is the means most frequently used.

> Heat is the most common type of sterilization for inanimate objects able to withstand high temperatures.

Two factors—*temperature* and *time*—determine the effectiveness of heat for sterilization. There is considerable variation from organism to organism in their susceptibility to heat; pathogens are usually more susceptible than nonpathogens. Also, the higher the temperature, the shorter the time required to kill the organisms. The **thermal death point (TDP)** of any particular species of microorganism is the lowest temperature that will kill all the organisms in a standardized pure culture within a specified period. The **thermal death time (TDT)** is the length of time necessary to sterilize a pure culture at a specified temperature.

In practical applications of heat for sterilization, one must consider the material in which a mixture of microorganisms and their spores may be found. Pus, feces, vomitus, mucus, and blood contain proteins that serve as a protective coating to insulate the pathogens; when these substances are present on bedding, bandages, surgical instruments, and syringes, very high temperatures are required to destroy vegetative (growing) microorganisms and spores. In practice, the most effective procedure is to wash away the protein debris with strong soap, hot water, and a disinfectant, and then sterilize the equipment or materials with heat.

---

[d]The term "hand hygiene" refers to handwashing; the use of alcohol-based gels, rinses, and foams; keeping fingernails clean and short; and not wearing artificial fingernails or rings.

Dry Heat. Dry-heat baking in a thermostatically controlled oven provides effective sterilization of metals, glassware, some powders, oils, and waxes. These items must be baked at 160° to 165°C for 2 hours or at 170° to 180°C for 1 hour. An ordinary oven of the type found in most homes may be used if the temperature remains constant. The effectiveness of dry-heat sterilization depends on how deeply the heat penetrates throughout the material, and the items to be baked must be positioned so that the hot air circulates freely among them.

Incineration (burning) is an effective means of destroying contaminated disposable materials. An incinerator must never be overloaded with moist or protein-laden materials, such as feces, vomitus, or pus, because the contaminating microorganisms within these moist substances may not be destroyed if the heat does not readily penetrate and burn them. Flaming the surface of metal forceps and wire bacteriologic loops is an effective way to kill microorganisms and, for many years, was a common laboratory procedure. Flaming is accomplished by briefly holding the end of the loop or forceps in the inner, hottest portion of a gas flame (Fig. 8-13). Open flames are dangerous, however, and, for this reason, are rarely used in modern microbiology laboratories, in which sterile, disposable, plastic inoculating loops are primarily used. Today, whenever wire inoculating loops are used, heat sterilization is usually accomplished using electrical heating devices (Fig. 8-13).

Moist Heat. Heat applied in the presence of moisture, as in boiling or steaming, is faster and more effective than dry heat, and can be accomplished at a lower temperature; thus, it is less destructive to many materials that otherwise would be damaged at higher temperatures. Moist heat causes proteins to coagulate (as occurs when eggs are hard boiled). Because cellular enzymes are proteins, they are inactivated by moist heat, leading to cell death.

The vegetative forms of most pathogens are quite easily destroyed by boiling for 30 minutes. Thus, clean articles made of metal and glass, such as syringes, needles, and simple instruments, may be disinfected by boiling for 30 minutes. Because the temperature at which water boils is lower at higher altitudes, water should always be boiled for longer times at high altitudes. Boiling is not always effective, however, because heat-resistant bacterial endospores, mycobacteria, and viruses may be present. The endospores of the bacteria that cause anthrax, tetanus, gas gangrene, and botulism, as well as hepatitis viruses, are especially heat resistant and often survive boiling. Also, because thermophiles thrive at high temperatures, boiling is not an effective means of killing them.

An **autoclave** is like a large metal pressure cooker that uses steam under pressure to completely destroy all microbial life (Fig. 8-14). The increased pressure raises the temperature above the temperature of boiling water (i.e., greater than 100°C), and forces the steam into the materials being sterilized. Autoclaving at a pressure of 15 psi, at a temperature of 121.5°C, for 20 minutes, kills vegetative microorganisms, bacterial endospores, and viruses, as long as they are not protected by pus, feces, vomitus, blood, or other proteinaceous substances. Some types of equipment and certain materials, such as rubber, which may be damaged by high temperatures, can be autoclaved at lower temperatures for longer periods. The timing must be carefully determined on the basis of contents and compactness of the load. All articles must be properly packaged and arranged within the autoclave to allow steam to penetrate each package completely. Cans should remain open, bottles covered loosely with foil or cotton, and instruments wrapped in cloth. Sealed containers should not be autoclaved.

> Autoclaves should be set to run 20 minutes at a pressure of 15 psi and a temperature of 121.5°C.

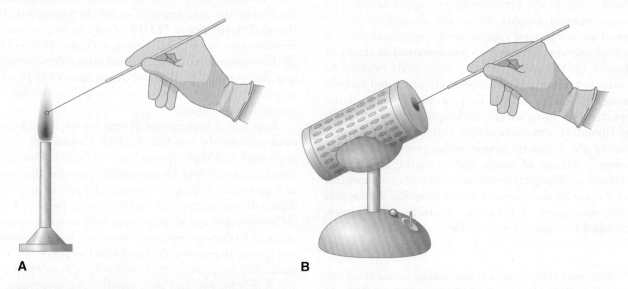

A   **B**

Figure 8-13. Dry-heat sterilization. A. Flaming a wire inoculating loop in a Bunsen burner flame. **B.** Sterilizing a wire inoculating loop using an electrical heating device.

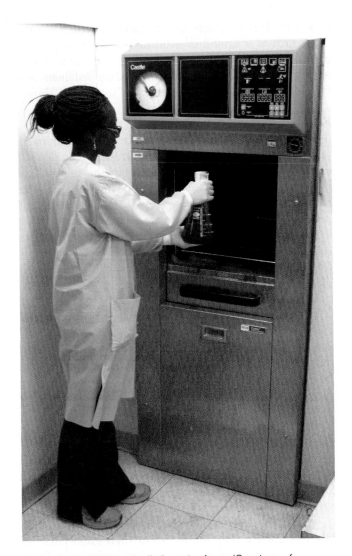

Figure 8-14. A large, built-in autoclave. (Courtesy of Dr. Robert Fader and Biomed Ed, Round Rock, TX.)

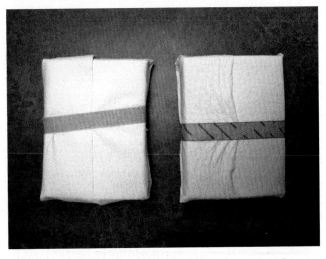

Figure 8-15. Autoclave tape. Left: Appearance of the tape before autoclaving. Right: Dark lines appear on the tape after autoclaving. The dark lines indicate that the proper temperature was achieved. (Courtesy of Dr. Robert Fader and Biomed Ed, Round Rock, TX.)

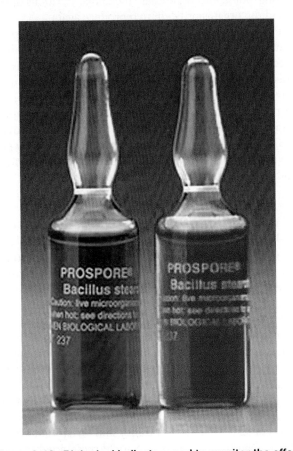

Figure 8-16. Biological indicator used to monitor the effectiveness of autoclaving. Sealed ampules containing bacterial spores suspended in a growth medium are placed within the load to be sterilized. Following sterilization, the ampules are incubated at 35°C. If the spores were killed, there will be no change in the color of the medium; it will remain purple. If the spores were not killed, germination will occur, and acid production by the bacteria will cause the pH indicator in the medium to change from purple to yellow. (Courtesy of Fisher Scientific.)

Pressure-sensitive autoclave tape (Fig. 8-15) and commercially available strips or solutions containing bacterial spores (Fig. 8-16) can be used as quality-control measures to ensure that autoclaves are functioning properly. Autoclave tape has diagonal markings that contain an ink that changes color (usually from beige to black) after exposure to proper autoclave temperature (121.5°C). After the spore strips or solutions are used, they are examined to see whether the spores were killed.

Home canning conducted without the use of a pressure cooker does not destroy the endospores of bacteria—notably the anaerobe, *Clostridium botulinum*. Occasionally, local newspapers report cases of food poisoning resulting from the ingestion of *C. botulinum* toxins in improperly canned fruits, vegetables, and meats. Botulism food poisoning is preventable by properly washing and pressure cooking (autoclaving) food.

An effective way to disinfect clothing, bedding, and dishes is to use hot water (greater than 60°C) with detergent or soap and to agitate the solution around the items.

This combination of heat, mechanical action, and chemical inhibition is deadly to most pathogens. The best way to remove microbes from a kitchen sponge is to rinse it, wring it out, and then microwave it for 30 to 60 seconds.[e]

Cold

Most microorganisms are not killed by cold temperatures and freezing, but their metabolic activities are slowed, greatly inhibiting their growth. Refrigeration merely slows the growth of most microorganisms; it does not completely inhibit growth. Slow freezing causes ice crystals to form within cells and may rupture the cell membranes and cell walls of some bacteria; hence, slow freezing should not be used as a way to preserve or store bacteria. Rapid freezing, using liquid nitrogen, is a good way to preserve foods, biologic specimens, and bacterial cultures. It places bacteria into a state of suspended animation. Then, when the temperature is raised above the freezing point, the organisms' metabolic reactions speed up and the organisms begin to reproduce again.

> Refrigeration cannot be relied upon to kill microorganisms; it merely slows their metabolism and their rate of growth.

Persons who are involved in the preparation and preservation of foods must be aware that thawing foods allow bacterial spores in the foods to germinate and microorganisms to resume growth. Consequently, refreezing of thawed foods is an unsafe practice, because it preserves the millions of microbes that might be present, leading to rapid deterioration of the food when it is rethawed. Also, if the endospores of *C. botulinum* or *Clostridium perfringens* were present, the viable bacteria would begin to produce the toxins that cause food poisoning.

Desiccation

For many centuries, foods have been preserved by drying. However, even when moisture and nutrients are lacking, many dried microorganisms remain viable, although they cannot reproduce. Foods, antisera, toxins, antitoxins, antibiotics, and pure cultures of microorganisms are often preserved by lyophilization—the combined use of freezing and drying (discussed previously).

In the hospital or clinical environment, healthcare professionals should keep in mind that dried viable pathogens may be present in dried matter, including blood, pus, fecal material, and dust that are found on floors, in bedding, on clothing, and in wound dressings. Should these dried materials be disturbed, such as by dry dusting, the microbes would be easily transmitted through the air or by contact. They would then grow rapidly if

> In a hospital setting, dried clinical specimens and dust may contain viable microorganisms.

they settled in a suitable moist, warm nutrient environment such as a wound or a burn. Therefore, important precautions that must be observed include wet mopping of floors, damp dusting of furniture, rolling bed linens and towels carefully, and proper disposal of wound dressings.

Radiation

The sun is not a particularly reliable disinfecting agent because it kills only those microorganisms that are exposed to direct sunlight. The rays of the sun include the long infrared (heat) rays, the visible light rays, and the shorter ultraviolet (UV) rays. The UV rays, which do not penetrate glass and building materials, are effective only in the air and on surfaces. They do, however, penetrate cells and, thus, can cause damage to DNA. When this occurs, genes may be so severely damaged that the cell dies (especially unicellular microorganisms) or is drastically changed.

In practice, a UV lamp (often called a germicidal lamp) is useful for reducing the number of microorganisms in the air. Its main component is a low-pressure mercury vapor tube. Such lamps are found in newborn nurseries, operating rooms, elevators, entryways, cafeterias, and classrooms, where they are incorporated into louvered ceiling fixtures designed to radiate UV light across the top of the room without striking people in the room. Sterility may also be maintained by having a UV lamp placed in a hood or cabinet containing instruments, paper and cloth equipment, liquid, and other inanimate articles. Many biologic materials, such as sera, antisera, toxins, and vaccines, are sterilized with UV rays.

Those whose work involves the use of UV lamps must be particularly careful not to expose their eyes or skin to the rays, because they can cause serious burns and cellular damage. Because UV rays do not penetrate cloth, metals, and glass, these materials may be used to protect persons working in a UV environment. It has been shown that skin cancer can be caused by excessive exposure to the UV rays of the sun; thus, extensive sun tanning is harmful.

X-rays and gamma and beta rays of certain wavelengths from radioactive materials may be lethal or cause mutations in microorganisms and tissue cells because they damage DNA and proteins within those cells. Studies performed in radiation research laboratories have demonstrated that these radiations can be used for the prevention of food spoilage, sterilization of heat-sensitive surgical equipment, preparation of vaccines, and treatment of some chronic diseases such as cancer, all of which are very practical applications for laboratory research. The US Food and Drug Administration approved the use of gamma rays (from cobalt-60) to process chickens and red meat in 1992 and 1997, respectively. Since then, gamma rays have been used by some food processing plants to kill pathogens (such as *Salmonella* and *Campylobacter* bacteria) in chickens; the chickens are labeled "irradiated" and marked with the green international symbol for irradiation (Fig. 8-17).

---

[e]To learn more about microbes in our food and kitchens, see "A Closer Look at Microbes in Our Food" and "A Closer Look at Inhibiting the Growth of Pathogens in Our Kitchens" on thePoint.

Figure 8-17. International symbol for irradiated food. (Courtesy of the United States Department of Agriculture.)

Ultrasonic Waves

In hospitals, medical clinics, and dental clinics, ultrasonic waves are a frequently used means of cleaning delicate equipment. Ultrasonic cleaners consist of tanks filled with liquid solvent (usually water); the short sound waves are then passed through the liquid. The sound waves mechanically dislodge organic debris on instruments and glassware. Glassware and other articles that have been cleansed in ultrasonic equipment must then be washed to remove the dislodged particles and solvent and are then sterilized by another method before they are used. Following cleaning of their instruments, most dental professionals sterilize them using steam under pressure (autoclave), chemical (formaldehyde) vapor, or dry heat (e.g., 160°C for 2 hours).

Filtration

Filters of various pore sizes are used to filter or separate cells, larger viruses, bacteria, and certain other microorganisms from the liquids or gases in which they are suspended. Filters with tiny pore sizes (called micropore filters) are used in laboratories to filter bacteria and viruses out of liquids. The variety of filters is large and includes sintered glass (in which uniform particles of glass are fused), plastic films, unglazed porcelain, asbestos, diatomaceous earth, and cellulose membrane filters. Small quantities of liquid can be filtered through a filter-containing syringe, but large quantities require larger apparatuses.

> Microbes, even those as small as viruses, can be removed from liquids using filters having appropriate pore sizes.

A cotton plug in a test tube, flask, or pipette is a good filter for preventing the entry of microorganisms. Dry gauze and paper masks prevent the outward passage of microbes from the mouth and nose, at the same time protecting the wearer from inhaling airborne pathogens and foreign particles that could damage the lungs. BSCs contain high-efficiency particulate air (HEPA) filters to protect workers from contamination. HEPA filters are also located in operating rooms and patient rooms to filter the air that enters or exits the room.

Gaseous Atmosphere

In limited situations, it is possible to inhibit growth of microorganisms by altering the atmosphere in which they are located. Because aerobes and microaerophiles require oxygen, they can be killed by placing them into an atmosphere devoid of oxygen or by removing oxygen from the environment in which they are living. Conversely, obligate anaerobes can be killed by placing them into an atmosphere containing oxygen or by adding oxygen to the environment in which they are living. For instance, wounds likely to contain anaerobes are lanced (opened) to expose them to oxygen. Another example is gas gangrene, a deep wound infection that causes rapid destruction of tissues. Gas gangrene is caused by various anaerobes in the genus *Clostridium*. In addition to debridement of the wound (removal of necrotic tissue) and the use of antibiotics, gas gangrene can be treated by placing the patient in a hyperbaric (increased pressure) oxygen chamber or in a room with high oxygen pressure. As a result of the pressure, oxygen is forced into the wound, providing oxygen to the oxygen-starved tissue and killing the clostridia.

Using Chemical Agents to Inhibit Microbial Growth

Disinfectants

Chemical disinfection refers to the use of chemical agents to inhibit the growth of pathogens, either temporarily or permanently. The mechanism by which various disinfectants kill cells varies from one type of disinfectant to another. Various factors affect the efficiency or effectiveness of a disinfectant (Fig. 8-18), and these factors must be taken into consideration whenever a disinfectant is used. These factors include the following:

- Prior cleaning of the object or surface to be disinfected.
- The organic load that is present, meaning the presence of organic matter (e.g., feces, blood, vomitus, pus) on the materials being treated.
- The bioburden, meaning the type and level of microbial contamination.
- The concentration of the disinfectant.
- The contact time, meaning the amount of time that the disinfectant must remain in contact with the organisms in order to kill them (see thePoint for "A Closer Look at Contact Time").
- The physical nature of the object being disinfected (e.g., smooth or rough surface, crevices, hinges).
- Temperature and pH.

Directions for preparing the proper dilution of a disinfectant must be followed carefully, because too weak or too strong a concentration is usually less effective than the

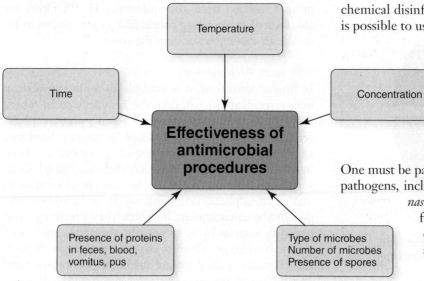

Figure 8-18. Factors that determine the effectiveness of any antimicrobial procedure.

proper concentration. (See Appendix 6 on thePoint: "Preparing Solutions and Dilutions.") The items to be disinfected must first be washed to remove any proteinaceous material in which pathogens may be hidden. Although the washed article may then be clean, it is not safe to use until it has been properly disinfected. Healthcare personnel need to understand an important limitation of chemical disinfection that many disinfectants that are effective against pathogens in the controlled conditions of the laboratory may be ineffective in the actual hospital or clinical environment. Furthermore, the stronger and more effective antimicrobial chemical agents are of limited usefulness because of their destructiveness to human tissues and certain other substances.

Almost all bacteria in the vegetative state, as well as fungi, protozoa, and most viruses, are susceptible to many disinfectants, although the mycobacteria that cause tuberculosis and leprosy, bacterial endospores, pseudomonads (*Pseudomonas* spp.), fungal spores, and hepatitis viruses are notably resistant (see Table 8-3). Therefore,

chemical disinfection should never be attempted when it is possible to use proper physical sterilization techniques.

The disinfectant most effective for each situation must be chosen carefully. Chemical agents used to disinfect respiratory therapy equipment and thermometers must destroy all pathogenic bacteria, fungi, and viruses that may be found in sputum and saliva. One must be particularly aware of the oral and respiratory pathogens, including *M. tuberculosis*; species of *Pseudomonas*, *Staphylococcus*, and *Streptococcus*; the various fungi that cause candidiasis, blastomycosis, coccidioidomycosis, and histoplasmosis; and all respiratory viruses.

Because most disinfection methods do not destroy all bacterial endospores that are present, any instrument or dressing used in the treatment of an infected wound or a disease caused by spore formers must be autoclaved or incinerated. Gas gangrene, tetanus, and anthrax are examples of diseases caused by spore formers that require the healthcare worker to take such precautions. Formaldehyde and ethylene oxide, when properly used, are highly destructive to spores, mycobacteria, and viruses. Certain articles are heat sensitive and cannot be autoclaved or safely washed before disinfection; such articles are soaked for 24 hours in a strong detergent and disinfectant solution, washed, and then sterilized in an ethylene oxide autoclave. The use of disposable equipment whenever possible in these situations helps to protect patients and healthcare personnel.

The effectiveness of a chemical agent depends to some extent on the physical characteristics of the article on which it is used. A smooth, hard surface is readily disinfected, whereas a rough, porous, or grooved surface is not. Thought must be given to selection of the most suitable germicide for cleaning patient rooms and all other areas where patients are treated.

The most effective antiseptic or disinfectant should be chosen for the specific purpose, environment, and pathogen or pathogens likely to be present. The characteristics of an ideal chemical antimicrobial agent include the following:

- It should have a wide or broad antimicrobial spectrum, meaning that it should kill a wide variety of microbes.
- It should be fast-acting, meaning that the contact time should be short.
- It should not be affected by the presence of organic matter (e.g., feces, blood, vomitus, pus).
- It must be nontoxic to human tissues and noncorrosive and nondestructive to materials on which it is used (for instance, if a tincture [e.g., alcohol–water solution] is being used, evaporation of the alcohol solvent can cause a 1% solution to increase to a 10% solution, and at this concentration, it may cause tissue damage).

Table 8-3	Degree of Resistance of Microbes to Disinfection and Sterilization
Level of Resistance	**Microbes**
High	Prions, bacterial spores, coccidia, mycobacteria
Intermediate	Nonlipid or extremely small viruses, fungi
Low	Vegetative bacteria, lipid or medium-sized viruses

Note: Coccidia is a category of protozoan parasites. Vegetative bacteria are bacteria that are actively metabolizing and multiplying (as opposed to spores, which are dormant and possess a thick spore coat).

- It should leave a residual antimicrobial film on the treated surface.
- It must be soluble in water and easy to apply.
- It should be inexpensive and easy to prepare, with simple, specific directions.
- It must be stable both as a concentrate and as a working dilution, so that it can be shipped and stored for reasonable periods.
- It should be odorless.

How do disinfectants kill microorganisms? Some disinfectants (e.g., surface-active soaps and detergents, alcohols, phenolic compounds) target and destroy cell membranes. Others (e.g., halogens, hydrogen peroxide, salts of heavy metals, formaldehyde, ethylene oxide) destroy enzymes and structural proteins. Others attack cell walls or nucleic acids. Some of the disinfectants that are commonly used in hospitals are discussed in Chapter 12.

The effectiveness of phenol as a disinfectant was demonstrated by Joseph Lister in 1867, when it was used to reduce the incidence of infections after surgical procedures.[f] The effectiveness of other disinfectants is compared with that of phenol using the *phenol coefficient test*. To perform this test, a series of dilutions of phenol and the experimental disinfectant are inoculated with the test bacteria, *Salmonella typhi* and *S. aureus*, at 37°C. The highest dilutions (lowest concentrations) that kill the bacteria after 10 minutes are used to calculate the phenol coefficient.

Antiseptics

Most antimicrobial chemical agents are too irritating and destructive to be applied to mucous membranes and skin. Those that may be used safely on human tissues are called antiseptics. An antiseptic merely reduces the number of organisms on a surface; it does not penetrate pores and hair follicles to destroy microorganisms residing there. To remove organisms lodged in pores and folds of the skin, healthcare personnel use an antiseptic soap and scrub with a brush. To prevent resident indigenous microbiota from contaminating the surgical field, surgeons wear sterile gloves on freshly scrubbed hands, and masks and hoods to cover their face and hair. Also, an antiseptic is applied at the site of the surgical incision to destroy local microorganisms.

> Antimicrobial chemical agents that can safely be applied to skin are called antiseptics.

Controversies Relating to the Use of Antimicrobial Agents in Animal Feed and Household Products

It has been estimated that farmers and ranchers use approximately 10 times the antibiotic tonnage as employed in human medicine. The reason is obvious: to cure or prevent infectious diseases in farm animals—infections that could lead to huge economic losses for farmers and ranchers. The problem is that when antibiotics are fed to an animal, the antibiotics kill any indigenous microbiota organisms that are susceptible to the antibiotics. But what survives? Any organisms that are resistant to the antibiotics. Having less competition now for space and nutrients, these drug-resistant organisms multiply and become the predominant organisms of the animal's indigenous microbiota. These drug-resistant organisms are then transmitted in the animal's feces or food products (e.g., eggs, milk, meat) obtained from the animal. Many multidrug-resistant *Salmonella* strains—strains that cause disease in animals and humans—developed in this manner. The use of antibiotic-containing animal feed is quite controversial. Microbiologists concerned about ever-increasing numbers of drug-resistant bacteria have, for years, been attempting to eliminate or drastically reduce the practice of adding antibiotics to animal feed. In April 2012, the US Food and Drug Administration announced a program calling for a voluntary halt to the use of antibiotics for growth promotion in animals being raised for food. Farmers and ranchers will require a prescription from a veterinarian before using antibiotics in such animals and will have to convince the veterinarian that their animals were either sick or at risk of getting a specific illness.

Another controversy concerns the antimicrobial agents that are being added to toys, cutting boards, hand soaps, antibacterial kitchen sprays, and many other household products. The antimicrobial agents in these products kill any organisms that are susceptible to these drugs, but what survives? Any organisms that are resistant to these agents. These drug-resistant organisms then multiply and become the predominant organisms in the home. Should a member of the household become infected with these drug-resistant and multidrug-resistant organisms, the infection will be more difficult to treat. For many years, concerned microbiologists have attempted to eliminate or drastically reduce the practice of adding antimicrobial agents to household products.

Another argument against the use of antimicrobial agents in the home concerns proper development of the immune system. Many scientists believe that children must be exposed to all sorts of microbes during their growth and development so that their immune systems will develop correctly and be capable of properly responding to pathogens in later years.[g] The use of household products containing antimicrobial agents

---

[f]Learn more about Joseph Lister in a Historical Note in Chapter 12.

[g]One scientist (Thomas McDade of Northwestern University) has stated that "Inflammatory networks may need the same type of microbial exposure early in life that have been part of the human environment for all of our evolutionary history to function optimally in adulthood." The American Society for Microbiology (ASM) has speculated that "Ultra-clean, ultra-hygienic environments early in life may contribute to higher levels of inflammation [that] individuals experience as adults, which in turn increases their risk for a wide range of diseases." (Microbe: 5, 98, 2010.)

might be eliminating the very organisms that are essential for proper maturation of the immune system.

ON thePoint

- Terms Introduced in This Chapter
- Review of Key Points
- A Closer Look:
- Hydrothermal Vents
- Barometric Pressure
- Contact Time
- Microbes in Our Food
- Inhibiting the Growth of Pathogens in Our Kitchens
- Increase Your Knowledge
- Critical Thinking
- Additional Self-Assessment Exercises

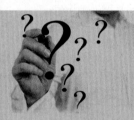

Self-Assessment Exercises

After studying this chapter, answer the following multiple-choice questions.

1. It would be necessary to use a tuberculocidal agent to kill a particular species of:

   a. *Clostridium*
   b. *Mycobacterium*
   c. *Staphylococcus*
   d. *Streptococcus*

2. Pasteurization is an example of what kind of technique?

   a. antiseptic technique
   b. disinfection
   c. sterilization
   d. surgical aseptic technique

3. The combination of freezing and drying is known as:

   a. desiccation
   b. lyophilization
   c. pasteurization
   d. tyndallization

4. Organisms that live in and around hydrothermal vents at the bottom of the ocean are:

   a. acidophilic, psychrophilic, and halophilic
   b. halophilic, alkaliphilic, and psychrophilic
   c. halophilic, psychrophilic, and piezophilic
   d. halophilic, thermophilic, and piezophilic

5. When placed into a hypertonic solution, a bacterial cell will:

   a. take in more water than it releases
   b. lyse
   c. shrink
   d. swell

6. To prevent *Clostridium* infections in a hospital setting, what kind of disinfectant should be used?

   a. fungicidal
   b. pseudomonicidal
   c. sporicidal
   d. tuberculocidal

7. Sterilization can be accomplished by use of:

   a. an autoclave
   b. antiseptics
   c. medical aseptic techniques
   d. pasteurization

8. The goal of medical asepsis is to kill _____, whereas the goal of surgical asepsis is to kill

   _____.

   a. all microorganisms . . . pathogens
   b. bacteria . . . bacteria and viruses
   c. nonpathogens . . . pathogens
   d. pathogens . . . all microorganisms

9. Which of the following types of culture media is selective *and* differential?

   a. blood agar
   b. MacConkey agar
   c. phenylethyl alcohol agar
   d. Thayer–Martin agar

10. All the following types of culture media are enriched and selective except:

    a. blood agar
    b. colistin–nalidixic acid agar
    c. phenylethyl alcohol agar
    d. Thayer–Martin agar

9

Inhibiting the Growth of Pathogens In Vivo using Antimicrobial Agents

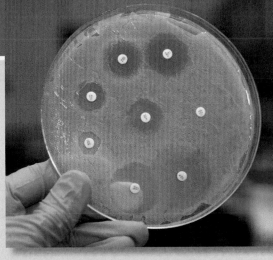

One of the methods used to determine if a particular bacterial strain is susceptible or resistant to various antimicrobial agents.

CHAPTER OUTLINE

LEARNING OBJECTIVES

After studying this chapter, you should be able to:

- Identify the characteristics of an ideal antimicrobial agent
- Compare and contrast chemotherapeutic agents, antimicrobial agents, and antibiotics as to their intended purpose
- State the five most common mechanisms of action of antimicrobial agents
- Differentiate between bactericidal and bacteriostatic agents
- State the difference between narrow-spectrum and broad-spectrum antimicrobial agents
- Identify the four most common mechanisms by which bacteria become resistant to antimicrobial agents
- State what the initials "MRSA" and "MRSE" stand for
- Define the following terms: β-lactam ring, β-lactam antibiotics, and β-lactamase
- Name two major groups of bacterial enzymes that destroy the β-lactam ring
- State six actions that clinicians and/or patients can take to help in the war against drug resistance
- Explain what is meant by empiric therapy
- List six factors that a clinician would take into consideration before prescribing an antimicrobial agent for a particular patient
- State three undesirable effects of antimicrobial agents

- Explain what is meant by a "superinfection," and cite three diseases that can result from superinfections
- Explain the difference between synergism and antagonism with regard to antimicrobial agents

Introduction

Chapter 8 contained information regarding the control of microbial growth in vitro. Another aspect of controlling the growth of microorganisms involves the use of drugs to treat (and, hopefully, to cure) infectious diseases; in other words, using drugs to control the growth of pathogens in vivo.

Although we most often hear the term *chemotherapy* used in conjunction with cancer (i.e., cancer chemotherapy), *chemotherapy* actually refers to the use of any chemical (drug) to treat any disease or condition. The chemicals (drugs) used to treat diseases are referred to as chemotherapeutic agents. By definition, a *chemotherapeutic agent* is *any* drug used to treat *any* condition or disease.

> A chemotherapeutic agent is *any* drug used to treat *any* condition or disease.

For thousands of years, people have been discovering and using herbs and chemicals to cure infectious diseases. Native witch doctors in Central and South America long ago discovered that the herb, ipecac, aided in the treatment of dysentery, and that a quinine extract of cinchona bark was effective in treating malaria. During the 16th and 17th centuries, the alchemists of Europe searched for ways to cure smallpox, syphilis, and many other diseases that were rampant during that period of history. Unfortunately, many of the mercury and arsenic chemicals that were used frequently caused more damage to the patient than to the pathogen.

The chemotherapeutic agents used to treat infectious diseases are collectively referred to as antimicrobial agents.[a] Thus, an *antimicrobial agent* is any chemical (drug) used to treat an infectious disease, either by inhibiting or by killing pathogens in vivo. Drugs used to treat bacterial diseases are called *antibacterial agents*, whereas those used to treat fungal diseases are called *antifungal agents*. Drugs used to treat protozoal diseases are called *antiprotozoal agents*, and those used to treat viral diseases are called *antiviral agents*.

> The chemotherapeutic agents used to treat infectious diseases are collectively referred to as antimicrobial agents.

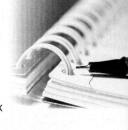

STUDY AID
Clarifying Drug Terminology

Imagine that all *chemotherapeutic agents* are contained within one very large wooden box. Within that large box are many smaller boxes. Each of the smaller boxes contains drugs to treat one particular category of diseases. For example, one of the smaller boxes contains drugs to treat cancer; these are called cancer chemotherapeutic agents. Another of the smaller boxes contains drugs to treat hypertension (high blood pressure). Another of the smaller boxes contains drugs to treat infectious diseases; these are called *antimicrobial agents*. Now imagine that the box containing antimicrobial agents contains even smaller boxes. One of these very small boxes contains drugs to treat bacterial diseases; these are called *antibacterial agents*. Another of these very small boxes contains drugs to treat fungal diseases; these are called *antifungal agents*. Other very small boxes contain drugs to treat protozoal diseases (*antiprotozoal agents*) and drugs to treat viral infections (*antiviral agents*). To appropriately treat a particular disease, a clinician[b] must select a drug from the appropriate box. To treat a fungal infection, for example, the clinician must select a drug from the box containing antifungal agents.

HISTORICAL NOTE
The Father of Chemotherapy

The true beginning of modern chemotherapy came in the late 1800s when Paul Ehrlich, a German chemist, began his search for chemicals (referred to as "magic bullets") that would destroy bacteria, yet would not damage normal body cells. By 1909, he had tested more than 600 chemicals, without success. Finally, in that year, he discovered an arsenic compound that proved effective in treating syphilis. Because this was the 606th compound Ehrlich had tried, he called it "Compound 606." The technical name for Compound 606 is arsphenamine, and the trade name was Salvarsan. Until the availability of penicillin in the early 1940s, Salvarsan and a related compound—Neosalvarsan—were used to treat syphilis. Ehrlich also found that rosaniline was useful for treating African trypanosomiasis.

---

[a]Technically, an antimicrobial agent is *any* chemical agent that kills or inhibits the growth of microbes. However, throughout this book, the term is used in reference to drugs that are used to treat infectious diseases.

[b]The term *clinician* is used throughout this book to refer to a physician or other healthcare professional, who is authorized to make diagnoses and prescribe medications.

> An antibiotic is a substance produced by a microorganism that is effective in killing or inhibiting the growth of other microorganisms.

Some antimicrobial agents are antibiotics. By definition, an *antibiotic* is a substance produced by a microorganism that is effective in killing or inhibiting the growth of other microorganisms. Although all antibiotics are antimicrobial agents, not all antimicrobial agents are antibiotics; therefore, the terms are not synonyms, and care should be taken to use the terms correctly.

Antibiotics are produced by certain moulds and bacteria, usually those that live in soil. The antibiotics produced by soil organisms give them a selective advantage in the struggle for the available nutrients in the soil. Penicillin and cephalosporins are examples of antibiotics produced by moulds; bacitracin, erythromycin, and chloramphenicol are examples of antibiotics produced by bacteria. Although originally produced by microorganisms, many antibiotics are now synthesized or manufactured in pharmaceutical laboratories. Also, many antibiotics

> Antibiotics are primarily antibacterial agents and are thus used to treat bacterial diseases.

have been chemically modified to kill a wider variety of pathogens or reduce side effects; these modified antibiotics are called *semisynthetic antibiotics*. Semisynthetic antibiotics include semisynthetic penicillins, such as ampicillin and carbenicillin. Antibiotics are primarily antibacterial agents and are thus used to treat bacterial diseases.

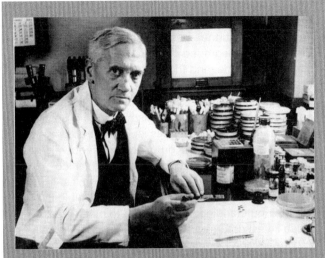

Figure 9-1. Alexander Fleming. (Courtesy of Calibuon at the English Wikibooks project.)

During World War II, two biochemists, **Sir Howard Walter Florey** and **Ernst Boris Chain**, purified penicillin and demonstrated its effectiveness in the treatment of various bacterial infections. By 1942, the US drug industry was able to produce sufficient penicillin for human use, and the search for other antibiotics began. (Earlier—in 1935—a chemist named **Gerhard Domagk** discovered that the red dye,

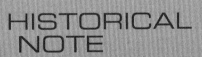

HISTORICAL NOTE

The First Antibiotics

In 1928, **Alexander Fleming** (Fig. 9-1), a Scottish bacteriologist, accidentally discovered the first antibiotic when he noticed that growth of contaminant *Penicillium notatum* mould colonies on his culture plates was inhibiting the growth of *Staphylococcus* bacteria (Fig. 9-2). Fleming gave the name "penicillin" to the inhibitory substance being produced by the mould. He found that broth cultures of the mould were not toxic to laboratory animals and that they destroyed staphylococci and other bacteria. He speculated that penicillin might be useful in treating infectious diseases caused by these organisms. As was stated by Kenneth B. Raper in 1978, "Contamination of his *Staphylococcus* plate by a mould was an accident; but Fleming's recognition of a potentially important phenomenon was no accident, for Pasteur's observation that 'chance favors the prepared mind' was never more apt than with Fleming and penicillin."

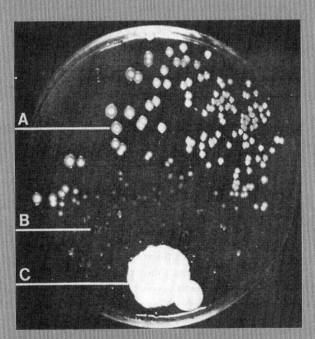

Figure 9-2. The discovery of penicillin by Alexander Fleming. A. Colonies of *S. aureus* (a bacterium) are growing well in this area of the plate. **B.** Colonies are poorly developed in this area of the plate because of an antibiotic (penicillin) being produced by the colony of *P. notatum* (a mould) shown at **(C)**. (This photograph originally appeared in the *British Journal of Experimental Pathology* in 1929.) (From Winn WC Jr, et al. *Koneman's Color Atlas and Textbook of Diagnostic Microbiology.* 6th ed. Philadelphia, PA: JB Lippincott; 2006.)

Prontosil, was effective against streptococcal infections in mice. Further research demonstrated that Prontosil was degraded or broken down in the body into sulfanilamide, and that sulfanilamide [a sulfa drug] was the effective agent. Although sulfanilamide is an antimicrobial agent, it is not an antibiotic because it is not produced by a microorganism.) In 1944, **Selman Waksman** and his colleagues isolated streptomycin (the first antituberculosis drug) and subsequently discovered antibiotics such as chloramphenicol, tetracycline, and erythromycin in soil samples. It was Waksman who first used the term "antibiotic." For their outstanding contributions to medicine, these investigators—Ehrlich, Fleming, Florey, Chain, Waksman, and Domagk—were all Nobel Prize recipients at various times.

Characteristics of an Ideal Antimicrobial Agent

The ideal antimicrobial agent should:

- Kill or inhibit the growth of pathogens
- Cause no damage to the host
- Cause no allergic reaction in the host
- Be stable when stored in solid or liquid form
- Remain in specific tissues in the body long enough to be effective
- Kill the pathogens before they mutate and become resistant to it

Unfortunately, most antimicrobial agents have some side effects, produce allergic reactions, or permit development of resistant mutant pathogens.

How Antimicrobial Agents Work

To be acceptable, an antimicrobial agent must inhibit or destroy the pathogen without damaging the host (i.e., the infected person). To accomplish this, the agent must target a metabolic process or structure possessed by the pathogen but not possessed by the host.

The five most common mechanisms of action of antimicrobial agents are as follows:

- Inhibition of cell wall synthesis
- Damage to cell membranes
- Inhibition of nucleic acid synthesis (either DNA or RNA synthesis)
- Inhibition of protein synthesis
- Inhibition of enzyme activity

Antibacterial Agents

Sulfonamide drugs inhibit production of folic acid (a vitamin) in those bacteria that require *p*-aminobenzoic acid (PABA) to synthesize folic acid. Because the sulfonamide molecule is similar in shape to the PABA molecule, bacteria attempt to metabolize sulfonamide to produce folic acid (Fig. 9-3). However, the enzymes that convert PABA to folic acid cannot produce folic acid from the sulfonamide molecule. Without folic acid, bacteria cannot produce certain essential proteins and finally die. Sulfa drugs, therefore, are called competitive inhibitors, that is, they inhibit growth of microorganisms by competing with an enzyme required to produce an essential metabolite. Sulfa drugs are *bacteriostatic*, meaning that they inhibit growth of bacteria (as opposed to a *bactericidal agent*, which kills bacteria). Cells of humans and animals do not synthesize folic acid from PABA; they get folic acid from the food they eat. Consequently, they are unaffected by sulfa drugs.

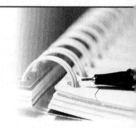

Bacteriostatic drugs inhibit growth of bacteria, whereas bactericidal agents kill bacteria.

STUDY AID
Spelling Tip

Note that the word bacteriostatic contains an "o," whereas the word bactericidal does not.

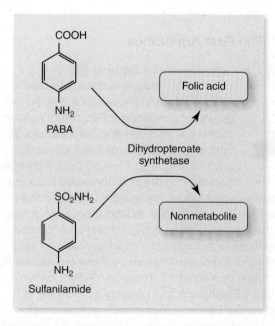

Figure 9-3. The effect of sulfonamide drugs. See text for details.

In most Gram-positive bacteria, including streptococci and staphylococci, penicillin interferes with the synthesis and cross-linking of peptidoglycan, a component of bacterial cell walls. Thus, by inhibiting cell wall synthesis, penicillin destroys the bacteria. Why doesn't penicillin also destroy human cells? Because human cells do not have cell walls.

There are other antimicrobial agents that have a similar action; they inhibit a specific step that is essential to the microorganism's metabolism and, thereby, cause its destruction. Antibiotics such as vancomycin, which destroys only Gram-positive bacteria, and colistin and nalidixic acid, which destroy only Gram-negative bacteria, are referred to as *narrow-spectrum antibiotics*. Those that destroy both Gram-positive and Gram-negative bacteria are called *broad-spectrum antibiotics*. Examples of broad-spectrum antibiotics are ampicillin, chloramphenicol, and tetracycline. Tables 9-1 and 9-2 contain information about some of the antimicrobial drugs most frequently used to treat bacterial infections.

> Narrow-spectrum antibiotics kill *either* Gram-positive or Gram-negative bacteria, whereas broad-spectrum antibiotics kill *both* Gram positives and Gram negatives.

Table 9-1 Antibacterial Agents Listed by Class or Category

Class/Category	Description/Source	Examples of Antibacterial Agents within the Class or Category
Penicillins[a]	Naturally occurring penicillins; produced by moulds in the genus *Penicillium*	Benzylpenicillin (penicillin G), phenoxymethyl penicillin (penicillin V)
	Semisynthetic penicillins: broad-spectrum aminopenicillins	Amoxicillin, ampicillin, bacampicillin, pivampicillin
	Semisynthetic penicillins: broad-spectrum carboxypenicillins	Carbenicillin, ticarcillin
	Semisynthetic penicillins: broad-spectrum ureidopenicillins	Azlocillin, mezlocillin, piperacillin
	Semisynthetic penicillins: penicillinase-resistant penicillins	Cloxacillin, dicloxacillin, methicillin, nafcillin, oxacillin
	Penicillin plus β-lactamase inhibitor	Amoxicillin–clavulanic acid (Augmentin), ampicillin–sulbactam (Unasyn), piperacillin–tazobactam (Zosyn), ticarcillin–clavulanic acid (Timentin)
Cephalosporins[a]	Derivatives of fermentation products of the mould, *Cephalosporium acremonium (now called Acremonium strictum)*	Narrow-spectrum (first-generation) cephalosporins: cephadroxil, cefazolin, cephalexin, cephalothin, cephaloridine, cephapirin, cephradine; first-generation cephalosporins have good activity against Gram-positive bacteria and relatively modest activity against Gram-negative bacteria
		Expanded-spectrum (second-generation) cephalosporins: cefaclor, cefamandole, cefonicid, cefuroxime, cefprozil, loracarbef; second-generation cephalosporins have increased activity against Gram-negative bacteria
		Cephamycins (second-generation cephalosporins): cefmetazole, cefotetan, cefoxitin
		Broad-spectrum (third-generation) cephalosporins: cefdinir, cefditoren, cefixime, cefoperazone, cefotaxime, cefpodoxime, ceftibuten, ceftizoxime, ceftriaxone; third-generation cephalosporins are less active against Gram-positive bacteria than first- and second-generation cephalosporins but are more active against members of the Enterobacteriaceae family and *P. aeruginosa*
		Extended-spectrum (fourth-generation) cephalosporins: cefepime, cefpirome; fourth-generation cephalosporins have increased activity against Gram-negative bacteria

(continued)

Table 9-1 Antibacterial Agents Listed by Class or Category (*Continued*)

Class/Category	Description/Source	Examples of Antibacterial Agents within the Class or Category
Monobactam[a]	Synthetic drug	Aztreonam
Carbapenems[a]	Imipenem is a semisynthetic derivative of thienamycin, produced by *Streptomyces* spp.	Ertapenem, imipenem, meropenem
Aminocyclitol	Produced by *Streptomyces spectabilis*	Spectinomycin, trospectinomycin
Aminoglycosides	Naturally occurring antibiotics or semisynthetic derivatives from *Micromonospora* spp. or *Streptomyces* spp.	Amikacin, gentamicin, kanamycin, neomycin, netilmicin, paromycin, sisomicin, streptomycin, tobramycin
Rifamycins	Semisynthetic antibiotics derived from compounds produced by *Streptomyces mediterranei*	Rifampin (rifampicin), rifabutin, rifaximin
Quinolones	Synthetic drugs	Cinoxacin, nalidixic acid, oxolinic acid
Fluoroquinolones	Synthetic drugs	Ciprofloxacin, cinoxacin, clinafloxacin, enoxacin, fleroxacin, gatifloxacin, gemifloxacin, levofloxacin, lomefloxacin, moxifloxacin, norfloxacin, ofloxacin, sparfloxacin, trovafloxacin
Macrolides	Erythromycin is produced by *Streptomyces erythraeus*; the others are natural analogs of erythromycin or semisynthetic antibiotics	Azithromycin, clarithromycin, dirithromycin, erythromycin
Ketolides	Semisynthetic derivative of erythromycin	Telithromycin
Tetracyclines	Tetracycline is produced by *Streptomyces rimosus*; the others are semisynthetic antibiotics	Chlortetracycline, oxytetracycline, demeclocycline, methacycline, doxycycline, minocycline, tetracycline
Lincosamides	Lincomycin was initially isolated from *Streptomyces lincolnnensis*; clindamycin is a semisynthetic antibiotic	Clindamycin, lincomycin
Glycopeptide	Produced by *Streptomyces orientales*	Vancomycin
Streptogramin	Produced by *Streptomyces* spp.	Quinupristin–dalfopristin
Oxazolidinone	Synthetic drug	Linezolid
Sulfonamides	Synthetic drugs derived from sulfanilamide	Sulfacetamide, sulfadiazine, sulfadoxine, sulfamethizole, sulfamethoxazole (SMX), sulfisoxazole, TMP–sulfamethoxazole (TMP–SMX or co-trimoxazole), trisulfapyrimidine (triple sulfa)
Trimethoprim (TMP)	Synthetic drug	Used alone or in combination with SMX
Polypeptides	Originally derived from *Bacillus polymyxa*	Polymyxins: polymyxin B, polymyxin E (colistin)
	Originally isolated from *Bacillus licheniformis* (formerly named *Bacillus subtilis*)	Bacitracin
Chloramphenicol	Originally produced by *Streptomyces venezuelae*	
Nitroimidazoles	Synthetic drug	Metronidazole, tinidazole
Nitrofurantoin	Synthetic drug	
Fosfomycin	Originally produced by *Streptomyces* spp.	

[a]β-Lactam antibiotics (i.e., antibiotics that contain a β-lactam ring).
Information Source: Yao JDC, Moellering RC Jr. Antibacterial agents. In: Murray PR, et al., eds. *Manual of Clinical Microbiology*. 9th ed. Washington, DC: ASM Press; 2007.

Table 9-2 Antibacterial Agents Listed by Mechanism of Action

Mode of Action	Agent	Spectrum of Activity	Bactericidal or Bacteriostatic
Inhibition of cell wall synthesis	Aztreonam	Gram-negative bacteria	Bactericidal
	Bacitracin (also disrupts cell membranes)	Broad spectrum[a]	Bactericidal
	Carbapenem	Broad spectrum	Bactericidal
	Cephalosporins	Broad spectrum	Bactericidal
	Daptomycin	Broad spectrum	Bactericidal
	Fosfomycin	Broad spectrum	Bactericidal
	Penicillins and semisynthetic penicillins	Broad spectrum	Bactericidal
	Vancomycin	Gram-positive bacteria	Bactericidal
Inhibition of protein synthesis	Aminoglycosides	Primarily Gram-negative bacteria and *S. aureus*; not effective against anaerobes	Bactericidal
	Chloramphenicol	Broad spectrum	Bacteriostatic
	Clindamycin	Most Gram-positive bacteria and some Gram-negative bacteria; highly active against anaerobes	Bacteriostatic or bactericidal, depending upon drug concentration and bacterial species
	Erythromycin and other macrolides	Most Gram-positive bacteria and some Gram-negative bacteria	Bacteriostatic (usually); bactericidal at higher concentrations
	Ketolides	Broad spectrum	Bacteriostatic
	Linezolid	Gram-positive bacteria	Bacteriostatic
	Mupirocin	Broad spectrum	Bacteriostatic
	Streptogramins	Primarily Gram-positive bacteria	Bactericidal
	Tetracyclines	Broad-spectrum and some intracellular bacterial pathogens	Bacteriostatic
Inhibition of nucleic acid synthesis	Rifampin	Gram-positive and some Gram-negative bacteria (e.g., *Neisseria meningitidis*)	Bactericidal
	Quinolones and fluoroquinolones (e.g., ciprofloxacin, levofloxacin, moxifloxacin)	Broad spectrum	Bactericidal
Destruction of DNA	Metronidazole	Effective against anaerobes	Bactericidal
Disruption of cell membranes	Polymyxin B and polymyxin E (colistin)	Gram-negative bacteria	Bactericidal
Inhibition of enzyme activity	Sulfonamides	Primarily Gram-positive bacteria and some Gram-negative bacteria	Bacteriostatic
	Trimethoprim	Gram-positive and many Gram-negative bacteria	Bacteriostatic

[a]Effective against both Gram-positive and Gram-negative bacteria, but spectrum may vary with the individual antimicrobial agent.

Antimicrobial agents work well against bacterial pathogens because the bacteria (being prokaryotic) have different cellular structures and metabolic pathways that can be disrupted or destroyed by drugs that do not damage the eukaryotic host's cells. As mentioned earlier, bactericidal agents kill bacteria, whereas bacteriostatic agents stop them from growing and dividing. Bacteriostatic agents should be used only in patients whose host defense mechanisms (see Chapters 15 and 16) are functioning properly (i.e., only in patients whose bodies are capable of killing the pathogen once its multiplication is stopped). Bacteriostatic agents should not be used in immunosuppressed or leukopenic patients (patients having an abnormally low number of white blood cells) because the host defense mechanisms of such patients would be unable to eliminate the nongrowing bacteria. Some of the mechanisms by which antibacterial agents kill or inhibit bacteria are shown in Table 9-2.

Virtually all of the antibacterial agents currently available either kill bacteria or inhibit their growth. Researchers are attempting to develop antibacterial agents that target bacterial virulence factors, rather than targeting the pathogens themselves. Bacterial virulence factors include various harmful substances, such as toxins and enzymes, produced by bacteria. Virulence factors are discussed in detail in Chapter 14.

Some Major Categories of Antibacterial Agents

Penicillins. Penicillins are referred to as β-lactam drugs because their molecular structure includes a four-sided ring structure known as a β-lactam ring (shown in Fig. 9-4).[c] Penicillins interfere with the synthesis of bacterial cell walls and have maximum effect on bacteria that are actively dividing. They are bactericidal drugs. Penicillin G and penicillin V are referred to as *natural penicillins* because they are produced and can be purified directly from cultures of *Penicillium* moulds. Natural penicillins are effective against some Gram-positive bacteria (especially *Streptococcus* spp.), some anaerobic bacteria, and some spirochetes. A few Gram-negative bacteria (e.g., *N. meningitidis* and some strains of *Haemophilus influenzae*) remain susceptible to natural penicillins. Some extended-spectrum penicillins (e.g., aminopenicillins and extended-spectrum penicillins) are used to treat infections caused by Gram-negative bacilli.

Cephalosporins. The cephalosporins are also β-lactam antibiotics and, like penicillin, are produced by moulds. Also like penicillins, cephalosporins interfere with cell wall synthesis and are bactericidal. The cephalosporins are classified as first-, second-, third-, fourth-, and fifth-generation cephalosporins. The first-generation agents are active primarily against Gram-positive bacteria. Second-generation

[c]The symbol "β" is the Greek letter "beta." The complete Greek alphabet can be found in Appendix D.

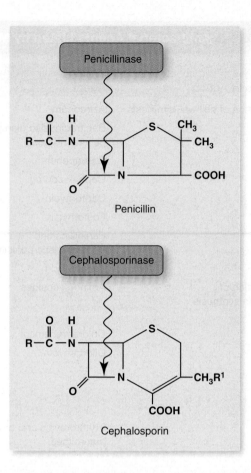

Figure 9-4. Sites of β-lactamase attack on penicillin and cephalosporin molecules. See text for details.

cephalosporins have increased activity against Gram-negative bacteria, and third-generation cephalosporins have even greater activity against Gram negatives (including *Pseudomonas aeruginosa*). Cefepime is an example of a fourth-generation cephalosporin with activity against both Gram positives and Gram negatives, including *P. aeruginosa*). Ceftaroline is a fifth-generation cephalosporin that has expanded activity against aerobic Gram-positive cocci, including methicillin-resistant *Staphylococcus aureus* (MRSA) and methicillin-resistant *Staphylococcus epidermidis* MRSE. Its activity against aerobic Gram-negative bacteria mimics that of the third-generation cephalosporins.

Carbapenems. Carbapenems, including imipenem, are among the most powerful antibacterial agents in use today. They target the cell envelope and have excellent activity against a broad spectrum of bacteria, including many aerobic Gram-positive bacteria, most aerobic Gram-negative bacteria, and most anaerobes.

Glycopeptides. Glycopeptides, including vancomycin, target the cell envelope. They have excellent activity against most aerobic and anaerobic Gram-positive bacteria. Unfortunately, these popular drugs have several drawbacks. Bacteria, especially enterococci, are becoming resistant to these drugs, and they have a number of toxic side effects.

Tetracyclines. Tetracyclines are broad-spectrum drugs that exert their effect by targeting bacterial ribosomes. They are bacteriostatic. Tetracyclines are effective against a wide variety of bacteria, including chlamydias, mycoplasmas, rickettsias, *Vibrio cholerae*, and spirochetes such as *Borrelia* spp. and *Treponema pallidum*.

Aminoglycosides. Aminoglycosides are bactericidal broad-spectrum drugs that inhibit bacterial protein synthesis. The major factor that limits their use is their toxicity. Aminoglycosides are effective against a wide variety of aerobic Gram-negative bacteria, but are ineffective against anaerobes. They are used to treat infections with members of the family Enterobacteriaceae (e.g., *Escherichia coli* and *Enterobacter*, *Klebsiella*, *Proteus*, *Serratia*, and *Yersinia* spp.), as well as *P. aeruginosa* and *Vibrio cholerae*.

Macrolides. Macrolides inhibit protein synthesis. They are considered bacteriostatic at lower doses and bactericidal at higher doses. The macrolides include erythromycin, clarithromycin, and azithromycin. They are effective against chlamydias, mycoplasmas, *T. pallidum*, and *Legionella* spp.

Fluoroquinolones. Fluoroquinolones are bactericidal drugs that inhibit DNA synthesis. The most commonly used fluoroquinolone, ciprofloxacin, is effective against members of the family Enterobacteriaceae and *P. aeruginosa*.

Multidrug Therapy

In some cases, a single antimicrobial agent is not sufficient to destroy all the pathogens that develop during the course of a disease; thus, two or more drugs may be used simultaneously to kill all the pathogens and to prevent resistant mutant pathogens from emerging. In tuberculosis, for example, in which multidrug-resistant strains of *Mycobacterium tuberculosis* are frequently encountered, four drugs (isoniazid, rifampin, pyrazinamide, and ethambutol) are routinely prescribed, and as many as 12 drugs may be required for especially resistant strains.

Synergism versus Antagonism

The use of two antimicrobial agents to treat an infectious disease sometimes produces a degree of pathogen killing that is far greater than that achieved by either drug alone. This is known as *synergism*. Synergism is a good thing! Many urinary, respiratory, and gastrointestinal infections respond particularly well to a combination of trimethoprim and sulfamethoxazole,

> When the use of two antimicrobial agents to treat an infectious disease produces a degree of pathogen killing that is far greater than that achieved by either drug alone, the phenomenon is known as synergism.

a combination referred to as co-trimoxazole; brand names include Bactrim and Septra.

There are situations, however, when two drugs are prescribed (perhaps by two different clinicians who are treating the patient's infection) that actually work against each other. This is known as *antagonism*. The extent of pathogen killing is less than that achieved by either drug alone. Antagonism is a bad thing!

> When the use of two drugs produces an extent of pathogen killing that is less than that achieved by either drug alone, the phenomenon is known as antagonism.

Antifungal Agents

It is much more difficult to use antimicrobial drugs against fungal and protozoal pathogens, because they are eukaryotic cells; thus, the drugs tend to be more toxic to the patient. Most antifungal agents work in one of three ways:

- By binding with cell membrane sterols (e.g., nystatin and amphotericin B)
- By interfering with sterol synthesis (e.g., clotrimazole and miconazole)
- By blocking mitosis or nucleic acid synthesis (e.g., griseofulvin and 5-flucytosine)

> Antifungal and antiprotozoal drugs tend to be more toxic to the patient because, like the infected human, they are eukaryotic organisms.

Examples of antifungal agents are shown in Table 9-3.

Antiprotozoal Agents

Antiprotozoal drugs are usually quite toxic to the host and work by (a) interfering with DNA and RNA synthesis (e.g., chloroquine, pentamidine, and quinacrine) or (b) interfering with protozoal metabolism (e.g., metronidazole; brand name Flagyl). Table 9-4 lists several antiprotozoal drugs and the protozoal diseases they are used to treat.

Antiviral Agents

Antiviral agents are the newest weapons in antimicrobial methodology. Until the 1960s, there were no drugs for the treatment of viral diseases. Antiviral agents are particularly difficult to develop and use because viruses are produced within host cells, but, as can be seen in Table 9-5, quite a few drugs have been found to be effective in certain viral infections.

Table 9-3 Antifungal Agents

Drug[a]	Fungal Disease(s) That the Drug Is Used to Treat
Amphotericin B	Aspergillosis, blastomycosis, invasive candidiasis, coccidioidomycosis, cryptococcosis, fusariosis, histoplasmosis, mucormycosis, paracoccidioidomycosis, penicilliosis, systemic sporotrichosis
Atovaquone	*Pneumocystis* pneumonia
Echinocandins	Aspergillosis, candidiasis
Fluconazole	Blastomycosis; oropharyngeal, esophageal, and invasive candidiasis; coccidioidomycosis, cryptococcosis, fusariosis, histoplasmosis, sporotrichosis
Flucytosine	Candidiasis, chromoblastomycosis, cryptococcosis
Griseofulvin	Dermatomycosis (less toxic drugs are available, however)
Itraconazole	Aspergillosis, blastomycosis, invasive candidiasis, coccidioidomycosis, cryptococcosis, histoplasmosis, paracoccidioidomycosis, penicilliosis, pseudallescheriasis, scedosporiosis, cutaneous or systemic sporotrichosis
Ketoconazole	Blastomycosis, coccidioidomycosis, histoplasmosis, paracoccidioidomycosis
Terbinafine	Dermatomycosis
Trimethoprim-	*Pneumocystis* pneumonia sulfamethoxazole
Voriconazole	Aspergillosis, invasive candidiasis, scedosporiasis

[a]This information is provided solely to acquaint readers of this book with the names of some antifungal agents and should not be construed as advice regarding recommended therapy.

Table 9-4 Antiprotozoal Agents

Drug[a]	Protozoal Disease(s) That the Drug Is Used to Treat
Amphotericin B	Primary amebic meningoencephalitis, mucocutaneous leishmaniasis
Artemisinin derivatives	Multidrug-resistant *Plasmodium falciparum* malaria
Benznidazole	American trypanosomiasis (Chagas disease)
Chloroquine phosphate or quinidine gluconate or quinine dihydrochloride	Malaria (except for chloroquine-resistant *P. falciparum* malaria and chloroquine-resistant *Plasmodium vivax* malaria)
Clindamycin plus quinine	Babesiosis
Diloxanide furoate	Amebiasis
Eflornithine	African trypanosomiasis (with or without CNS involvement)
Furazolidone	Giardiasis
Halofantrine	Chloroquine-resistant *P. falciparum* malaria
Iodoquinol	Amebiasis, balantidiasis, *Dientamoeba fragilis* infection
Mefloquine	Chloroquine-resistant *P. falciparum* and *P. vivax* malaria
Melarsoprol	African trypanosomiasis (with CNS involvement)
Metronidazole	Amebiasis, giardiasis, trichomoniasis
Nifurtimox	American trypanosomiasis (Chagas disease)
Nitazoxanide	Giardiasis in children and cryptosporidiosis
Paromomycin	Amebiasis, cryptosporidiosis, *D. fragilis* infection, cutaneous leishmaniasis
Pentamidine isethionate	African sleeping sickness (without CNS involvement), leishmaniasis
Primaquine phosphate	Malaria
Proguanil hydrochloride	Malaria
Pyrimethamine plus sulfadiazine	*P. falciparum* malaria, toxoplasmosis

Table 9-4 Antiprotozoal Agents (*Continued*)

Drug[a]	Protozoal Disease(s) That the Drug Is Used to Treat
Quinacrine hydrochloride	Giardiasis
Quinidine gluconate	*P. falciparum* malaria
Quinine	Malaria
Spiramycin	Toxoplasmosis
Stibogluconate sodium	Visceral, cutaneous, and mucocutaneous leishmaniasis
Suramin	African trypanosomiasis (with no CNS involvement)
Tetracycline hydrochloride	Balantidiasis, *D. fragilis* infection; can be used with quinine or quinidine for *P. falciparum* malaria
Tinidazole	Amebiasis, giardiasis, trichomoniasis
Trimethoprim–sulfamethoxazole	Cyclosporiasis, isosporiasis

CNS, central nervous system.

[a]This information is provided solely to acquaint the reader with the names of some antiprotozoal agents and should not be construed as advice regarding recommended therapy.

The first antiviral agent effective against human immunodeficiency virus (HIV) (the causative agent of acquired immune deficiency syndrome or acquired immunodeficiency syndrome [AIDS])—zidovudine (also known as azidothymidine [AZT])—was introduced in 1987. A variety of additional drugs for the treatment of HIV infection were introduced subsequently. Certain of these antiviral agents are administered simultaneously, in combinations referred to as "cocktails." Unfortunately, such cocktails are quite expensive, and some strains of HIV have become resistant to some of the drugs.

Drug Resistance

"Superbugs"

These days, it is quite common to hear about drug-resistant bacteria, or "superbugs," as they have been labeled by the press (Fig. 9-5). Although "superbug" can refer to an organism that is resistant to only one antimicrobial agent, the term usually refers to multidrug-resistant organisms (i.e., organisms that are resistant to more than one antimicrobial agent). Infections caused

Table 9-5 Antiviral Agents

Virus/Viral Infection(S)	Antiviral Agents[a]
Herpes simplex infections	Acyclovir, cidofovir, famciclovir, fomivirsen, foscarnet, ganciclovir, penciclovir, valacyclovir, valganciclovir, vidarabine
Influenza virus types A and B	Oseltamivir, ribavirin, zanamivir
Hepatitis B virus	Adefovir, entecavir, peginterferon α-2a, lamivudine, telbivudine, tenofovir
Hepatitis C virus	Peginterferon α-2a, ribavirin
Human cytomegalovirus	Cidofovir, foscarnet, ganciclovir
Varicella-zoster virus	Acyclovir, famciclovir, valacyclovir
HIV: nucleoside/-tide analog reverse transcriptase inhibitors	Abacavir, didanosine, emtricitabine, lamivudine, stavudine, tenofovir, zalcitabine, zidovudine (AZT, ZDV)
HIV: non-nucleoside reverse transcriptase inhibitors	Delavirdine, efavirenz, etravirine, nevirapine
HIV: protease inhibitors	Amprenavir, atazanavir, indinavir, lopinavir, nelfinavir, ritonavir, saquinavir
HIV: fusion inhibitor	Enfuvirtide
HIV: integrase inhibitor	Raltegravir

[a]This information is provided solely to acquaint the reader with the names of some antiviral agents and should not be construed as advice regarding recommended therapy.
Modified from Harvey RA, et al. *Lippincott's Illustrated Reviews: Microbiology*. 3rd ed. Philadelphia, PA: Lippincott Williams & Wilkins; 2013.

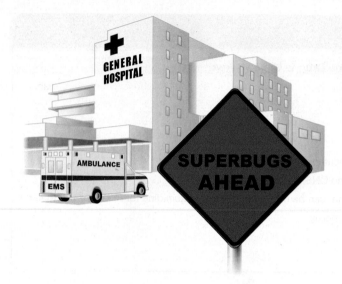

Figure 9-5. Fictitious caution sign. This sign warns those who are about to enter that hospitals are notorious havens for multidrug-resistant microbes ("superbugs"). (Courtesy of Dr. Pat Hidy and Biomed Ed, Round Rock, TX.)

by superbugs are much more difficult to treat. Especially troublesome superbugs are listed in Table 9-6.

It is important to note that bacteria are not the only microbes that have developed resistance to drugs. Certain viruses (including HIV, herpes simplex viruses, and influenza viruses), fungi (both yeasts and moulds),

parasitic protozoa, and helminths have also developed resistance to drugs. Parasitic protozoa that have become drug-resistant include strains of *P. falciparum*, *Trichomonas vaginalis*, *Leishmania* spp., and *Giardia lamblia*.

How Bacteria Become Resistant to Drugs

How do bacteria become resistant to antimicrobial agents? Some bacteria are naturally resistant to a particular antimicrobial agent because they lack the specific target site for that drug (e.g., mycoplasmas have no cell walls and are, therefore, resistant to any drugs that interfere with cell wall synthesis). Other bacteria are naturally resistant because the drug is unable to cross the organism's cell wall or cell membrane and, thus, cannot reach its site of action (e.g., ribosomes). Such resistance is known as *intrinsic resistance*.

It is also possible for bacteria that were once susceptible to a particular drug to become resistant to it; this is called *acquired resistance*. Bacteria usually acquire resistance to antibiotics and other antimicrobial agents by one of four mechanisms, each of which is shown in Table 9-7 and briefly described here:

> Although the term *superbug* most often refers to multidrug-resistant bacteria, other types of microbes (e.g., viruses, fungi, protozoa) have also become multidrug-resistant.

Table 9-6 Especially Troublesome "Superbugs"

Bacteria	Discussion
MRSA and MRSE (Fig. 9-6)	These strains are resistant to all antistaphylococcal drugs except vancomycin and several recently developed drugs (e.g., linezolid, tigecycline, quinupristin-dalfopristin, daptomycin, ceftaroline). Some strains of *S. aureus*, called vancomycin-intermediate *S. aureus* (VISA), have developed resistance to the usual dosages of vancomycin, necessitating the use of higher doses to treat infections caused by these organisms. Recently, strains of *S. aureus* (called vancomycin-resistant *S. aureus* or VRSA strains) have been isolated that are resistant to even the highest practical doses of vancomycin. *S. aureus* is a very common cause of healthcare-associated infections[a] (Fig. 9-6). *S. epidermidis* is not as virulent or versatile as *S. aureus*, but this organism does cause many hospital-associated infections (especially urinary tract infections and infections associated with foreign objects, such as intravenous catheters, prosthetic heart valves, and prosthetic joints). Most strains of *S. epidermidis* are resistant to penicillin, and many strains are resistant to the antistaphylococcal penicillins.
Streptococcus pyogenes and *Streptococcus pneumoniae*	*S. pyogenes* and *S. pneumoniae* are very important human pathogens, in that they cause a wide variety of infectious diseases. Strains of *S. pyogenes* that are resistant to macrolide antibiotics have emerged, but fortunately, all strains of *S. pyogenes* remain susceptible to penicillin. The same is not true for *S. pneumoniae*. Many strains of *S. pneumoniae* have developed resistance to penicillin and other beta-lactam antibiotics.
Vancomycin-resistant *Enterococcus* spp. (VRE)	These strains are resistant to most antienterococcal drugs, including vancomycin. *Enterococcus* spp. are common causes of healthcare-associated infections, especially urinary tract infections.
P. aeruginosa	*P. aeruginosa* infections are very common and especially difficult to treat. Strains of *P. aeruginosa* have a variety of resistance mechanisms, including a relatively impermeable outer membrane and multiple efflux pumps. Aminopenicillins, macrolides, and most cephalosporins are ineffective against *P. aeruginosa*.
Clostridium difficile	*C. difficile* is a major cause of hospital-associated diarrheal disease. Strains of *C. difficile* have become resistant to clindamycin, ciprofloxacin, and levofloxacin.

Table 9-6 Especially Troublesome "Superbugs" (*Continued*)

Bacteria	Discussion
Acinetobacter baumannii	Infections caused by multidrug-resistant strains of *A. baumannii* were first reported in military personnel stationed in Iraq and Afghanistan. Some strains were resistant to all drugs tested.
Klebsiella pneumoniae	Carbapenemase-producing strains of *K. pneumoniae* produce a β-lactamase that destroys penicillins, cephalosporins, aztreonam, carbapenemes, and other antibiotics.
Multidrug-resistant *M. tuberculosis* (MDR-TB)	MDR-TB strains are resistant to the two most effective first-line therapeutic drugs—isoniazid and rifampin. Extensively drug-resistant strains, called XDR-TB, are also resistant to the most effective second-line therapeutic drugs—fluoroquinolones and at least one of the following: amikacin, kanamycin, capreomycin. Some drug-resistant strains of *M. tuberculosis* are resistant to *all* antitubercular drugs and combinations of these drugs. Patients infected with these strains may require removal of a lung or section of a lung—just as in the preantibiotic days—and many will die. Tuberculosis remains one of the major killers worldwide.
Multidrug-resistant strains of *Burkholderia cepacia*, *E. coli, Neisseria gonorrhoeae, Ralstonia pickettii, Salmonella* spp., *Shigella* spp., *Stenotrophomonas maltophilia,* and *H. influenzae*	

[a]The term *healthcare-associated infections* refers to infections acquired by individuals while they are hospitalized or within other types of healthcare facilities. Healthcare-associated infections are discussed in detail in Chapter 12.

- Before a drug can enter a bacterial cell, molecules of the drug must first bind (attach) to proteins on the surface of the cell; these protein molecules are called *drug-binding sites*. A chromosomal mutation can result in an alteration in the structure of the drug-binding site, so that the drug is no longer able to bind to the cell. If the drug cannot bind to the cell, it cannot enter the cell, and the organism is, therefore, resistant to the drug.
- To enter a bacterial cell, a drug must be able to pass through the cell wall and cell membrane. A chromosomal mutation can result in an alteration in the structure of the cell membrane, which in turn can change the permeability of the membrane. If the drug is no longer able to pass through the cell membrane, it cannot reach its target (e.g., a ribosome or the DNA of the cell), and the organism is now resistant to the drug.
- Another way in which bacteria become resistant to a certain drug is by developing the ability to produce an enzyme that destroys or inactivates the drug. Because enzymes are coded for by genes, a bacterial cell would have to acquire a new gene for the cell to be able to produce an enzyme that it never before produced. The primary way in which bacteria acquire new genes is by conjugation (Chapter 7). Often, a plasmid containing such a gene is transferred from one bacterial cell (the donor cell) to another bacterial cell (the recipient cell) during conjugation. For example, many bacteria have become resistant to penicillin because they have acquired the gene for penicillinase production during conjugation. (Penicillinase is described in the following section.) A plasmid containing multiple genes for drug resistance is called a *resistance factor* (R-factor). A recipient cell that receives an R-factor becomes multidrug-resistant (i.e., it becomes a superbug). Bacteria can also acquire new genes by transduction (whereby bacteriophages carry bacterial DNA from one bacterial cell to another) and transformation (the uptake of naked DNA from the environment). (Transduction and transformation were discussed in Chapter 7.)
- A fourth way in which bacteria become resistant to drugs is by developing the ability to produce multidrug-resistance (MDR) pumps (also known as MDR transporters or efflux pumps). An MDR pump enables the cell to pump drugs out of the cell before the drugs can damage or kill the cell. The genes encoding these pumps are often located on plasmids that bacteria receive during conjugation. Bacteria receiving such plasmids become multidrug-resistant (i.e., they become resistant to several drugs).

> Bacteria can acquire resistance to antimicrobial agents as a result of chromosomal mutation or the acquisition of new genes by transduction, transformation, and, most commonly, conjugation.

Thus, bacteria can acquire resistance to antimicrobial agents as a result of chromosomal mutation or the acquisition of new genes by transduction, transformation, and, most commonly, conjugation.

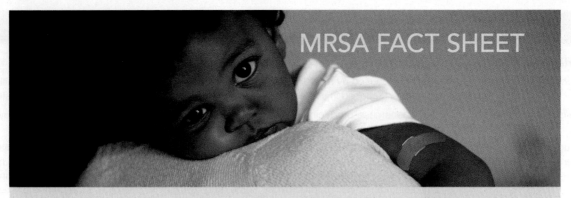

MRSA FACT SHEET

What is MRSA?

MRSA is methicillin-resistant *Staphylococcus aureus*, a potentially dangerous type of staph bacteria that is resistant to certain antibiotics and may cause skin and other infections. As with all regular staph infections, recognizing the signs and receiving treatment for MRSA skin infections in the early stages reduces the chances of the infection becoming severe. MRSA is spread by:

> Having direct contact with another person's infection
> Sharing personal items, such as towels or razors, that have touched infected skin
> Touching surfaces or items, such as used bandages, contaminated with MRSA

What are the signs and symptoms?

Most staph skin infections, including MRSA, appear as a bump or infected area on the skin that may be:

> Red
> Swollen
> Painful
> Warm to the touch
> Full of pus or other drainage
> Accompanied by a fever

What if I suspect an MRSA skin infection?

Cover the area with a bandage and contact your healthcare professional. It is especially important to contact your healthcare professional if signs and symptoms of an MRSA skin infection are accompanied by a fever.

How are MRSA skin infections treated?

Treatment for MRSA skin infections may include having a healthcare professional drain the infection and, in some cases, prescribe an antibiotic. Do not attempt to drain the infection yourself – doing so could worsen or spread it to others. If you are given an antibiotic, be sure to take all of the doses (even if the infection is getting better), unless your healthcare professional tells you to stop taking it.

How can I protect my family from MRSA skin infections?

> Know the signs of MRSA skin infections and get treated early
> Keep cuts and scrapes clean and covered
> Encourage good hygiene such as cleaning hands regularly
> Discourage sharing of personal items such as towels and razors

 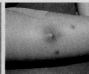

© Bernard Cohen, MD, Dermatlas; www.dermatlas.org   http://phil.cdc.gov

For more information, please call 1-800-CDC-INFO or visit www.cdc.gov/MRSA.

Developed with support from the CDC Foundation through an educational grant from Pfizer Inc.

Figure 9-6. MRSA fact sheet. (From the Centers for Disease Control and Prevention, http://www.cdc.gov/mrsa)

β-Lactamases

At the heart of every penicillin and cephalosporin molecule is a double-ringed structure, which in penicillins resembles a "house and garage" (see Fig. 9-4).

The "garage" is called the β-lactam ring. Some bacteria produce enzymes that destroy the β-lactam ring; these enzymes are known as β-lactamases. When the β-lactam ring is destroyed, the antibiotic no longer works. Thus, an organism that produces a β-lactamase is resistant to antibiotics containing the β-lactam ring (collectively referred to as β-lactam antibiotics or β-lactams).

> A β-lactam antibiotic is an antibiotic that contains a β-lactam ring in its molecular structure.

There are two types of β-lactamases: penicillinases and cephalosporinases. *Penicillinases* destroy the β-lactam ring in penicillins; thus, an organism that produces penicillinase

Table 9-7 Mechanisms by Which Bacteria Become Resistant to Antimicrobial Agents

Mechanism	Effect
A chromosomal mutation that causes a change in the structure of a drug-binding site	The drug cannot bind to the bacterial cell
A chromosomal mutation that causes a change in cell membrane permeability	The drug cannot pass through the cell membrane and thus cannot enter the cell
Acquisition (by conjugation, transduction, or transformation) of a gene that enables the bacterium to produce an enzyme that destroys or inactivates the drug	The drug is destroyed or inactivated by the enzyme
Acquisition (by conjugation, transduction, or transformation) of a gene that enables the bacterium to produce an MDR pump	The drug is pumped out of the cell before it can damage or kill the cell

is resistant to penicillins. *Cephalosporinases* destroy the β-lactam ring in cephalosporins; thus, an organism that produces cephalosporinase is resistant to cephalosporins. Some bacteria produce both types of β-lactamases.

To combat the effect of β-lactamases, drug companies have developed special drugs that combine a β-lactam antibiotic with a β-lactamase inhibitor (e.g., clavulanic acid, sulbactam, or tazobactam). The β-lactam inhibitor irreversibly binds to and inactivates the β-lactamase, thus enabling the companion drug to enter the bacterial cell and disrupt cell wall synthesis. Some of these special combination drugs are

> Penicillinases and cephalosporinases are examples of β-lactamases; they destroy the β-lactam ring in penicillins and cephalosporins, respectively.

- Clavulanic acid (clavulanate) combined with amoxicillin (brand name, Augmentin)
- Clavulanic acid (clavulanate) combined with ticarcillin (Timentin)
- Sulbactam combined with ampicillin (Unasyn)
- Tazobactam combined with piperacillin (Zosyn)

Some Strategies in the War against Drug Resistance

- Education is crucial—education of healthcare professionals and, in turn, education of patients.
- Patients should never pressure clinicians to prescribe antimicrobial agents. Parents must stop demanding

antibiotics every time they have a sick child. The majority of sore throats and many respiratory infections are caused by viruses, and viruses are unaffected by antibiotics. Because viruses are not killed by antibiotics, patients and parents should not expect antibiotics when they or their children have viral infections. Instead of demanding antibiotics from clinicians, they should be asking *why* one is being prescribed.

- It is important that clinicians not allow themselves to be pressured by patients. They should prescribe antibiotics only when warranted (i.e., only when there is a demonstrated need for them). Whenever possible, clinicians should collect a specimen for culture and have the Clinical Microbiology Laboratory perform susceptibility testing (Chapter 13) to determine which antimicrobial agents are likely to be effective.
- Clinicians should prescribe an inexpensive, narrow-spectrum drug whenever the laboratory results demonstrate that such a drug effectively kills the pathogen. According to Dr. Stuart B. Levy,[d] by some estimates, at least half of current antibiotic use in the United States is inappropriate—antibiotics are either not indicated at all or incorrectly prescribed as the wrong drug, the wrong dosage, or the wrong duration. One study showed that antibiotics were prescribed in 68% of acute respiratory tract visits, and of those, 80% were unnecessary according to CDC guidelines.[e] Table 9-8 lists upper respiratory infections that typically do not benefit from antibiotics. Taking antibiotics for these viral infections will not cure the infections, will not keep other individuals from catching the illness, and will not help the patient feel better.
- Patients must take their antibiotics in the exact manner in which they are prescribed. Healthcare professionals should emphasize this to patients and do a better job explaining exactly how medications should be taken.
- It is critical that clinicians prescribe the appropriate amount of antibiotic necessary to cure the infection. Then, unless instructed otherwise, patients must take *all* their pills—even after they are feeling better. Again, this must be explained and emphasized. If treatments are cut short, there is selective killing of only the most susceptible members of a bacterial population. The more resistant variants are left behind to multiply and cause a new infection.
- Patients should always destroy any excess medications and should never keep antibiotics in their medicine cabinet. Antimicrobial agents, including antibiotics, should be taken only when prescribed and only under a clinician's supervision.

[d]Levy SB. *The Antibiotic Paradox: How the Misuse of Antibiotics Destroys Their Curative Powers.* 2nd ed. Cambridge, MA: Perseus Publishing; 2002.

[e]Scott JG, et al. Antibiotic use in acute respiratory infections and the ways patients pressure physicians for a prescription. *J Fam Pract* 2001;50(10):853–858.

Table 9-8	Viral Infections for Which Antibiotic Treatment Is Deemed Inappropriate		
Infection	**Usually Caused by Viruses**	**Usually Caused by Bacteria**	**Antibiotic Needed**
Cold	Yes	No	No
Flu	Yes	No	No
Chest cold (in otherwise healthy children and adults)	Yes	No	No
Sore throats (other than strep throat)	Yes	No	No
Bronchitis (in otherwise healthy children and adults)	Yes	No	No
Runny nose (with green or yellow mucus)	Yes	No	No
Fluid in the middle ear	Yes	No	No

Source: The Centers for Disease Control and Prevention, Atlanta, GA.

- Unless prescribed by a clinician, antibiotics should never be used in a prophylactic manner—such as to avoid "traveler's diarrhea" when traveling to a foreign country. Taking antibiotics in that manner actually *increases* the chances of developing traveler's diarrhea. The antibiotics kill some of the beneficial indigenous intestinal microbes, eliminating the competition for food and space, making it easier for pathogens to gain a foothold.
- Healthcare professionals must practice good infection prevention and control procedures (Chapter 12). Frequent and proper handwashing is essential to prevent the transmission of pathogens from one patient to another. Healthcare professionals should monitor for important pathogens (such as MRSA) within healthcare settings and always isolate patients infected with multidrug-resistant pathogens.

Empiric Therapy

In some cases, a clinician must initiate therapy before laboratory results are available. This is referred to as *empiric therapy*. In an effort to save the life of a patient, it is sometimes necessary for the clinician to "guess" the most likely pathogen and the drug most likely to be effective. It will be an "educated guess," based on the clinician's prior experiences with the particular type of infectious disease that the patient has. Before writing a prescription for a certain antimicrobial agent, several factors must be taken into consideration by the clinician; some of these are in the following list:

- If the laboratory has reported the identity of the pathogen, the clinician can refer to a "pocket chart" that is available in most hospitals. This pocket chart, which is technically known as an antibiogram, is published by the Clinical Microbiology Laboratory; it usually contains antimicrobial susceptibility test data that have been accumulated during the past year. The pocket chart provides important information regarding drugs to which various bacterial pathogens were susceptible and resistant (Fig. 9-7).
- Is the patient allergic to any antimicrobial agents? Obviously, it would be unwise to prescribe a drug to which the patient is allergic.
- What is the age of the patient? Certain drugs are contraindicated in very young or very old patients.
- Is the patient pregnant? Certain drugs are known to be or suspected to be teratogenic (i.e., they cause birth defects).
- Is the patient an inpatient or outpatient? Certain drugs can be administered only intravenously and, therefore, cannot be prescribed for outpatients.
- If the patient is an inpatient, the clinician must prescribe a drug that is available in the hospital pharmacy (i.e., a drug that is listed in the hospital formulary).
- What is the site of the patient's infection? If the patient has cystitis (urinary bladder infection), the clinician might prescribe a drug that concentrates in the urine. Such a drug is rapidly removed from the blood by the kidneys, and high concentrations of the drug are achieved in the urinary bladder. To treat a brain abscess, the clinician would select a drug capable of crossing the blood–brain barrier.
- What other medications is the patient taking or receiving? Some antimicrobial agents will cross-react with certain other drugs, leading to a drug interaction that could be harmful to the patient.
- What other medical problems does the patient have? Certain antimicrobial agents are known to have toxic side effects (e.g., nephrotoxicity, hepatotoxicity, ototoxicity). For example, a clinician would not prescribe a nephrotoxic drug to a patient who has prior kidney damage.
- Is the patient leukopenic or immunocompromised? If so, it would be necessary to use a bactericidal agent to treat the patient's bacterial infection, rather than a bacteriostatic agent. Recall that bacteriostatic agents should be used only in patients whose host defense mechanisms

AEROBIC GRAM-NEGATIVE BACTERIA	No.	ampicillin	amp/sulbactam	pip/tazo	aztreonam	ertapenem	imipenem	cefazolin	cefuroxime	ceftriaxone	ceftazidime	cefepime	ciprofloxacin	gentamicin	tobramycin	amikacin	trimeth/sulfa	tetracycline	nitrofurantoin*
Escherichia coli	1843	46	53	96	95	100	100	86	90	95	95	97	67	90	90	100	71	70	96
Klebsiella pneumoniae	772	0	75	89	90	94	94	85	82	90	90	91	88	92	91	99	84	82	57
Klebsiella oxytoca	100	0	55	84	83	99	99	45	74	85	93	96	88	96	97	99	88	78	93
Enterobacter aerogenes	84	0	38	77	73	90	90	0	0	71	71	87	79	86	83	99	83	93	30
Enterobacter cloacae	196	0	24	76	68	99	99	0	0	69	70	93	94	93	94	99	89	90	26
Citrobacter freundii	72	0	55	83	79	99	99	0	0	72	77	97	82	88	92	100	79	64	96
Citrobacter koseri	39	0	97	97	97	100	100	97	97	100	100	100	97	100	100	100	97	92	83
Serratia marcescens	67	0	0	81	88	100	100	0	0	85	85	100	93	94	90	94	87	29	0
Proteus mirabilis	376	73	80	98	98	100	97	82	96	99	99	100	58	87	88	99	70	0	0
Morganella morganii	68	0	23	100	96	100	100	0	0	90	85	100	51	81	93	100	56	0	0
Pseudomonas aeruginosa	685			90	68		80				83	75	66	74	92	88			
Stenotrophomonas maltophilia	78										37						100		
Acinetobacter baumannii	48		47		0					42	52	52	48	53	65	85	50		
Haemophilus influenzae	39**	70	100						100		100		100				76		

*Urine only

** Represents inpatient and outpatient isolates

Figure 9–7. Pocket chart for aerobic Gram-negative bacteria. Illustrated here is the type of chart that clinicians carry in their pockets for use as a quick reference whenever empiric therapy is necessary. The pocket chart, which is prepared by the medical facility's Clinical Microbiology Laboratory, shows the percentage of particular organisms that were susceptible to the various drugs that were tested. The following is an example of how the pocket chart is used. A clinician is informed that *P. aeruginosa* has been isolated from his or her patient's blood culture, but the antimicrobial susceptibility testing results on that isolate will not be available until the following day. Because therapy must be initiated immediately, the clinician refers to the pocket chart and sees that tobramycin is the most appropriate drug to use (of the 685 strains of *P. aeruginosa* tested, 92% were susceptible to tobramycin). (As mentioned in the text, other factors would be taken into consideration by the clinician *before* prescribing tobramycin for this patient.) According to the pocket chart, which drug would be the second choice, if tobramycin is no longer available in the hospital pharmacy? Answer: piperacillin/tazobactam (90%). (Note: This chart is included for educational purposes only. It should not actually be used in a clinical setting.)

Although the patient's weight will influence the dosage of a particular drug, it is usually not taken into consideration when deciding which drug to prescribe.

are functioning properly (i.e., only in patients whose bodies are capable of killing the pathogen once its multiplication is stopped). A leukopenic patient has too few white blood cells to kill the pathogen, and the immune system of an immunocompromised patient would be unable to kill the pathogen.

• The cost of the various drugs is also a major consideration. Whenever possible, clinicians should prescribe less costly, narrow-spectrum drugs, rather than expensive, broad-spectrum drugs.

Undesirable Effects of Antimicrobial Agents

Listed below are some of the many reasons why antimicrobial agents should not be used indiscriminately.

• Whenever an antimicrobial agent is administered to a patient, any organisms within that patient that are susceptible to the agent will die, but resistant ones will survive. This is referred to as selecting for resistant organisms (Fig. 9-8). The resistant organisms then multiply, become dominant, and can be transmitted to other people. To prevent the overgrowth of resistant organisms, sometimes several drugs, each with a different mode of action, are administered simultaneously.

• The patient may become allergic to the agent. For example, penicillin G in low doses often sensitizes those who are prone to allergies; when these persons receive a second dose of penicillin at some later date, they may have a severe reaction known as anaphylactic shock, or they may break out in hives.

• Many antimicrobial agents are toxic to humans, and some are so toxic that they are administered only for serious diseases for which no other agents are available. One such drug is chloramphenicol, which, if given in high doses for a long period, may cause a very severe type of anemia called aplastic anemia. Another is streptomycin, which can damage the auditory nerve and cause deafness. Other drugs are hepatotoxic or nephrotoxic, causing liver or kidney damage, respectively.

Prolonged antibiotic use can lead to population explosions of microorganisms that are resistant to the antibiotic(s) being used. Such overgrowths are known as "superinfections."

• With prolonged use, broad-spectrum antibiotics may destroy the indigenous microbiota of the mouth, intestine, or vagina. The person no longer has the protection of the indigenous microbiota

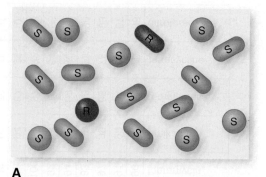

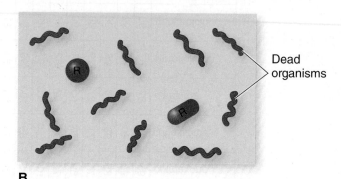

Dead organisms

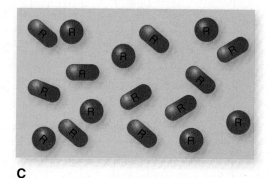

Figure 9-8. Selecting for drug-resistant organisms. A. Indigenous microbiota of a patient before initiation of antibiotic therapy. Most members of the population are susceptible (indicated by S) to the antibiotic to be administered; very few are resistant (indicated by R). **B.** After antibiotic therapy has been initiated, the susceptible organisms are dead; only a few resistant organisms remain. **C.** As a result of decreased competition for nutrients and space, the resistant organisms multiply and become the predominant organisms in the patient's indigenous microbiota. (The same type of selection process occurs when farm animals are fed antibiotic-containing feed and when antimicrobial-containing products [e.g., toys, cutting boards] are used in our homes. Both of these topics were discussed in Chapter 8.)

and thus becomes much more susceptible to infections caused by opportunists or secondary invaders. The resultant overgrowth by such organisms is referred to as a *superinfection*. A superinfection can be thought of as a "population explosion" of organisms that are usually present only in small numbers. For example, the prolonged use of oral antibiotics can result in a superinfection of *Clostridium difficile* in the colon, which can lead to such diseases as antibiotic-associated diarrhea and pseudomembranous colitis. Yeast vaginitis often follows antibacterial therapy because many bacteria of the vaginal microbiota were destroyed, leading to a superinfection of the indigenous yeast, *Candida albicans.*

Concluding Remarks

In recent years, microorganisms have developed resistance at such a rapid pace that many people, including many scientists, are beginning to fear that science is losing the war against pathogens. Some strains of pathogens have arisen that are resistant to all known drugs; examples include certain strains of *M. tuberculosis* (the bacterium that causes tuberculosis), *Plasmodium* spp. (the protozoa that cause malaria), and *S. aureus* (the bacterium that causes many different types of infections, including pneumonia and postsurgical wound infections). To win the war against drug resistance, more prudent use of currently available drugs, the discovery of new drugs, and the development of new vaccines will all be necessary. Unfortunately, as someone once said, "When science builds a better mousetrap, nature builds a better mouse." To learn more about antibiotic resistance, the book by Dr. Stuart Levy (previously cited) is highly recommended.

Fortunately, antimicrobial agents are not the only in vivo weapons against pathogens. Operating within our bodies are various systems that function to kill pathogens and protect us from infectious diseases. These systems, collectively referred to as host defense systems, are discussed in Chapters 15 and 16.

SOMETHING TO THINK ABOUT

"Initially hailed as 'magic bullets,' [antibiotics] are now used so often that success threatens their long-term utility. Unfortunately, the natural mutability of microbes enables pathogens to develop bullet-proof shields that make antibiotic treatments increasingly ineffective. Our failure to adequately address resistance problems may ultimately push the control of infectious diseases back to the pre-penicillin era." (From Drlica K and David S. Perlin. *Antibiotic Resistance: Understanding and Responding to an Emerging Crisis.* Upper Saddle River, NJ: Pearson Education, Inc; 2011.)

ON **thePoint**

- Terms Introduced in This Chapter
- Review of Key Points
- Increase Your Knowledge
- Critical Thinking
- Additional Self-Assessment Exercises

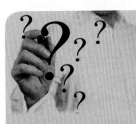

Self-Assessment Exercises

After studying this chapter, answer the following multiple-choice questions.

1. Which of the following is *least* likely to be taken into consideration when deciding which antibiotic to prescribe for a patient?
   a. patient's age
   b. patient's underlying medical conditions
   c. patient's weight
   d. other medications that the patient is taking

2. Which of the following is *least* likely to lead to drug resistance in bacteria?
   a. a chromosomal mutation that alters cell membrane permeability
   b. a chromosomal mutation that alters the shape of a particular drug-binding site
   c. receiving a gene that codes for an enzyme that destroys a particular antibiotic
   d. receiving a gene that codes for the production of a capsule

3. Which of the following is *not* a common mechanism by which antimicrobial agents kill or inhibit the growth of bacteria?
   a. damage to cell membranes
   b. destruction of capsules
   c. inhibition of cell wall synthesis
   d. inhibition of protein synthesis

4. Multidrug therapy is always used when a patient is diagnosed as having:
   a. an infection caused by MRSA
   b. diphtheria
   c. strep throat
   d. tuberculosis

5. Which of the following terms or names has *nothing* to do with the use of two drugs simultaneously?
   a. antagonism
   b. Salvarsan
   c. Septra
   d. synergism

6. Which of the following is *not* a common mechanism by which antifungal agents work?
   a. by binding with cell membrane sterols
   b. by blocking nucleic acid synthesis
   c. by dissolving hyphae
   d. by interfering with sterol synthesis

7. Which of the following scientists discovered penicillin?
   a. Alexander Fleming
   b. Paul Ehrlich
   c. Selman Waksman
   d. Sir Howard Walter Florey

8. Which of the following scientists is considered to be the "Father of Chemotherapy"?
   a. Alexander Fleming
   b. Paul Ehrlich
   c. Selman Waksman
   d. Sir Howard Walter Florey

9. All the following antimicrobial agents work by inhibiting cell wall synthesis except:
   a. cephalosporins
   b. chloramphenicol
   c. penicillin
   d. vancomycin

10. All the following antimicrobial agents work by inhibiting protein synthesis except:
    a. chloramphenicol
    b. erythromycin
    c. imipenem
    d. tetracycline

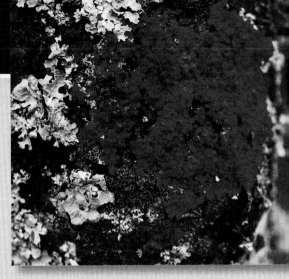

Several types of lichen growing on the bark of a tree.

10

Microbial Ecology and Microbial Biotechnology

CHAPTER OUTLINE

LEARNING OBJECTIVES

After studying this chapter, you should be able to:

- Define ecology, human ecology, and microbial ecology
- List three categories of symbiotic relationships
- Differentiate between mutualism and commensalism and give an example of each
- Cite an example of a parasitic relationship
- Discuss the beneficial and harmful roles of the indigenous microbiota of the human body
- Describe biofilms and their impact on human health
- Outline the nitrogen cycle; include the meanings of the terms nitrogen fixation, nitrification, denitrification, and ammonification in the description
- Name 10 foods that require microbial activity for their production
- Define biotechnology and cite four examples of how microbes are used in industry
- Define bioremediation and cite an example

Introduction

The science of *ecology* is the systematic study of the interrelationships that exist between organisms and their environment. If you were to take a course in human ecology, you would study the interrelationships between humans and the world around them—the nonliving world as well as the living world. *Microbial ecology* is the study of the numerous interrelationships between microbes and the world around them; how microbes interact with other microbes, how microbes interact with organisms other than microbes, and how microbes interact with the nonliving world around them. Interactions between microorganisms and animals, plants, other microbes, soil, and our atmosphere have far-reaching effects on our lives. We are all aware of the diseases caused by pathogens (see Chapters 17 to 21), but this is only one example of many ways that microbes interact with humans. Most relationships between humans and microbes are beneficial rather than harmful. Although the "bad guys" get most of the attention in the news media, our microbial allies far outnumber our microbial enemies.

> Microbial ecology is the study of the numerous interrelationships between microbes and the world around them.

Microbes interact with humans in many ways and at many levels. The most intimate association that we have with microbes is their presence both on and within our bodies. Additionally, microbes play important roles in agriculture, various industries, disposal of industrial and toxic wastes, sewage treatment, and water purification. Microbes are essential in the fields of biotechnology, bioremediation, genetic engineering, and gene therapy (genetic engineering and gene therapy were discussed in Chapter 7).

Symbiotic Relationships Involving Microorganisms

Symbiosis

Symbiosis, or a *symbiotic relationship*, is defined as the living together or close association of two dissimilar organisms (usually two different species). The organisms that live together in such a relationship are referred to as *symbionts*. Some symbiotic relationships (called mutualistic relationships) are beneficial to *both* symbionts, others (commensalistic relationships) are beneficial to only one

> Symbiosis is defined as the living together or close association of two dissimilar organisms (usually two different species).

symbiont, and others (parasitic relationships) are harmful to one symbiont. Many microbes participate in symbiotic relationships. Various symbiotic relationships involving microbes are discussed in subsequent sections; some are illustrated in Figure 10-1.

Neutralism

The term *neutralism* is used to describe a symbiotic relationship in which neither symbiont is affected by the relationship. In other words, neutralism reflects a situation in which different microorganisms occupy the same ecologic niche, but have absolutely no effect on each other.

Commensalism

A symbiotic relationship that is beneficial to one symbiont and of no consequence (i.e., is neither beneficial nor harmful) to the other is called *commensalism*. Many of the organisms in the indigenous microbiota of humans are considered to be commensals. The relationship is of obvious benefit to the microorganisms (they are provided nutrients and "housing"), but the microorganisms have no effect on the host. A *host* is defined as a living organism that harbors another living organism. One example

> Commensalism is a symbiotic relationship that is beneficial to one symbiont and of no consequence (i.e., is neither beneficial nor harmful) to the other.

of a commensal, illustrated in Figure 10-1, is the tiny mite called *Demodex*, which lives within hair follicles and sebaceous glands, especially those of the eyelashes and eyebrows.

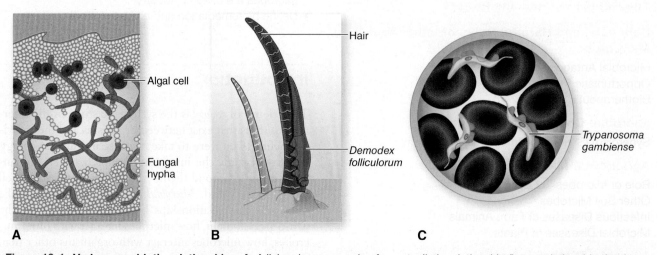

Figure 10-1. Various symbiotic relationships. A. A lichen is an example of a mutualistic relationship (i.e., a relationship that is beneficial to both symbionts). **B.** The tiny *Demodex* mites that live in human hair follicles are examples of commensals. **C.** The flagellated protozoan that causes African sleeping sickness is a parasite (*RBC*, red blood cell).

Mutualism

Mutualism is a symbiotic relationship that is beneficial to both symbionts (i.e., the relationship is mutually beneficial). Humans have a mutualistic relationship with many of the microorganisms of their indigenous microbiota.

> Mutualism is a symbiotic relationship that is beneficial to both symbionts (i.e., the relationship is mutually beneficial).

An example is the intestinal bacterium *Escherichia coli*, which obtains nutrients from food materials ingested by the host and produces vitamins (such as vitamin K) that are used by the host. Vitamin K is a blood-clotting factor that is essential to humans. Also, some members of our indigenous microbiota prevent colonization by pathogens and overgrowth by opportunistic pathogens (discussed further in a following section entitled "Microbial Antagonism").

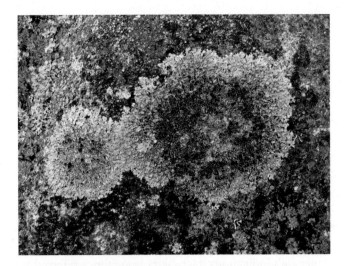

Figure 10-2. Lichens on a rock in Maine. (Courtesy of Biomed Ed, Round Rock, TX.)

The lichens that you see as colored patches on rocks and tree trunks are further examples of mutualism (Fig. 10-2). As discussed in Chapter 5, a lichen is composed of an alga (or a cyanobacterium) and a fungus, living so closely together that they appear to be one organism. The fungus uses some of the energy that the alga produces by photosynthesis (recall that fungi are not photosynthetic), and the chitin in the fungal cell walls protects the alga from desiccation. Thus, both symbionts benefit from the relationship.

Parasitism

Parasitism is a symbiotic relationship that is beneficial to one symbiont (the parasite) and detrimental to the other symbiont (the host). Being detrimental to the host does not necessarily mean that the parasite causes disease. In some cases, a host can harbor a parasite, without the parasite causing harm to the host. "Smart'" parasites do not cause disease, but rather take only the nutrients they need to exist. The especially "dumb" parasites kill their hosts; then they must either find a new host or die. Nonetheless, certain parasites always cause disease, and some

> Parasitism is a symbiotic relationship that is beneficial to one symbiont (the parasite) and detrimental to the other symbiont (the host).

cause the death of the host. For example, the protozoan illustrated in Figure 10-1—*Trypanosoma gambiense*—is the parasite that causes African sleeping sickness, a human disease that often causes death of the host. Parasites are discussed further in Chapter 21.

A change in conditions can cause one type of symbiotic relationship to shift to another type. For example, conditions can cause a mutualistic or commensalistic relationship between humans and their indigenous microbiota to shift to a parasitic, disease-causing (pathogenic) relationship. Recall that many of the microbes of our indigenous microbiota are opportunistic pathogens

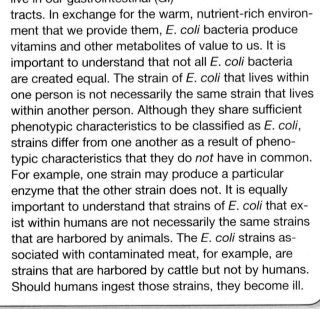

A Bit More About *E. coli*

We normally live in harmony with the *E. coli* bacteria that live in our gastrointestinal (GI) tracts. In exchange for the warm, nutrient-rich environment that we provide them, *E. coli* bacteria produce vitamins and other metabolites of value to us. It is important to understand that not all *E. coli* bacteria are created equal. The strain of *E. coli* that lives within one person is not necessarily the same strain that lives within another person. Although they share sufficient phenotypic characteristics to be classified as *E. coli*, strains differ from one another as a result of phenotypic characteristics that they do *not* have in common. For example, one strain may produce a particular enzyme that the other strain does not. It is equally important to understand that strains of *E. coli* that exist within humans are not necessarily the same strains that are harbored by animals. The *E. coli* strains associated with contaminated meat, for example, are strains that are harbored by cattle but not by humans. Should humans ingest those strains, they become ill.

As another example of a mutualistic relationship, consider the protozoa that live in the intestine of termites. Termites eat wood, but they cannot digest wood. Fortunately for them, the protozoa that live in their intestinal tract break down the large molecules in wood into smaller molecules that can be absorbed and used as nutrients by the termites. In turn, the termite provides food and a warm, moist place for the protozoa to live. Without these protozoa, the termites would die of starvation.

(opportunists), awaiting the opportunity to cause disease. Conditions that may enable an opportunist to cause disease include burns, lacerations, surgical procedures, or diseases that debilitate (weaken) the host or interfere with host defense mechanisms. Immunosuppressed individuals are particularly susceptible to opportunistic pathogens. Opportunists can also cause disease in otherwise healthy persons if they gain access to the blood, urinary bladder, lungs, or other organs and tissues of those individuals.

Indigenous Microbiota of Humans

A person's indigenous microbiota (sometimes referred to as the *human microbiome* or *human bioneme)* includes all of the microbes (bacteria, fungi, protozoa, and viruses) that

> A person's indigenous microbiota includes all of the microbes (bacteria, fungi, protozoa, and viruses) that reside on and within that person.

reside on and within that person (Fig. 10-3). It has been estimated that our bodies are composed of about 10 trillion cells (including nerve cells, muscle cells, and epithelial cells), and that we have about 10 times that many microbes that live on and within our bodies (10 × 10 trillion = 100 trillion). It has also been estimated that our indigenous microbiota is composed of as many as 10,000 different species!

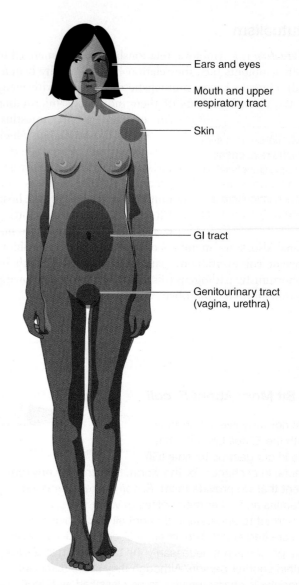

Figure 10-3. **Areas of the body where most of the indigenous microbiota reside.**

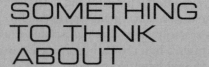

SOMETHING TO THINK ABOUT

"I would like to point out that we depend on more than the activity of some 30,000 genes encoded in the human genome. Our existence is critically dependent on the presence of upwards of 1000 bacterial species (the exact number is unknown because many are uncultivable) living in and on us; the oral cavity and gastrointestinal tracts contain particularly rich and active populations. Thus, if truth be known, human life depends on an additional 2 to 4 million genes, mostly uncharacterized. Until the synergistic activities between humans (and other animals) with their obligatory commensals have been elucidated, an understanding of human biology will remain incomplete." (Julian Davies, *Science Magazine*, 2001; 291:2316.)

A fetus has no indigenous microbiota. During and after delivery, a newborn is exposed to many microorganisms from its mother, food, air, and virtually everything that touches the infant. Both harmless and helpful microbes take up residence on the baby's skin, at all body openings, and on mucous membranes that line the digestive tract (mouth to anus) and the genitourinary (GU) tract. These moist, warm environments provide excellent conditions for growth. Conditions for proper growth (moisture, pH, temperature, nutrients) vary throughout the body; thus, the types of resident microbiota differ from one anatomic site to another. Blood, lymph, spinal fluid, and most internal tissues and organs are normally free of microorganisms (i.e., they are sterile). Table 10-1 lists microorganisms frequently found on and within the human body.

Table 10-1 Anatomic Locations of Bacteria and Yeasts Found as Indigenous Microbiota of Humans

	Skin	Mouth	Nose and Nasopharynx	Oropharynx	GI Tract	GU Tract
Anaerobic Gram-negative cocci	−	+	−	−	−	−
Anaerobic Gram-positive cocci	−	+	−	+	+	+
Bacteroides spp.	±	+	−	+	+	+
Candida spp.	+	±	−	−	−	+
Clostridium spp.	+	−	−	−	+	+
Diphtheroids	+	−	+	+	−	+
Enterobacteriaceae[a]	−	−	−	−	+	±
Enterococcus spp.	−	±	±	−	+	+
Fusobacterium spp.	−	±	±	+	+	−
Haemophilus spp.	−	−	+	+	−	−
Lactobacillus spp.	+	+	−	−	−	+
Micrococcus spp.	+	−	−	−	−	−
Neisseria meningitidis	−	−	±	±	−	−
Prevotella/Porphyromonas spp.	−	+	−	+	−	−
Staphylococcus spp.	+	+	+	+	+	+
Streptococcus spp.	±	+	+	+	−	−

+, commonly present; ±, less commonly present; −, absent.

[a]Sometimes referred to as enteric bacilli (includes *Escherichia*, *Klebsiella*, and *Proteus* spp.).

In addition to the resident microbiota, transient microbes take up temporary residence on and within humans. The body is constantly exposed to microorganisms from the external environment; these transient microbes are frequently attracted to moist, warm body areas. These microbes are only temporary for many reasons: they may be washed from external areas by bathing; they may not be able to compete with the resident microbiota; they may fail to survive in the acidic or alkaline environment of the site; they may be killed by substances produced by resident microbiota; or they may be flushed away by bodily excretions or secretions (such as urine, feces, tears, and sweat). Many microbes are unable to colonize (inhabit) the human body because they do not find the body to be a suitable host.

Destruction of the resident microbiota disturbs the delicate balance established between the host and its microorganisms. For example, prolonged therapy with certain antibiotics often destroys many of the intestinal microbiota. Diarrhea is usually the result of such an imbalance, which in turn leaves the body more susceptible to secondary invaders. When the number of usual resident microbes is greatly reduced, opportunistic invaders can more easily establish themselves within those areas. One important opportunist usually found in small numbers near body openings is the yeast, *Candida albicans*, which, in the absence of sufficient numbers of other resident microbiota, may grow unchecked in the mouth, vagina, or lower intestine, causing the disease *candidiasis* (also known as moniliasis). Such an overgrowth or population explosion of an organism that is usually present in low numbers is referred to as a *superinfection*.

Microbiota of the Skin

The resident microbiota of the skin consists primarily of bacteria and fungi—as many as 300 different species, depending on the anatomical location. The number of different types of microbes varies greatly from body part to body part and from person to person. Although the skin is constantly exposed to air, many of the bacteria that live on the skin are anaerobes; in fact, anaerobes actually outnumber aerobes on the skin. Anaerobes live in the deeper layers of skin, hair follicles, and sweat and sebaceous glands. The most common bacteria on the skin are species of *Staphylococcus* (especially *S. epidermidis* and other coagulase-negative staphylococci[a]), *Corynebacterium*, and *Propionibacterium*. The number and variety of microorganisms present on the skin depend on many factors, such as the

> The most common bacteria on the skin are *Staphylococcus*, *Corynebacterium*, and *Propionibacterium* spp.

- Anatomical location
- Amount of moisture present
- pH
- Temperature
- Salinity (saltiness)
- Presence of chemical wastes such as urea and fatty acids
- Presence of other microbes, which may be producing toxic substances

Moist, warm conditions in hairy areas of the body where there are many sweat and oil glands, such as under the arms and in the groin area, stimulate the growth of many different microorganisms. Dry, calloused areas of skin have few bacteria, whereas moist folds between the toes and fingers support many bacteria and fungi. The surface of the skin near mucosal openings of the body (the mouth, eyes, nose, anus, and genitalia) is inhabited by bacteria present in various excretions and secretions.

Frequent washing with soap and water removes most of the potentially harmful transient microbes harbored in sweat, oil, and other secretions from moist body parts, as well as the dead epithelial cells on which they feed. Proper hygiene also serves to remove odorous organic materials present in sweat, sebum (sebaceous gland secretions), and microbial metabolic by-products. Healthcare professionals must be particularly careful to keep their skin and clothing as free of transient microbes as possible to help prevent personal infections and to avoid transferring pathogens to patients. These individuals should always keep in mind that most infections after burns, wounds, and surgery result from the growth of resident or transient skin microbiota in these susceptible areas.

Microbiota of the Ears and Eyes

The middle ear and inner ear are usually sterile, whereas the outer ear and the auditory canal contain the same types of microbes as are found on the skin. When a person coughs, sneezes, or blows his or her nose, these microbes may be carried along the eustachian tube and into the middle ear where they can cause infection. Infection can also develop in the middle ear when the eustachian tube does not open and close properly to maintain correct air pressure within the ear.

---

[a]Coagulase is an enzyme that causes clot formation. In the Clinical Microbiology Laboratory, the coagulase test is used to differentiate *Staphylococcus aureus* (which produces coagulase and is referred to as being coagulase-positive) from other species of *Staphylococcus* (which do not produce coagulase and are referred to as being coagulase-negative).

The external surface of the eye is lubricated, cleansed, and protected by tears, mucus, and sebum. Thus, continual production of tears and the presence of the enzyme lysozyme and other antimicrobial substances found in tears greatly reduce the numbers of indigenous microbiota organisms found on the eye surfaces.

Microbiota of the Respiratory Tract

The respiratory tract can be divided into the upper respiratory tract and the lower respiratory tract. The upper respiratory tract consists of the nasal passages and the throat (pharynx). The lower respiratory tract consists of the larynx (voice box), trachea, bronchi, bronchioles, and lungs.

The nasal passages and throat have an abundant and varied population of microbes, because these areas provide moist, warm mucous membranes that furnish excellent conditions for microbial growth. Many microorganisms found in the healthy nose and throat are harmless. Others are opportunistic pathogens, which have the potential to cause disease under certain circumstances. Some people—known as healthy *carriers*—harbor virulent (disease-causing) pathogens in their nasal passages or throats, but do not have the diseases associated with them, such as diphtheria, meningitis, pneumonia, and whooping cough. Although these carriers are unaffected by these pathogens, carriers can transmit them to susceptible persons.

The lower respiratory tract is usually free of microbes because the mucous membranes and lungs have defense mechanisms (described in Chapter 15) that efficiently remove invaders.

Microbiota of the Oral Cavity (Mouth)

The anatomy of the oral cavity (mouth) affords shelter for numerous anaerobic and aerobic bacteria. Anaerobic microorganisms flourish in gum margins, crevices between the teeth, and deep folds (crypts) on the surface of the tonsils. Bacteria thrive especially well in particles of food and in the debris of dead epithelial cells around the teeth. Food remaining on and between teeth provides a rich nutrient medium for growth of many oral bacteria. Carelessness in dental hygiene allows growth of these bacteria, with development of dental caries (tooth decay), gingivitis (gum disease), and more severe periodontal diseases.

The list of microbes that have been isolated from healthy human mouths reads like a manual of the major groups of microbes. It includes Gram-positive and Gram-negative bacteria (both cocci and bacilli), spirochetes, and sometimes yeasts, mouldlike organisms, protozoa, and viruses. The bacteria include species of *Actinomyces*, *Bacteroides*, *Borrelia*, *Corynebacterium*, *Fusobacterium*,

The most common organisms in the indigenous micro- biota of the mouth are various spe- cies of α-hemolytic streptococci.

Haemophilus, *Lactobacillus*, *Neis- seria*, *Porphyromonas*, *Prevotella*, *Propionibacterium*, *Staphylococ- cus*, *Streptococcus*, *Treponema*, and *Veillonella*. The most common organisms in the indigenous microbiota of the mouth are various species of α-hemolytic streptococci. The bacterium most often implicated in the formation of dental plaque is *Streptococcus mutans*.

Microbiota of the GI Tract

The GI tract (or digestive tract) consists of a long tube with many expanded areas designed for digestion of food, absorption of nutrients, and elimination of undigested materials. Excluding the oral cavity and pharynx, which have already been discussed, the GI tract includes the esophagus, stomach, small intestine, large intestine (co- lon), and anus. Accessory glands and organs of the GI system include the salivary glands, pancreas, liver, and gallbladder.

Gastric enzymes and the extremely acidic pH (ap- proximately pH 1.5) of the stomach usually prevent growth of indigenous microbiota, and most transient microbes (i.e., microbes consumed in foods and bever- ages) are killed as they pass through the stomach. There is one bacterium—a Gram-negative bacillus named *He- licobacter pylori*—that lives in some people's stomachs and is a common cause of ulcers. A few microbes, enveloped by food particles, manage to pass through the stomach during periods of low acid concentration. Also, when the amount of acid is reduced in the course of diseases such as stomach cancer, certain bacteria may be found in the stomach.

Few microbes usually exist in the upper portion of the small intestine (the duodenum) because bile inhibits their growth, but many are found in the lower parts of the small intestine (the jejunum and ileum).

The colon contains the largest number and variety of microorganisms of any colonized area of the body. It has been estimated that as many as 500 to 600 differ- ent species—primarily bacteria—live there. Because the colon is anaerobic, the bacte- ria living there are obligate, aerotolerant, and facultative anaerobes. Bacteria found in the GI tract include species of *Actinomyces*, *Bacteroides*, *Clostrid- ium*, *Enterobacter*, *Enterococcus*, *Escherichia*, *Klebsiella*, *Lactobacillus*, *Proteus*, *Pseudomonas*, *Staphylococcus*, and *Streptococcus*.

The colon contains as many as 500 to 600 different species—primarily bacteria.

Also, many fungi, protozoa, and viruses can live in the colon. Many of the microbes of the colon are opportun- ists, causing disease only when they gain access to other areas of the body (e.g., urinary bladder, bloodstream, or

lesion of some type), or when the usual balance among the microorganisms is upset. *E. coli* is a good example. All humans have *E. coli* bacteria in their colon. They are op- portunists, usually causing us no problems at all, but they can cause urinary tract infections (UTIs) when they gain access to the urinary bladder. In fact, *E. coli* is the most common cause of UTIs.

Many microbes are removed from the GI tract as a result of defecation. It has been estimated that about 50% of the fecal mass consists of bacteria.

Microbiota of the GU Tract

The GU tract (or urogenital tract) consists of the uri- nary tract (kidneys, ureters, urinary bladder, and urethra) and the various parts of the male and female reproductive systems.

The healthy kidney, ureters, and urinary bladder are sterile. However, the distal urethra (the part of the ure- thra farthest from the urinary bladder) and the external opening of the urethra harbor many microbes, including bacteria, yeasts, and viruses. As a rule, these microbes do not invade the bladder because the urethra is periodi- cally flushed by acidic urine. Frequent urination helps to prevent UTIs. However, persistent, recurring UTIs often develop when there is an obstruction or narrow- ing of the urethra, which allows the invasive organisms to multiply. The most frequent causes of urethral infection (urethritis)—*Chlamydia trachomatis*, *Neisseria gonorrhoeae*, and mycoplasmas—are easily introduced into the urethra by sexual intercourse.

The reproductive systems of both men and women are usually sterile, with the exception of the vagina; here, the microbiota varies with the stage of sexual develop- ment. During puberty and after menopause, vaginal se- cretions are alkaline, supporting the growth of various diphtheroids, streptococci, staphylococci, and coliforms (*E. coli* and closely related enteric Gram-negative ba- cilli). Through the childbearing years, vaginal secre- tions are acidic (pH 4.0–5.0), encouraging the growth mainly of lactobacilli, along with a few α-hemolytic streptococci, staphylococci, diphtheroids, and yeasts. Bacteria found in the vagina include species of *Actino- myces*, *Bacteroides*, *Corynebacterium*, *Klebsiella*, *Lactobacil- lus*, *Mycoplasma*, *Proteus*, *Pseudomonas*, *Staphylococcus*, and *Streptococcus*.

The metabolic by-products of lactobacilli, especially lactic acid, inhibit growth of the bacteria associated with bacterial vaginosis (BV). Factors that lead to a decrease in the number of lactobacilli in the vaginal microbi- ota can lead to an overgrowth of other bacteria (e.g., *Bacteroides* spp., *Mobiluncus* spp., *Gardnerella vaginalis*, and anaerobic cocci), which in turn can lead to bacterial vaginosis (BV). Likewise, a decrease in the number of lactobacilli can lead to an overgrowth of yeasts, which in turn can lead to yeast vaginitis.

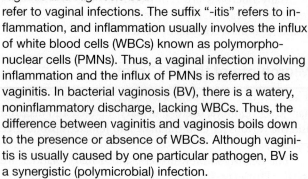

"Vaginitis" versus "Vaginosis"

The similarly sounding terms *vaginitis* and *vaginosis* both refer to vaginal infections. The suffix "-itis" refers to inflammation, and inflammation usually involves the influx of white blood cells (WBCs) known as polymorphonuclear cells (PMNs). Thus, a vaginal infection involving inflammation and the influx of PMNs is referred to as vaginitis. In bacterial vaginosis (BV), there is a watery, noninflammatory discharge, lacking WBCs. Thus, the difference between vaginitis and vaginosis boils down to the presence or absence of WBCs. Although vaginitis is usually caused by one particular pathogen, BV is a synergistic (polymicrobial) infection.

The Human Microbiome Project

The Human Microbiome Project (HMP) is a US National Institutes of Health initiative that was launched in 2008 with a 5-year mission to generate resources enabling comprehensive characterization of the human microbiome and analysis of its role in human health and disease. As of October 2012, approximately 5,000 samples had been collected from 129 men and 113 women. Body sites sampled included the mouth, nose, skin, lower intestine (stool samples), and vagina. HMP researchers have calculated that more than 10,000 microbial species occupy the human ecosystem and that they have identified between 81% and 99% of the genera. The following extracts are from a 2012 journal article:[b]

- "Studies of the human microbiome have revealed that even healthy individuals differ remarkably in the microbes that occupy habitats such as the gut, skin, and vagina."
- "Much of this diversity remains unexplained, although diet, environment, host genetics, and early microbial exposure have all been implicated."

Other interesting findings (according to Wikipedia):

- "Microbes contribute more genes responsible for human survival than humans' own genes. It is estimated that bacterial protein genes are 360 times more abundant than human genes."
- "Microbial metabolic activities—for example, digestion of fats—are not always provided by the same bacterial species."

[b]The Human Microbiome Project Consortium. Structure, function and diversity of the healthy human microbiome. *Nature* 2012; 486:207–214.

- "Components of the human microbiome change over time, affected by a patient disease state and medication. However, the microbiome eventually returns to a state of equilibrium, even though the composition of bacterial types has changed."

Beneficial and Harmful Roles of Indigenous Microbiota

Humans derive many benefits from their indigenous microbiota, some of which have already been mentioned. Some nutrients, particularly vitamins K and B_{12}, pantothenic acid, pyridoxine, and biotin, are obtained from secretions of certain intestinal bacteria. Evidence also indicates that indigenous microbes provide a constant source of irritants and antigens to stimulate the immune system. This causes the immune system to respond more readily by producing antibodies to foreign invaders and substances, which in turn enhances the body's protection against pathogens. The mere presence of large numbers of microorganisms at certain anatomic locations is beneficial, in that they prevent pathogens from colonizing those locations.

> Certain of our intestinal bacteria are beneficial to us in that they produce useful vitamins and other nutrients.

Microbial Antagonism

The term *microbial antagonism* means "microbes versus microbes" or "microbes against microbes." Many of the microbes of our indigenous microbiota serve a beneficial role by preventing other microbes from becoming established in or colonizing a particular anatomic location. For example, the huge numbers of bacteria in our colons accomplish this by occupying space and consuming nutrients. "Newcomers" (including pathogens that we have ingested) cannot gain a foothold because of the intense competition for space and nutrients.

> Many members of our indigenous microbiota serve a beneficial role by preventing other microbes from becoming established in or colonizing a particular anatomic location.

Other examples of microbial antagonism involve the production of antibiotics and bacteriocins. As discussed in Chapter 9, many bacteria and fungi produce antibiotics. Recall that an antibiotic is a substance produced by one microorganism that kills or inhibits the growth of another microorganism. (Actually, the term antibiotic is usually reserved for those substances produced by bacteria and fungi that have been found useful in treating infectious diseases.) Some bacteria produce proteins called bacteriocins which kill other bacteria. An example is colicin, a bacteriocin produced by *E. coli*.

Opportunistic Pathogens

As you know, many members of the indigenous microbiota of the human body are opportunistic pathogens (opportunists), which can be thought of as organisms that are hanging around, waiting for the opportunity to cause infections. Take *E. coli*, for example. Huge numbers of *E. coli* live in our intestinal tract, causing us no problems whatsoever on a day-to-day basis. They do possess the potential to be pathogenic, however, and can cause serious infections should they find their way to a site such as the urinary bladder, the bloodstream, or a wound. Other especially important opportunistic pathogens in the human indigenous microbiota include other members of the family *Enterobacteriaceae*, *S. aureus*, and *Enterococcus* spp.

> Opportunistic pathogens (opportunists) can be thought of as organisms that are hanging around, awaiting the opportunity to cause infections.

Biotherapeutic Agents

When the delicate balance among the various species in the population of indigenous microbiota is upset by antibiotics, other types of chemotherapy, or changes in pH, many complications may result. Certain microorganisms may flourish out of control, such as *C. albicans* in the vagina, leading to yeast vaginitis. Also, diarrhea and pseudomembranous colitis may occur as a result of overgrowth of *Clostridium difficile* in the colon. Cultures of *Lactobacillus* in yogurt or in medications may be prescribed to reestablish and stabilize the microbial balance. Bacteria and yeasts used in this manner are called *biotherapeutic agents* (or probiotics).[c] Other microorganisms that have been used as biotherapeutic agents include *Bifidobacterium* spp., nonpathogenic *Enterococcus* spp., and *Saccharomyces* spp. (yeasts).

> Bacteria and yeasts that are ingested to reestablish and stabilize the microbial balance within our bodies are called biotherapeutic agents or probiotics.

Microbial Communities (Biofilms)

We often read about one particular microbe as being the cause of a certain disease or as playing a specific role in nature. In reality, it is rare to find an ecologic niche in which only one type of microbe is present or only one microbe is causing a particular effect. In nature, microbes are often organized into what are known as *biofilms*—complex and persistent communities of assorted microbes. Bacterial biofilms are virtually everywhere; examples include dental plaque, the slippery coating on a rock in a stream, and the slime that accumulates on the inner walls of various types of pipes and tubing. A bacterial biofilm consists of a variety of different species of bacteria plus a gooey extracellular matrix that the bacteria secrete, composed of polysaccharides, proteins, and nucleic acids. The bacteria grow in tiny clusters—called *microcolonies*—that are separated by a network of water channels. The fluid that flows through these channels bathes the microcolonies with dissolved nutrients and carries away waste products.

> In nature, microbes are often organized into complex and persistent communities of assorted organisms called biofilms.

Biofilms have medical significance. They form on bones, heart valves, tissues, and inanimate objects such as artificial heart valves, catheters, and prosthetic implants (Fig. 10-4). Biofilms have been implicated in diseases such as endocarditis, cystic fibrosis, middle ear infections, kidney stones, periodontal disease, and prostate infections. It has been estimated that perhaps as many as 60% of human infections are due to biofilms. Microbes commonly associated with biofilms on indwelling medical devices include the yeast *Candida albicans* and bacteria such as *S. aureus*, coagulase-negative staphylococci, *Enterococcus* spp., *Klebsiella pneumoniae*, and *Pseudomonas aeruginosa*.

> Biofilms have been implicated in diseases such as endocarditis, cystic fibrosis, middle ear infections, kidney stones, periodontal disease, and prostate infections.

Dental plaque consists of a community of microorganisms attached to various proteins and glycoproteins adsorbed onto tooth surfaces. If the plaque is not

---

[c] Probiotics should not be confused with prebiotics. Whereas probiotics are microorganisms, prebiotics are food ingredients with the capacity to improve health when metabolized by intestinal bacteria.

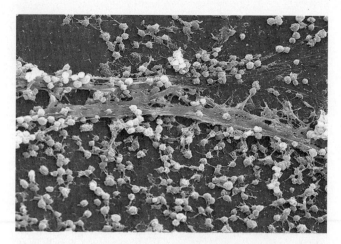

Figure 10-4. Scanning electron micrograph of a *S. aureus* biofilm inside the lumen of an indwelling catheter. (Courtesy of Janice Carr and the CDC.)

removed, substances produced by these organisms can penetrate the tooth enamel, leading to cavities, and eventually causing soft tissue disease.

Biofilms are very resistant to antibiotics, disinfectants, and certain types of host defense mechanisms. Antibiotics that, in the laboratory, have been shown to be effective against pure cultures of organisms within biofilms may be ineffective against those same organisms within an actual biofilm. Let us take penicillin as an example. Penicillin is an antibiotic that prevents bacteria from producing cell walls. In the laboratory, penicillin may kill actively growing cells of a particular organism, but it does not kill any cells of that organism within the biofilm that are not growing (i.e., that are not actively building cell walls). Also, any penicillinases (discussed in Chapter 9) being produced by organisms within the biofilm will inactivate the penicillin molecule, and will thus protect other organisms within the biofilm from the effects of penicillin. Therefore, some bacteria that are present within the biofilm protect other species of bacteria within the biofilm. Biofilms are also protected from antimicrobial agents as a result of decreased penetration or diffusion of the agents into the biofilms.

Another example of how bacteria within a biofilm cooperate with each other involves nutrients. In some biofilms, bacteria of different species cooperate to break down nutrients that any single species cannot break down by itself. In some cases, one species within a biofilm feeds on the metabolic wastes of another.

Biofilms are resistant to certain types of host defense mechanisms. For example, it is difficult for leukocytes to penetrate biofilms, and those that do penetrate seem less efficient at phagocytizing bacteria within the biofilm. Although the macrophages and leukocytes cannot ingest the bacteria, they do become activated and secrete toxic compounds that cause damage to nearby healthy host tissues. This phenomenon has

> Bacteria within biofilms are protected from antibiotics and certain types of host defense mechanisms.

been referred to as *frustrated phagocytosis*. The biofilms also appear to suppress the ability of phagocytes to kill any biofilm bacteria that they do manage to ingest.

Research has shown that bacteria within biofilms produce many different types of proteins that those same organisms do not produce when they are grown in pure culture. Some of these proteins are involved in the formation of the extracellular matrix and microcolonies. It is thought that bacteria in biofilms can communicate with each other. Experiments with *P. aeruginosa* have demonstrated that when a sufficient number of cells accumulate, the concentration of certain signaling molecules becomes high enough to trigger changes in the activity of dozens of genes. Whereas in the past, scientists studied ways to control individual species of bacteria, they are now concentrating their efforts on ways to attack and control biofilms.

Synergism (Synergistic Infections)

Sometimes, two (or more) microorganisms may "team up" to produce a disease that neither could cause by itself. This is referred to as *synergism* or a *synergistic relationship*. The diseases are referred to as *synergistic infections*, polymicrobial infections, or mixed infections. For example, certain oral bacteria can work together to cause a serious oral disease called acute necrotizing ulcerative gingivitis (ANUG; also known as Vincent disease and "trench mouth"). Similarly, the disease known as BV is the result of the combined efforts of several different species of bacteria.

> When two or more microbes "team up" to produce a disease that neither could cause by itself, the phenomenon is referred to as synergism or a synergistic relationship, and the diseases they cause are referred to as synergistic infections, polymicrobial infections, or mixed infections.

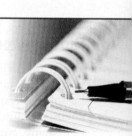

STUDY AID

Different Uses of the Term Synergism

As was just explained, *synergism* can refer to the combined effects of more than one type of bacteria, as in synergistic infections. In this case, synergism is a bad thing! However, as you learned in Chapter 9, synergism can also refer to the beneficial effects of using two antibiotics simultaneously. With respect to antibiotic use, a synergistic effect is a good thing, because many more pathogens are killed by using a particular combination of two drugs than would be killed if either drug was used alone.

Agricultural Microbiology

There are many uses for microorganisms in agriculture. They are used extensively in the field of genetic engineering to create new or genetically altered plants. Such genetically engineered plants might grow larger, be better tasting, or be more resistant to insects, plant diseases, or extremes in temperature. Some microorganisms are used as pesticides. Many microorganisms are decomposers, which return minerals and other nutrients to soil. In addition, microorganisms play major roles in elemental cycles, such as the carbon, oxygen, nitrogen, phosphorous, and sulfur cycles.

Role of Microbes in Elemental Cycles

Bacteria are exceptionally adaptable and versatile. They are found on the land, in all waters, in every animal and plant, and even inside other microorganisms (in which case they are referred to as *endosymbionts*). Some bacteria and fungi serve a valuable function by recycling back into the soil the nutrients from dead, decaying animals and plants, as was briefly discussed in Chapter 1. Free-living fungi and bacteria that decompose dead organic matter into inorganic materials are called saprophytes. The inorganic nutrients that are returned to the soil are used by chemotrophic bacteria and plants for synthesis of biologic molecules necessary for their growth. The plants are eaten by animals, which eventually die and are recycled again with the aid of saprophytes. The cycling of elements by microorganisms is sometimes referred to as biogeochemical cycling.

Good examples of the cycling of nutrients in nature are the nitrogen, carbon, oxygen, sulfur, and phosphorus cycles, in which microorganisms play very important roles. In the nitrogen cycle (Fig. 10-5), free atmospheric nitrogen gas (N_2) is converted by *nitrogen-fixing bacteria* and cyanobacteria into ammonia (NH_3) and the ammonium ion (NH_4^+). Then, chemolithotrophic soil bacteria, called *nitrifying bacteria*, convert ammonium ions into nitrite ions (NO_2^-) and nitrate ions (NO_3^-). Plants then use the nitrates to build plant proteins; these proteins are eaten by animals, which then use them to build animal proteins. Excreted nitrogen-containing animal waste products (such as urea in urine) are converted by certain bacteria to ammonia by a process known as *ammonification*. Also, dead plant and animal nitrogen-containing debris and fecal material are transformed by saprophytic fungi and bacteria into ammonia, which in turn is converted into nitrites and nitrates for recycling by plants. To replenish the free nitrogen in the air, a group of bacteria called *denitrifying bacteria* convert nitrates to atmospheric nitrogen gas (N_2). The cycle goes on and on.

> The nitrogen cycle involves nitrogen-fixing bacteria, nitrifying bacteria, and denitrifying bacteria.

Some nitrogen-fixing bacteria (e.g., *Rhizobium* and *Bradyrhizobium* spp.) live in and near the root nodules of plants called legumes, such as alfalfa, clover, peas, soybeans, and peanuts (Fig. 10-6). These plants are often used in crop-rotation techniques by farmers to return nitrogen compounds to the soil for use as nutrients by cash crops. Nitrifying soil bacteria include *Nitrosomonas*, *Nitrosospira*, *Nitrosococcus*, *Nitrosolobus*, and *Nitrobacter* spp. Denitrifying bacteria include certain species of *Pseudomonas* and *Bacillus*.

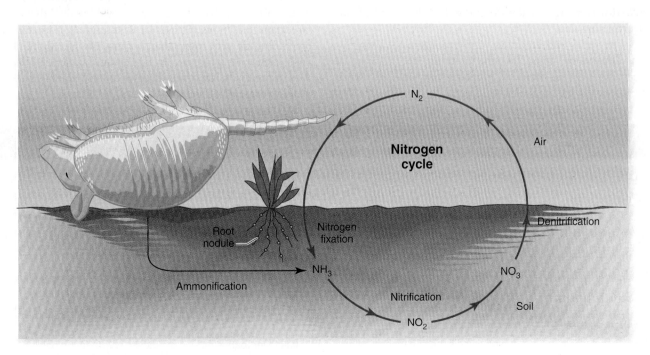

Figure 10-5. The nitrogen cycle. See text for details.

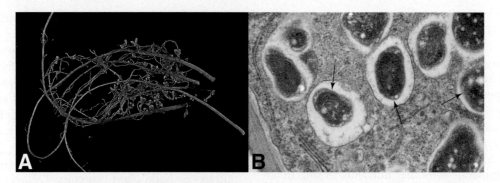

Figure 10-6. Root nodules of legumes. A. Soybean root nodules, which contain nitrogen-fixing *Rhizobium* bacteria. **B.** Nitrogen-fixing bacteria (*arrows*) can be seen in this cross section of a soybean root nodule. (Courtesy of **(A)** http://en.wikipedia.org and **(B)** http://commons.wikimedia.org.)

Other Soil Microbes

In addition to the bacteria that play essential roles in elemental cycles, there are a multitude of other microbes in soil—bacteria (including cyanobacteria), fungi (primarily moulds), algae, protozoa, viruses, and viroids. Many of the soil microorganisms are decomposers.

A variety of human pathogens live in soil, including various *Clostridium* spp. (e.g., *Clostridium tetani*, the causative agent of tetanus; *Clostridium botulinum*, the causative agent of botulism; and the various *Clostridium* spp. that cause gas gangrene). The spores of *Bacillus anthracis* (the causative agent of anthrax) may also be present in soil, where they can remain viable for many years. Various yeasts (e.g., *Cryptococcus neoformans*) and fungal spores present in soil may cause human diseases after inhalation of the dust that results from overturning dirt.

> The spores of many human pathogens can be found in soil, including those of *Clostridium* spp., *B. anthracis*, and *Cryptococcus neoformans*.

The types and amounts of microorganisms living in soil depend on many factors, including the amount of decaying organic material, available nutrients, moisture content, amount of oxygen available, pH, temperature, and the presence of waste products of other microbes.

Infectious Diseases of Farm Animals

Farmers, ranchers, and agricultural microbiologists are concerned about the many infectious diseases of farm animals—diseases that may be caused by a wide variety of pathogens (e.g., viruses, bacteria, protozoa, fungi, and helminths). Not only is there the danger that some of these diseases could be transmitted to humans (discussed in Chapter 11), but these diseases are also of obvious economic concern to farmers and ranchers. Fortunately, vaccines are available to prevent many of these diseases. Although a discussion of these diseases is beyond the scope of this introductory microbiology book, it is important for microbiology students to be aware of their existence. (Likewise, microbiology students should realize that there are many infectious diseases of wild animals, zoo animals, and domestic pets; topics that, because of space limitations, also cannot be addressed in this book.) Table 10-2 lists a few of the many infectious diseases of farm animals and the causative agents of those diseases.

> Microbes cause many diseases of farm animals, wild animals, zoo animals, and domestic pets.

Table 10-2 Infectious Diseases of Farm Animals

Category	Diseases
Prion diseases	Diseases of the nervous system such as bovine spongiform encephalopathy ("mad cow disease") and scrapie
Viral diseases	Blue tongue (sore muzzle), bovine viral diarrhea (BVD), equine encephalomyelitis (sleeping sickness), equine infectious anemia, foot-and-mouth disease, infectious bovine rhinotracheitis, influenza, rabies, swine pox, vesicular stomatitis, warts
Bacterial diseases	Actinomycosis ("lumpy jaw"), anthrax, blackleg, botulism, brucellosis ("Bang disease"), campylobacteriosis, distemper (strangles), erysipelas, foot rot, fowl cholera, leptospirosis, listeriosis, mastitis, pasteurellosis, pneumonia, redwater (bacillary hemoglobinuria), salmonellosis, tetanus ("lock jaw"), tuberculosis, vibriosis
Fungal diseases	Ringworm
Protozoal diseases	Anaplasmosis, bovine trichomoniasis, cattle tick fever (babesiosis), coccidiosis, cryptosporidiosis

Microbial Diseases of Plants

Microbes cause thousands of different types of plant diseases, often resulting in huge economic losses. Most plant diseases are caused by fungi, viruses, viroids, and bacteria. Not only are living plants attacked and destroyed, but microbes (primarily fungi) also cause the rotting of stored grains and other crops. Plant diseases have interesting names such as blights, cankers, galls, leaf spots, mildews, mosaics, rots, rusts, scabs, smuts, and wilts. Three especially infamous plant diseases are Dutch elm disease (which, since its importation into the United States in 1930, has destroyed about 70% of the elm trees in North America), late blight of potatoes (which resulted in the Great Potato Famine in Ireland, 1845–1849), and wheat rust (which destroys tons of wheat annually). Table 10-3 lists the names of a few of the many plant diseases caused by microorganisms.

> Microbes cause thousands of different types of plant diseases, with names such as blights, cankers, galls, leaf spots, mildews, mosaics, rots, rusts, scabs, smuts, and wilts.

SOMETHING TO THINK ABOUT

"As our planet warms, a world locked in permafrost will come alive, and researchers worry the tiny inhabitants of the frozen soil will start churning out greenhouse gases, magnifying global warming."

"'Nobody has looked at what happens to microbes when the permafrost thaws,' said Janet Jansson, a senior staff scientist at Lawrence Berkeley National Laboratory in California. She led a study that recorded what happened when chunks of Alaskan permafrost thawed for the first time in 1,200 years. 'We now have a picture, there wasn't really one before,' said Jansson, who along with her colleagues sequenced the genetic material of microbes within frozen and thawed permafrost. Along the way, they also discovered a new-to-science microbe and sequenced its entire genetic blueprint or genome."

"Permafrost is pretty much what it sounds like — soil that has been frozen for thousands or even hundreds of thousands of years — and it is packed with the dead plants and other once-living things present when the permafrost formed. Rising global temperatures thaw this organic matter, allowing microbes to begin breaking it down. In the process, they release greenhouse gases containing carbon. Scientists are particularly worried this process could pump a great deal of methane, which contains carbon and is a potent world warmer, into the atmosphere."

"Because there is a lot of carbon tucked away in the permafrost, scientists have feared the melting of it could aggravate global warming. Arctic permafrost, for example, is estimated to contain more than 250 times the greenhouse gas emissions from the United States in 2009." (Parry W. Frozen microscopic worlds come alive as Earth warms. Nov. 2011. Complete article is at http://www.livescience.com/16898-arctic-microbes-permafrost-climate-change.html.)

Table 10-3 Examples of Plant Diseases Caused by Microbes

Disease	Pathogen	Disease	Pathogen
Bean mosaic disease	Virus	Late blight of potatoes	Fungus (a water mould)
Black spot of roses	Fungus	Mushroom root rot	Fungus
Blue mould of tobacco	Fungus (a water mould)	Potato spindle tuber	Viroid
Brown patch of lawns	Fungus	Powdery mildews	Fungi
Chestnut blight	Fungus	Tobacco mosaic disease	Virus
Citrus exocortis	Viroid	Various leaf spots	Bacteria and fungi
Cotton root rot	Fungus	Various rots	Fungi
Crown gall	Bacteria	Various rusts	Fungi
Downy mildew of grapes	Fungus (a water mould)	Various smuts	Fungi
Dutch elm disease	Fungus	Wheat mosaic disease	Virus
Ergot	Fungus	Wheat rust	Fungus

Microbial Biotechnology

The United Nations Convention on Biological Diversity defines biotechnology as "any technological application that uses biological systems, living organisms, or derivatives thereof, to make or modify products or processes for specific use." Although not all areas of biotechnology involve microbes, microbes are used in many aspects of biotechnology. Some examples are listed here:

- **Production of therapeutic proteins.** Human genes are introduced (usually by transformation) into bacteria and yeasts. Such genetically engineered microorganisms have been used to produce therapeutic proteins such as human insulin, human growth hormone, human tissue plasminogen activator, interferon, and hepatitis B vaccine.
- **Production of DNA vaccines.** DNA vaccines (also called gene vaccines) are presently only experimental. To prepare a DNA vaccine, a particular pathogen gene (let us use as an example the gene that codes for a specific protein on a pathogen's surface) is inserted into a plasmid (*E. coli* plasmids have been used). Copies of the plasmid are then injected (usually intramuscularly) into a person's tissue. After cells within that tissue internalize the plasmids, the cells produce copies of the gene product (the pathogen's surface protein in this example). The person's immune system then produces antibodies against that gene product, and the antibodies protect the person from infection with that pathogen. The various ways in which antibodies protect us from pathogens are discussed in Chapter 16.
- **Production of vitamins.** Bacteria can be used as sources of vitamins B_2 (riboflavin), B_7 (biotin), B_9 (folic acid), B_{12}, and K_2.
- **Use of microbial metabolites as antimicrobial agents and other types of therapeutic agents.** Penicillins and cephalosporins are examples of antibiotics produced by fungi. Bacitracin, chloramphenicol, erythromycin, polymyxin B, streptomycin, tetracycline, and vancomycin are examples of antibiotics produced by bacteria. Recall that antibiotics were discussed in Chapter 9. Other microbial metabolites have been used as anticancer drugs, immunosuppressants, and herbicides.
- **Agricultural applications.**
  - Certain microbial metabolites have microbicidal, herbicidal, insecticidal, or nematocidal activities. For example, a soil bacterium named *Bacillus subtilis* secretes compounds with antifungal, antibacterial, and insecticidal activities.
  - Bacterial plasmids are used to introduce foreign genes into plants. Plants containing foreign genes are referred to as transgenic plants. Transgenic plants have been produced that are tolerant of or resistant to harsh environments, herbicides, insect pests, and

viral, bacterial, fungal, and nematode pathogens. For example, *Bacillus thuringiensis* is a bacterium that produces toxins capable of killing various plant pathogens (e.g., caterpillar larvae). The genes that code for these toxins can be introduced into plants, thus protecting the plants from damage caused by these larvae. Tobacco, cotton, and tomato plants have been protected in this manner.

> Biotechnology is defined as "any technological application that uses biological systems, living organisms, or derivatives thereof, to make or modify products or processes for specific use."

- **Food technology.**
  - Microorganisms are used in the production of foods such as acidophilus milk, bread, butter, cocoa, coffee, cottage cheese, cultured buttermilk, fish sauces, green olives, kimchi (from cabbage), meat products (e.g., country-cured hams, sausage, salami), olives, pickles, poi (fermented taro root), sauerkraut, sour cream, soy sauce, tofu, various ripened cheeses (e.g., Brie, Camembert, Cheddar, Colby, Edam, Gouda, Gruyere, Limburger, Muenster, Parmesan, Romano, Roquefort, Swiss), vinegar, and yogurt.
  - Yeasts are used in the production of alcoholic beverages, such as ale, beer, bourbon, brandy, cognac, rum, rye whiskey, sake (rice wine), Scotch whiskey, vodka, and wine.
  - Microbes are used in the commercial production of amino acids (e.g., alanine, aspartate, cysteine, glutamate, glycine, histidine, lysine, methionine, phenylalanine, tryptophan) for use in the food industry.
  - Algae and fungi are used as a source of single-cell protein for animal and human consumption.
- **Production of chemicals.** Microbes can be used in the large-scale production of acetic acid, acetone, butanol, citric acid, ethanol, formic acid, glycerol, isopropanol, and lactic acid, as well as biofuels such as hydrogen and methane.
- **Biomining.** Microbes have been used in the mining of arsenic, cadmium, cobalt, copper, nickel, uranium, zinc, and other metals by a process known as leaching or bioleaching.
- **Bioremediation.** The term *bioremediation* refers to the use of microorganisms to clean up various types of wastes, including industrial wastes and other pollutants (e.g., herbicides and pesticides). Some of the microbes used in this manner have been genetically engineered to digest specific wastes. For example, genetically engineered, petroleum-digesting bacteria were used to clean up the 11 million–gallon oil spill in Prince William Sound, Alaska, in 1989. At a government defense plant in Savannah River, Georgia, scientists have used naturally occurring bacteria known as methanotrophs to remove highly toxic solvents such as trichloroethylene and tetrachloroethylene (collectively referred to as TCEs) from the soil. The methanotrophs, which normally consume

methane in the environment, were more or less "tricked" into decomposing the TCEs. In addition, microbes are used extensively in composting, sewage treatment, and water purification (see Chapter 11).

- **Other.**
  - Microbial enzymes used in industry include amylases, cellulase, collagenase, lactase, lipase, pectinase, and proteases.
  - Two amino acids produced by microbes are used in the artificial sweetener called aspartame (NutraSweet).

ON thePoint

- Terms Introduced in This Chapter
- Review of Key Points
- A Closer Look: How Bacteria Communicate with Each Other
- Increase Your Knowledge
- Critical Thinking
- Additional Self-Assessment Exercises

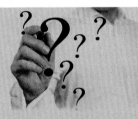

Self-Assessment Exercises

After studying this chapter, answer the following multiple-choice questions.

1. A symbiont could be a(n):
   a. commensal
   b. opportunist
   c. parasite
   d. all of the above

2. The greatest number and variety of indigenous microbiota of the human body live in or on the:
   a. colon
   b. genitourinary tract
   c. mouth
   d. skin

3. *Escherichia coli* living in the human colon can be considered to be a(n):
   a. endosymbiont
   b. opportunist
   c. symbiont in a mutualistic relationship
   d. all of the above

4. Which of the following sites of the human body does not have indigenous microbiota?
   a. bloodstream
   b. colon
   c. distal urethra
   d. vagina

5. Which of the following would be present in highest numbers in the indigenous microbiota of the human mouth?
   a. α-hemolytic streptococci
   b. β-hemolytic streptococci
   c. *Candida albicans*
   d. *Staphylococcus aureus*

6. Which of the following would be present in highest numbers in the indigenous microbiota of the skin?
   a. *C. albicans*
   b. coagulase-negative staphylococci
   c. *Enterococcus* spp.
   d. *E. coli*

7. The indigenous microbiota of the external ear canal is most like the indigenous microbiota of the:
   a. colon
   b. mouth
   c. skin
   d. distal urethra

8. Which of the following are *least* likely to play a role in the nitrogen cycle?
   a. indigenous microbiota
   b. nitrifying and denitrifying bacteria
   c. nitrogen-fixing bacteria
   d. bacteria living in the root nodules of legumes

9. Microorganisms are used in which of the following industries?
   a. antibiotic
   b. chemical
   c. food, beer, and wine
   d. all of the above

10. The term that best describes a symbiotic relationship in which two different microorganisms occupy the same ecologic niche, but have absolutely no effect on each other is:
    a. commensalism
    b. mutualism
    c. neutralism
    d. parasitism

11

Epidemiology and Public Health

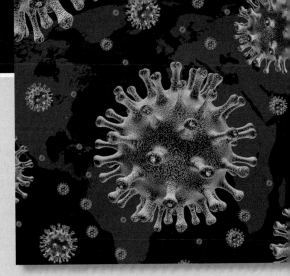

Artist rendering of a worldwide viral pandemic.

CHAPTER OUTLINE

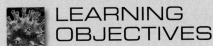

LEARNING OBJECTIVES

After studying this chapter, you should be able to:

- Define epidemiology
- Differentiate between infectious, communicable, and contagious diseases; cite an example of each
- Differentiate between the incidence of a disease and the prevalence of a disease
- Distinguish between sporadic, endemic, nonendemic, epidemic, and pandemic diseases
- Name three diseases that are currently considered to be pandemics
- List, in the proper order, the six components of the chain of infection
- Identify three examples of living reservoirs and three examples of nonliving reservoirs
- List five modes of infectious disease transmission
- List four examples of potential biological warfare (BW) or bioterrorism agents
- Outline the steps involved in water treatment
- Explain what is meant by a coliform count and state its importance

Epidemiology

Introduction

Both **pathology** and **epidemiology** can be loosely defined as the study of disease, but they involve different aspects of disease. A pathologist studies the structural and functional manifestations of disease and is involved in diagnosing diseases in individuals, whereas an *epidemiologist* studies the factors that determine the frequency, distribution, and determinants of diseases in human populations. With respect to infectious diseases, these factors include the characteristics of various pathogens; susceptibility of different human populations resulting from overcrowding, lack of immunization, nutritional status, inadequate sanitation procedures, and other factors; locations (reservoirs) where pathogens are lurking; and the various ways in which infectious diseases are transmitted. It could be said that epidemiologists are concerned with the who, what, where, when, and why of infectious diseases: Who becomes infected? What pathogens are causing the infections? Where do the pathogens come from? When do certain diseases occur? Why do some diseases occur in certain places but not in others? How are pathogens transmitted? Do some diseases occur only at certain times of the year? If so, why? Epidemiologists also develop ways to prevent, control, or eradicate diseases in populations. Epidemiologists are concerned with *all* types of diseases—not just infectious diseases. However, only infectious diseases are discussed in this chapter.

> Epidemiology is the study of factors that determine the frequency, distribution, and determinants of diseases in human populations, and ways to prevent, control, or eradicate diseases in populations.

and figure out how to stop them. Data collection and statistical analysis of data are among the many duties of epidemiologists.

Epidemiologists have various educational backgrounds. Some are physicians, with specialization in epidemiology or public health. Others have a Doctor of Philosophy degree (PhD or DPhil), a Master of Science or Master of Public Health degree (MS or MPH), or a Bachelor of Science degree (e.g., RN degree) plus specialized training in epidemiology. Many epidemiologists are employed at public health agencies and healthcare institutions. The Centers for Disease Control and Prevention (CDC) employs many epidemiologists and offers a 2-year postgraduate course to train health professionals as Epidemic Intelligence Service (EIS) officers. EIS officers, many of whom are employed at state health departments, conduct epidemiologic investigations, research, and public health surveillance. To learn more about the EIS, visit this CDC web site: http://www.cdc.gov/eis.

Epidemiologic Terminology

It sometimes seems like epidemiologists speak a language all their own. They frequently use terms such as communicable, contagious, and zoonotic diseases; the incidence, morbidity rate, prevalence, and mortality rate of a particular disease; and adjectives such as sporadic, endemic, epidemic, and pandemic to describe the status of a particular infectious disease in a given population. The following sections briefly examine these terms.

Communicable and Contagious Diseases

As previously stated, an infectious disease (infection) is a disease that is caused by a pathogen. If the infectious disease is transmissible from one human to another (ie., person to person), it is called a **communicable disease**. Although it might seem like splitting hairs, a **contagious disease** is defined as a communicable disease that is *easily transmitted* from one person to another. Example: Assume that you are in the front row of a movie theater. One person seated in the back row has gonorrhea and another has influenza, both of which are communicable diseases. The person with influenza is coughing and sneezing throughout the movie, creating an aerosol of influenza viruses. Thus, even though you are seated far away from the person with influenza, you might very well develop influenza as a result of inhalation of the aerosols produced by that person. Influenza is a contagious disease. On the other hand, you would not contract gonorrhea as a result of your movie-going experience. Gonorrhea is not a contagious disease.

SPOTLIGHTING

Epidemiologists

Epidemiologists are scientists who specialize in the study of disease and injury patterns (incidence and distribution patterns) in populations and ways to prevent or control diseases and injuries. Epidemiologists study virtually all types of diseases, including heart, hereditary, communicable, and zoonotic diseases and cancer. In some ways, epidemiologists are like disease detectives, gathering and piecing together clues to determine what causes a particular disease, why it occurs only at certain times, and why certain people in a population get the disease while others do not. Quite often, epidemiologists are called on to track down the cause of epidemics

Zoonotic Diseases

Infectious diseases that humans acquire from animal sources are called **zoonotic diseases** or **zoonoses** (sing., zoonosis). These diseases are discussed later in this chapter.

Incidence and Morbidity Rate

The **incidence** of a particular disease is defined as the number of new cases of that disease in a defined population during a specific time period; for example, the number of new cases of hantavirus pulmonary syndrome (HPS) in the United States during 2012. The incidence of a disease is similar to the **morbidity rate** for that disease, which is usually expressed as the number of new cases of a particular disease that occurred during a specified time period per a specifically defined population (usually per 1,000, 10,000, or 100,000 population), for example, the number of new cases of a particular disease in 2012 per 100,000 U.S. population.

STUDY AID

Infectious versus Communicable Diseases

Infectious diseases (infections) are diseases caused by pathogens. **Communicable diseases** are infectious diseases that can be transmitted from one human to another (i.e., person to person). **Contagious diseases** are communicable diseases that are *easily* transmitted from one person to another.

Prevalence

There are two types of **prevalence**: period prevalence and point prevalence. The **period prevalence** of a particular disease is the number of cases of the disease existing in a given population during a specific time period (e.g., the total number of cases of gonorrhea that existed in the U.S. population during 2012). The **point prevalence** of a particular disease is the number of cases of the disease existing in a given population at a particular moment in time (e.g., the number of cases of malaria in the U.S. population at this moment).

Mortality Rate

Mortality refers to death. The **mortality rate** (also known as the *death rate*) is the ratio of the number of people who died of a particular disease during a specified time period per a specified population (usually per 1,000, 10,000, or 100,000 population); for example, the number of people who died of a particular disease in 2012 per 100,000 U.S. population.

Sporadic Diseases

A **sporadic disease** is a disease that occurs only occasionally (sporadically) within the population of a particular geographic area. In the United States, sporadic diseases include botulism, cholera, gas gangrene, plague, tetanus, and typhoid fever. Quite often, certain diseases occur only sporadically because they are kept under control as a result of immunization programs and sanitary conditions. It is possible for outbreaks of these controlled diseases to occur, however, whenever vaccination programs and other public health programs are neglected.

> A sporadic disease is a disease that occurs only occasionally (sporadically) within the population of a particular geographic area, whereas an endemic disease is a disease that is always present within that population.

Endemic Diseases

Endemic diseases are diseases that are always present within the population of a particular geographic area. The number of cases of the disease may fluctuate over time, but the disease never dies out completely. Endemic infectious diseases of the United States include bacterial diseases such as tuberculosis (TB); staphylococcal and streptococcal infections; sexually transmitted diseases (STDs) such as gonorrhea and syphilis; and viral diseases such as the common cold, influenza, chickenpox, and mumps. In some parts of the United States, plague (caused by a bacterium called *Yersinia pestis*) is endemic among rats, prairie dogs, and other rodents, but is not endemic among humans. Plague in humans is only occasionally observed in the United States, and is, therefore, a sporadic disease. The actual incidence of an endemic disease at any particular time depends on a balance among several factors, including the environment, genetic susceptibility of the population, behavioral factors, number of people who are immune, virulence of the pathogen, and reservoir or source of infection.

Epidemic Diseases

Endemic diseases may on occasion become **epidemic diseases**. An epidemic (or outbreak) is defined as a greater than usual number of cases of a disease in a particular region, usually occurring within a relatively short period of time. An epidemic does not necessarily involve a large number of people, although it might. If a dozen people develop staphylococcal food poisoning shortly after their return from a church picnic, then that constitutes an epidemic—a small one, to be sure, but an epidemic nonetheless.

> Epidemic diseases are diseases that occur in a greater than usual number of cases in a particular region and usually occur within a relatively short period of time.

HISTORICAL NOTE

The Broad Street Pump

In the mid-19th century, a British physician by the name of John Snow designed and conducted an epidemiologic investigation of a cholera outbreak in London. He carefully compared households affected by cholera with households that were unaffected and concluded that the primary difference between them was their source of drinking water. At one point in his investigation, he ordered the removal of the handle of the Broad Street water pump, thus helping to end an epidemic that had killed more than 500 people. People were unable to pump (and, therefore, unable to drink) the contaminated water. He published a paper, *On the Communication of Cholera by Impure Thames Water,* in 1884, and a book, *On the Mode of Communication of Cholera,* in 1885. He concluded that cholera was spread via fecally contaminated water. The water at the Broad Street pump was being contaminated with sewage from the adjacent houses (Fig. 11-1). Snow is considered by many to be the "Father of Epidemiology."

Listed here are a few of the epidemics that have occurred in the United States within the past 40 years:

- **1976.** An epidemic of a respiratory disease (Legionnaires disease or legionellosis) occurred during an American Legion convention in Philadelphia, Pennsylvania. It resulted in approximately 220 hospitalizations and 34 deaths. The pathogen (a Gram-negative bacillus named *Legionella pneumophila*) was present in the water being circulated through the air-conditioning system of the hotel where the affected Legionnaires were staying. Aerosols of the organism were inhaled by occupants of some of the rooms in the hotel. Subsequent epidemics of legionellosis have occurred in other hotels, hospitals, cruise ships, and supermarkets. The supermarket outbreaks were associated with the misting of vegetables. Virtually all epidemics of legionellosis have involved contaminated water or colonized water pipes and aerosols containing the pathogen.

- **1992–1993.** An epidemic involving *Escherichia coli* O157:H7-contaminated hamburger meat occurred in the Pacific northwest. It resulted in approximately 500 diarrheal cases, 45 cases of kidney failure as a result of hemolytic uremic syndrome, and the death of several young children. *E. coli* O157:H7 is a particularly virulent serotype of *E. coli*; it is also known as enterohemorrhagic *E. coli*. In this epidemic, the source of the *E. coli* was cattle feces. The ground beef used to make the hamburgers had been contaminated with cattle feces during the slaughtering process. The hamburgers had not been cooked long enough, or at a high-enough temperature, to kill the bacteria.

- **1993.** An epidemic of HPS occurred on Native American reservations in the Four Corners region (where the borders of Colorado, New Mexico, Arizona, and Utah all meet). It resulted in approximately 50 to 60 cases, including 28 deaths. The particular hantavirus strain (now called *Sin Nombre virus*) was present in the urine and feces of deer mice, some of which had gained entrance to the homes of villagers. Aerosols of the virus were produced when residents swept up house dust containing the rodent droppings. The pathogen was then inhaled by individuals in those homes.

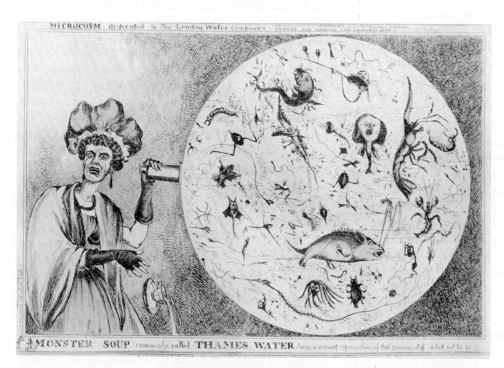

Figure 11-1. *Thames Water,* an etching by William Heath, c. 1828. This etching is a satire on the contamination of the water supply. A London commission reported in 1828 that the Thames River water at Chelsea was "charged with the contents of the great common-sewers, the drainings of the dunghills and laystalls, [and] the refuse of hospitals, slaughterhouses, and manufactures." (Zigrosser C. *Medicine and the Artist [Ars Medica].* New York, NY: Dover Publications, Inc.; 1970. By permission of the Philadelphia Museum of Art.)

- **1993.** An epidemic of cryptosporidiosis (a diarrheal disease) occurred in Milwaukee, Wisconsin. It resulted from drinking water that was contaminated with the oocysts of *Cryptosporidium parvum* (a protozoan parasite). This epidemic is described more fully later in this chapter.
- **2002–2003.** An epidemic of West Nile virus (WNV) infections occurred throughout the United States in 2002, resulting in more than 4,100 human cases and 284 deaths. The 2002 WNV epidemic was the largest recognized arboviral meningoencephalitis epidemic in the Western Hemisphere and the largest WNV meningoencephalitis epidemic ever recorded. However, the 2003 WNV epidemic was even worse, with a total of 9,862 cases and 264 deaths. WNV epidemics occur each year in the United States.
- **2012.** A multistate outbreak of fungal meningitis was linked to contaminated lots of an injectable steroid. The outbreak led to 32 deaths among 438 cases. The patients were infected with a mold called *Exserohilum rostratum*, which is usually associated with soils and plants.

    Other 2012 epidemics included a country-wide WNV outbreak and a hantavirus outbreak in Yosemite National Park. As of December 11, 2012, a total of 5,387 cases of WNV disease in people, including 243 deaths, had been reported to the CDC. Of these, 2,734 (51%) were classified as neuroinvasive disease (such as meningitis or encephalitis) and 2,653 (49%) were classified as non-neuroinvasive disease. The 5,387 cases was the highest number of WNV disease cases reported to the CDC through the second week in December since 2003. A third of all cases were reported from Texas. The hantavirus outbreak resulted in 10 confirmed cases (including 3 deaths). Nine of the 10 individuals with hantavirus infection stayed in Yosemite's tent cabins; the tenth person hiked and camped elsewhere in Yosemite National Park.
- **Waterborne disease outbreaks.** Such outbreaks occur annually in the United States, associated with both drinking water and water that is not intended for drinking ("recreational water"). The CDC (described later in the chapter) have presented data associated with 36 drinking water disease outbreaks and 134 recreational water outbreaks that occurred during 2007 and 2008.[a] Of the 32 drinking water outbreaks where etiologic agents were identified, 21 were associated with bacteria, 5 with viruses, 3 with parasites, 1 with a chemical, 1 with both bacteria and viruses, and 1 with both bacteria and parasites. Of the 105 recreational water outbreaks where etiologic agents were identified, 68 were caused by parasites, 22 by bacteria, 5 by viruses, 9 by chemicals or toxins, and 1 by multiple etiology types. *Cryptosporidium* (a protozoan parasite) was confirmed as the etiologic agent of 45% of the recreational water outbreaks.
- **Foodborne disease outbreaks, 2009–2010.** Known pathogens cause an estimated 9.4 million foodborne illnesses per year in the United States. According to the CDC,[b] during 2009–2010, a total of 1,527 foodborne disease outbreaks were reported, resulting in 29,444 cases of illness, 1,184 hospitalizations, and 23 deaths. Among the 790 outbreaks with a single laboratory-confirmed etiologic agent, norovirus was the most commonly reported, accounting for 491 of the outbreaks. *Salmonella* was second, accounting for 243 of outbreaks. Some of the other pathogens associated with foodborne outbreaks during 2009–2010 were Shiga-toxin producing *E. coli* (60 outbreaks), *Clostridium perfringens* (57 outbreaks), *Campylobacter* (40 outbreaks), *Bacillus* (25 outbreaks), and *Staphylococcus* enterotoxin (19 outbreaks). The food commodities most often implicated were beef, dairy, fish, and poultry. One *Salmonella* infection was the most common infection reported and was associated with the largest number of hospitalizations and deaths. One national outbreak of *Salmonella* infections in 2010 was caused by contaminated eggs, which led to a massive recall of approximately 500 million eggs.

These and other epidemics have been identified through constant surveillance and accumulation of data by the CDC. Epidemics usually follow a specific pattern, in which the number of cases of a disease increases to a maximum and then decreases rapidly, because the number of susceptible and exposed individuals is limited.

Epidemics may occur in communities that have not been previously exposed to a particular pathogen. People from populated areas who travel into isolated communities frequently introduce a new pathogen to susceptible inhabitants of that community, after which the disease spreads rapidly. Over the years, there have been many such examples. The syphilis epidemic in Europe in the early 1500s might have been caused by a highly virulent spirochete carried back from the West Indies by Columbus' men in 1492. Also, measles, smallpox, and TB introduced to Native Americans by early explorers and settlers almost destroyed many tribes.

In communities in which normal sanitation practices are relaxed, allowing fecal contamination of water supplies and food, epidemics of typhoid fever, cholera, giardiasis, and dysentery often occur. Visitors to these communities should be aware that they are especially susceptible to these diseases, because they never developed a natural immunity by being exposed to them during childhood.

Influenza ("flu") epidemics occur in many areas during certain times of the year and involve most of the population because the immunity developed in prior years is usually temporary. Thus, the disease recurs each year among those who are not revaccinated or naturally resistant to the infection. Epidemics of influenza cause approximately 20,000 deaths per year in the United

---

[a]*Morbidity and Mortality Weekly Report (MMWR) Surveillance Summaries* 60 (SS12): 1–68, 2011.

[b]*Morbidity and Mortality Weekly Report (MMWR)* 60 (03); 41–47, 2013.

States. According to the World Health Organization (WHO), the 2009 pandemic of swine flu (also known as H1N1) killed more than 18,000 people worldwide. The CDC reported that 22 million Americans had contracted the virus, that 98,000 required hospitalization, and about 3,900 died of H1N1-related causes.

Since 1976, Ebola virus has caused a number of severe epidemics of hemorrhagic fever, primarily in African countries. The largest outbreaks have occurred in Uganda (425 cases with 224 deaths in 2000–2001), Zaire (318 cases with 280 deaths in 1976), the Democratic Republic of Congo (315 cases with 250 deaths in 1995; 264 cases with 187 deaths in 2007), and Sudan (284 cases with 151 deaths in 1976). Between 25% and 90% of infected patients have died in these epidemics. According to a 2012 article,[c] the likely source of the virus is Ethiopian epauletted fruit bats.

In a hospital setting, a relatively small number of infected patients can constitute an epidemic. If a higher than usual number of patients on a particular ward should suddenly become infected by a particular pathogen, this would constitute an epidemic, and the situation must be brought to the attention of the Hospital Infection Control Committee (discussed in Chapter 12).

Pandemic Diseases

A **pandemic disease** is a disease that is occurring in epidemic proportions in many countries simultaneously—sometimes worldwide. The 1918 Spanish flu pandemic was the most devastating pandemic of the 20th century and is the catastrophe against which all modern pandemics are measured. That pandemic killed more than 20 million people worldwide, including 500,000 in the United States. Almost every nation on Earth was affected. Influenza pandemics are often named for the point of origin or first recognition, such as the Taiwan flu, Hong Kong flu, London flu, Port Chalmers flu, and the Russian flu.

> A pandemic disease is a disease that is occurring in epidemic proportions in many countries simultaneously—sometimes worldwide.

According to the WHO, infectious diseases are responsible for approximately half the deaths that occur in developing countries; approximately half of those are caused by three infectious diseases—human immunodeficiency virus/acquired immunodeficiency syndrome (HIV/AIDS), TB, and malaria—each of which is currently occurring in pandemic proportions. Collectively, these three diseases cause more than 300 million illnesses and more than 5 million deaths per year.

> Collectively, HIV/AIDS, TB, and malaria cause more than 300 million illnesses and more than 5 million deaths per year.

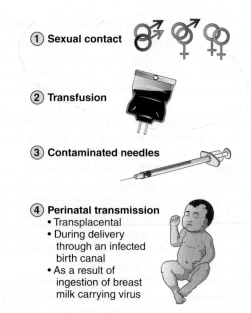

Figure 11-2. Common modes of HIV transmission. (Redrawn from Harvey RA, et al. *Lippincott's Illustrated Reviews: Microbiology*. 3rd ed. Philadelphia, PA: Lippincott Williams & Wilkins; 2013.)

1. Sexual contact
2. Transfusion
3. Contaminated needles
4. Perinatal transmission
   • Transplacental
   • During delivery through an infected birth canal
   • As a result of ingestion of breast milk carrying virus

HIV/AIDS. Although the first documented evidence of HIV infection in humans can be traced to an African serum sample collected in 1959, it is possible that humans were infected with HIV before that date. The AIDS epidemic began in the United States around 1979, but the epidemic was not detected until 1981. It was not until 1983 that HIV—the virus that causes AIDS—was discovered. HIV is thought to have been transferred to humans from other primates (chimpanzees in the case of HIV-1, and sooty mangabeys [a type of Old World monkey] in the case of HIV-2). Common modes of HIV transmission are shown in Figure 11-2. AIDS can take 10 to 15 years to develop, following HIV infection. Additional information about AIDS can be found in Chapter 18. The following statistics, which should prove sobering to anyone who thought that AIDS was "on the run," were obtained from the WHO and CDC web sites (http://www.who.int/; http://www.cdc.gov):

• HIV has claimed more than 25 million lives over the past three decades.
• The total number of people living with HIV, worldwide, in 2011 was estimated to be 34.2 million. Over 60% of people living with HIV are in sub-Saharan Africa. Table 11-1 shows the distribution of HIV-infected individuals in 2010.
• An estimated 2.5 million people worldwide acquired HIV infection in 2011.
• The global AIDS pandemic killed an estimated 1.7 million people worldwide in 2011 (over 4,650 AIDS deaths per day).
• In 2010, an estimated 47,129 people in the United States were diagnosed with HIV infection. In that same year, an estimated 33,015 people throughout the United States were diagnosed with AIDS.

[c]Hammer J. Smithsonian, Nov. 2012: 24–34.

Table 11-1 Estimated Number of People Living with HIV Infection/AIDS in 2010

Geographic Area	Estimated Number
Sub-Saharan Africa	22.9 million
South and Southeast Asia	4.0 million
Latin America	1.5 million
Eastern Europe and Central Asia	1.5 million
East Asia	790,000
North America	1.3 million
Western and Central Europe	840,000
North Africa and Middle East	470,000
Caribbean	200,000
Oceania	54,000

Source: WHO, Geneva (http://www.who.int).

- Since the epidemic began, an estimated 1,129,127 people in the United States have been diagnosed with AIDS.
- An estimated 17,774 people with AIDS in the United States died in 2009, and nearly 619,400 people with AIDS in the United States have died since the epidemic began.
- According to the CDC, an estimated 1.2 million people in the United States are currently living with HIV infection. One in five of those people are unaware of their infection.

HISTORICAL NOTE

AIDS in the United States

It has been stated that the AIDS epidemic in the United States officially began with publication of the June 5, 1981, issue of *Morbidity and Mortality Weekly Report*. That issue contained a report of five cases of *Pneumocystis carinii* pneumonia (PCP) in male patients at the UCLA Medical Center. The PCP infections were later shown to be the result of a disease syndrome, which in September 1982 was named acquired immunodeficiency syndrome or AIDS. It was not until 1983 that the virus that causes AIDS—now called human immunodeficiency virus or HIV—was discovered. By the end of 2009, a total of 619,400 Americans (more than those who had died in World Wars I and II combined) had died of AIDS. (Note: *P. carinii* is now called *Pneumocystis jiroveci*.)

Tuberculosis. Another current pandemic is TB. To complicate matters, many strains of *Mycobacterium tuberculosis* (the bacterium that causes TB) have developed resistance to the drugs that are used to treat TB. TB caused by these strains is known as *multidrug-resistant tuberculosis* (MDR-TB), or in some cases, *extensively drug-resistant tuberculosis* (XDR-TB). Some strains of *M. tuberculosis* have developed resistance to every drug and every combination of drugs that has ever been used to treat TB. MDR-TB and XDR-TB are present in virtually all regions of the world, including the United States. According to the WHO, China and the countries of the former Soviet Union have the highest occurrence rates of MDR-TB. Additional information about TB can be found in Chapter 19. The following statistics were obtained from the WHO and CDC web sites:

- Among infectious diseases, TB is second only to HIV/AIDS as the greatest killer worldwide due to a single infectious agent.
- TB is a worldwide pandemic. In 2010, the largest number of new TB cases occurred in Asia, accounting for 60% of new cases globally. However, sub-Saharan Africa carried the greatest proportion of new cases per population with over 270 cases per 100,000 population in 2010.
- In 2010, 8.8 million people fell ill with TB and 1.4 million died of TB.
- Over 95% of TB deaths occur in low- and middle-income countries, and TB is among the top three causes of death for women aged 15 to 44.
- In 2009, there were about 10 million orphan children as a result of TB deaths among parents.
- MDR-TB is present in virtually all countries surveyed.
- About one-third of the world's population has latent TB, which means people who have been infected by TB bacteria but are not (yet) ill with disease and cannot transmit the disease.
- In 2010, about half a million children (0–14 years of age) fell ill with TB, and approximately 64,000 children died of the disease.
- TB is a leading killer among people infected with HIV, causing one quarter of all deaths. Worldwide, about 200,000 people with HIV die of TB every year, most of them in Africa.
- In 2011, 10,528 new U.S. cases of TB were reported to the CDC. The number of reported TB cases in 2011 was the lowest recorded since national reporting began in 1953. The CDC reported a total of 529 U.S. TB deaths in 2009.

Malaria. Malaria is the fifth leading cause of death from infectious diseases worldwide (after respiratory infections, HIV/AIDS, diarrheal diseases, and TB). The following statistics were obtained from the WHO and CDC web sites. Additional information about malaria can be found in Chapter 21.

- About half the world's population (3.3 billion people) live in areas at risk of malaria transmission in 109 countries and territories.

- A total of 35 countries (30 in sub-Saharan Africa and 5 in Asia) account for 98% of global malaria deaths.
- Worldwide, there were about 216 million cases of malaria in 2010.
- In 2010, malaria caused an estimated 655,000 deaths worldwide, with most cases occurring among African children. Malaria is the second leading cause of death from infectious diseases in Africa, after HIV/AIDS. In Africa, every minute a child dies of malaria.
- On average, 1,500 cases of malaria are reported each year in the United States.
- During 2010, 1,773 new U.S. cases of malaria were reported to the CDC.
- Mosquito-borne malaria does occur in the United States, but only rarely. Between 1957 and 2009, 63 such outbreaks have occurred. In virtually all cases, the mosquito vectors became infected by biting persons who had acquired malaria outside the United States.

Interactions between Pathogens, Hosts, and Environments

Whether or not an infectious disease occurs depends on many factors, some of which are listed here:

1. Factors pertaining to the pathogen:
   - The virulence of the pathogen (Virulence will be discussed in Chapter 14; for now, think of virulence as a measure or degree of pathogenicity; some pathogens are more virulent than others.)
   - A way for the pathogen to enter the body (i.e., Is there a portal of entry?)
   - The number of organisms that enter the body (i.e., Will there be a sufficient number to cause infection?)
2. Factors pertaining to the host (i.e., the person who may become infected):
   - The person's health status (e.g., Is the person hospitalized? Does he or she have any underlying illnesses? Has the person undergone invasive medical or surgical procedures or catheterization? Does he or she have any prosthetic devices?)
   - The person's nutritional status
   - Other factors pertaining to the susceptibility of the host (e.g., age, lifestyle [behavior], socioeconomic level, occupation, travel, hygiene, substance abuse, immune status [immunizations or previous experience with the pathogen])
3. Factors pertaining to the environment:
   - Physical factors such as geographic location, climate, heat, cold, humidity, and season of the year.
   - Availability of appropriate reservoirs (discussed later in this chapter), intermediate

hosts (discussed in Chapter 21), and vectors (discussed later in this chapter)
- Sanitary and housing conditions; adequate waste disposal; adequate health care
- Availability of potable (drinkable) water

> Whether or not an infectious disease occurs depends on many factors, including those pertaining to the pathogen, those pertaining to the host, and those pertaining to the environment.

Chain of Infection

There are six components in the infectious disease process (also known as the *chain of infection*). They are illustrated in Figure 11-3 and are briefly described here:

1. There must first be a pathogen. As an example, let us assume that the pathogen is a cold virus.
2. There must be a source of the pathogen (i.e., a reservoir). In Figure 11-3, the infected person on the right ("Andy") is the reservoir. Andy has a cold.
3. There must be a portal of exit (i.e., a way for the pathogen to escape from the reservoir). When Andy blows his nose, cold viruses get onto his hands.
4. There must be a mode of transmission (i.e., a way for the pathogen to travel from Andy to another person). In Figure 11-3, the cold virus is being transferred by direct contact between Andy and his friend ("Bob")—by shaking hands.

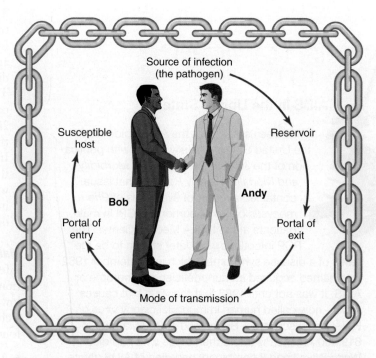

Figure 11-3. The six components in the infectious disease process, also known as the chain of infection.

5. There must be a portal of entry (i.e., a way for the pathogen to gain entry into Bob). When Bob rubs his nose, the cold virus is transferred from his hand to the mucous membranes of his nose.

6. There must be a susceptible host. For example, Bob would not be a susceptible host (and would, therefore, not develop a cold) if he had previously been infected by that particular cold virus and had developed immunity to it.

> The six components in the chain of infection are (a) a pathogen, (b) a reservoir of infection, (c) a portal of exit, (d) a mode of transmission, (e) a portal of entry, and (f) a susceptible host.

Strategies for Breaking the Chain of Infection

To prevent infections from occurring, measures must be taken to break the chain of infection at some point (link) in the chain. Strategies for breaking the chain of infection are discussed in detail in Chapter 12. Some of the broad goals are to

- eliminate or contain the reservoirs of pathogens or curtail the persistence of a pathogen at the source
- prevent contact with infectious substances from exit pathways
- eliminate means of transmission
- block exposure to entry pathways
- reduce or eliminate the susceptibility of potential hosts

Some of the specific methods of breaking the chain of infection are

- practicing effective hand hygiene procedures
- maintaining good nutrition and adequate rest and reduce stress
- obtaining immunizations against common pathogens
- practicing insect and rodent control measures
- practicing proper patient isolation procedures
- ensuring proper decontamination of surfaces and medical instruments
- disposing sharps and infectious wastes properly
- using gloves, gowns, masks, respirators, and other personal protective equipment, whenever appropriate to do so
- using needle safety devices during blood collection

Reservoirs of Infection

The sources of microbes that cause infectious diseases are many and varied. They are known as **reservoirs of infection** or simply **reservoirs**. A reservoir is any site where the pathogen can multiply or merely survive until it is transferred to a host. Reservoirs may be living hosts or inanimate objects or materials (Fig. 11-4).

> Reservoirs of infection may be living hosts or inanimate objects or materials.

Living Reservoirs

Living reservoirs include humans, household pets, farm animals, wild animals, certain insects, and certain arachnids (ticks and mites). The human and animal reservoirs may or may not be experiencing illness caused by the pathogens they are harboring.

Human Carriers

The most important reservoirs of human infectious diseases are other humans—people with infectious diseases as well as carriers. A **carrier** is a person who is colonized with a particular pathogen, but the pathogen is not currently causing disease in that person. However, the pathogen can be transmitted from the carrier to others, who may then become ill. There are several types of carriers. **Passive carriers** carry the pathogen without ever having had the disease. An **incubatory carrier** is a person who is capable of transmitting a pathogen during the incubation period of a particular infectious disease. **Convalescent carriers** harbor and can transmit a particular pathogen

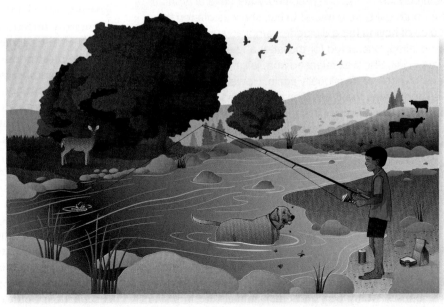

Figure 11-4. Reservoirs of infection include soil, dust, contaminated water, contaminated foods, insects, and infected humans, domestic animals, and wild animals.

while recovering from an infectious disease (i.e., during the convalescent period). **Active carriers** have completely recovered from the disease, but continue to harbor the pathogen indefinitely (see the following "Historical Note" for an example). Respiratory secretions or feces are usually the vehicles by which the pathogen is transferred, either directly from the carrier to a susceptible individual or indirectly through food or water. Human carriers are very important in the spread of staphylococcal and streptococcal infections as well as in the spread of hepatitis, diphtheria, dysentery, meningitis, and STDs.

> A carrier is a person who is colonized with a particular pathogen, but the pathogen is not currently causing disease in that person.

HISTORICAL NOTE

"Typhoid Mary": An Infamous Carrier

Mary Mallon was a domestic employee—a cook—who worked in the New York City area in the early 1900s. She had recovered from typhoid fever earlier in life. Although no longer ill, she was a carrier. *Salmonella typhi*, the causative agent of typhoid fever, was still living in her gallbladder and passing in her feces. Apparently, her hygienic practices were inadequate, and she would transport the *Salmonella* bacteria via her hands from the restroom to the kitchen, where she then unwittingly introduced them into foods that she prepared. After several typhoid fever outbreaks were traced to her, she was offered the choice of having her gallbladder removed surgically or being jailed. She opted for the latter and spent several years in jail. She was released from jail after promising never to cook professionally again. However, the lure of the kitchen was too great. She changed her name and resumed her profession in various hotels, restaurants, and hospitals. As in the past, "everywhere that Mary went, typhoid fever was sure to follow." She was again arrested and spent her remaining years quarantined in a New York City hospital. She died in 1938 at the age of 70.

Animals

As previously stated, infectious diseases that humans acquire from animal sources are called zoonotic diseases or zoonoses. Many pets and other animals are important reservoirs of zoonoses. Zoonoses are acquired by direct contact with the animal, by inhalation or ingestion of the pathogen, or by injection of the pathogen by an arthropod vector. Measures for the control of zoonotic diseases include the use of personal protective equipment when handling animals, animal vaccinations, proper use of pesticides, isolation or destruction of infected animals, and proper disposal of animal carcasses and waste products.

> Zoonotic diseases (zoonoses) are infectious diseases that humans acquire from animal sources.

Examples of Zoonoses. Dogs, cats, bats, skunks, and other animals are known reservoirs of rabies. The rabies virus is usually transmitted to a human through the saliva that is injected when one of these rabid animals bites the human. Cat and dog bites often transfer bacteria from the mouths of these animals into tissues, where severe infections may result. Toxoplasmosis, a protozoan disease caused by *Toxoplasma gondii*, can be contracted by ingesting oocysts from cat feces that are present in litter boxes or sand boxes, as well by ingesting cysts that are present in infected raw or undercooked meats. Toxoplasmosis may cause severe brain damage to, or death of, the fetus when contracted by a woman during her first trimester (first 3 months) of pregnancy. The diarrheal disease, salmonellosis, is frequently acquired by ingesting *Salmonella* bacteria from the feces of turtles, other reptiles, and poultry. A variant form of Creutzfeldt-Jakob (CJ) disease in humans, called variant CJ disease, may be acquired by ingestion of prion-infected beef from cows with bovine spongiform encephalopathy (BSE or "mad cow disease"). Persons skinning rabbits can become infected with the bacterium *Francisella tularensis* and develop tularemia. Contact with dead animals or animal hides could result in the inhalation of the spores of *Bacillus anthracis*, leading to inhalation anthrax, or the spores could enter a cut, leading to cutaneous anthrax. Ingestion of the spores could lead to gastrointestinal anthrax. Psittacosis or "parrot fever" is a respiratory infection that may be acquired from infected birds (usually parakeets and parrots).

The most prevalent zoonotic infection in the United States is Lyme disease (discussed under "Arthropods"), one of many arthropod-borne zoonoses. (Arthropod-borne diseases are diseases that are transmitted by arthropods.) Other zoonoses that occur in the United States include anthrax, brucellosis, campylobacteriosis, cryptosporidiosis, echinococcosis, ehrlichiosis, HPS, leptospirosis, pasteurellosis, plague, psittacosis, Q fever, rabies, ringworm, spotted fever rickettsiosis, salmonellosis, toxoplasmosis, tularemia, and various viral encephalitides (e.g., Western equine encephalitis, Eastern equine encephalitis, St. Louis encephalitis, California encephalitis, WNV encephalitis). Some of the more than 200 known zoonoses are listed in Table 11-2. Consult Chapter 12 on thePoint for a discussion of healthcare-associated zoonoses.

> There are over 200 known zoonoses— diseases that can be transmitted from animals to humans.

Table 11-2 Examples of Zoonotic Diseases

Category	Disease	Pathogen	Animal Reservoir(s)	Mode of Transmission
Viral diseases	Avian influenza ("bird flu")	An influenza virus	Birds	Direct or indirect contact with infected birds
	Equine encephalitis	Various arboviruses	Birds, small mammals	Mosquito bite
	HPS	Hantaviruses	Rodents	Inhalation of contaminated dust or aerosols
	Lassa fever	Lassa virus	Wild rodents	Inhalation of contaminated dust or aerosols
	Marburg disease	Marburg virus	Monkeys	Contact with blood or tissues from infected monkeys
	Rabies	Rabies virus	Rabid dogs, cats, skunks, foxes, wolves, raccoons, coyotes, bats	Animal bite or inhalation
	Yellow fever	Yellow fever virus	Monkeys	*Aedes aegypti* mosquito bite
	WNV encephalitis	WNV	Birds	Mosquito bite
Bacterial diseases	Anthrax	*B. anthracis*	Cattle, sheep, goats	Inhalation, ingestion, entry through cuts, contact with mucous membranes
	Bovine TB	*Mycobacterium bovis*	Cattle	Ingestion
	Brucellosis	*Brucella* spp.	Cattle, swine, goats	Inhalation, ingestion of contaminated milk, entry through cuts, contact with mucous membranes
	Campylobacter infection	*Campylobacter* spp.	Wild mammals, cattle, sheep, pets	Ingestion of contaminated food and water
	Cat-scratch disease	*Bartonella henselae*	Domestic cats	Cat scratch, bite, or lick
	Ehrlichiosis	*Ehrlichia* spp.	Deer, mice	Tick bite
	Endemic typhus	*Rickettsia typhi*	Rodents	Flea bite
	Leptospirosis	*Leptospira* spp.	Cattle, rodents, dogs	Contact with contaminated animal urine
	Lyme disease	*B. burgdorferi*	Deer, rodents	Tick bite
	Pasteurellosis	*Pasteurella multocida*	Oral cavities of animals	Bites, scratches
	Plague	*Y. pestis*	Rodents	Flea bite
	Psittacosis (ornithosis, parrot fever)	*Chlamydophila psittaci*	Parrots, parakeets, other pet birds, pigeons, poultry	Inhalation of contaminated dust and aerosols
	Relapsing fever	*Borrelia* spp.	Rodents	Tick bite
	Rickettsial pox	*Rickettsia akari*	Rodents	Mite bite
	Rocky Mountain spotted fever	*Rickettsia rickettsii*	Rodents, dogs	Tick bite
	Salmonellosis	*Salmonella* spp.	Poultry, livestock, reptiles	Ingestion of contaminated food, handling reptiles
	Scrub typhus	*Orientia tsutsugamushi*	Rodents	Mite bite
	Tularemia	*F. tularensis*	Wild mammals	Entry through cuts, inhalation, tick or deer fly bite
	Q fever	*Coxiella burnetii*	Cattle, sheep, goats	Tick bite, air, mild contact with infected animals
Fungal diseases	Tinea (ringworm) infections	Various dermatophytes	Various animals including dogs	Contact with infected animals

(continued)

	Examples of Zoonotic Diseases (Continued)			
Category	**Disease**	**Pathogen**	**Animal Reservoir(s)**	**Mode of Transmission**
Protozoal diseases	African trypanosomiasis	Subspecies of *Trypanosoma brucei*	Cattle, wild game animals	Tsetse fly bite
	American trypanosomiasis (Chagas disease)	*Trypanosoma cruzi*	Numerous wild and domestic animals, including dogs, cats, and wild rodents	Trypomastigotes in the feces of reduviid bug are rubbed into bite wound or the eye
	Babesiosis	*Babesia microti*	Deer, mice, voles	Tick bite
	Leishmaniasis	*Leishmania* spp.	Rodents, dogs	Sandfly bite
	Toxoplasmosis	*T. gondii*	Cats, pigs, sheep, rarely cattle	Ingestion of oocysts in cat feces or cysts in raw or undercooked meat
Helminth diseases	Echinococcosis (hydatid disease)	*Echinococcus granulosis*	Dogs	Ingestion of eggs
	Dog tapeworm infection	*Dipylidium caninum*	Dogs, cats	Ingestion of flea containing the larval stage
	Rat tapeworm infection	*Hymenolepis diminuta*	Rodents	Ingestion of beetle containing the larval stage

Arthropods

Technically, arthropods are animals, but they are being discussed here separately from other animals because, as a group, they are so commonly associated with human infections. Many different types of arthropods serve as reservoirs of infection, including insects (e.g., mosquitoes, biting flies, lice, fleas) and arachnids (e.g., mites, ticks). When involved in the transmission of infectious diseases, these arthropods are referred to as **vectors**. The arthropod vector may first take a blood meal from an infected person or animal and then transfer the pathogen to a healthy individual. Take Lyme disease, for example, which is the most common arthropod-borne disease in the United States. First, a tick takes a blood meal from an infected deer or mouse (Fig. 11-5). The tick is now infected with *Borrelia burgdorferi*, the spirochete that causes Lyme disease. Sometime later, the tick takes a blood meal from a human and, in the process, injects the bacteria into the human. Ticks are especially notorious vectors. In the United States, there are at least 10 infectious diseases that are transmitted by ticks (see the adjacent "Study Aid"). Other arthropod-borne infectious diseases are listed in Table 11-3. Chapter 21 contains additional information about arthropods.

Nonliving Reservoirs

Nonliving or inanimate reservoirs of infection include air, soil, dust, food, milk, water, and fomites (defined later in the chapter). Air can become contaminated by dust or respiratory secretions of humans expelled into the air by breathing, talking, sneezing, and coughing. The most highly contagious diseases include colds and influenza, in which the respiratory viruses can be transmitted through the air on droplets of respiratory tract secretions. Air currents and air vents can transport respiratory pathogens throughout healthcare facilities and other buildings. Dust particles can carry

> Air, soil, dust, food, milk, water, and fomites are examples of nonliving or inanimate reservoirs of infection.

STUDY AID

Tick-Borne Diseases of the United States

Viral diseases:

Colorado tick fever
Powassan virus encephalitis

Bacterial diseases:

Human granulocytic ehrlichiosis
Human monocytic ehrlichiosis
Lyme disease
Q fever
Spotted fever rickettsiosis
Tick-borne relapsing fever
Tularemia

Protozoal disease:

Babesiosis

(In addition to serving as vectors in these infectious diseases, ticks can cause tick paralysis.)

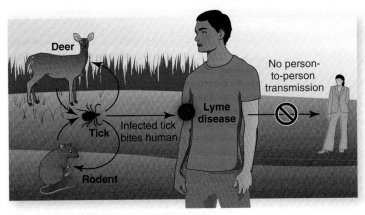

Figure 11-5. Transmission of Lyme disease.

spores of certain bacteria and dried bits of human and animal excretions containing pathogens. Bacteria cannot multiply in the air, but can easily be transported by airborne particles to a warm, moist, nutrient-rich site, where they can multiply. Also, some fungal respiratory diseases (e.g., histoplasmosis) are frequently transferred

by dust containing yeasts or spores. Soil contains the spores of the *Clostridium* species that cause tetanus, botulism, and gas gangrene. Any of these diseases can follow the introduction of spores into an open wound.

Food and milk may be contaminated by careless handling, which allows pathogens to enter from soil, dust particles, dirty hands, hair, and respiratory secretions. If these pathogens are not destroyed by proper processing and cooking, food poisoning can develop. As stated previously, foodborne diseases cause approximately 76 million illnesses, 325,000 hospitalizations, and 5,000 deaths per year in the United States. Diseases frequently transmitted through foods and water are amebiasis (caused by the ameba, *Entamoeba histolytica*), botulism (caused by the bacterium, *Clostridium botulinum*), cholera (caused by the bacterium, *Vibrio cholerae*), *C. perfringens* food poisoning, infectious hepatitis (caused by hepatitis A virus), staphylococcal food poisoning, typhoid fever (caused by the bacterium, *Salmonella typhi*), and trichinosis (a helminth disease, caused by ingesting *Trichinella spiralis* larvae in pork). Other common foodborne and waterborne pathogens are listed in Table 11-4.

Human and animal fecal matter from outhouses, cesspools, and feed lots is often carried into water supplies. Improper disposal of sewage and inadequate treatment of drinking water contribute to the spread of fecal and soil pathogens. **Fomites** are inanimate objects capable of transmitting pathogens. Fomites found within healthcare settings include patients' gowns, bedding, towels, eating and drinking utensils, and hospital equipment, such as bedpans, stethoscopes, latex gloves, electronic thermometers, and electrocardiographic electrodes, which become contaminated by pathogens from the respiratory tract, intestinal tract, or the skin of patients. Even telephones, doorknobs, and computer keyboards can serve as fomites. Great care must be taken by healthcare personnel to prevent transmission of pathogens from living and nonliving reservoirs to hospitalized patients.

Table 11-3 Arthropods That Serve as Vectors of Human Infectious Diseases

Vectors	Disease(s)
Black flies (*Simulium* spp.)	Onchocerciasis ("river blindness") (H)
Cyclops spp.	Fish tapeworm infection (H), guinea worm infection (H)
Fleas	Dog tapeworm infection (H), endemic typhus (B), murine typhus (B), plague (B)
Lice	Epidemic relapsing fever (B), epidemic typhus (B), trench fever (B)
Mites	Rickettsial pox (B), scrub typhus (B)
Mosquitoes	Dengue fever (V), filariasis ("elephantiasis") (H), malaria (P), viral encephalitis (V), yellow fever (V)
Reduviid bugs	American trypanosomiasis (Chagas disease) (P)
Sand flies (*Phlebotomus* spp.)	Leishmaniasis (P)
Ticks	Babesiosis (P), Colorado tick fever (V), ehrlichiosis (B), Lyme disease (B), relapsing fever (B), spotted fever rickettsiosis (B), tularemia (B)
Tsetse flies (*Glossina* spp.)	African trypanosomiasis (P)

B, bacterial disease; P, protozoal disease; H, helminth disease; V, viral disease.

Modes of Transmission

Healthcare professionals must be thoroughly familiar with the sources (reservoirs) of potential pathogens and pathways for their transfer. A hospital staphylococcal epidemic may begin when aseptic conditions are relaxed and when a *Staphylococcus aureus* carrier transmits the pathogen to susceptible patients (e.g., babies, surgical patients, debilitated persons). Such an infection could quickly spread throughout the entire hospital population.

The five principal modes by which transmission of pathogens occurs are contact (either direct or indirect), droplet, airborne, vehicular, and vector transmission

Table 11-4 Pathogens Commonly Transmitted via Food and Water[a]

Pathogen	Vehicle	Comments
Campylobacter jejuni (bacterium)	Chickens	
C. parvum (protozoan)	Drinking water	Highly resistant to disinfectants used to purify drinking water
Cyclospora cayetanensis (protozoan)	Drinking water, raspberries	
E. coli O157:H7 (bacterium)	Meats, produce contaminated by manure in growing fields (e.g., sprouts), drinking water	
Giardia lamblia (also called *Giardia intestinalis*) (protozoan)	Drinking water	Moderately resistant to disinfectants used to purify drinking water
Listeria monocytogenes (bacterium)	Soft cheeses and deli meats	
Salmonella enteritidis (bacterium)	Eggs	
Salmonella typhimurium DT-104 (bacterium)	Unpasteurized milk	Resistant to many antibiotics
Shigella spp. (bacteria)	Drinking water	

[a]Additional pathogens transmitted in food and water are mentioned in the text.

(Fig. 11-6 and Table 11-5). Droplet transmission involves the transfer of pathogens via infectious droplets (particles 5 μm in diameter or larger). Droplets may be generated by coughing, sneezing, and even talking. Airborne transmission involves the dispersal of droplet

> The five principal modes by which transmission of pathogens occurs are contact (either direct or indirect), droplet, airborne, vehicular, and vector transmission.

nuclei, which are the residue of evaporated droplets, and are smaller than 5 μm in diameter. Vehicular transmission involves contaminated inanimate objects ("vehicles"), such as food, water, dust, and fomites. Vectors include various types of biting insects and arachnids.

Communicable diseases—infectious diseases that are transmitted from person to person—are most commonly transmitted in the following ways:

- **Direct skin-to-skin contact.** For example, the common cold virus is frequently transmitted from the hand of someone who just blew his or her nose to another person by hand shaking. Within hospitals, this mode of transfer is particularly prevalent, which is why it is so important for healthcare professionals to wash their hands before and after every patient contact. Frequent handwashing will prevent the transfer of pathogens from one patient to another.

- **Direct mucous membrane-to-mucous membrane contact by kissing or sexual intercourse.** Most STDs are transmitted in this manner. STDs include syphilis, gonorrhea, and infections caused by *Chlamydia*, herpes virus, and HIV. Chlamydial genital infections are especially common in the United States; in fact, they are the most common nationally notifiable infectious diseases in the United States. (Nationally notifiable infectious diseases are discussed later in this chapter.)

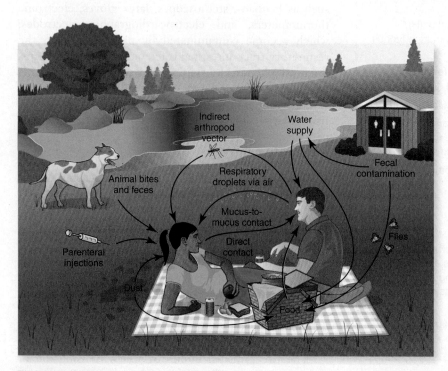

Figure 11-6. Modes of disease transmission.

Table 11-5 Common Routes of Transmission of Infectious Diseases

Route of Exit	Route of Transmission or Entry	Diseases
Skin	Skin discharge → air → respiratory tract	Chickenpox, colds, influenza, measles, staph and strep infections
	Skin to skin	Impetigo, eczema, boils, warts, syphilis
Respiratory secretions	Aerosol droplet inhalation	Colds, influenza, pneumonia, mumps, measles, chickenpox, TB
	Nose or mouth → hand or object → nose	
Gastrointestinal secretions	Feces → hand → mouth	Gastroenteritis, hepatitis, salmonellosis, shigellosis, typhoid fever, cholera, giardiasis, amebiasis
	Stool → soil, food, or water → mouth	
Saliva	Direct salivary transfer	Herpes cold sore, infectious mononucleosis, strep throat
Genital secretions	Urethral or cervical secretions	Gonorrhea, herpes, *Chlamydia* infection
	Semen	Cytomegalovirus infection, AIDS, syphilis, warts
Blood	Transfusion or needlestick injury	Hepatitis B, cytomegalovirus infection, malaria, AIDS
	Insect bite	Malaria relapsing fever
Zoonotic	Animal bite	Rabies
	Contact with animal carcasses	Tularemia, anthrax
	Arthropod	Spotted fever rickettsiosis, Lyme disease, typhus, viral encephalitis, yellow fever, malaria, plague

- **Indirect contact via airborne droplets of respiratory secretions, usually produced as a result of sneezing or coughing.** Most contagious airborne diseases are caused by respiratory pathogens carried to susceptible people in droplets of respiratory secretions. Some respiratory pathogens may settle on dust particles and be carried long distances through the air and into a building's ventilation or air-conditioning system. Improperly cleaned inhalation therapy equipment can easily transfer these pathogens from one patient to another. Diseases that may be transmitted in this manner include colds, influenza, measles, mumps, chickenpox, smallpox, and pneumonia.
- **Indirect contact via food and water contaminated with fecal material.** Many infectious diseases are transmitted by restaurant food handlers who fail to wash their hands after using the restroom.
- **Indirect contact via arthropod vectors.** Arthropods such as mosquitoes, flies, fleas, lice, ticks, and mites can transfer various pathogens from person to person.
- **Indirect contact via fomites that become contaminated by respiratory secretions, blood, urine, feces, vomitus, or exudates from hospitalized patients.** Fomites such as stethoscopes and latex gloves are sometimes the vehicles by which pathogens are transferred from one patient to another. Examples of fomites are shown in Figure 11-7.

- **Indirect contact via transfusion of contaminated blood or blood products from an ill person or by *parenteral injection* (injection directly into the bloodstream) using nonsterile syringes and needles.** One reason why disposable sterile tubes, syringes, and various other types of single-use hospital equipment have become very popular is that they are effective in preventing blood-borne infections (e.g., hepatitis, syphilis, malaria, AIDS, systemic staphylococcal infections) that result from reuse of equipment. Individuals using illegal intravenous drugs commonly transmit these diseases to each other by sharing needles and syringes, which easily become contaminated with the blood of an infected person.

Public Health Agencies

Public health agencies at all levels constantly strive to prevent epidemics and to identify and eliminate any that do occur. One way in which healthcare personnel participate in this massive program is by reporting cases of communicable diseases to the proper agencies. They also help by educating the public, explaining how diseases are transmitted, explaining proper sanitation procedures, identifying and attempting to eliminate reservoirs of infection, carrying out measures to isolate diseased

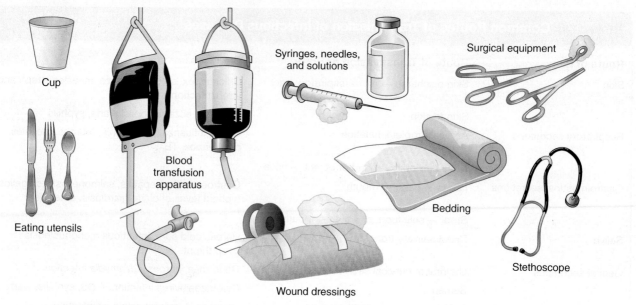

Figure 11-7. Various medical instruments and apparatus that may serve as inanimate vectors of infection (fomites).

persons, participating in immunization programs, and helping to treat sick persons. Through these measures, smallpox and poliomyelitis have been totally or nearly eliminated in most parts of the world.

The World Health Organization

The WHO, a specialized agency of the United Nations, was founded in 1948. Its missions are to promote technical cooperation for health among nations, carry out programs to control and eradicate diseases, and improve the quality of human life. When an epidemic strikes, such as the 2000 Ebola outbreak in Uganda, teams of epidemiologists are sent to the site to investigate the situation and assist in bringing the outbreak under control. Because of this assistance, many countries have been successful in their fight to control smallpox, diphtheria, malaria, trachoma, and numerous other diseases. At one time, smallpox killed about 40% of those infected and caused scarring and blindness in many others. In 1980, the WHO announced that smallpox had been completely eradicated from the face of the Earth; hence, routine smallpox vaccination is no longer required.[d] More recently, the WHO has been attempting to eradicate polio and dracunculiasis (Guinea worm infection); to eliminate leprosy, neonatal tetanus, and Chagas disease; and to control onchocerciasis ("river blindness"). WHO's definitions of control, elimination, and eradication of disease are presented in Table 11-6. The WHO is currently

Table 11-6 WHO Definitions of Epidemiologic Terms Relating to Infectious Diseases	
Term	**Definition**
Control of an infectious disease	Ongoing operations or programs aimed at reducing the incidence or prevalence of that disease
Elimination of an infectious disease	The reduction of case transmission to a predetermined very low level (e.g., to a level below one case per million population)
Eradication of an infectious disease	Achieving a status where no further cases of that disease occur anywhere and where continued control measures are unnecessary

attempting to eradicate polio. Thus far, polio has been eradicated from the Western Hemisphere (including the United States). Certification of total eradication requires that no wild poliovirus be found through optimal surveillance for at least 3 years.

The Centers for Disease Control and Prevention

In the United States, a federal agency called the U.S. Department of Health and Human Services administers the Public Health Service and CDC, which assist state and local health departments in the application of all aspects of epidemiology. Many microbiologists and epidemiologists work at the CDC headquarters in Atlanta, Georgia.

---

[d]Because smallpox virus is a potential bioterrorism agent, public health authorities have authorized the manufacture and stockpiling of smallpox vaccine, to be administered in the event of an emergency.

Microbiologists at the CDC are able to work with the most dangerous pathogens known to science because of the elaborate containment facilities that are located there. CDC epidemiologists travel to areas of the United States and elsewhere in the world, wherever and whenever an epidemic is occurring, to investigate and attempt to control the epidemic.

When the CDC was first established as the Communicable Disease Center in Atlanta, Georgia, in 1946, its focus was communicable diseases. The two most important infectious diseases in the United States at that time were malaria and typhus. Since then, the CDC's scope has been expanded greatly, and the organization now consists of approximately two dozen offices, centers, and institutes. The CDC's overall mission is "collaborating to create the expertise, information, and tools that people and communities need to protect their health—through health promotion, prevention of disease, injury and disability, and preparedness for new health threats" (http://www.cdc.gov). The CDC seeks to accomplish its mission by working with partners throughout the nation and the world to

- monitor health,
- detect and investigate health problems,
- conduct research to enhance prevention,
- develop and advocate sound public health policies,
- implement prevention strategies,
- promote healthy behaviors,
- foster safe and healthful environments, and
- provide leadership and training.

One of the CDC offices—the Office of Infectious Diseases—coordinates the activities of three National Centers:

- National Center for Immunization and Respiratory Diseases
- National Center for Emerging and Zoonotic Infectious Diseases
- National Center for HIV/AIDS, Viral Hepatitis, STD, and TB Prevention

Certain infectious diseases, referred to as nationally notifiable diseases, must be reported to the CDC by all 50 states whenever they are diagnosed.[e] (As of January 2010, there were approximately 65 nationally notifiable diseases; most of them are discussed in Chapters 18 through 21.) Ten of the most common nationally notifiable infectious diseases in the United States are listed in Table 11-7. Note that 3 of the 4 most commonly reported diseases in 2010 are sexually transmitted (chlamydial infections, gonorrhea, and syphilis) and 2 of the top 10 diseases are vaccine-preventable (pertussis and chickenpox).

---

[e]A notifiable disease is one for which regular, frequent, and timely information regarding individual cases is considered necessary for the prevention and control of the disease. Notifiable disease reporting protects the public's health by ensuring the proper identification and follow-up of cases.

Table 11-7 Ten of the Most Common Nationally Notifiable Infectious Diseases in the United States, 2010

Ranking	Disease	Number of U.S. Cases Reported (2010)
1	Genital chlamydial infections	1,307,893
2	Gonorrhea	309,341
3	Salmonellosis	54,424
4	Syphilis (all stages)	45,834
5	HIV diagnosis	35,741
6	Lyme disease	30,158
7	Pertussis (whooping cough)	27,550
8	Giardiasis	19,811
9	*Streptococcus pneumoniae*, invasive disease, drug resistant	16,569
10	Varicella (chickenpox)	15,427

Source: The Centers for Disease Control (CDC), Atlanta, GA (http://www.cdc.gov).

The CDC prepares a weekly publication entitled *Morbidity and Mortality Weekly Report* (*MMWR*), which contains timely information about infectious disease outbreaks in the United States and other parts of the world, as well as cumulative statistics regarding the number of cases of nationally notifiable infectious diseases that have occurred in the United States during the current year. Students of the health sciences are encouraged to read *MMWR*, which is accessible at the CDC web site (http://www.cdc.gov).

Through the efforts of these public health agencies, working with local physicians, nurses, other healthcare professionals, educators, and community leaders, many diseases are no longer endemic in the United States. Some of the diseases that no longer pose a serious threat to U.S. communities include cholera, diphtheria, malaria, polio, smallpox, and typhoid fever.

The prevention and control of epidemics is a never-ending community goal. To be effective, it must include measures to

- increase host resistance through the development and administration of vaccines that induce active immunity and maintain it in susceptible persons;
- ensure that persons who have been exposed to a pathogen are protected against the disease (e.g., through injections of γ-globulin or antisera);

- segregate, isolate, and treat those who have contracted a contagious infection to prevent the spread of pathogens to others;
- identify and control potential reservoirs and vectors of infectious diseases; this control may be accomplished by prohibiting healthy carriers from working in restaurants, hospitals, nursing homes, and other institutions where they may transfer pathogens to susceptible people and by instituting effective sanitation measures to control diseases transmitted through water supplies, sewage, and food (including milk).

Four of the pathogens most often discussed as potential BW and bioterrorism agents are *B. anthracis, C. botulinum,* smallpox virus (*Variola major*), and *Y. pestis,* the causative agents of anthrax, botulism, smallpox, and plague, respectively.

> Four of the most commonly discussed pathogens that are potential BW and bioterrorism agents are *B. anthracis, C. botulinum, V. major,* and *Y. pestis.*

Bioterrorism and Biological Warfare Agents

Sad to say, pathogenic microbes sometimes wind up in the hands of terrorists and extremists who want to use them to cause harm to others. In times of war, the use of microbes in this manner is called **biological warfare** (BW), and the microbes are referred to as **biological warfare agents**. However, the danger does not exist solely during times of war. The possibility that members of terrorist or radical hate groups might use pathogens to create fear, chaos, illness, and death always exists. These people are referred to as biological terrorists or bioterrorists, and the specific pathogens they use are referred to as **bioterrorism agents**.

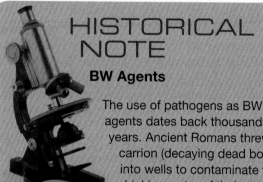

HISTORICAL NOTE

BW Agents

The use of pathogens as BW agents dates back thousands of years. Ancient Romans threw carrion (decaying dead bodies) into wells to contaminate the drinking water of their enemies. In the Middle Ages, the bodies of plague victims were catapulted over city walls in an attempt to infect the inhabitants of the cities. Early North American explorers provided Native Americans with blankets and handkerchiefs that were contaminated with smallpox and measles viruses.

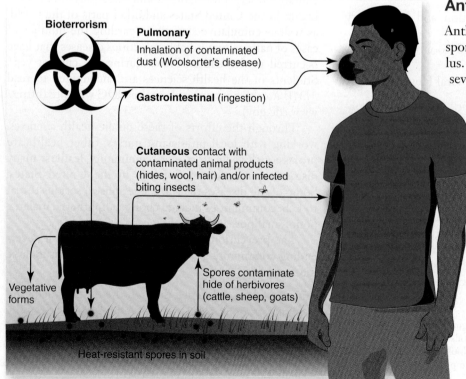

Figure 11-8. Modes of anthrax transmission.

Anthrax

Anthrax is caused by *B. anthracis,* a spore-forming, Gram-positive bacillus. People can develop anthrax in several ways (Fig. 11-8), resulting in three forms of the disease: cutaneous anthrax, inhalation anthrax, and gastrointestinal anthrax. Anthrax infections involve marked hemorrhaging and serous effusions (fluid that has escaped from blood or lymphatic vessels) in various organs and body cavities and are frequently fatal. Of the three forms of anthrax, inhalation anthrax is the most severe, followed by gastrointestinal anthrax and then cutaneous anthrax. Patients with cutaneous anthrax develop lesions called eschars (Fig. 11-9). Bioterrorists could disseminate *B. anthracis* spores via aerosols or contamination of food supplies. In the fall

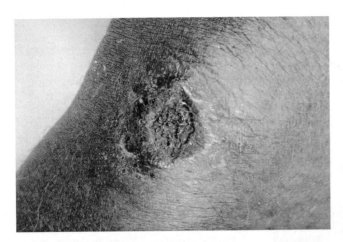

Figure 11-9. Black anthrax lesion (eschar) on a patient's forearm. The name of the disease comes from the Greek word *anthrax*, which means "coal," in reference to the black skin lesions of anthrax. (Courtesy of James H. Steele and the CDC.)

of 2001, letters containing *B. anthracis* spores were mailed to several politicians and members of the news media. According to the CDC, a total of 22 cases of anthrax resulted: 11 cases of inhalation anthrax (with 5 fatalities) and 11 cases of cutaneous anthrax (with no fatalities). Undoubtedly, many additional cases were prevented as a result of prompt prophylactic (preventative) antibiotic therapy.

Botulism

Botulism is a potentially fatal microbial intoxication, caused by botulinal toxin, a neurotoxin produced by *C. botulinum*. *C. botulinum* is a spore-forming, anaerobic, Gram-positive bacillus. Botulinal toxin may cause nerve damage, visual difficulty, respiratory failure, flaccid paralysis of voluntary muscles, brain damage, coma, and death within a week if untreated. Respiratory failure is the usual cause of death. Bioterrorists could add botulinal toxin to water supplies or food. Botulinal toxin is odorless and tasteless, and only a tiny quantity of the toxin need be ingested to cause a potentially fatal case of botulism. Botulism can also result from entry of *C. botulinum* spores into open wounds.

Smallpox

Smallpox is a serious, contagious, and sometimes fatal viral disease. Patients experience fever, malaise, headache, prostration, severe backache, a characteristic skin rash (Fig. 11-10), and occasional abdominal pain and vomiting. Smallpox can become severe, with bleeding into the skin and mucous membranes, followed by death. The last case of smallpox in the United States was in 1949, and the last naturally occurring case in the world was in Somalia in 1977. Since 1980, when the WHO announced that smallpox had been eradicated, most people no longer received smallpox vaccinations. Thus, throughout the world, huge numbers of people are highly susceptible to the virus.

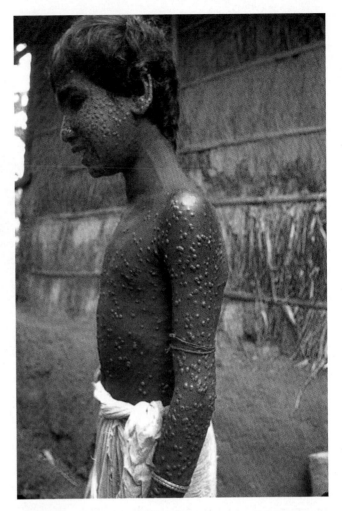

Figure 11-10. Child with smallpox. (Courtesy of Jean Roy and the CDC.)

Although there are no reservoirs for smallpox virus in nature, preserved samples of the virus exist in a few medical research laboratories worldwide. There is always the

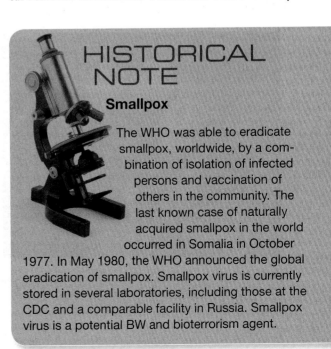

HISTORICAL NOTE

Smallpox

The WHO was able to eradicate smallpox, worldwide, by a combination of isolation of infected persons and vaccination of others in the community. The last known case of naturally acquired smallpox in the world occurred in Somalia in October 1977. In May 1980, the WHO announced the global eradication of smallpox. Smallpox virus is currently stored in several laboratories, including those at the CDC and a comparable facility in Russia. Smallpox virus is a potential BW and bioterrorism agent.

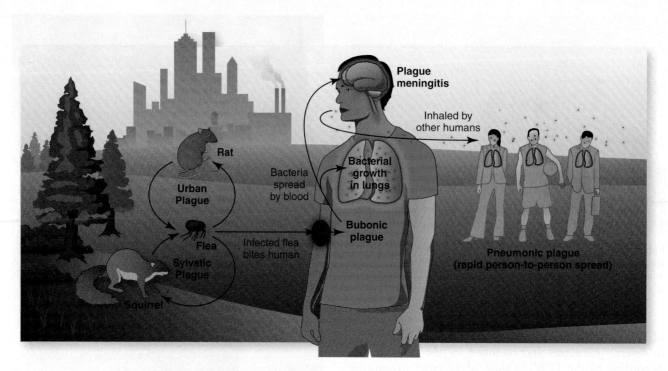

Figure 11-11. **Epidemiology and pathology of plague.**

danger that smallpox virus, or any of the other pathogens mentioned here, could fall into the wrong hands.

Plague

Plague is caused by *Y. pestis*, a Gram-negative coccoba-cillus. Plague is predominantly a zoonosis and is usually transmitted to humans by flea bite (Fig. 11-11). Plague can manifest itself in several ways: bubonic plague, septi-cemic plague, pneumonic plague, and plague meningitis.

Bubonic plague is named for the swollen, inflamed, and tender lymph nodes (buboes) that develop. Pneumonic plague, which is highly communicable, involves the lungs. It can result in localized outbreaks or devastating epidemics. Septicemic plague may cause septic shock, meningitis, or death. Patients with plague are depicted in Figure 11-12. Bioterrorists could disseminate *Y. pestis* via aerosols, resulting in numerous severe and potentially fatal pulmonary infections. Pneumonic plague can be transmitted from person to person.

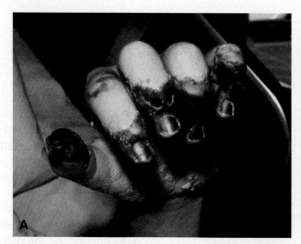
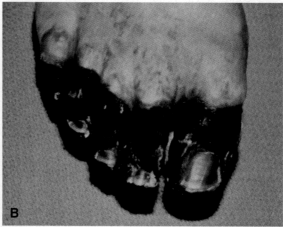

Figure 11-12. **Gangrenous hand (A) and foot (B) of patients with plague.** ([A] Courtesy of Dr. Jack Poland and the CDC. [B] Courtesy of William Archibald and the CDC.)

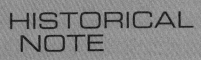

HISTORICAL NOTE

The Black Death

During the Middle Ages, plague was referred to as the black death because of the darkened, bruised appearance of the corpses. The blackened skin and foul smell were the result of cell necrosis and hemorrhaging into the skin. Plague probably dates back from 1000 or more years BC. In the past 2,000 years, the disease has killed millions of people—perhaps hundreds of millions. Huge plague epidemics occurred in Asia and Europe, including the European plague epidemic of 1348 to 1350, which killed about 44% of the population (40 million of 90 million people). The last major plague epidemic in Europe occurred in 1721. Plague still occurs, but the availability of insecticides and antibiotics has greatly reduced the incidence of this dreadful disease. Human plague is very rare in the United States (only two cases in 2010).

The CDC has classified the etiologic agents of anthrax, botulism, smallpox, and plague as Category A bioterrorism agents (see Table 11-8 for the definition of Category A agents).

Table 11-8 contains a listing of potential bioterrorism agents that, according to the CDC, pose the greatest threats to civilians—pathogens with which public health agencies must be prepared to cope.

To minimize the danger of potentially deadly microorganisms falling into the wrong hands, the U.S. Antiterrorism and Effective Death Penalty Act of 1996 makes the CDC responsible for controlling shipment of select agents—pathogens and toxins—deemed most likely to be used as BW agents. Authorities must constantly be on the alert for possible theft of these pathogens from biological supply houses and legitimate laboratories. In addition, vaccines, antitoxins, and other antidotes must be available wherever the threat of the use of these biological agents is high, as in various potential war zones.

All clinical microbiology laboratories should be staffed with persons familiar with the likely agents of bioterrorism and trained to detect, identify, and safely handle these agents. What individuals can do to prepare for bioterrorist attacks is discussed in "Preparing for a Bioterrorist Attack" on thePoint.

Table 11-8 Critical Biological Agent Categories for Public Health Preparedness

Category	Biological Agent(s)	Disease
Category A: These agents pose a risk to national security because they • can be easily disseminated or transmitted from person to person; • result in high mortality rates and have the potential for major public health impact; • might cause public panic and social disruption; and • require special action for public health preparedness.	*B. anthracis*	Anthrax
	C. botulinum	Botulism
	Y. pestis	Plague
	V. major	Smallpox
	F. tularensis	Tularemia
	Filoviruses (e.g., Ebola, Marburg) and arenaviruses (e.g., Lassa, Machupol)	Viral hemorrhagic fevers
Category B: These agents include those that • are moderately easy to disseminate; • result in moderate morbidity rates and low mortality rates; and • require specific enhancements of CDC's diagnostic capacity and enhanced disease surveillance.	*Brucella* species	Brucellosis
	Epsilon toxin of *C. perfringens*	
	Food safety threats (e.g., *Salmonella* spp., *E. coli* O157:H7, *Shigella* spp.)	

(continued)

Table 11-8 **Critical Biological Agent Categories for Public Health Preparedness (Continued)**

Category	Biological Agent(s)	Disease
	Burkholderia mallei	Glanders
	Burkholderia pseudomallei	Melioidosis
	C. psittaci	Psittacosis
	C. burnetii	Q fever
	Ricin toxin from castor beans	
	Staphylococcal enterotoxin B	
	Rickettsia prowazekii	Typhus fever
	Encephalitis viruses (e.g., Venezuelan equine encephalitis virus; eastern equine encephalitis virus; western equine encephalitis virus)	Encephalitis
	Water safety threats (e.g., *V. cholerae*, *C. parvum*)	
Category C: These are emerging pathogens that could be engineered for mass dissemination in the future because of • availability; • ease of production and dissemination; and • potential for high morbidity and mortality rates and major health impact.	Emerging infectious diseases such as Nipah virus and hantavirus	

Source: http://emergency.cdc.gov/agent/agentlist-category.asp

Water Supplies and Sewage Disposal

Water is the most essential resource necessary for the survival of humanity. The main sources of community water supplies are surface water from rivers, natural lakes, and reservoirs, as well as groundwater from wells. However, two general types of water pollution (i.e., chemical pollution and biological pollution) are present in our society, making it increasingly difficult to provide safe water supplies.

Chemical pollution of water occurs when industrial installations dump waste products into local waters without proper pretreatment, when pesticides are used indiscriminately, and when chemicals are expelled in the air and carried to earth by rain ("acid rain"). The main source of biological pollution is waste products of humans—fecal material and garbage—that swarm with pathogens. The causative agents of cholera, typhoid fever, bacterial and amebic dysentery, giardiasis, cryptosporidiosis, infectious hepatitis, and poliomyelitis can all be spread through contaminated water.

Waterborne epidemics today are the result of failure to make use of available existing knowledge and technology. In those countries that have established safe sanitary procedures for water purification and sewage disposal, outbreaks of typhoid fever, cholera, and dysentery occur only rarely.

In spring 1993, a waterborne epidemic of cryptosporidiosis (a diarrheal disease) affected more than 400,000 people in Milwaukee, Wisconsin. This was the largest waterborne epidemic that has ever occurred in the United States. The oocysts of *C. parvum* (a protozoan parasite) were present in cattle feces, which, when the winter snow melted, were washed off Wisconsin's numerous dairy farms into Lake Michigan. Milwaukee uses the water of Lake Michigan as its drinking water supply. Although the lake water had been treated, the tiny oocysts passed through the filters that were being used at that time. Thus, the *Cryptosporidium* oocysts were present in the city's drinking water, and people became infected when they drank the water. The epidemic caused the death of more than 100 immunosuppressed individuals.

> The largest waterborne epidemic to occur in the United States was an outbreak of cryptosporidiosis in Milwaukee, Wisconsin, in 1993, which affected more than 400,000 people.

Sources of Water Contamination

Rainwater falling over large areas collects in lakes and rivers and, thus, is subject to contamination by soil microbes and raw fecal material. For example, an animal feed lot located near a community water supply source harbors innumerable pathogens, which are washed into lakes and rivers. A city that draws its water from

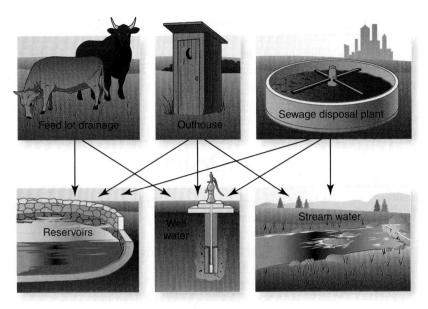

Figure 11-13. Sources of water contamination.

a local river, processes it, and uses it, but then dumps inadequately treated sewage into the river at the other side of town, may be responsible for a serious health problem in another city downstream on the same river. The city downstream must then find some way to rid its water supply of the pathogens. In many communities, untreated raw sewage and industrial wastes are dumped directly into local waters. Also, a storm or a flood may result in contamination of the local drinking water with sewage (Fig. 11-13).

Groundwater from wells also can become contaminated. To prevent such contamination, the well must be dug deep enough to ensure that the surface water is filtered through soil before it reaches the level of the well. Outhouses, septic tanks, and cesspools must be situated in such a way that surface water passing through these areas does not carry fecal microbes directly into the well water. With the growing popularity of trailer homes, a new problem has arisen because of trailer sewage disposal tanks that are located too near a water supply. In some very old cities, where cracked underground water pipes lie alongside leaking sewage pipes, sewage can enter the water pipes, thus contaminating the water just before it enters people's homes.

Water Treatment

Water must be properly treated to make it safe for human consumption. It is interesting to trace many steps involved in such treatment (Fig. 11-14). The water first is filtered to remove large pieces of debris such as twigs and leaves. Next, the water remains in a holding tank, where additional debris settles to the bottom of the tank; this phase of the process is known as **sedimentation** or **settling**. Alum (aluminum potassium sulfate) is then added to coagulate smaller pieces of debris, which

then settle to the bottom; this phase is known as **coagulation** or **flocculation**. The water is then filtered through sand or diatomaceous earth filters to remove the remaining bacteria, protozoan cysts and oocysts, and other small particles. In some water treatment facilities, charcoal filters or membrane filtration systems are also used. Membrane filtration will remove tiny *Giardia lamblia* cysts and *C. parvum* oocysts. Finally, chlorine gas or sodium hypochlorite is added to a final concentration of 0.2 to 1.0 ppm; this kills most remaining bacteria. In some water treatment facilities, ozone (O_3) treatment or ultraviolet light may be used in place of chlorination.

Small communities in rural areas may be financially unable to construct water treatment plants that incorporate all of these steps. Some may rely on chlorination alone. Unfortunately, the levels of chlorine routinely used for water treatment do not kill some pathogens, such as *Giardia* cysts and *Cryptosporidium* oocysts. Other communities use all the water treatment steps, but fail to use filters having a small enough pore size to trap tiny pathogens such as *Cryptosporidium* oocysts (which are about 4–6 μm in diameter).

In the laboratory, water can be tested for fecal contamination by checking for the presence of coliform bacteria (**coliforms**). Coliforms are *E. coli* and other lactose-fermenting members of the family Enterobacteriaceae, such as *Enterobacter* and *Klebsiella* spp. These bacteria normally live in the intestinal tracts of animals and humans; thus, their presence in drinking water is an indication that the water was fecally

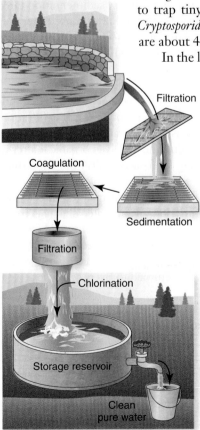

Figure 11-14. Steps in water treatment. (See text for details.)

Water is considered potable (safe to drink) if it contains 1 coliform or less per 100 mL of water.

contaminated. With respect to the presence of coliforms, water is considered potable (safe to drink) if it contains 1 coliform or less per 100 mL of water.

If one is unsure about the purity of drinking water, boiling it for 20 minutes destroys most pathogens that are present. It can then be cooled and consumed. Boiling will kill *Giardia* cysts and *Cryptosporidium* oocysts, but there are some bacterial spores and viruses that can withstand long periods of boiling. The most common causes of waterborne outbreaks in the United States are *G. lamblia*, *C. parvum*, *E. coli* O157:H7, *Shigella*, and norovirus.

Sewage Treatment

Raw sewage consists mainly of water, fecal material (including intestinal pathogens), and garbage and bacteria from the drains of houses and other buildings. When sewage is adequately treated in a disposal plant, the water it contains can be returned to lakes and rivers to be recycled.

Primary Sewage Treatment

In the sewage disposal plant, large debris is first filtered out (called screening), skimmers remove floating grease and oil, and floating debris is shredded or ground. Then, solid material settles out in a primary sedimentation tank. Flocculating substances can be added to cause other solids to settle out. The material that accumulates at the bottom of the tank is called **primary sludge**.

Secondary Sewage Treatment

The liquid (called primary effluent) then undergoes secondary treatment, which includes aeration or trickling filtration. The purpose of aeration is to encourage the growth of aerobic microbes, which oxidize the dissolved organic matter to CO_2 and H_2O. Trickling filters accomplish the same thing (i.e., conversion of dissolved organic matter to CO_2 and H_2O by microbes), but in a different manner. After either aeration or trickling filtration, the activated sludge is transferred to a settling tank, where any remaining solid material settles out. The remaining liquid (called secondary effluent) is filtered and disinfected (usually by chlorination), so that the effluent water can be returned to rivers or oceans.

Tertiary Sewage Treatment

In some desert cities, where water is in short supply, the effluent water from the sewage disposal plant is further treated (referred to as tertiary sewage treatment), so that it can be returned directly to the drinking water system; this is a very expensive process. Tertiary sewage treatment involves the addition of chemicals, filtration (using fine sand or charcoal), chlorination, and sometimes distillation.

In other cities, effluent water is used to irrigate lawns; however, it is expensive to install a separate water system for this purpose. In some communities, the sludge is heated to kill bacteria, then dried and used as fertilizer.

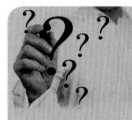

ON **thePoint**

- Terms Introduced in This Chapter
- Review of Key Points
- A Closer Look
  - Preparing for a Bioterrorist Attack
- Increase Your Knowledge
- Critical Thinking
- Additional Self-Assessment Exercises

Self-Assessment Exercises

After studying this chapter, answer the following multiple-choice questions.

1. Which of the following terms best describes chlamydial genital infection in the United States?
   a. arthropod-borne disease
   b. epidemic disease
   c. pandemic disease
   d. sporadic disease

2. Which of the following are considered reservoirs of infection?
   a. carriers
   b. contaminated food and drinking water
   c. rabid animals
   d. all of the above

3. The most common nationally notifiable infectious disease in the United States is:
   a. chlamydial genital infections
   b. gonorrhea
   c. the common cold
   d. TB

4. Which of the following arthropods is the vector of Lyme disease?

   a. flea
   b. mite
   c. mosquito
   d. tick

5. The most common zoonotic disease in the United States is:

   a. Lyme disease
   b. plague
   c. rabies
   d. Rocky Mountain spotted fever

6. Which one of the following organisms is *not* one of the four most likely potential BW or bioterrorism agents?

   a. *B. anthracis*
   b. Ebola virus
   c. *V. major*
   d. *Y. pestis*

7. All of the following are major steps in the treatment of a community's drinking water except:

   a. boiling
   b. filtration
   c. flocculation
   d. sedimentation

8. The largest waterborne epidemic ever to occur in the United States occurred in which of the following cities?

   a. Chicago
   b. Los Angeles
   c. Milwaukee
   d. New York City

9. Typhoid fever is caused by a species of:

   a. *Campylobacter*
   b. *Escherichia*
   c. *Salmonella*
   d. *Shigella*

10. Which of the following associations is incorrect?

    a. ehrlichiosis—tick
    b. malaria—mosquito
    c. plague—flea
    d. Spotted fever rickettsiosis—mite

12

Healthcare Epidemiology

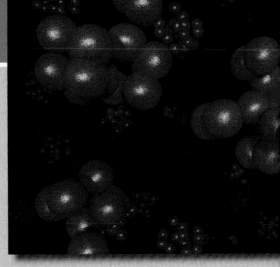

Artist rendering of *Staphylococcus* bacteria, which frequently lurk in healthcare facilities.

CHAPTER OUTLINE

LEARNING OBJECTIVES

After studying this chapter, you should be able to:

- Differentiate between healthcare-associated, community-acquired, and iatrogenic infections
- List the seven pathogens that most commonly cause healthcare-associated infections
- State the four most common types of healthcare-associated infections
- List six types of patients who are especially vulnerable to healthcare-associated infections
- State the three major contributing factors in healthcare-associated infections
- Differentiate between medical and surgical asepsis
- State the most important and effective way to reduce the number of healthcare-associated infections
- Differentiate between Standard Precautions and Transmission-Based Precautions, and state the three types of Transmission-Based Precautions
- Describe the types of patients placed in Protective Environments
- Cite three important considerations in the handling of each of the following in healthcare settings: food, eating utensils, fomites, and sharps

- List six responsibilities of an Infection Control Committee
- Explain three ways in which the Clinical Microbiology Laboratory participates in infection control

Introduction

Healthcare epidemiology can be defined as the study of the occurrence, determinants, and distribution of health and disease within healthcare settings. Health and disease are the result of complex interactions between pathogens, patients, and the healthcare environment. Although the primary focus of healthcare epidemiology is on infection control and preventing healthcare-associated infections (HAIs), healthcare epidemiology includes any activities designed to study and improve patient-care outcomes. These activities include surveillance measures; risk reduction programs focused on device and procedure management; policy development and implementation; education of healthcare personnel in infection control practices and procedures; cost–benefit assessment of prevention and control programs; and any measures designed to eliminate or contain reservoirs of infection, interrupt the transmission of infection, and protect patients, healthcare workers, and visitors against infection and disease.

> Healthcare epidemiology can be defined as the study of the occurrence, determinants, and distribution of health and disease within healthcare settings.

The importance of microbiology to those who work in health-related occupations can never be overemphasized. Whether working in a hospital, medical or dental clinic, long-term care facility, rehabilitation center, or hospice, or caring for sick persons in their homes, all healthcare professionals must follow standardized procedures to prevent the spread of infectious diseases. Thoughtless or careless actions when providing patient care can cause serious infections that otherwise could have been prevented.

Healthcare-Associated Infections

Definitions

Infectious diseases (infections) can be divided into two categories, depending on where the person became infected: (a) infections that are acquired *within* hospitals or other healthcare facilities (called **healthcare-associated infections** or HAIs)[a] and (b) infections that are acquired *outside* of healthcare facilities (called **community-acquired infections**). A hospitalized patient could have either type of infection. According to the Centers for Disease Control and Prevention (CDC), community-acquired infections are those that are present or incubating at the time of hospital admission. All other infections are considered HAIs, including those that erupt within 14 days of hospital discharge.

> Community-acquired infections are those that are present or incubating at the time of hospital admission. All other infections are considered HAIs, including those that erupt within 14 days of hospital discharge.

The term "healthcare-associated infection" should not be confused with the term "iatrogenic infection" (iatrogenic literally meaning "physician-induced"). An iatrogenic infection is an infection that results from medical or surgical treatment (i.e., an infection that is *caused* by a surgeon, another physician, or some other healthcare worker). Examples of iatrogenic infections are surgical site infections and urinary tract infections (UTIs) that result from urinary catheterization of patients. Iatrogenic infections are a type of HAI, but not all HAIs are iatrogenic infections.

> An iatrogenic infection is an infection that results from medical or surgical treatment—an infection that is *caused* by a surgeon, another physician, or some other healthcare worker.

Frequency of HAIs

It is sad to think that a patient who enters a hospital for one problem could develop an infection while in the hospital and perhaps die of that infection. However, this is an all too common occurrence. In 2002, the estimated number of HAIs in U.S. hospitals was approximately 1.7 million (roughly 5% of hospitalized patients).[b] The estimated number of deaths in 2002 associated with HAIs was 98,987 (approximately 6% of the patients having HAIs). Of these, the greatest number of deaths (35,967) was caused by pneumonia. HAIs cause significant increases in excess hospital stays and costs for additional treatment.

> In the United States, approximately 5% of hospitalized patients develop HAIs.

Pathogens Most Often Involved in HAIs

The hospital environment harbors many pathogens and potential pathogens. Some live on and in healthcare professionals, other hospital employees, visitors to the

---

[a]The CDC recommends use of the term "healthcare-associated infections" for infections acquired within any type of healthcare facility. The term replaces the older term "hospital-acquired infections," and its synonym, "nosocomial infections."

[b]Information source: Klevens RM, et al. 2002. Estimating healthcare-associated infections and deaths in U.S. hospitals. *Public Health Reports* 2007;122:160-166.

hospital, and patients themselves. Others live in dust or wet or moist areas such as sink drains, showerheads, whirlpool baths, mop buckets, flower pots, and even food from the kitchen. To make matters worse, the bacterial pathogens that are present in hospital settings are usually drug-resistant strains and, quite often, are multidrug-resistant.

The following bacteria account for ~84% of all HAIs in the United States[c]:

- Gram-positive cocci:
  Staphylococcus aureus (including methicillin-resistant strains of *Staphylococcus aureus* [MRSA]) (~15%)
  Coagulase-negative staphylococci (~15%)
  Enterococcus spp. (including vancomycin-resistant enterococci [VRE]) (~12%)
- Gram-negative bacilli:
  Escherichia coli (10%)
  Pseudomonas aeruginosa (~8%)
  Klebsiella pneumoniae (~6%)
  Enterobacter spp. (~5%)
  Acinetobacter baumannii (~3%)
  Klebsiella oxytoca (~2%)

Although some of the pathogens that cause HAIs originate in the external environment, many come from the patients themselves—their own indigenous microbiota that enter a surgical incision or otherwise gain entrance to areas of the body other than those where they normally reside. Urinary catheters, for example, provide a "superhighway" for indigenous microbiota of the distal urethra to gain access to the urinary bladder.

Approximately 70% of HAIs involve drug-resistant bacteria, which are common in hospitals, nursing homes, and other healthcare settings as a result of the many antimicrobial agents in use there. The drugs place selective pressure on the microbes, meaning that only those that are resistant to the drugs will survive. These resistant organisms then multiply and predominate (refer back to Fig. 9-8).

> Approximately 70% of HAIs involve drug-resistant bacteria.

Pseudomonas infections are especially difficult to treat, as are infections caused by multidrug-resistant *Mycobacterium tuberculosis* (MDR-TB), VRE, MRSA, and methicillin-resistant strains of *Staphylococcus epidermidis* (MRSE). Bacteria are not the only pathogens that have become drug resistant, however. Viruses (such as human immunodeficiency virus [HIV]), fungi (such as various *Candida* spp.), and protozoa (such as malarial parasites) have also developed drug resistance.

In 2001, the CDC launched a campaign to prevent antimicrobial resistance in healthcare settings. Table 12-1 contains the 12 steps that the CDC recommended to prevent antimicrobial resistance among hospitalized adults.

Modes of Transmission

The three principal routes by which pathogens involved in HAIs are transmitted are contact, droplet, and airborne.

Contact Transmission

There are two types of contact transmission:

- In direct contact transmission, pathogens are transferred from one infected person to another person without a contaminated intermediate object or person.
- Indirect contact transmission happens when pathogens are transferred via a contaminated intermediate object or person.

Droplet Transmission

In droplet transmission, respiratory droplets carrying pathogens transmit infection when they travel from the respiratory tract of an infectious individual (e.g., by sneezing or coughing) to susceptible mucosal surfaces of a recipient. Droplets traditionally have been defined as being larger than 5 μm in size.

Airborne Transmission

Airborne transmission occurs with dissemination of either airborne droplet nuclei or small particles containing pathogens. Traditionally, airborne droplets are defined as being less than or equal to 5 μm in size.

> The three most common modes of transmission in healthcare settings are contact, droplet, and airborne transmission.

Most Common Types of HAIs

According to the CDC,[d] the four most common types of HAIs in U.S. hospitals are the following:

1. **UTIs**, which represent about 32% of all HAIs and cause about 13% of the deaths associated with HAIs;
2. **surgical site infections**, which represent about 22% of all HAIs and cause about 8% of the deaths associated with HAIs;
3. **lower respiratory tract infections (primarily pneumonia)**, which represent about 15% of HAIs

---

[c]Hidron AI, et al. Antimicrobial-resistant pathogens associated with healthcare-associated infections: annual summary of data reported to the National Healthcare Safety Network at the Centers for Disease Control and Prevention, 2006-2007. *Infect Control Hosp Epidemiol.* 2008;29:996-1011.

[d]Much of the information in this chapter is from Siegel JD, et al. *Guidelines for Isolation Precautions: Preventing Transmission of Infectious Agents in Healthcare Settings.* Centers for Disease Control and Prevention, Atlanta, GA: 2007. Additional information can be obtained in the CDC-HICPA Guidelines for Environmental Infection Control in Healthcare Facilities (June 2003) at www.cdc.gov/ncidod/hip/enviro/guide.htm. HICPA stands for the Healthcare Infection Control Practices Advisory Committee.

Table 12-1	**Twelve Steps to Prevent Antimicrobial Resistance among Hospitalized Adults**
Prevent infection	
Step 1. Vaccinate	Give influenza vaccine and *Streptococcus pneumoniae* vaccine to at-risk patients before discharge. Healthcare workers should receive the influenza vaccine annually.
Step 2. Get the catheters out	Use catheters only when essential. Use the correct catheter. Use proper insertion and catheter-care protocols. Remove catheters when they are no longer essential.
Diagnose and treat infection effectively	
Step 3. Target the pathogen	Culture the patient. Target empiric therapy to likely pathogens and your facility's antibiogram information. Target definitive therapy to known pathogens and antimicrobial susceptibility test results.
Step 4. Access the experts	Consult infectious disease experts for patients with serious infections.
Use antimicrobials wisely	
Step 5. Practice antimicrobial control	Engage in local antimicrobial control efforts.
Step 6. Use local data	Know your facility's antibiogram. Know your patient population.
Step 7. Treat infection, not contamination	Use proper antisepsis for blood and other cultures. Culture the blood, not the skin or catheter hub. Use proper methods to obtain and process all cultures.
Step 8. Treat infection, not colonization	Treat pneumonia, not the tracheal aspirate. Treat bacteremia, not the catheter tip or hub. Treat UTI, not the indwelling catheter.
Step 9. Know when to say "no" to vancomycin	Treat infection, not contaminants or colonization. Fever in a patient with an intravenous catheter is not a routine indication for vancomycin.
Step 10. Stop antimicrobial treatment	When infection is cured. When cultures are negative and infection is unlikely. When infection is not diagnosed.
Prevent transmission	
Step 11. Isolate the pathogen	Use standard infection control precautions. Contain infectious body fluids. (Follow Airborne, Droplet, and Contact Precautions.) When in doubt, consult infection control experts.
Step 12. Break the chain of contagion	Stay home when you (the healthcare worker) are sick. Keep your hands clean. Set an example.

Source: The Centers for Disease Control (CDC), Atlanta, GA.

and cause about 36% of the deaths associated with HAIs;

4. **bloodstream infections (septicemia)**, which represent about 14% of HAIs and cause about 31% of the deaths associated with HAIs.

> The most common type of HAI in the United States is UTI, followed, in order, by surgical site, lower respiratory tract, and bloodstream infections.

Other common HAIs are the gastrointestinal diseases caused by *Clostridium difficile*, which are referred to as *C. difficile*-**associated diseases**. *C. difficile* (often referred to as "*C. diff*") is an anaerobic, spore-forming, Gram-positive bacillus. It is a common member of the indigenous microbiota of the colon, where it exists in relatively small numbers. Although *C. difficile* produces two types of toxins (an enterotoxin and a cytotoxin), the concentrations of these toxins are too low to cause disease when only small numbers of *C. difficile* are present. However, superinfections of *C. difficile* can

> *Clostridium difficile* is a common cause of healthcare-associated gastrointestinal infections.

occur when a patient receives oral antibiotics that kill off susceptible members of the gastrointestinal microbiota (superinfections are described in Chapter 9). *C. difficile*, which is resistant to many orally administered antibiotics, then increases in number, leading to increased concentrations of the toxins. The enterotoxin causes a disease known as **antibiotic-associated diarrhea** (AAD). The cytotoxin causes a disease known as **pseudomembranous colitis** (PMC), in which sections of the lining of the colon slough off, resulting in bloody stools. Both AAD and PMC are common in hospitalized patients.

Healthcare-associated zoonoses are another recognized problem in hospitals (see "Healthcare-Associated Zoonoses" on thePoint). Recall that zoonoses are diseases that are transmissible from animals to humans.

Patients Most Likely to Develop HAIs

Patients most likely to develop HAIs are immunosuppressed patients—patients whose immune systems have been weakened by age, underlying diseases, or medical or surgical treatments. Contributing factors include an aging population; increasingly aggressive medical and therapeutic interventions; and an increase in the number of implanted prosthetic devices, organ transplantations, xenotransplantations (the transplantation of animal organs or tissues into humans), and vascular and urinary catheterizations. The highest infection rates are in intensive care unit (ICU) patients. HAI rates are three times higher in adult and pediatric ICUs than elsewhere in the hospital. Listed here are the most vulnerable patients in a hospital setting:

- elderly patients,
- women in labor and delivery,
- premature infants and newborns,
- surgical and burn patients,
- patients with diabetes or cancer,
- patients with cystic fibrosis,
- patients having an organ transplant,
- patients receiving treatment with steroids, anticancer drugs, antilymphocyte serum, or radiation,
- immunosuppressed patients (i.e., patients whose immune systems are not functioning properly),
- patients who are paralyzed or are undergoing renal dialysis or urinary catheterization,
- patients with indwelling devices such as endotracheal tubes, central venous and arterial catheters, and synthetic implants.

> Immunosuppressed patients are especially likely to develop HAIs.

Major Factors Contributing to HAIs

The three major factors that combine to cause HAIs (Fig. 12-1) are

1. an ever-increasing number of drug-resistant pathogens,
2. the failure of healthcare personnel to follow infection control guidelines,
3. an increased number of immunocompromised patients.

Additional contributing factors are

> The three major causes of HAIs are drug-resistant bacteria, the failure of healthcare personnel to follow infection control guidelines, and an increased number of immunocompromised patients.

- the indiscriminate use of antimicrobial agents, which has resulted in an increase in the number of drug-resistant and multidrug-resistant pathogens;
- a false sense of security about antimicrobial agents, leading to a neglect of aseptic techniques and other infection control procedures;
- lengthy, more complicated types of surgery;
- overcrowding of hospitals and other healthcare facilities, as well as shortages of staff;
- increased use of less-highly trained healthcare workers, who are often unaware of infection control procedures;

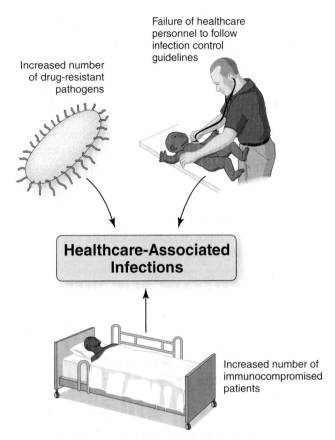

Figure 12-1. The three major contributing factors in HAIs.

- increased use of anti-inflammatory and immunosuppressant agents, such as radiation, steroids, anticancer chemotherapy, and antilymphocyte serum;
- overuse and improper use of indwelling medical devices.

Indwelling medical devices that support or monitor basic body functions contribute greatly to the success of modern medical treatment. However, by bypassing normal defensive barriers, these devices provide microbes access to normally sterile body fluids and tissues. The risk of bacterial or fungal infection is related to the degree of debilitation of the patient and the design and management of the device. It is advisable to discontinue the use of urinary catheters, vascular catheters, respirators, and hemodialysis on individual patients as soon as medically feasible.

What Can Be Done to Reduce the Number of HAIs?

It is critical for all healthcare workers to be aware of the problem of HAIs and to take appropriate measures to minimize the number of such infections that occur within healthcare facilities. The primary way to reduce

> The primary way to reduce the number of HAIs is strict compliance with infection control guidelines.

the number of HAIs is strict compliance with infection control guidelines (these guidelines are described in a subsequent section).

Handwashing is the single most important measure to reduce the risks of transmitting pathogens from one patient to another or from one anatomic site to another on the same patient. Handwashing, as it specifically pertains to healthcare personnel, is discussed later in the chapter ("Standard Precautions"). Presented here are commonsense, everyday, handwashing guidelines that pertain to everyone:

Wash your hands before you:

- Prepare or eat food
- Treat a cut or wound or tend to someone who is sick
- Insert or remove contact lenses

Wash your hands after you:

- Use the restroom
- Handle uncooked foods, particularly raw meat, poultry, or fish
- Change a diaper
- Cough, sneeze, or blow your nose
- Touch a pet, particularly reptiles and exotic animals
- Handle garbage
- Tend to someone who is sick or injured

Wash your hands in the following manner:

- Use warm or hot running water
- Use soap
- Wash all surfaces thoroughly, including wrists, palms, back of hands, fingers, and under fingernails (preferably with a nail brush)
- Rub hands together for at least 10 to 15 seconds
- When drying, begin with your forearms and work toward your hands and fingertips, and pat your skin rather than rubbing to avoid chapping and cracking

> Handwashing is the single most important measure to reduce the risks of transmitting pathogens from one patient to another or from one anatomic site to another on the same patient.

(These handwashing guidelines were originally published by the Bayer Corporation and the American Society for Microbiology.)

Other means of reducing the incidence of HAIs include disinfection and sterilization techniques, air filtration, use of ultraviolet lights, isolation of especially infectious patients, and wearing gloves, masks, and gowns whenever appropriate.

Infection Control

The term **infection control** pertains to the numerous measures that are taken to prevent infections from occurring within healthcare settings. These preventive measures include actions taken to eliminate or contain reservoirs of infection, interrupt the transmission of pathogens, and protect persons (patients, employees, and visitors) from becoming infected—in short, they are ways to break various links in the chain of infection (refer back to Fig. 11-3).

> Infection control measures are designed to break various links in the chain of infection.

Ever since the discoveries and observations of Joseph Lister and Ignaz Semmelweis (see the following "Historical Notes") in the 19th century, it has been known that wound contamination is not inevitable and that pathogens can be prevented from reaching vulnerable areas, a concept referred to as **asepsis**. Asepsis, which literally means *without infection*, includes any actions (referred to as aseptic techniques) taken to prevent infection or break the chain of infection. Such actions include general cleanliness, frequent and thorough handwashing, isolation of infected patients, disinfection, and sterilization. The techniques used to achieve asepsis depend on the site, circumstances, and environment. There are two main types or categories of asepsis: medical asepsis and surgical asepsis.

> Aseptic techniques are actions taken to prevent infection or break the chain of infection.

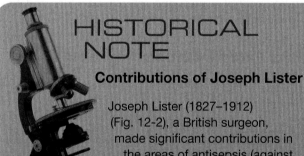

HISTORICAL NOTE

Contributions of Joseph Lister

Joseph Lister (1827–1912) (Fig. 12-2), a British surgeon, made significant contributions in the areas of antisepsis (against infection) and asepsis (without infection). During the 1860s, he instituted the practice of using phenol (carbolic acid) as an antiseptic to reduce microbial contamination of open surgical wounds. Lister routinely applied a dilute phenol solution to all wounds and insisted that anything coming in contact with the wounds (e.g., surgeons' hands, surgical instruments, and wound dressings) be immersed in phenol. In 1870, he instituted the practice of performing surgical procedures within a phenol mist. Although this practice probably killed microbes that were present in the air, it proved unpopular with the surgeons and nurses who inhaled the irritating phenol mist. Later contributions by Lister included such aseptic techniques as steam sterilization of surgical instruments; the use of sterile masks, gloves, and gowns by members of the surgical team; and the use of sterile drapes and

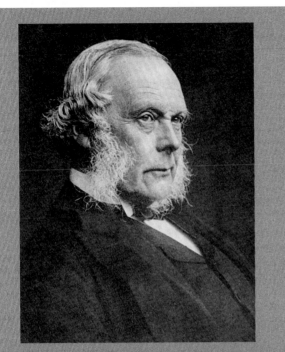

Figure 12-2. Joseph Lister. (Courtesy of Wikipedia Commons.)

gauze sponges in the operating room. Lister's antiseptic and aseptic techniques greatly reduced the incidence of surgical wound infections and surgical mortality. Because phenol is quite caustic and toxic, it was later replaced by other antiseptics.

Medical Asepsis

Once basic cleanliness is achieved, it is not difficult to maintain asepsis. Medical asepsis, or clean technique, involves procedures and practices that reduce the number and transmission of pathogens. Medical asepsis includes all the precautionary measures necessary to prevent direct transfer of pathogens from person to person and indirect transfer of pathogens through the air or on instruments, bedding, equipment, and other inanimate objects (fomites). Medical aseptic techniques include frequent and thorough handwashing; personal grooming; wearing of clean masks, gloves, and gowns when appropriate; proper cleaning of supplies and equipment; disinfection; proper disposal of needles, contaminated materials, and infectious waste; and sterilization.

> Medical asepsis is a clean technique. Its goal is to exclude pathogens.

Disinfection

General principles of disinfection were discussed in Chapter 8. Principles of disinfection as they pertain to the healthcare environment are discussed in this section.[e]

---

[e]Much of the information in this section is from Rutala WA, et al. *Guideline for Disinfection and Sterilization in Healthcare Facilities*. Atlanta, GA: Centers for Disease Control and Prevention; 2008.

Categories of Disinfectants. A few disinfectants will kill bacterial spores with prolonged exposure times (3–12 hours); these are referred to as **chemical sterilants**. Other disinfectants used within healthcare settings are categorized as high-level, intermediate-level, and low-level disinfectants. **High-level disinfectants** kill all microbes (including viruses),[f] except large numbers of bacterial spores. **Intermediate-level disinfectants** might kill mycobacteria, vegetative bacteria, most viruses, and most fungi, but do not necessarily kill bacterial spores. **Low-level disinfectants** kill most vegetative bacteria, some fungi, and some viruses within 10 minutes of exposure. Disinfectants commonly used in healthcare settings are shown in Table 12-2.

Spaulding System for Classification of Instruments and Items for Patient Care. More than 30 years ago, Earle H. Spaulding devised a system of classifying instruments and items for patient care according to the degree of risk for infection that was involved. This system is still used to determine how these items are to be disinfected or sterilized.

- **Critical items**. Critical items confer a high risk for infection if they are contaminated with *any* microbe. Thus, such objects must be sterile. Critical items include surgical instruments, cardiac and urinary catheters, implants, and ultrasound probes used in sterile body cavities. Items in this category should be purchased as sterile or be sterilized using steam (preferably), ethylene oxide gas, hydrogen peroxide gas plasma, or liquid chemical sterilants.

- **Semicritical items**. Semicritical items contact mucous membranes or nonintact skin and require high-level disinfection. These include respiratory therapy and anesthesia equipment, some endoscopes, laryngoscope blades, esophageal manometry probes, cytoscopes, anorectal manometry catheters, and diaphragm fitting rings. They minimally require high-level disinfection using glutaraldehyde, hydrogen peroxide, ortho-phthalaldehyde, or peracetic acid with hydrogen peroxide.

- **Noncritical items**. Noncritical items are those that come in contact with intact skin, but not mucous membranes. Such items are divided into two subcategories: noncritical patient-care items (e.g., bedpans, blood pressure cuffs, crutches, computers) and noncritical environmental surfaces (e.g., bed rails, some food utensils, bedside tables, patient furniture, floors). Low-level disinfectants may be used for noncritical items. Any of the following disinfectants may be used for noncritical items: 70% to 90% ethyl or isopropyl alcohol, sodium hypochlorite (household bleach diluted 1:500), phenolic germicidal detergent solution, iodophor germicidal detergent solution, and quaternary ammonium germicidal detergent solution.

---

[f]Viruses can be inactivated by some disinfectants, but are not really "killed." Recall that viruses are not actually "alive" to begin with.

Table 12-2 Disinfectants Commonly Used in Hospitals

Disinfectant	Mode of Action and Spectrum	Uses
Alcohols (e.g., 60%–90% solutions of ethyl, isopropyl, and benzyl alcohols)	Cause denaturation of proteins; bactericidal, tuberculocidal, fungicidal, virucidal, but not sporicidal	For disinfection of thermometers, rubber stoppers, external surfaces of stethoscopes, endoscopes, and certain other equipment
Chorine and chlorine compounds (Clorox, Halazone, hypochlorites, Warexin)	Thought to cause inhibition of key enzymatic reactions, protein denaturation, and inactivation of nucleic acids; bactericidal, tuberculocidal, fungicidal, virucidal, sporicidal	For disinfection of countertops, floors, blood spills, needles, syringes; water treatment
Formaldehyde (formalin is 37% formaldehyde by weight)	Alters the structure of proteins and purine bases; bactericidal, tuberculocidal, fungicidal, virucidal, sporicidal	Limited uses because of irritating fumes, pungent odor, and potential carcinogenicity; used for preserving anatomic specimens
Glutaraldehyde	Interferes with DNA, RNA, and protein synthesis; bactericidal, fungicidal, virucidal, sporicidal; relatively slow tuberculocidal activity	For disinfection of medical equipment such as endoscopes, tubing, dialyzers, and anesthesia and respiratory therapy equipment; has a pungent odor and is irritating to eyes, throat, and nose; may cause respiratory irritation, asthma, rhinitis, and contact dermatitis
Hydrogen peroxide	Produces destructive free radicals that attack membrane lipids, DNA, and other essential cell components; bactericidal, tuberculocidal, fungicidal, virucidal, sporicidal	For disinfection of inanimate surfaces; limited clinical use; contact with eyes may cause serious eye damage
Iodine (iodine solutions or tinctures) and iodophors (e.g., povidone-iodine, Wescodyne, Betadine, Isodine, Ioprep, Surgidine)	Thought to disrupt protein and nucleic acid structure and synthesis; bactericidal, tuberculocidal, virucidal; may require prolonged contact times to be fungicidal and sporicidal	Primarily for use as antiseptics; also for disinfection of rubber stoppers, thermometers, endoscopes
Ortho-phthalaldehyde	Mode of action unknown; bactericidal, tuberculocidal, fungicidal, virucidal, sporicidal	Stains skin, clothing, environmental surfaces; limited clinical use
Peracetic acid (peroxyacetic acid)	Thought to disrupt cell wall permeability and alter the structure of proteins; bactericidal, tuberculocidal, fungicidal, virucidal, sporicidal	Used in an automated machine to chemically sterilize immersible medical, surgical, and dental instruments, including endoscopes and arthroscopes; concentrate can cause serious eye and skin damage
Combination of peracetic acid and hydrogen peroxide	Mode of action as described above for hydrogen peroxide and peracetic acid; bactericidal, tuberculocidal, fungicidal, virucidal, but not sporicidal	For disinfection of hemodialyzers
Phenol (carbolic acid) and phenolics (e.g., xylenols, o-phenylphenol, hexylresorcinol, hexachlorophene, cresol, Lysol)	Disrupts cell walls and inactivates essential enzyme systems; bactericidal, tuberculocidal, fungicidal, virucidal, but not sporicidal	For decontamination of the hospital environment, including laboratory surfaces, and for noncritical medical and surgical items; residual disinfectant on porous surfaces may cause tissue irritation
Quaternary ammonium compounds (a variety of organically substituted ammonium compounds, such as dodecyldimethyl ammonium chloride)	Inactivate energy-producing enzymes, denaturation of disruption of cell membranes; bactericidal, fungicidal, and virucidal to lipophilic viruses; generally not tuberculocidal, sporicidal, or virucidal to hydrophilic viruses	For disinfection of noncritical surfaces such as floors, furniture, and walls; should not be used as antiseptics

Additional information about disinfectants can be found in CDC's Guideline for Disinfection and Sterilization in Healthcare Facilities, 2008, available on the CDC web site: http://www.cdc.gov.

Surgical Asepsis

Surgical asepsis, or sterile technique, includes practices used to render and keep objects and areas sterile (i.e., free of microbes). Note the differences between medical and surgical asepsis:

- Medical asepsis is a clean technique, whereas surgical asepsis is a sterile technique.
- The goal of medical asepsis is to exclude pathogens, whereas the goal of surgical asepsis is to exclude all microbes.

> Surgical asepsis is a sterile technique. Its goal is to exclude all microbes.

Surgical aseptic techniques are practiced in operating rooms, in labor and delivery areas, and during invasive procedures. For example, invasive procedures, such as drawing blood, injecting medications, urinary catheter insertion, cardiac catheterization, and lumbar punctures, must be performed using strict surgical aseptic precautions. Other surgical aseptic techniques include surgical scrubbing of hands and fingernails before entering the operating room; wearing sterile masks, gloves, caps, gowns, and shoe covers; using sterile solutions and dressings; using sterile drapes and creating a sterile field; and using heat-sterilized surgical instruments. Methods of sterilization were discussed in Chapter 8.

SPOTLIGHTING

Perfusionists

As stated in the American Medical Association's Health Care Careers Directory (available at http://www.ama-assn.org under "Education"), "A perfusionist is a skilled allied health professional, qualified by academic and clinical education, who operates extracorporeal circulation equipment during any medical situation in which it is necessary to support or temporarily replace the patient's circulatory or respiratory function. Perfusionists serve as members of an open-heart, surgical team responsible for the selection, setup, and operation of a mechanical device, commonly referred to as the heart-lung machine."

"During open heart surgery, when the patient's heart is immobilized and cannot function in a normal fashion while the operation is being performed, the patient's blood is diverted and circulated outside the body through the heart-lung machine and returned again to the patient. In effect, the machine assumes the function of both the heart and lungs."

"The perfusionist is responsible for operating the machine during surgery, closely monitoring the altered circulatory process, taking appropriate corrective action when abnormal situations arise, and keeping both the surgeon and anesthesiologist fully informed."

"In addition to the operation of the heart-lung machine during surgery, perfusionists often function in supportive roles for other medical specialties in operating mechanical devices to assist in the conservation of blood and blood products during surgery, and provide extended, long-term support of patients' circulation outside of the operating room environment."

Information concerning educational requirements and programs, certification, and salary is available at the AMA web site.

Hair at the surgical site must be clipped using an electric shaver and the patient's skin must be thoroughly cleansed and scrubbed with soap and antiseptic. If the surgery is to be extensive, the surrounding area is covered with a sterile plastic film or sterile cloth drapes so that a sterile surgical field is established. The surgeon and all surgical assistants must scrub their hands for 5 to 10 minutes with a disinfectant soap and cover their clothes, mouth, and hair, because these might shed microbes onto the operative site. These coverings include sterile gloves, gowns, caps, masks, and shoe covers (Fig. 12-3). All instruments, sutures, and dressings must be sterile. They are handled only while wearing sterile masks and gloves. As soon as these items become contaminated, they must be thoroughly cleaned and sterilized for reuse or disposed of properly. All needles, syringes, and other sharp items of equipment ("sharps") must be disposed of by placing them into appropriate puncture-proof "sharps containers."

Floors, walls, and all equipment in the operating room must be thoroughly cleaned and disinfected before

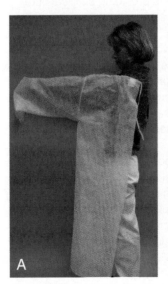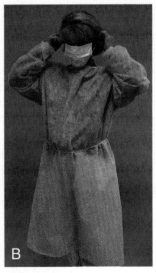

Figure 12-3. Healthcare professional donning PPE. A. Sterile gown. **B.** Mask. **C.** Gloves. (From McCall RE, Tankersley CM. *Phlebotomy Essentials.* 5th ed. Philadelphia, PA: Lippincott Williams & Wilkins; 2012.)

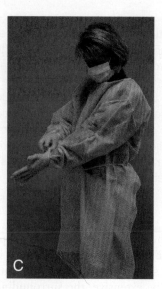

Figure 12-3. (*Continued*)

and after each use. Proper ventilation must be maintained to ensure that fresh, filtered air is circulated throughout the room at all times.

SPOTLIGHTING
Surgical Technologists

As stated in the American Medical Association's Health Care Careers Directory (available at http://www.ama-assn.org under "Education"), "Surgical technologists are allied health professionals working with surgeons and other medical practitioners providing surgical care to patients in a variety of settings as integral members of the health care team."

"Surgical technologists work under the supervision of the surgeon to ensure that the operating room or environment is safe, equipment functions properly, and operative procedure is conducted under conditions that maximize patient safety. They handle the instruments, supplies, and necessary equipment during the surgical procedure."

"Surgical technologists possess expertise in the theory and application of sterile and aseptic technique combined with the knowledge of human anatomy, surgical procedures, and implementation tools and technologies to facilitate a physician's performance of invasive therapeutic and diagnostic procedures."

Specific duties of surgical technologists in the first scrub role, the assistant circulating role, and the second assisting role can be found on the AMA web site, as can information concerning educational requirements and programs, certification, and salary.

Regulations Pertaining to Healthcare Epidemiology and Infection Control

In the United States, there are many different regulations that pertain to healthcare epidemiology and infection control—so many, in fact, that it is not possible to discuss them all in a book this size. One of the most important of these regulations was published in 2001 by the Occupational Safety and Health Administration (OSHA). It is entitled the Bloodborne Pathogen Standard (29 CFR 1910.1030). This standard requires facilities having employees who have occupational exposure to blood or other potentially infectious materials to prepare and update a written plan called the Exposure Control Plan. This plan is designed to eliminate or minimize employee exposure to pathogens. Other topics addressed in 29 CFR 1910.1030 are:

- Postexposure follow-up
- Recordkeeping for bloodborne pathogens
- Needlestick injuries and other sharps
- Universal precautions
- Latex allergy
- Bloodborne illnesses such as HIV, hepatitis B virus (HBV), and hepatitis C virus (HCV)
- Labeling and signs

(29 CFR 1910.1030 can be found on the OSHA web site: http://www.osha.gov)

Standard Precautions

In a healthcare setting, one is not always aware of which patients are infected with HIV, HBV, HCV, or other communicable pathogens. Thus, to prevent transmission of pathogens within healthcare settings, two levels of safety precautions have been developed by the CDC: Standard Precautions and Transmission-Based Precautions. Standard Precautions combine the major features of Universal Precautions and Body Substance Isolation Precautions,[g] and are intended to be applied to the care of *all* patients in *all* healthcare settings, regardless of the suspected or confirmed presence of an infectious agent. Transmission-Based Precautions (discussed in a subsequent section), on the other hand, are enforced only for certain specific types of infections.

Implementation of Standard Precautions constitutes the primary strategy for the prevention of healthcare-associated transmission of infectious agents between patients and healthcare personnel. Standard Precautions

> Standard Precautions are to be applied to the care of ALL patients in ALL healthcare settings, regardless of the suspected or confirmed presence of an infectious agent.

[g]Universal Precautions (published in 1985, 1987, and 1988) pertained to blood and body fluids, whereas Body Substance Isolation Precautions (published in 1987) were designed to reduce the risk of transmission of pathogens from moist body substances.

Implementation of Standard Precautions constitutes the primary strategy for the prevention of healthcare-associated transmission of infectious agents between patients and healthcare personnel.

are based on the principle that all blood, body fluids, secretions, excretions except sweat, nonintact skin, and mucous membranes may contain transmissible infectious agents. Standard Precautions provide infection prevention guidelines regarding hand hygiene; wearing of gloves, gowns, masks, eye protection; respiratory hygiene/ cough etiquette; safe injection practices; lumbar puncture; cleaning of patient-care equipment; environmental control (including cleaning and disinfection); handling of soiled linens; handling and disposal of used needles and other sharps; resuscitation devices; and patient placement. OSHA guidelines are designed to protect healthcare personnel, whereas Standard Precautions will protect *both* healthcare personnel and their patients from becoming infected with HIV, HBV, HCV, and many other pathogens. The sign shown in Figure 12-4 summarizes the most important aspects of Standard Precautions.

STANDARD PRECAUTIONS
FOR INFECTION CONTROL

Assume that every person is potentially infected or colonized with an organism that could be transmitted in the healthcare setting.

Hand Hygiene
Avoid unnecessary touching of surfaces in close proximity to the patient.

When hands are visibly dirty, contaminated with proteinaceous material, or visibly soiled with blood or body fluids, wash hands with soap and water.

If hands are not visibly soiled, or after removing visible material with soap and water, decontaminate hands with an alcohol-based hand rub. Alternatively, hands may be washed with an antimicrobial soap and water.

Perform hand hygiene:
    Before having direct contact with patients.
    After contact with blood, body fluids or excretions, mucous membranes, nonintact skin, or wound dressings.
    After contact with a patient's intact skin (e.g., when taking a pulse or blood pressure or lifting a patient).
    If hands will be moving from a contaminated body site to a clean body site during patient care.
    After contact with inanimate objects (including medical equipment) in the immediate vicinity of the patient.
    After removing gloves.

Personal protective equipment (PPE)
Wear PPE when the nature of the anticipated patient interaction indicates that contact with blood or body fluids may occur.

Before leaving the patient's room or cubicle, remove and discard PPE.

Gloves
Wear gloves when contact with blood or other potentially infectious materials, mucous membranes, nonintact skin, or potentially contaminated intact skin (e.g., of a patient incontinent of stool or urine) could occur.

Remove gloves after contact with a patient and/or the surrounding environment using proper technique to prevent hand contamination. Do not wear the same pair of gloves for the care of more than one patient.

Change gloves during patient care if the hands will move from a contaminated body site (e.g., perineal area) to a clean body site (e.g., face).

Gowns
Wear a gown to protect skin and prevent soiling or contamination of clothing during procedures and patient-care activities when contact with blood, body fluids, secretions, or excretions is anticipated.

Wear a gown for direct patient contact if the patient has uncontained secretions or excretions.

Remove gown and perform hand hygiene before leaving patient's environment.

Mouth, nose, eye protection
Use PPE to protect the mucous membranes of the eyes, nose and mouth during procedures and patient-care activities that are likely to generate splashes or sprays of blood, body fluids, secretions and excretions.

During aerosol-generating procedures wear one of the following: a face shield that fully covers the front and sides of the face, a mask with attached shield, or a mask and goggles.

Respiratory Hygiene/Cough Etiquette
Educate healthcare personnel to contain respiratory secretions to prevent droplet and fomite transmission of respiratory pathogens, especially during seasonal outbreaks of viral respiratory tract infections.

Offer masks to coughing patients and other symptomatic persons (e.g., persons who accompany ill patients) upon entry into the facility.

Patient-Care equipment and instruments/devices
Wear PPE (e.g., gloves, gown), according to the level of anticipated contamination, when handling patient-care equipment and instruments/devices that are visibly soiled or may have been in contact with blood or body fluids.

Care of the environment
Include multi-use electronic equipment in policies and procedures for preventing contamination and for cleaning and disinfection, especially those items that are used by patients, those used during delivery of patient care, and mobile devices that are moved in and out of patient rooms frequently (e.g., daily).

Textiles and laundry
Handle used textiles and fabrics with minimum agitation to avoid contamination of air, surfaces and persons.

SPR7 · ©2007 Brevis Corporation · www.brevis.com

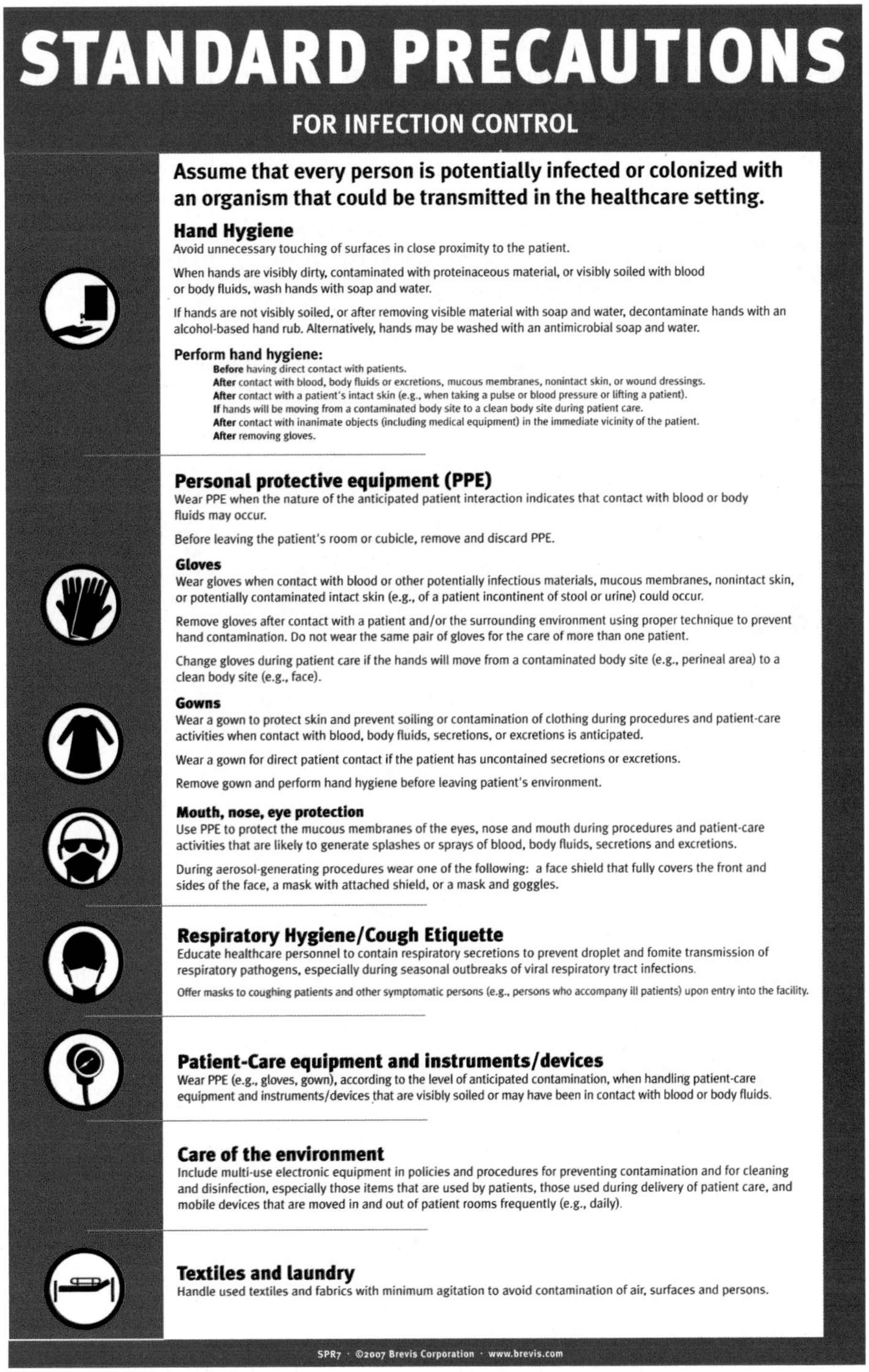

Figure 12-4. ▶ **Standard Precautions sign.** (From McCall RE, Tankersley CM. *Phlebotomy Essentials*. 5th ed. Philadelphia, PA: Lippincott Williams & Wilkins; 2012. Courtesy of the Brevis Corp., Salt Lake City, UT.)

Vaccinations

Because healthcare personnel are at particular risk for several vaccine-preventable infectious diseases, the Immunization Action Coalition (www.vaccineinformation.org) recommends that they receive the following vaccines:

- Hepatitis B vaccine
- Influenza (annually)
- Measles–mumps–rubella (MMR)
- Varicella (chickenpox)
- Tetanus–diphtheria–pertussis (Tdap)
- Meningococcal vaccine (for microbiologists who are routinely exposed to isolates of *Neisseria meningitidis*)

> The most important and most basic technique in preventing and controlling infections and preventing the transmission of pathogens is handwashing.

Hand Hygiene

It cannot be said too often: the most important and most basic technique in preventing and controlling infections and preventing the transmission of pathogens is handwashing. Because contaminated hands are a prime cause of cross-infection (i.e., transmission of pathogens from one patient to another), healthcare personnel caring for hospitalized patients must wash their hands thoroughly between patient contacts (i.e., before and after each patient contact). In addition, hands should be washed between tasks and procedures on the same patient to prevent cross-contamination of different body sites. Hands must be washed after touching blood, body fluids, secretions, excretions, and contaminated items, even when gloves are worn. Hands must be washed immediately after gloves are removed.

A plain (nonantimicrobial) soap may be used for routine handwashing, but an antimicrobial or antiseptic agent should be used in certain circumstances (e.g., before entering an operating room or to control outbreaks within the hospital). Figure 12-5 contains the step-by-step instructions for effective handwashing. According to the CDC, alcohol-based handrubs that do not require the use of water can be used in place of handwashing when hands are not visibly soiled. The volume of handrub to be used varies from product to product; thus, manufacturer's directions must be followed. Artificial fingernails and rings should not be worn by healthcare personnel who provide direct patient care.

Step		Explanation/Rationale

① Stand back so that you do not touch the sink.

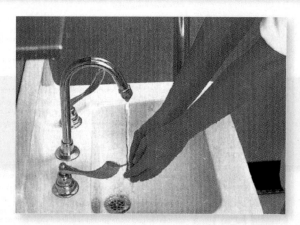

The sink may be contaminated.

② Turn on the faucet and wet hands under warm running water.

Water should not be too hot or too cold and hands should be wet before applying soap to minimize drying, chapping, or cracking of hands from frequent handwashing.

③ Apply soap and work up a lather.

A good lather is needed to reach all surfaces.

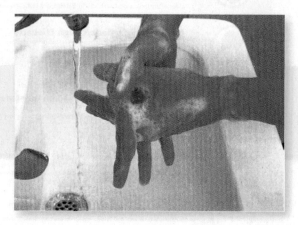

④ Scrub all surfaces, including between the fingers and around the knuckles.

Scrubbing is necessary to dislodge microorganisms from surfaces, especially between fingers and around knuckles.

⑤ Rub your hands together vigorously.

Friction helps loosen dead skin, dirt, debris, and microorganisms. (Steps 4–5 should take at least 15 seconds, about the time it takes to sing the ABC song.)

Figure 12-5. Proper hand washing technique. (From McCall RE, Tankersley CM. *Phlebotomy Essentials.* 5th ed. Philadelphia, PA: Lippincott Williams & Wilkins; 2008.)

Step	Explanation/Rationale

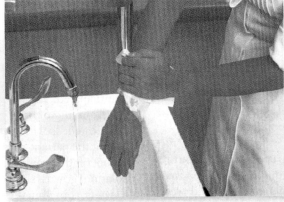

6. Rinse your hands in a downward motion from wrists to fingertips.

Rinsing with the hands downward allows contaminants to be flushed from the hands and fingers into the sink rather than flowing back up the arm or wrist.

7. Dry hands with a clean paper towel.

Hands must be dried thoroughly and gently to prevent chapping or cracking. Reusable towels can be a source of contamination.

8. Use a clean paper towel to turn off the faucet unless it is foot or motion activated.

Clean hands should not touch contaminated faucet handles.

Images from Molle EA, Kronenberger J, West-Stack C. Lippincott Williams & Wilkins' Clinical Medical Assisting, 2nd ed. Baltimore: Lippincott Williams & Wilkins, 2005.

Figure 12-5. (*Continued*)

HISTORICAL NOTE

The Father of Handwashing

Ignaz Philipp Semmelweis (1818–1865) has been referred to as the "Father of Handwashing," the "Father of Hand Disinfection," and the "Father of Hospital Epidemiology." Semmelweis, a Hungarian physician, was employed in the maternity department of a large Viennese hospital during the 1840s. Many of the women whose babies were delivered in one of the hospital's clinics became ill and died of a disease known as puerperal fever (also known as childbed fever), the cause of which was unknown at the time. (It is now known that puerperal fever is caused by *Streptococcus pyogenes*.) Semmelweis observed that physicians and medical students often went directly from an autopsy room to the obstetrics clinic to assist in the delivery of a baby. Although they washed their hands with soap and water upon entering the clinic, Semmelweis noted that their hands still had a disagreeable odor. He concluded that the puerperal fever that the women later developed was caused by "cadaverous particles" present on the hands of the physicians and students. In May 1847, Semmelweis instituted a policy that stated that "all students or doctors who enter the wards for the purpose of making an examination must wash their hands thoroughly in a solution of chlorinated lime that will be placed in convenient basins near the entrance of the wards." Thereafter, the maternal mortality rate dropped dramatically. This was the first evidence that cleansing contaminated hands with an antiseptic agent reduces HAIs more effectively than handwashing with plain soap and water. It is interesting to note that Oliver Wendell Holmes (1809–1894), an American physician, had concluded some years earlier that puerperal fever was spread by healthcare workers' hands. However, the recommendations Holmes made in his historical essay of 1843, entitled *The Contagiousness of Puerperal Fever*, met with opposition (as did Semmelweis' recommendations) and had little impact on obstetric practices of the time.

HELPFUL HINTS: HANDWASHING

To make sure that you have washed your hands sufficiently, rub your soapy hands and interlaced fingers together for as long as it takes you to sing the birthday song ("Happy Birthday to You") twice through, or all verses of "Twinkle, Twinkle, Little Star" once. Alternatively, you could use a quick-drying alcohol foam, gel, or lotion. Studies have shown that these convenient products are at least as effective as old-fashioned soap and water. They are quick, they dry in about 15 seconds, and by using them, you eliminate the possibility of someone overhearing you singing off key!

Personal Protective Equipment

There are many components of personal protective equipment (PPE). The most common are listed here.

Gloves. Gloves can protect both patients and healthcare personnel from exposure to infectious materials that may be carried on hands. Healthcare personnel should wear gloves when

- anticipating direct contact with blood or body fluids, mucous membranes, nonintact skin, and other potentially infectious materials,
- having direct contact with patients who are colonized or infected with pathogens transmitted by the contact route,
- handling or touching visibly or potentially contaminated patient-care equipment and environmental surfaces.

Gloves must be changed between tasks and procedures on the same patient whenever there is risk of transferring microorganisms from one body site to another. Always remove gloves promptly after use and before going to another patient. Thoroughly wash your hands immediately after removing gloves; there is always the possibility that the gloves contained small tears in them or that your hands became contaminated while removing the gloves. Figure 12-6 illustrates the proper method of glove removal.

> PPE includes gloves, gowns, masks, eye protection, and respiratory protection.

Isolation Gowns. Isolation gowns are worn in conjunction with gloves and with other PPE when indicated. Gowns are usually the first piece of PPE to be donned. They protect the healthcare worker's arms and exposed body areas and prevent contamination of clothing with blood, body fluids, and other potentially infectious material. When applying Standard Precautions, an isolation gown is worn only if contact with blood or body fluid is anticipated. However, when Contact Precautions are used, donning of both gown and gloves upon room entry is indicated. Isolation gowns should be removed before leaving the patient-care area to prevent possible contamination of the environment outside the patient's room. Isolation gowns should be removed in a manner that prevents contamination of clothing or skin. The outer, "contaminated," side of the gown is turned inward and rolled into a bundle, and then discarded into a designated container for waste or linen to contain contamination.

Masks. Masks are used for three primary purposes in healthcare settings:

1. They are worn by healthcare personnel to protect them from contact with infectious material from patients.

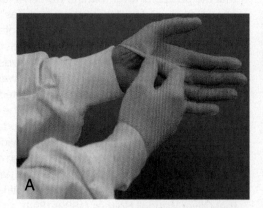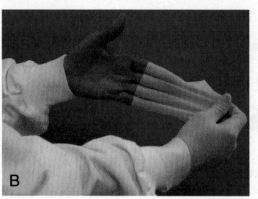

Figure 12-6. Proper procedure for glove removal. A. The wrist of one glove is grasped with the opposite gloved hand. **B.** The glove is pulled inside out, over, and off the hand. **C.** With the first glove held in the gloved hand, the fingers of the nongloved hand are slipped under the wrist of the remaining glove without touching the exterior surfaces. **D.** The glove is then pulled inside out over the hand so that the first glove lies within the second glove, with no exterior glove surfaces exposed. **E.** Contaminated gloves ready to be placed into the proper biohazardous waste receptacle. (From McCall RE, Tankersley CM. *Phlebotomy Essentials*. 5th ed. Philadelphia, PA: Lippincott Williams & Wilkins; 2012.)

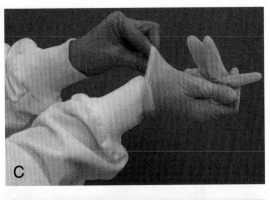
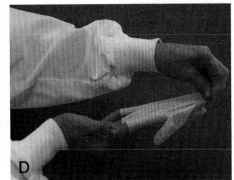
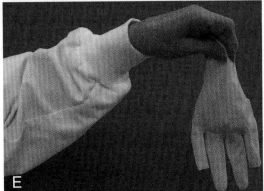

Figure 12-6. (*Continued*)

2. They are worn by healthcare personnel when engaged in procedures requiring sterile technique to protect patients from exposure to pathogens that may be present in a healthcare worker's mouth or nose.
3. They are placed on coughing patients to limit potential dissemination of infectious respiratory secretions from the patient to others.

Eye Protection. Types of eye protection include goggles and disposable or nondisposable face shields. Masks may be used in combination with goggles, or a face shield may be used instead of a mask and goggles. Even when Droplet Precautions are not indicated, eye, nose, and mouth protection are necessary when it is likely that there will be a splash or spray of any respiratory secretions or other body fluids. Eye protection and masks are removed after gloves are removed.

Respiratory Protection. Respiratory protection requires the use of a respirator with N95 or higher filtration to prevent inhalation of infectious particles (Fig. 12-7).[h] Do not confuse masks with particulate

respirators. Respirators are recommended when working with patients with tuberculosis, severe acute respiratory syndrome (SARS), and smallpox, and during the performance of aerosol-generating procedures on patients with avian or pandemic influenza.

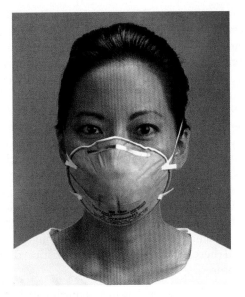

Figure 12-7. The type N95 respirator. See text for details. (From McCall RE, Tankersley CM. *Phlebotomy Essentials.* 5th ed. Philadelphia, PA: Lippincott Williams & Wilkins; 2012. Courtesy of 3M Occupational Health and Environmental Safety Division, St. Paul, MN.)

[h]N95 respirators are tight-fitting, adjustable masks that are designed to protect against small droplets of respiratory fluids and other airborne particles in addition to all the protection afforded by surgical masks. The designation "N95" refers to the fact that this product filters at least 95% of airborne particles.

Patient-Care Equipment

Organic material (e.g., blood, body fluids, secretions, excretions) must be removed from medical equipment, instruments, and devices prior to high-level disinfection and sterilization because residual proteinaceous material reduces the effectiveness of disinfection and sterilization processes. All such equipment and devices must be handled in a manner that will protect healthcare workers and the environment from potentially infectious material. Cleaning and disinfection must include computer keyboards and personal digital assistants (PDAs). Whenever possible, the use of dedicated medical equipment, such as stethoscopes, blood pressure cuffs, and electronic thermometers, reduces the potential for transmission. Items such as commodes, intravenous pumps, and ventilators must be thoroughly cleaned and disinfected before use by or on another patient.

Environmental Control

The hospital must have, and employees must comply with, adequate procedures for the routine care, cleaning, and disinfection of environmental surfaces such as bedrails, bedside tables, commodes, doorknobs, sinks, and any other surfaces and equipment in close proximity to patients.

Linens

Textiles such as bedding, towels, and patient gowns that have become soiled with blood, body fluids, secretions, or excretions must be handled, transported, and laundered in a safe manner. Soiled textiles must not be shaken, must not come in contact with the healthcare worker's body or clothing, and must be contained in a laundry bag or designated bin.

Disposal of Sharps

Needlestick injuries and injuries resulting from broken glass and other sharps are the primary manner in which healthcare workers become infected with pathogens such as HIV, HBV, and HCV. Thus, Standard Precautions include guidelines regarding the safe handling of such items. Needles and other sharp devices must be handled in a manner that prevents injury to the user and to others who may encounter the device during or after a procedure. Accidents can be prevented by employing safer techniques (such as by not recapping needles), by disposing of used needles in appropriate sharps disposal containers, and by using safety-engineered sharp devices. Safety devices may be an integral part of the needle (including butterfly needles), the evacuated tube holder, or the syringe.

Listed here are desirable characteristics of needle safety features:

- It is as simple to use as possible, requiring little training to use it effectively.
- It is an integral part of the device, not an accessory.
- It provides a barrier between the hands of the healthcare worker and the needle after its use.

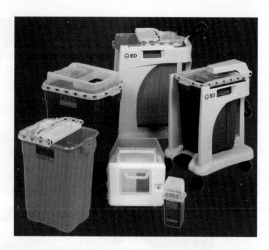

Figure 12-8. Several types of sharps containers. (From McCall RE, Tankersley CM. *Phlebotomy Essentials*. 5th ed. Philadelphia: Lippincott Williams & Wilkins; 2012. Courtesy of Becton Dickinson, Franklin Lakes, NJ.)

- It allows the worker's hands to remain behind the needle at all times.
- It is in effect before disassembly and remains in effect after disposal to protect users and trash handlers and for environmental safety.

Contaminated needles and other contaminated sharps must not be bent, recapped, or removed, and shearing or breaking of needles is prohibited. All contaminated needles, lancets, scalpel blades, and other sharps must be disposed of immediately after use, by placing them in special containers known as sharps containers. This is true whether or not the sharp contains a safety feature. Sharps containers are rigid, puncture resistant, leak proof, disposable, and clearly marked with a biohazard label (Figs. 12-8 and 12-9). Sharps containers must be easily accessible to all personnel needing them and must be located in all areas where needles are commonly used, as in areas where blood is drawn, including patient rooms, emergency rooms, ICUs, and surgical suites. When full, sharps containers are properly disposed of as biohazardous waste.

Figure 12-9. Biohazard symbol. (From McCall RE, Tankersley CM. *Phlebotomy Essentials*. 5th ed. Philadelphia, PA: Lippincott Williams & Wilkins; 2012.)

Transmission-Based Precautions

Within a healthcare setting, pathogens are transmitted by three major routes: contact, droplet, and airborne. Transmission-Based Precautions are used for patients who are known or suspected to be infected or colonized with highly transmissible or epidemiologically important pathogens for which additional safety precautions *beyond* Standard Precautions are required to interrupt transmission within hospitals. There are three types of Transmission-Based Precautions, which may be used either singly or in combination: Contact Precautions, Droplet Precautions, and Airborne Precautions. It is very important to understand that Transmission-Based Precautions are to be used *in addition to* the Standard Precautions already being used. Infectious diseases requiring Transmission-Based Precautions are listed in Table 12-3.

> The three types of Transmission-Based Precautions are used *in addition to* Standard Precautions.

Contact Precautions

Contact transmission is the most important and frequent mode of transmission of HAIs. Contact Precautions are used for patients known or suspected to be infected or colonized with epidemiologically important pathogens that can be transmitted by direct or indirect contact. Examples include multidrug-resistant bacteria, *C. difficile*-associated diseases, respiratory syncytial virus (RSV) infection in children, scabies, impetigo, chickenpox or shingles, and viral hemorrhagic fevers. Contact Precautions are summarized on the sign shown in Figure 12-10. Infectious diseases requiring Contact Precautions are listed in Table 12-3.

> Contact transmission is the most important and frequent mode of transmission of HAIs.

Droplet Precautions

Technically, droplet transmission is a form of contact transmission. However, in droplet transmission, the mechanism of transfer is quite different than in either

Table 12-3 Infectious Diseases Requiring Transmission-Based Precautions	
Type of Transmission-Based Precautions	**Infectious Diseases or Conditions**[a]
Contact precautions	Acute viral (hemorrhagic) conjunctivitis; adenovirus pneumonia; any acute respiratory infectious disease in infants and young children; adverse events following vaccinia vaccination; aseptic meningitis in infants and young children; bronchiolitis; chickenpox; *C. difficile* gastroenteritis; congenital rubella in children <1 year of age; cutaneous diphtheria; decubitus ulcer; disseminated shingles in any patient; localized shingles in immunocompromised patients; extrapulmonary tuberculosis with draining lesion; gastroenteritis due to adenovirus, *Campylobacter*, cholera, *Cryptosporidium*; enterohemorrhagic O157:H7 *E. coli*, giardiasis, norovirus, rotavirus, *Salmonella*, *Shigella*, *Vibrio parahemolyticus* or *Yersinia enterocolitica* in diapered or incontinent persons; group A streptococcus infections if skin lesions contain head lice; human metapneumovirus infection; impetigo; infection or colonization with multidrug-resistant organisms; major draining abscesses; major wound infections; monkeypox; poliomyelitis; respiratory parainfluenza virus infection in infants and young children; RSV infection in infants, young children, and immunocompromised adults; rotavirus gastroenteritis; severe mucocutaneous herpes simplex infections; neonatal herpes simplex infections; scabies; SARS; smallpox; staphylococcal furunculosis in infants and young children; staphylococcal scalded skin syndrome (Ritter diseases); major staphylococcal or streptococcal disease of skin, wounds, or burns; type A or type E viral hepatitis in diapered or incontinent patients; viral hemorrhagic fevers due to Lassa, Ebola, Marburg, or Crimean-Congo fever viruses
Droplet precautions	Adenovirus infection in infants and young children; adenovirus pneumonia; epiglottitis or meningitis caused by *Haemophilus influenzae* type b; group A streptococcus infections (major skin, wound, or burn infections; pharyngitis in infants and young children; scarlet fever in infants and young children; serious invasive disease); influenza; meningitis or pneumonia caused by *N. meningitidis*; mumps; *Mycoplasma* pneumonia; parvovirus B19 skin infection; pertussis (whooping cough); pharyngeal diphtheria; pneumonic plague; rhinovirus infection; rubella (German measles); SARS; viral hemorrhagic fevers due to Lassa, Ebola, Marburg, or Crimean-Congo fever viruses
Airborne precautions	Chickenpox, confirmed or suspected pulmonary or laryngeal tuberculosis; extrapulmonary tuberculosis with draining lesions; disseminated shingles in any patient; localized shingles in immunocompromised patients, measles (rubeola); monkeypox; SARS; smallpox

[a]This is not an all-inclusive list of diseases. Information source: 2007 Guideline for Isolation Precautions: Preventing Transmission of Infectious Agents in Healthcare Settings. (available at www.cdc.gov/ncidod/dhgp/pdf/isolation2007.pdf).

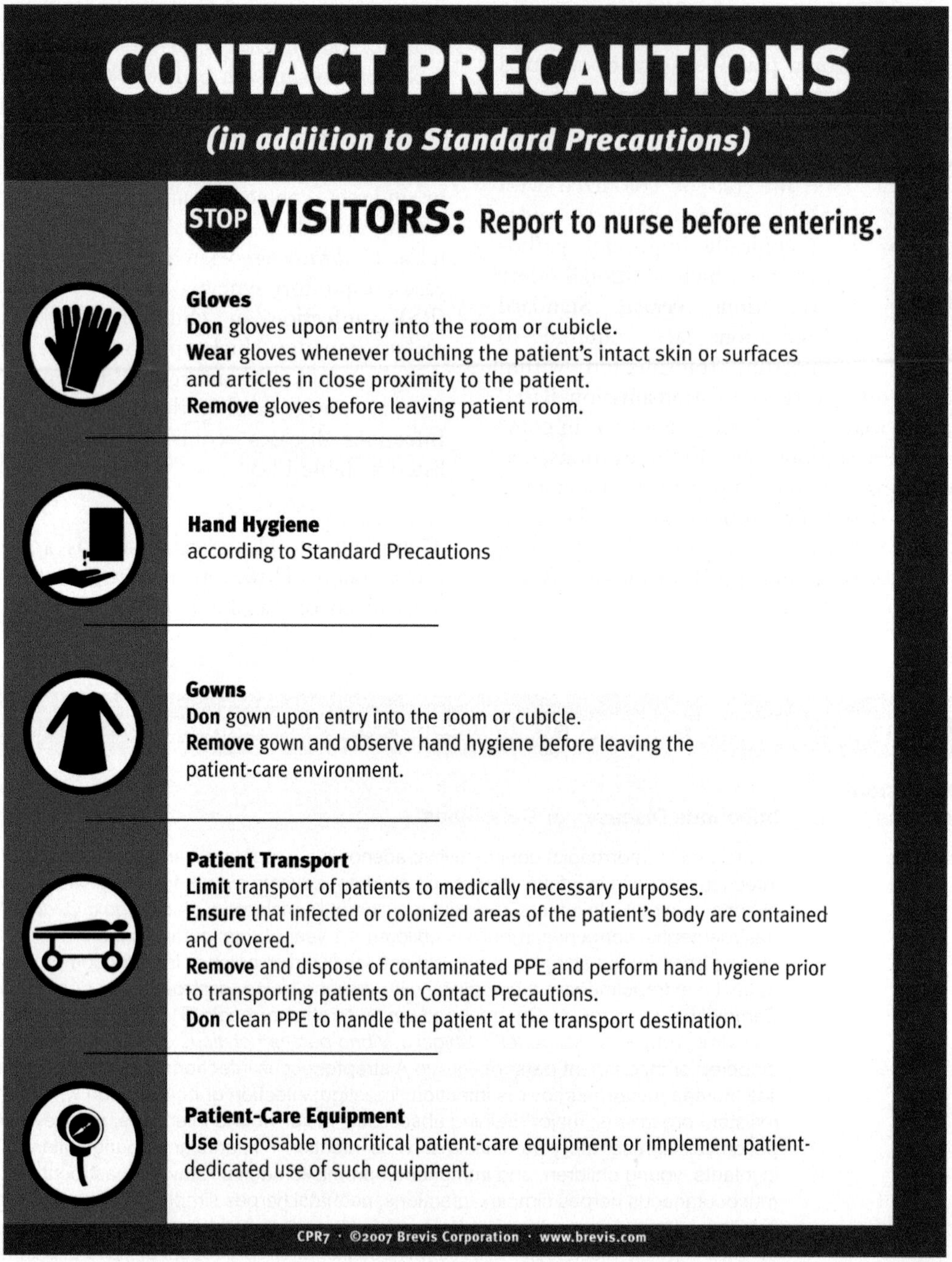

CONTACT PRECAUTIONS
(in addition to Standard Precautions)

STOP VISITORS: Report to nurse before entering.

Gloves
Don gloves upon entry into the room or cubicle.
Wear gloves whenever touching the patient's intact skin or surfaces and articles in close proximity to the patient.
Remove gloves before leaving patient room.

Hand Hygiene
according to Standard Precautions

Gowns
Don gown upon entry into the room or cubicle.
Remove gown and observe hand hygiene before leaving the patient-care environment.

Patient Transport
Limit transport of patients to medically necessary purposes.
Ensure that infected or colonized areas of the patient's body are contained and covered.
Remove and dispose of contaminated PPE and perform hand hygiene prior to transporting patients on Contact Precautions.
Don clean PPE to handle the patient at the transport destination.

Patient-Care Equipment
Use disposable noncritical patient-care equipment or implement patient-dedicated use of such equipment.

CPR7 · ©2007 Brevis Corporation · www.brevis.com

Figure 12-10. Contact Precautions sign. (From McCall RE, Tankersley CM. *Phlebotomy Essentials.* 5th ed. Philadelphia, PA: Lippincott Williams & Wilkins; 2012. Courtesy of the Brevis Corp., Salt Lake City, UT.)

direct or indirect contact transmission. Droplets are produced primarily as a result of coughing, sneezing, and talking, as well as during hospital procedures such as suctioning and bronchoscopy. Transmission occurs when droplets (larger than 5 μm in diameter) containing microbes are propelled a short distance through the air and become deposited on another person's conjunctiva, nasal mucosa, or mouth. Because of

> Droplet Precautions are used for particles that are larger than 5 μm in diameter.

their size, droplets do not remain suspended in the air. Droplet Precautions must be used for patients known or suspected to be infected with microbes transmitted by droplets that can be generated in the ways previously mentioned. Droplet Precautions are summarized on the sign shown in Figure 12-11. Infectious diseases requiring Droplet Precautions are listed in Table 12-3.

Airborne Precautions

Airborne transmission involves either airborne droplet nuclei or dust particles containing a pathogen. Airborne

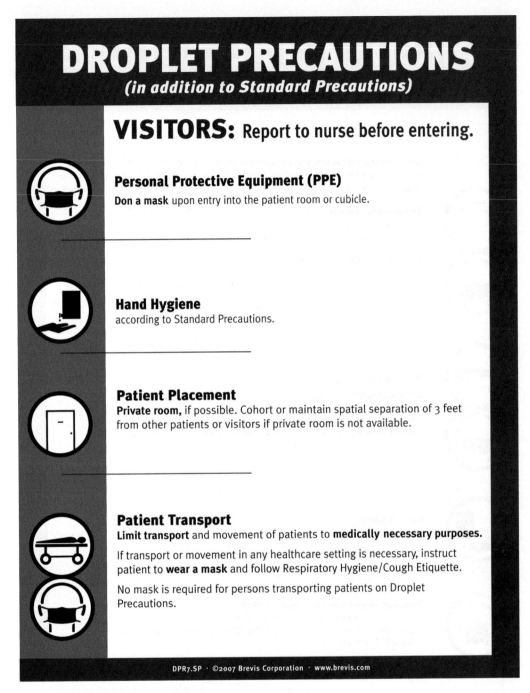

DROPLET PRECAUTIONS
(in addition to Standard Precautions)

VISITORS: Report to nurse before entering.

Personal Protective Equipment (PPE)
Don a mask upon entry into the patient room or cubicle.

Hand Hygiene
according to Standard Precautions.

Patient Placement
Private room, if possible. Cohort or maintain spatial separation of 3 feet from other patients or visitors if private room is not available.

Patient Transport
Limit transport and movement of patients to **medically necessary purposes.**

If transport or movement in any healthcare setting is necessary, instruct patient to **wear a mask** and follow Respiratory Hygiene/Cough Etiquette.

No mask is required for persons transporting patients on Droplet Precautions.

DPR7.SP · ©2007 Brevis Corporation · www.brevis.com

Figure 12-11. Droplet Precautions sign. (From McCall RE, Tankersley CM. *Phlebotomy Essentials*. 5th ed. Philadelphia, PA: Lippincott Williams & Wilkins; 2012. Courtesy of the Brevis Corp., Salt Lake City, UT.)

droplet nuclei are small-particle residues (5 µm or less in diameter) of evaporated droplets containing microbes; because of their small size, they remain suspended in air for long periods. Airborne Precautions are summarized on the sign shown in Figure 12-12. Airborne Precautions apply to patients known or suspected to be infected with epidemiologically important pathogens that can be transmitted by the airborne route. Infectious diseases requiring Airborne Precautions are listed in Table 12-3.

> Airborne Precautions are used when particles are 5 µm or less in diameter.

Patient Placement

Whenever possible, single-patient rooms are used for patients who might contaminate the hospital environment or who do not (or cannot be expected to) assist in maintaining appropriate hygiene or environmental control. Single rooms are always indicated for patients placed

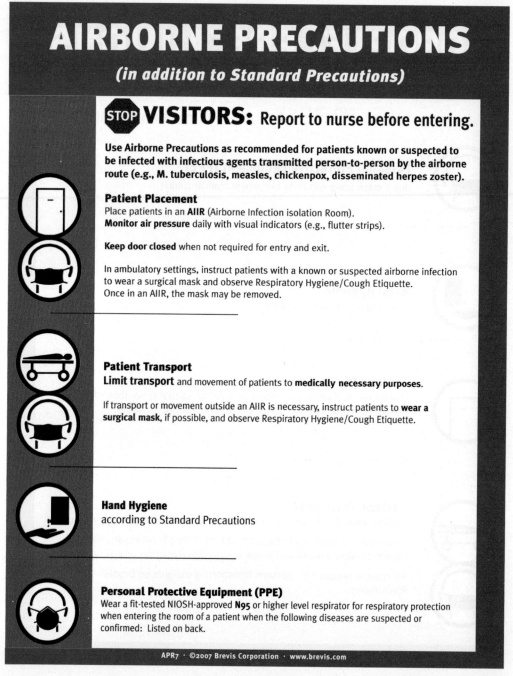

Figure 12-12. Airborne Precautions sign. (From McCall RE, Tankersley CM. *Phlebotomy Essentials*. 5th ed. Philadelphia, PA: Lippincott Williams & Wilkins; 2012. Courtesy of the Brevis Corp., Salt Lake City, UT.)

on Airborne Precautions and are preferred for patients requiring Contact or Droplet Precautions.

Airborne Infection Isolation Rooms

The preferred placement for patients who are infected with pathogens that are spread via airborne droplet nuclei, and therefore require Airborne Precautions, is in an airborne infection isolation room (AIIR). An AIIR (Fig. 12-13) is a single-patient room that is equipped with special air handling and ventilation systems. AIIRs are under negative pressure to prevent room air from entering the corridor when the door is opened, and air that is evacuated from such rooms passes through high-efficiency particulate air (HEPA) filters to remove pathogens. Standard and Airborne Precautions are strictly enforced.

> AIIRs are under negative pressure, and air that is evacuated from these rooms passes through HEPA filters.

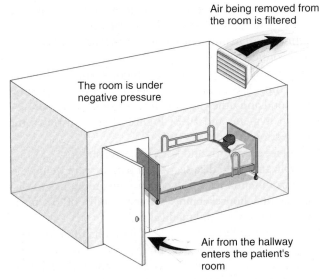

Figure 12-13. Airborne infection isolation room. See text for details.

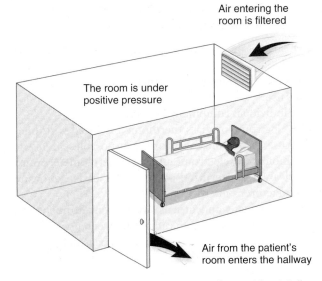

Figure 12-14. Protective environment. See text for details.

Protective Environments

Certain patients are especially vulnerable to infection, particularly to invasive environmental fungal infections. Examples of such patients are patients with severe burns, those who have leukemia, patients who have received a transplant (such as a hematopoietic stem cell transplant), immunosuppressed persons, those receiving radiation treatments, leukopenic patients (those having abnormally low white blood cell counts), and premature infants. These patients can be protected by placing them in a Protective Environment (sometimes referred to as protective isolation or positive pressure isolation). The Protective Environment is a well-sealed single-patient room in which vented air entering the room is passed through HEPA filters. The room is under positive pressure to prevent corridor air from entering when the door is opened (Fig. 12-14). Strategies to minimize dust include scrubbable surfaces rather than upholstery and carpet. Crevices and sprinkler heads are routinely cleaned. Appropriate Standard and Transmission-Based Precautions are strictly enforced.

> Protective Environments are rooms that are under positive pressure, and vented air that enters these rooms passes through HEPA filters.

Handling Food and Eating Utensils

Contaminated food provides an excellent environment for the growth of pathogens. Most often, human carelessness, especially neglecting the practice of handwashing, is responsible for this contamination. Foodborne pathogens and the diseases they cause are discussed in Chapter 11. Regulations for safe handling of food and eating utensils are not difficult to follow. They include the following:

- Using high-quality, fresh food
- Properly refrigerating and storing food
- Properly washing, preparing, and cooking food
- Properly disposing of uneaten food
- Thoroughly washing hands and fingernails before handling food and after visiting a restroom
- Properly disposing of nasal and oral secretions in tissues and then thoroughly washing hands and fingernails
- Covering hair and wearing clean clothes and aprons
- Providing periodic health examinations for kitchen workers
- Prohibiting anyone with a respiratory or gastrointestinal disease from handling food or eating utensils
- Keeping all cutting boards and other surfaces scrupulously clean
- Rinsing and then washing cooking and eating utensils in a dishwasher in which the water temperature is greater than 80°C

According to the CDC, the combination of hot water and detergents used in dishwashers is sufficient to decontaminate dishware and eating utensils; no special precautions are needed.

Handling Fomites

As previously described, fomites are any nonliving or inanimate objects other than food that may harbor and transmit microbes. Examples of fomites in healthcare settings are patients' gowns, bedding, towels, and eating and drinking utensils; and hospital equipment such as bedpans, stethoscopes, latex gloves, electronic thermometers, and electrocardiographic electrodes that become contaminated by pathogens from the respiratory tract, intestinal tract, or the skin of patients. Telephones and computer keyboards in patient-care areas can also serve as fomites. Transmission of pathogens by fomites can be prevented by observing the following rules:

- Use disposable equipment and supplies wherever possible
- Disinfect or sterilize equipment as soon as possible after use
- Use individual equipment for each patient
- Use electronic or glass thermometers fitted with one-time use, disposable covers or use disposable, single-use thermometers; electronic and glass thermometers must be cleaned or sterilized on a regular basis, following manufacturer's instructions
- Empty bedpans and urinals, wash them in hot water, and store them in a clean cabinet between uses
- Place bed linen and soiled clothing in bags to be sent to the laundry

Medical Waste Disposal

Materials or substances that are harmful to health are referred to as biohazards (short for biologic hazards). They must be identified by a biohazard symbol, which was shown in Figure 12-9. According to OSHA standards, medical wastes must be disposed of properly. These standards include the following:

- Any receptacle used for decomposable solid or liquid waste or refuse must be constructed so that it does not leak and must be maintained in a sanitary condition. This receptacle must be equipped with a solid, tight-fitting cover, unless it can be maintained in a sanitary condition without a cover.
- All sweepings, solid or liquid wastes, refuse, and garbage shall be removed to avoid creating a menace to health and shall be removed as often as necessary to maintain the place of employment in a sanitary condition.
- The medical facility's infection control program must address the handling and disposal of potentially contaminated items.

Disposal of sharps was discussed earlier in the chapter.

Infection Control in Dental Healthcare Settings

In 2003, the CDC published a set of infection control guidelines applicable to dental healthcare settings, entitled *Guidelines for Infection Control in Dental Healthcare Settings, 2003* (www.cdc.gov/oralhealth/infectioncontrol/guidelines/index.htm). Students in dental-related programs, such as dental assistant, dental hygienist, and dental laboratory technician programs should familiarize themselves with these guidelines. Listed here are some of the major considerations addressed in the CDC publication:

- Development of a written infection control program that includes policies, procedures, and guidelines for education and training of dental healthcare personnel,

immunizations, exposure prevention and postexposure management, work restriction caused by medical conditions, and maintenance of records, data management, and confidentiality

- Preventing transmission of bloodborne pathogens, including HBV vaccination and preventing exposures to blood and other potentially infectious materials
- Hand hygiene and PPE; Figure 12-15 illustrates the protection afforded by PPE
- Contact dermatitis and latex hypersensitivity
- Sterilization and disinfection of patient-care items
- Environmental infection control, including use of disinfectants, housekeeping services, spills of blood or body substances, and medical waste
- Special considerations, such as dental handpieces, dental radiology, aseptic technique for parenteral medications, oral-surgical procedures, handling of biopsy specimens and extracted teeth, dental laboratory, and patients with tuberculosis

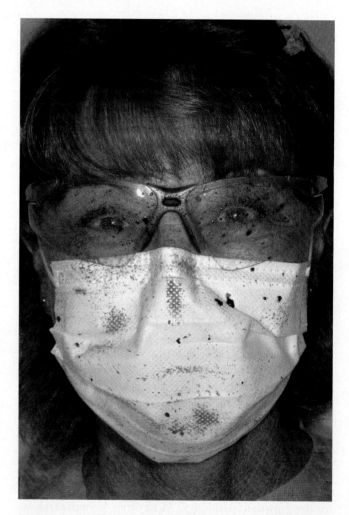

Figure 12-15. Dental hygienist wearing appropriate PPE. A red dye was used to simulate a patient's saliva that can spatter onto a hygienist's face, mask, and protective eyewear during a polishing procedure. (From Molinari JA, Harte JA. *Cotton's Practical Infection Control in Dentistry*. 3rd ed. Philadelphia, PA: Lippincott Williams & Wilkins; 2010.)

SPOTLIGHTING

Dental Assistants and Dental Hygienists

As stated in the American Medical Association's Health Care Careers Directory (available at http://www.ama-assn.org under "Education"), "Dental assistants increase the efficiency of the dental care team by aiding dentists in the delivery of oral health care. Dental assistants are responsible for

- Helping patients feel comfortable before, during, and after treatment.
- Assisting the dentist during treatment.
- Exposing and processing dental radiographs (x-rays). (Some states require additional education and/or examinations to perform this function.)
- Recording the patient's medical history and taking blood pressure and pulse.
- Preparing and sterilizing instruments and equipment for the dentist's use.
- Providing patients with oral care instructions following such procedures as surgery or placement of a restoration (filling).
- Teaching patients proper brushing and flossing techniques.
- Making impressions of patients' teeth for study casts. (Most states require additional education and/or examination to perform this function.)
- Performing various administrative and scheduling tasks."

"Dental hygienists provide dental hygiene services as they work with dentists in the delivery of dental care to patients. Patient services rendered by dental hygienists frequently include the following:

- Performing patient screening procedures, such as assessing oral health conditions, reviewing health and dental history, and taking blood pressure, pulse, and temperature; oral cancer screening; head and neck inspection; and dental charting.
- Exposing and developing dental radiographs.
- Removing calculus and plaque (hard and soft deposits) from teeth.
- Applying preventive materials to teeth (e.g., sealants and fluorides).
- Teaching patients appropriate oral hygiene techniques.
- Counseling patients regarding proper nutrition and its impact on oral health.
- Making impressions of patients' teeth for study casts.
- Administration of anesthesia (depending upon state regulations).

Information concerning educational requirements and programs, certification, and salary is available at the AMA web site."

Infection Control Committees and Infection Control Professionals

All healthcare facilities should have some type of formal infection control program in place. Its functions will vary slightly from one type of healthcare facility to another. In a hospital setting, the infection control program is usually under the jurisdiction of the hospital's Infection Control Committee (ICC) or Epidemiology Service. The ICC is composed of representatives from most of the hospital's departments, including medical and surgical services, pathology, nursing, hospital administration, risk management, pharmacy, housekeeping, food services, and central supply. The chairperson is usually an Infection Control Professional (ICP), such as a physician (e.g., an epidemiologist or infectious disease specialist), an infection control nurse, a microbiologist, or some other person knowledgeable about infection control.

> A hospital's infection control program is usually under the jurisdiction of the hospital's ICC or Epidemiology Service.

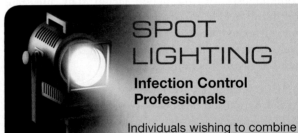

SPOT LIGHTING

Infection Control Professionals

Individuals wishing to combine their interest in detective work with a career in medicine might consider a career as an ICP. ICPs include physicians (infectious disease specialists or epidemiologists), nurses, clinical laboratory scientists (medical technologists), and microbiologists. Most ICPs are nurses, many having baccalaureate degrees and some with Master of Science degrees. In addition to having strong clinical skills, ICPs require knowledge and expertise in such areas as epidemiology, microbiology, infectious disease processes, statistics, and computers. To be effective, they must be part detective, part diplomat, part administrator, and part educator. In addition, ICPs function as role models, patient advocates, and consultants.

Within the hospital, ICPs provide valuable services that minimize the risks of infection and spread of disease, thereby aiding patients, healthcare professionals, and visitors. The ICP is the key person in implementing and facilitating the institution's infection control program. The ICP is often the head of the hospital's ICC and, as such, is responsible for scheduling, organizing, and conducting ICC meetings. At these meetings, medical records are reviewed of all patients suspected of having incurred a hospital-associated infection since the previous meeting. The committee discusses possible or known causes of such infections and ways to prevent them from occurring in the future. The ICP receives timely information from the clinical microbiology laboratory (CML) concerning possible outbreaks of infection within the hospital and is responsible for rapidly organizing a team to investigate these outbreaks. ICPs are also responsible for educating healthcare personnel about infection risk, prevention, and control.

The primary responsibilities of an ICP are as follows:

- Possess knowledge of infectious diseases processes, reservoirs, incubation periods, periods of communicability, and susceptibility of patients
- Conduct surveillance and epidemiologic investigations
- Prevent/control the transmission of pathogens to include strategies for hand hygiene, antisepsis, cleaning, disinfection, sterilization, patient-care settings, patient placement, medical waste disposal, and implementation of outbreak control measures
- Manage the facility's infection control program
- Communicate with the public, facility staff, and state and local health departments concerning infection control-related issues
- Evaluate new medical products that could be associated with increased infection risk

The ICC periodically reviews the hospital's infection control program and the incidence of HAIs. It is a policy-making and review body that may take drastic action (e.g., instituting quarantine measures) when epidemiologic circumstances warrant. Other ICC responsibilities include patient surveillance, environmental surveillance, investigation of outbreaks and epidemics, and education of the hospital staff regarding infection control.

Although every department of the hospital endeavors to maintain aseptic conditions, the total environment is constantly bombarded with microbes from outside the hospital. These must be controlled for the protection of the patients. Hospital personnel (usually ICPs) entrusted with this aspect of healthcare diligently and constantly work to maintain the proper environment. In the event of an epidemic, the ICP notifies city, county, and state health authorities, so they can assist in ending the epidemic.

Role of the Microbiology Laboratory in Healthcare Epidemiology

Listed here are some of the ways in which CML personnel participate in healthcare epidemiology and infection control:

- By monitoring the types and numbers of pathogens isolated from hospitalized patients. In most hospitals,

such monitoring is accomplished using computers and appropriate software programs.
- By performing antimicrobial susceptibility testing, detecting emerging resistance patterns, and preparing and distributing periodic cumulative antimicrobial susceptibility summary reports (see information on "pocket charts" in Chapter 9).
- By notifying the appropriate ICP should an unusual pathogen or an unusually high number of isolates of a common pathogen be detected. The ICP will then initiate an investigation of the outbreak.
- By processing environmental samples, including samples from hospital employees that have been collected from within the affected ward(s), with the goal of pinpointing the exact source of the pathogen that is causing the outbreak. Examples of environmental samples include air samples, nasal swabs from healthcare personnel, and swabs of sink drains, whirlpool tubs, respiratory therapy equipment, bed rails, and ventilation grates and ducts.
- By performing biochemical, immunological, and molecular identification and typing procedures to compare various isolates of the same species. *Example:* Assume that there is an epidemic of *Klebsiella pneumoniae* infections on the pediatric ward and that *K. pneumoniae* has been isolated from a certain environmental sample collected on that ward. How do CML personnel determine that the *K. pneumoniae* that has been isolated from the environmental sample is the same strain of *K. pneumoniae* that has been isolated from the patients? Traditionally, the two most commonly used methods have been biotype and antibiogram. If the two strains produce the same biochemical test results, they are said to have the same biotype. If they produce the same susceptibility and resistance patterns when antimicrobial susceptibility testing is performed, they are said to have the same antibiogram. Having the same biotype and antibiogram is evidence (but not absolute proof) that they are the same strain. Because of the limitations of phenotypic methods (such as biotypes and antibiograms), however, most hospitals are currently using what is known as molecular epidemiology, in which genotypic (as opposed to phenotypic) typing methods are used. Most often, these methods involve genotyping of plasmid or chromosomal DNA. Genotypic methods provide more accurate data than do phenotypic methods. If the two isolates of *K. pneumoniae* in the given example have exactly the same genotype (i.e., possess exactly the same genes), they are the same strain; therefore, the source of the epidemic has been found. Action will then be taken to eliminate the source.

> A hospital's CML participates in that hospital's infection control program in various ways.

Conclusions

An HAI can add several weeks to a patient's hospital stay and may lead to serious complications and even death. From an economic viewpoint, insurance companies rarely reimburse hospitals and other healthcare facilities for the costs associated with HAIs. Insurance companies take the position that HAIs are the fault of the healthcare facility and, therefore, that the facility should bear any additional patient costs related to such infections. Sadly, cross-infections transmitted by hospital personnel, including physicians, are all too common; this is particularly true when hospitals and clinics are overcrowded and the staff is overworked. However, HAIs can be avoided through proper education and disciplined compliance with infection control practices.

All healthcare workers must fully comprehend the problem of HAIs, must be completely knowledgeable about infection control practices, and must personally do everything in their power to prevent HAIs from occurring.

ON thePoint

- Terms Introduced in This Chapter
- Review of Key Points
- Spotlighting the Nursing Profession
- A Closer Look:
  - Florence Nightingale
  - Healthcare-Associated Zoonoses
  - Infection Control Professionals
  - Donning PPE
  - Removing PPE
- Increase Your Knowledge
- Critical Thinking
- Additional Self-Assessment Exercises

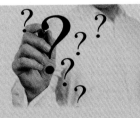

Self-Assessment Exercises

After studying this chapter, answer the following multiple-choice questions.

1. An HAI is one that:
   a. develops during hospitalization or erupts within 14 days of hospital discharge
   b. develops while the patient is hospitalized
   c. is acquired in the community
   d. the patient has at the time of hospital admission

2. An example of a fomite would be:
   a. a drinking glass used by a patient
   b. bandages from an infected wound
   c. soiled bed linens
   d. all of the above

3. Which of the following Gram-positive bacteria is most likely to be the cause of an HAI?
   a. *Clostridium difficile*
   b. *Staphylococcus aureus*
   c. *Streptococcus pneumoniae*
   d. *Streptococcus pyogenes*

4. Which of the following Gram-negative bacteria is least likely to be the cause of an HAI?
   a. a *Klebsiella* species
   b. a *Salmonella* species
   c. *Escherichia coli*
   d. *Pseudomonas aeruginosa*

5. A Protective Environment would be appropriate for a patient:
   a. infected with MRSA
   b. with leukopenia
   c. with pneumonic plague
   d. with tuberculosis

6. Which of the following is not part of Standard Precautions?
   a. handwashing between patient contacts
   b. placing a patient in a private room having negative air pressure
   c. properly disposing of needles, scalpels, and other sharps
   d. wearing gloves, masks, eye protection, and gowns when appropriate

7. A patient suspected of having tuberculosis has been admitted to the hospital. Which one of the following is not appropriate?
   a. Droplet Precautions
   b. an AIIR
   c. Standard Precautions
   d. use of a type N95 respirator by healthcare professionals who are caring for the patient

8. Which of the following statements about medical asepsis is false?
   a. Disinfection is a medical aseptic technique
   b. Handwashing is a medical aseptic technique
   c. Medical asepsis is considered a clean technique
   d. The goal of medical asepsis is to exclude all microbes from an area

9. Which of the following statements about an AIIR is false?

    a. Air entering the room is passed through HEPA filters
    b. The room is under negative air pressure
    c. An AIIR is appropriate for patients with meningococcal meningitis, whooping cough, or influenza
    d. Transmission-Based Precautions will be necessary

10. Contact Precautions are required for patients with:

    a. *Clostridium difficile*-associated diseases
    b. infections caused by multidrug-resistant bacteria
    c. viral hemorrhagic fevers
    d. all of the above

13

Diagnosing Infectious Diseases

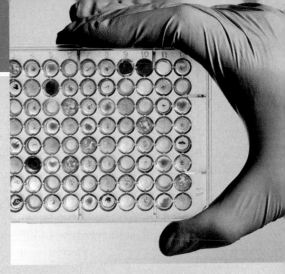

Example of a biochemical "minisystem" used to identify bacteria in the Clinical Microbiology Laboratory.

 ## CHAPTER OUTLINE

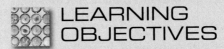 ## LEARNING OBJECTIVES

After studying this chapter, you should be able to:

- Discuss the role of healthcare professionals in the collection and transport of clinical specimens
- List the types of clinical specimens that are submitted to the Clinical Microbiology Laboratory for the diagnosis of infectious diseases
- Discuss general precautions that must be observed during the collection and handling of clinical specimens
- Describe the proper procedures for obtaining blood, urine, cerebrospinal fluid (CSF), sputum, throat swabs, wound specimens, GC cultures, and fecal specimens for submission to the Clinical Microbiology Laboratory
- State the information that must be included on specimen labels and laboratory test requisitions
- Outline the organization of the Pathology Department and the Clinical Microbiology Laboratory
- Compare and contrast the anatomical and clinical pathology divisions of the Pathology Department
- Identify the various types of personnel that work in anatomical and clinical pathology

Introduction

The proper diagnosis of an infectious disease requires (a) taking a complete patient history, (b) conducting a thorough physical examination of the patient, (c) carefully evaluating the patient's signs and symptoms, and (d) implementing the proper selection, collection, transport, and processing of appropriate clinical specimens.

The latter topics—those involving clinical specimens—are discussed in this chapter. The other topics are beyond the scope of this book.

Clinical Specimens

The various types of specimens, such as blood, urine, feces, and CSF, that are collected from patients and used to diagnose or follow the progress of infectious diseases are referred to as *clinical specimens*. The most common types of clinical specimens that are sent to the hospital's microbiology laboratory (hereafter referred to as the Clinical Microbiology Laboratory or CML) are listed in Table 13-1. It is extremely important that these specimens are of the highest possible quality and that they are collected in a manner that does not jeopardize either the patient or the person collecting the specimen.

> The clinical specimens that are used to diagnose infectious diseases must be of the highest possible quality.

Role of Healthcare Professionals in the Submission of Clinical Specimens

A close working relationship among the members of the healthcare team is essential for the proper diagnosis of infectious diseases. When a clinician suspects that a patient has a particular infectious disease, appropriate clinical specimens must be obtained and certain diagnostic tests requested. The doctor, nurse, medical technologist (MT), or other qualified healthcare professional must select the appropriate specimen, collect it properly, and then transport it properly to the CML for processing (Fig. 13-1). Laboratory findings must then be conveyed to the attending clinician as quickly as possible to facilitate the prompt diagnosis and treatment of the infectious disease. Although laboratory professionals do not themselves make diagnoses, they make laboratory observations and generate test results that assist clinicians to correctly diagnose infectious diseases and initiate appropriate therapy.

> Laboratory professionals make laboratory observations and generate test results that are used by clinicians to diagnose infectious diseases and initiate appropriate therapy.

Healthcare professionals who collect and transport clinical specimens should exercise extreme caution during the collection and transport of clinical specimens to avoid sticking themselves with needles, cutting themselves with other types of sharps, or coming in contact with any type of specimen. Healthcare personnel who collect clinical specimens must strictly adhere to the safety policies known as Standard Precautions (discussed in detail in Chapter 12). According to the Clinical and Laboratory Standards Institute (CLSI), "All specimens should be collected or transferred into a leakproof primary container with a secure closure. Care should be taken by the person collecting the specimen not to contaminate the outside of the primary container. Within the institution, the primary container should be placed into a second container, which will contain the specimen if the primary container breaks

Table 13-1   Types of Clinical Specimens Submitted to the CML

Type of Specimen	Type(s) of Infectious Disease That the Specimen Is Used to Diagnose	Type of Specimen	Type(s) of Infectious Disease That the Specimen Is Used to Diagnose
Blood	B, F, P, V	"Scotch tape prep"	P
Bone marrow	B	Skin scrapings	F
Bronchial and bronchoalveolar washes	V	Skin snip	P
CSF	B, F, P, V	Sputum	B, F, P
Cervical and vaginal swabs	B	Synovial (joint) fluid	B
Conjunctival swab or scraping	B, V	Throat swabs	B, V
Feces and rectal swabs	B, P, V	Tissue (biopsy and autopsy) specimens	B, F, P, V
Hair clippings	F	Urethral discharge material	B
Nail (fingernail and toenail) clippings	F	Urine	B, P, V
Nasal swabs	B	Urogenital secretions (e.g., vaginal discharge material, prostatic secretions)	B, P
Pus from a wound or abscess	B	Vesicle fluid or scraping	V

B, bacterial infections; F, fungal infections; P, parasitic infections; V, viral infections.

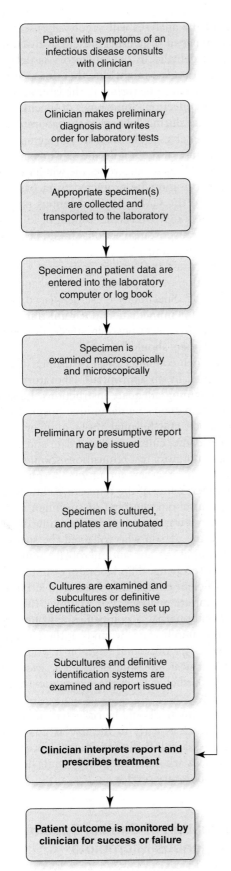

Figure 13-1. **Diagrammatic representation of the steps involved in the diagnosis of infectious diseases.** (Modified from Winn WC Jr, et al. *Koneman's Color Atlas and Textbook of Diagnostic Microbiology.* 6th ed. Philadelphia, PA: Lippincott Williams & Wilkins; 2006.)

or leaks in transit to the laboratory" (CLSI Document M29-A3, 2005). Within the laboratory, all specimens are handled carefully, following Standard Precautions and ultimately disposed of as infectious waste.

Importance of High-Quality Clinical Specimens

Specimens submitted to the CML must be of the highest possible quality. High-quality clinical specimens are required to achieve accurate, *clinically relevant laboratory results*—meaning results that *truly* provide information about the patient's infectious disease. **It has often been stated that the quality of the laboratory work performed in a CML can be only as good as the quality of the specimens it receives.** It is impossible for a CML to obtain and report high-quality test results if the laboratory receives poor-quality specimens or the wrong types of specimens.

> High-quality clinical specimens are required to achieve accurate, clinically relevant laboratory results.

The three components of specimen quality are (a) proper specimen selection (i.e., the correct type of specimen must be submitted), (b) proper specimen collection, and (c) proper transport of the specimen to the laboratory. The laboratory must provide written guidelines regarding specimen selection, collection, and transport in the form of a manual. Although the name of the manual varies from one institution to the next, it is referred to in this book as the "Laboratory Policies and Procedures Manual" (or the "Lab P&P Manual" for short).

> The laboratory must provide written instructions for the proper selection, collection, and transport of clinical specimens.

Copies of the Lab P&P Manual must be available to every ward, floor, clinic, and department. Often, it is accessible through the hospital's computer system. **Although the laboratory provides guidelines, it is the person who collects the specimen who is ultimately responsible for its quality.**

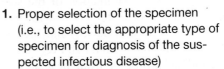
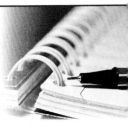

STUDY AID

Three Components of Specimen Quality

1. Proper selection of the specimen (i.e., to select the appropriate type of specimen for diagnosis of the suspected infectious disease)
2. Proper collection of the specimen
3. Proper transport of the specimen to the laboratory

It would not be feasible in a book of this size to provide a complete discussion of the proper methods for selecting, collecting, and transporting all types of clinical specimens. Only a few important concepts are discussed here. See "Specimen Quality and Clinical Relevance" on thePoint for additional details.

When clinical specimens are improperly collected and handled, (a) the etiologic agent (causative agent) may not be found or may be destroyed, (b) overgrowth by indigenous microbiota may mask the pathogen, and/or (c) contaminants may interfere with the identification of pathogens and the diagnosis of the patient's infectious disease.

Proper Selection, Collection, and Transport of Clinical Specimens

When collecting clinical specimens for microbiology, the following general precautions should be taken:

- The specimen must be properly selected. That is, it must be the appropriate type of specimen for diagnosis of the suspected infectious disease.
- The specimen must be properly and carefully collected. Whenever possible, specimens must be collected in a manner that will eliminate or minimize contamination of the specimen with indigenous microbiota.
- The material should be collected from a site where the suspected pathogen is most likely to be found and where the least contamination is likely to occur.
- Whenever possible, specimens should be obtained before antimicrobial therapy has begun. If this is not possible, the laboratory should be informed as to which antimicrobial agent(s) the patient is receiving.
- The acute stage of the disease—when the patient is experiencing the symptoms of the disease—is the appropriate time to collect most specimens. Some viruses, however, are more easily isolated during the prodromal or onset stage of disease.
- Specimen collection should be performed with care and tact to avoid harming the patient, causing discomfort, or causing undue embarrassment. If the patient is to collect the specimen, such as sputum or urine, the patient must be given clear and detailed collection instructions.
- A sufficient quantity of the specimen must be obtained to provide enough material for all required diagnostic tests. The amount of specimen to collect should be specified in the Lab P&P Manual.
- All specimens should be placed or collected into a sterile container to prevent contamination of the specimen by indigenous microbiota and airborne microbes. Appropriate types of collection devices and specimen containers should be specified in the Lab P&P Manual.
- Specimens should be protected from heat and cold and promptly delivered to the laboratory so that the results of the analyses will validly represent the number and types of organisms present at the time of collection. If delivery to the laboratory is delayed, some delicate pathogens might die; therefore, certain types of specimens must be rushed to the laboratory immediately after collection. Some types of specimens must be placed on ice during delivery to the laboratory, whereas other specimens should never be refrigerated or placed on ice because of the fragile and sensitive nature of the pathogens. Obligate anaerobes die when exposed to air and therefore must be protected from oxygen during transport to the CML. Any indigenous microbiota in the specimen may overgrow, inhibit, or kill pathogens. Specimen transport instructions should be contained in the Lab P&P Manual.
- Specimens must be handled with great care to avoid contamination of the patients, couriers, and healthcare professionals. Specimens must be placed in a sealed plastic bag for immediate and careful transport to the laboratory. Whenever possible, sterile, disposable specimen containers should be used.
- The specimen container must be properly labeled and accompanied by an appropriate laboratory test requisition containing adequate instructions. Labels should contain the patient's name, unique hospital identification number, and hospital room number; requesting clinician's name; culture site; and date and time of collection. Laboratory test requisitions should contain the patient's name, age, sex, and unique hospital identification number; name of the requesting clinician; specific information about the type of specimen and the site from which it was collected; date and time of collection; initials of the person who collected the specimen; and information about any antimicrobial agent(s) that the patient is receiving. The laboratory should always be given sufficient clinical information to aid in performing appropriate analyses. For example, the laboratory test requisition that accompanies a wound specimen should not merely state "wound"; rather, it should state the specific *type* of wound (e.g., burn wound, dog bite wound, surgical site infection, etc.), the anatomical site, and whether it is on the left side or right side, if applicable.
- Ideally, specimens should be collected and delivered to the laboratory as early in the day as possible to give CML professionals sufficient time to process the material, especially when the hospital or clinic does not have 24-hour laboratory service.

Contamination of Clinical Specimens with Indigenous Microbiota

As mentioned in Chapter 1, vast numbers of microbes live on and in the human body. Usually, they are collectively referred to as indigenous microbiota (or the human microbiome). Clinical specimens must be collected in a manner that eliminates, or at least reduces, contamination of the specimens with members of the indigenous microbiota. Recall that many members of our indigenous microbiota are opportunistic pathogens. Thus, when present in specimens, these organisms *might* merely be contaminants, but it is also possible that they are causing an infection.

Types of Clinical Specimens Usually Required to Diagnose Infectious Diseases

Specific techniques for the collection and transport of clinical specimens vary from institution to institution and are contained in the institution's Lab P&P Manual. Only a few of the most important considerations are mentioned here.

Blood

The study of blood is known as hematology. Blood consists of a mixture of cells and fluid (Fig. 13-2). Within the human body, the liquid portion of blood is called *plasma*; it makes up about 55% of the volume of blood. When a blood specimen is allowed to clot, the liquid portion is called *serum*. (Thus, serum is plasma that no longer contains clotting factors.) The cells (also referred to as *cellular elements* or *formed elements*) make up about 45% of the volume of blood. The various blood cells include red blood cells (RBCs or erythrocytes), white blood cells (WBCs

> Within the body, the liquid portion of blood is called plasma, but if a blood specimen is allowed to clot, the liquid portion is called *serum*.

or leukocytes), and platelets (or thrombocytes). The three major categories of WBCs are granulocytes, monocytes, and lymphocytes. Lymphocytes are discussed in detail in Chapter 16. The three types of granulocytes are neutrophils, basophils, and eosinophils.

As it circulates throughout the body, blood is usually sterile. However, blood sometimes contains bacteria. The presence of bacteria in the bloodstream (*bacteremia*) may indicate a disease, although temporary or transient bacteremias may occur after oral surgery, tooth extraction, or even aggressive tooth brushing that causes bleeding. Bacteremia may occur during certain stages of many infectious diseases. These diseases include bacterial meningitis, typhoid fever and other *Salmonella* infections, pneumococcal pneumonia, urinary infections, endocarditis, brucellosis, tularemia, plague, anthrax, syphilis, and wound infections caused by β-hemolytic streptococci, staphylococci, and other invasive bacteria. Bacteremia should not be confused with septicemia. *Septicemia* is a serious disease characterized by chills, fever, prostration, and the presence of bacteria or their toxins in the bloodstream. The most severe types of septicemia are those caused by Gram-negative bacilli, owing to the endotoxin that is released from their cell walls. Endotoxin can induce fever and septic shock, which can be fatal. To diagnose either bacteremia or septicemia, it is recommended that at least three blood cultures be collected during a 24-hour period.

> Bacteremia— the presence of bacteria in the bloodstream—may or may not be a sign of disease. Septicemia, on the other hand, is a disease.

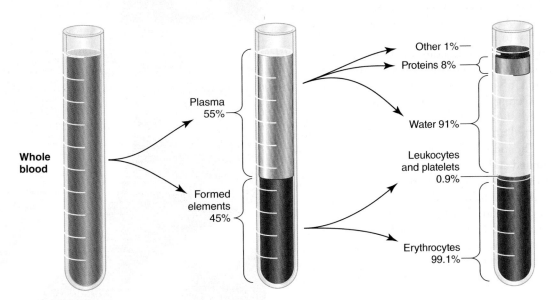

Figure 13-2. Composition of whole blood. Following centrifugation, the layer of WBCs and platelets— referred to as the buffy coat—lies above the RBCs. (Redrawn from Cohen BJ. *Memmler's The Human Body in Health and Disease*. 11th ed. Philadelphia, PA: Lippincott Williams & Wilkins; 2009.)

STUDY AID

-Emias

The suffix *-emia* refers to the bloodstream, often the presence of something in the bloodstream. **Toxemia** refers to the presence of toxins in the bloodstream; bacteremia, the presence of bacteria; **fungemia,** the presence of fungi; **viremia,** the presence of viruses; **parasitemia,** the presence of parasites. **Septicemia**, however, is an actual disease, quite often a serious, life-threatening disease. Septicemia is defined as chills, fever, prostration (extreme fatigue), and the presence of bacteria or their toxins in the bloodstream. **Meningococcemia** is a specific type of septicemia, in which the bloodstream contains *Neisseria meningitidis* (also known as *meningococci*). **Leukemia** is also a disease—actually, there are several different types of leukemias. In all types, there is a proliferation of abnormal WBCs (*leukocytes*) in the blood. Some types of leukemia are known to be caused by viruses.

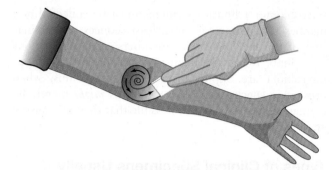

Figure 13-3. Proper method of preparing the venipuncture site when obtaining blood for culture. (Redrawn from McCall RE, Tankersley CM. *Phlebotomy Essentials*. 5th ed. Philadelphia, PA: Lippincott Williams & Wilkins; 2012.)

to insertion of the needle. Then an appropriate volume of blood is injected; the amount will depend on the type of blood culture being used. Following the venipuncture procedure, the iodophor should be removed from the skin using alcohol. The blood culture bottle(s) should be transported promptly to the laboratory for incubation at 37°C. Blood culture specimens should never be refrigerated.

To prevent contamination of the blood specimen with indigenous skin microbes, extreme care must be taken to use aseptic technique when collecting blood for culture. The person drawing the blood must wear sterile gloves, and gloves must be changed between patients.

Blood for culture is usually obtained from a vein located at the antecubital fossa.[a] After locating a suitable vein, the skin at the site is disinfected with 70% isopropyl alcohol and then with an iodophor. (It should be noted that the protocol for skin disinfection varies from one medical facility to another. For example, some facilities use isopropyl alcohol or tincture of iodine alone; some use povidone-iodine or chlorhexadine alone; some use a combination of ethyl alcohol and povidone-iodine.) When disinfecting the site, a concentric swabbing motion is used, starting at the point at which the needle is to be inserted and working outward from that point (Fig. 13-3). The iodophor is then allowed to dry. A tourniquet is applied and the appropriate amount of blood is withdrawn (Fig. 13-4). It is important not to touch the site after it has been disinfected.

Traditionally, blood has been injected into a pair of blood culture bottles (one aerobic bottle and one anaerobic bottle), but there are many different types of blood culture systems currently available (Fig. 13-5). The rubber tops of blood culture bottles must be disinfected prior

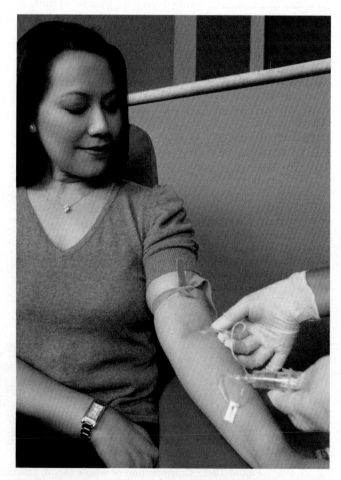

Figure 13-4. Blood being extracted from a patient's antecubital vein during a phlebotomy procedure. (Courtesy of Amanda Mills and the CDC.)

---

[a]The antecubital fossa is located on the inner part of the arm, opposite the bend of the elbow. The major superficial veins in this area are referred to as antecubital veins.

Urine

Urine is ordinarily sterile while it is in the urinary bladder. However, during urination, it becomes contaminated by indigenous microbiota of the distal urethra (the portion of the urethra farthest from the bladder). Contamination can be reduced by collecting a *clean-catch, midstream urine* (CCMS urine). "Clean-catch" refers to the fact that the area around the external opening of the urethra is cleansed by washing with soap and rinsing with water before urinating. This removes the indigenous microbiota that live in this area. "Midstream" refers to the fact that the initial portion of the urine stream is directed into a toilet or bedpan, and then the urine stream is directed into a sterile container. Thus, the microbes that live in the distal urethra are flushed out of the urethra by the initial portion of the urine stream, into the toilet or bedpan, rather than into the specimen container. In some circumstances, the clinician may prefer to collect a catheterized specimen or use the suprapubic needle aspiration technique to obtain a sterile sample of urine. In the latter technique, a needle is inserted through the abdominal wall into the urinary bladder, and a syringe is used to withdraw urine from the bladder. To prevent continued bacterial growth, all urine specimens must be processed within 30 minutes of collection, or refrigerated at 4°C until they can be analyzed. Refrigerated urine specimens should be cultured within 24 hours. Failure to refrigerate a urine specimen will cause an inflated colony count (described later), which could lead to an incorrect diagnosis of a urinary tract infection (UTI).

> The ideal specimen for a urine culture is a clean-catch, midstream urine specimen.

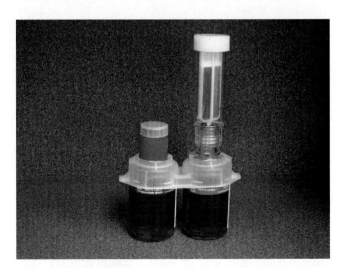

Figure 13-5. An example of a commercial blood culture system. The Septi-Chek blood culture system, manufactured by BD Biosciences, Franklin Lakes, NJ. The system consists of two bottles; an aerobic bottle and an anaerobic bottle. The aerobic bottle to the right is a biphasic system, consisting of a broth-containing vial with an attached agar-coated plastic paddle. (Courtesy of Dr. Robert Fader and Biomed Ed, Round Rock, TX.)

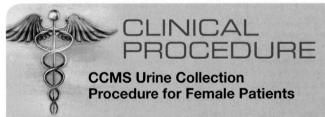

CLINICAL PROCEDURE

CCMS Urine Collection Procedure for Female Patients

Purpose: To instruct a female in how to properly collect a CCMS urine specimen.

Equipment: Requisition, specimen label, sterile urine container, special sterile antiseptic wipes, and copy of written instructions.

Step	Rationale
1. Wash hands thoroughly.	Aids in infection control and helps avoid contamination of the site while cleaning.
2. Remove the lid of the container, being careful not to touch the inside of the cover or the container.	The lid and container must remain sterile for accurate interpretation of results.
3. Stand in a squatting position over the toilet.	Facilitates cleaning and downward flow of urine.
4. Separate the folds of skin around the urinary opening.	Allows proper cleaning of the area.

Step	Rationale
5. Cleanse the area on either side and around the opening with the special wipes, using a fresh wipe for each area and wiping from front to back. Discard used wipes in the trash.	Antiseptic solution in the wipe removes bacteria from area. Front-to-back motion carries bacteria away from the site.
6. While keeping the skin folds separated, void into the toilet for a few seconds.	Separation of the folds maintains site antisepsis. Voiding the first portion of urine into the toilet washes away the antiseptic and microbes remaining in the urinary opening.
7. Touching only the outside and without letting it touch the genital area, bring the urine container into the urine stream until a sufficient amount of urine (30–100 mL) is collected.	Bringing the urine container into the stream without touching the genital area helps ensure sterility of the specimen. An adequate amount of urine is needed to perform the test.
8. Void the remaining urine into the toilet	Only 30–100 mL of urine is needed for the test.
9. Cover the specimen with the lid provided, touching only the outside surfaces of the lid and container.	The lid and container must remain sterile, and the specimen must be covered to maintain sterility and protect others from exposure to the contents.
10. Clean any urine off the outside of the container with an antiseptic wipe.	Aids in infection control.
11. Wash hands.	Aids in infection control.
12. Hand specimen to phlebotomist or place where instructed if already labeled.	Follow facility protocol.

CCMS Urine Collection Procedure for Male Patients

Purpose: To instruct a male in how to properly collect a CCMS urine specimen.
Equipment: Requisition, specimen label, sterile urine container, special sterile antiseptic wipes, and copy of written instructions.

Step	Rationale
1. Wash hands thoroughly.	Aids in infection control and helps avoid contamination of the site while cleaning.
2. Remove the lid of the container, being careful not to touch the inside of the cover or the container.	The lid and container must remain sterile for accurate interpretation of results.

Step	Rationale
3. Wash the end of the penis with the special wipe (or soapy water), beginning at the urethral opening and working away from it in a circular motion (the foreskin of an uncircumcised male must first be retracted). Repeat the procedure with a clean wipe.	The foreskin must be retracted to allow thorough cleaning of the penis. Antiseptic solution in the wipe removes bacteria from the area. Wiping away from the urinary opening carries microbes away from the site.
4. Keeping the foreskin retracted, if applicable, void into the toilet for a few seconds.	Keeping the foreskin retracted maintains site antisepsis. Voiding the first portion of urine into the toilet washes away the antiseptic and microbes remaining in the urinary opening.
5. Touching only the outside and without letting it touch the penis, bring the urine container into the urine stream until a sufficient amount of urine (30–100 mL) is collected.	Bringing the urine container into the stream without touching the penis helps ensure sterility of the specimen. An adequate amount of urine is needed to perform the test.
6. Void the remaining urine into the toilet.	Only 30–100 mL of urine is needed for the test.
7. Cover the specimen with the lid provided, touching only the outside surfaces of the lid and container.	The lid and container must remain sterile, and the specimen must be covered to maintain sterility and protect others from exposure to the contents.
8. Clean any urine spilled on the outside of the container with an antiseptic wipe.	Aids in infection control.
9. Wash hands.	Aids in infection control.
10. Hand specimen to phlebotomist or place where instructed if already labeled.	Follow facility protocol.

From McCall RE, Tankersley CM. *Phlebotomy Essentials.* 5th ed. Philadelphia, PA: Lippincott Williams & Wilkins; 2012.

There are actually three parts to a urine culture: (a) a colony count, (b) isolation and identification of the pathogen, and (c) antimicrobial susceptibility testing. The colony count is a way of estimating the number of viable bacteria that are present in the urine specimen. A calibrated loop is used to perform the colony count. A *calibrated loop* is a bacteriologic loop that has

> A complete urine culture consists of a colony count, isolation and identification of the pathogen, and antimicrobial susceptibility testing.

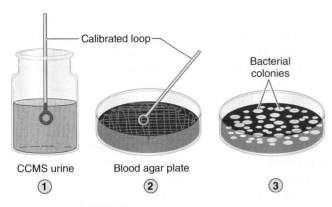

Figure 13-6. Obtaining a urine colony count. 1. A calibrated loop is dipped into a CCMS urine specimen. **2.** The volume of urine contained within the calibrated loop is spread over the entire surface of a blood agar plate, which is then incubated overnight at 37°C. **3.** The colonies are counted after the plate is removed from the incubator. (See text for additional details.)

been manufactured so that it contains a precise volume of urine. There are two types of calibrated loops: those calibrated to contain 0.01 mL of fluid, and those calibrated to contain 0.001 mL of fluid. The calibrated loop is dipped into the CCMS urine specimen. Then the volume of urine within the calibrated loop is inoculated over the entire surface of a blood agar plate, which is then incubated overnight at 37°C (Fig. 13-6). After incubation, the colonies are counted, and this number is then multiplied by the dilution factor (either 100 or 1,000) to obtain the number of colony-forming units (CFU) per milliliter of urine.[b] (The dilution factor is 100 if a 0.01-mL calibrated loop was used, or 1,000 if a 0.001-mL calibrated loop was used.) **Example:** If the number of colonies is 300 and a 0.001-mL calibrated loop was used, then the colony count is 300 × 1,000 or 300,000 (3×10^5) CFU/mL.

A CFU count that is 100,000 (1×10^5) CFU/mL or higher is indicative of a UTI, although high colony counts may also be caused by contamination of the urine specimen with indigenous microbiota during specimen collection or failure to refrigerate the specimen between collection and transport to the laboratory. The mere presence of bacteria in the urine (*bacteriuria*) is not significant, as urine always becomes contaminated with bacteria during urination (voiding). However, the presence of two or more bacteria per × 1,000 microscopic field of a Gram-stained urine smear is indicative of a UTI with 100,000 (10^5) or more CFU per milliliter.

Cerebrospinal Fluid (CSF)

Meningitis, encephalitis, and meningoencephalitis are rapidly fatal diseases that can be caused by various microbes, including bacteria, fungi, protozoa, and viruses.

---

[b]A CFU is a viable bacterial cell, capable of dividing and producing a colony. Thus, the number of CFUs represents the number of viable bacteria that were present in the urine specimen at the time the specimen was inoculated onto the blood agar plate.

Meningitis is inflammation or infection of the membranes (meninges) that surround the brain and spinal column. *Encephalitis* is inflammation or infection of the brain. *Meningoencephalitis* is inflammation or infection of both the brain and the meninges. To diagnose these diseases, CSF must be collected into a sterile tube by a lumbar puncture (spinal tap) under surgically aseptic conditions (Fig.13-7). This technically difficult procedure is performed by a physician. CSF specimens must be rushed to the laboratory and must not be refrigerated. Refrigeration might kill any fragile pathogens present in the specimen.

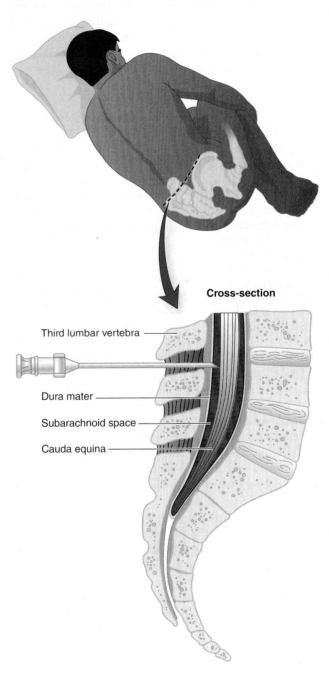

Figure 13-7. Technique of lumbar puncture. (Redrawn from Taylor C, et al. *Fundamentals of Nursing*. 2nd ed. Philadelphia, PA: JB Lippincott; 1993.)

Because of the extremely serious nature of central nervous system (CNS) infections, the CSF will be treated as a STAT (emergency) specimen in the CML, and a workup of the specimen will be initiated immediately.[c] Information obtained as a result of examining a Gram stain of the spinal fluid sediment will be reported by telephone to the clinician immediately; this is what is known as a *preliminary report*. Preliminary reports are laboratory reports that are communicated (usually by telephone) to the requesting clinician before the availability of the final report. Preliminary reports containing CSF Gram stain observations frequently enable clinicians to make diagnoses and initiate therapy, and often save patients' lives.

> CSF specimens are treated as STAT (emergency) specimens in the CML, where workup of the specimens is initiated immediately upon receipt.

Sputum

Sputum is pus that accumulates deep within the lungs of a patient with pneumonia, tuberculosis, or other lower respiratory infection. Laboratory workup of a good-quality sputum specimen can provide important information about a patient's lower respiratory infection. Unfortunately, many of the sputum specimens that are submitted to the CML are actually saliva. Owing to the presence of indigenous oral microbes, a laboratory workup of a patient's saliva will not provide clinically relevant information about the patient's lower respiratory infection and will be a waste of time, effort, and money. This situation can be avoided if someone (most often, a nurse) takes a moment to explain to the patient what is required. (For example, "The next time you cough up some of that thick, greenish material from your lungs, Mr. Smith, please spit it into this container.") If proper mouth hygiene is maintained, the sputum will not be severely contaminated with indigenous oral microbes. If tuberculosis is suspected, extreme care in collecting and handling the specimen should be exercised because one could easily be infected with the pathogens. Usually, sputum specimens may be refrigerated for several hours without loss of the pathogens.

> Laboratory workup of a good-quality sputum specimen can provide important information about a patient's lower respiratory infection, whereas workup of a patient's saliva cannot.

The clinician may wish to obtain a better quality specimen by bronchial aspiration through a bronchoscope or by a process known as transtracheal aspiration. Needle biopsy of the lungs may be necessary for diagnosis of *Pneumocystis jiroveci* pneumonia (as in patients with acquired immunodeficiency syndrome [AIDS] and for certain other pathogens). Although once classified as a protozoan, *P. jiroveci* is currently considered to be a fungus.

Throat Swabs

Routine throat swabs are collected to determine whether a patient has strep throat (*Streptococcus pyogenes* pharyngitis). If any other pathogen (e.g., *Neisseria gonorrhoeae* or *Corynebacterium diphtheriae*) is suspected by the clinician to be causing the patient's pharyngitis, a specific culture for that pathogen must be noted on the laboratory test requisition, so that the appropriate culture media will be inoculated. There is an art to the proper collection of a throat swab, as described in the following box.

> If a clinician suspects a pathogen other than *S. pyogenes* to be causing a patient's pharyngitis, that information must be included on the laboratory test requisition.

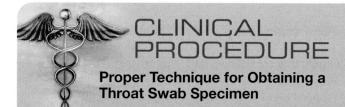

CLINICAL PROCEDURE

Proper Technique for Obtaining a Throat Swab Specimen

Purpose: To provide instruction in how to properly collect a throat culture specimen.
Equipment: Requisition, specimen label, sterile container with swab and transport medium.

Step	Rationale
1. Wash hands and put on gloves. The phlebotomist may wish to wear a mask and goggles. Follow facility protocol.	Aids in infection control. Throat culture collection can cause the patient to have a gag reflex or cough.
2. Open container and remove swab in an aseptic manner.	Swab sterility must be maintained for accurate interpretation of results.
3. Stand back or to the side of the patient.	Helps avoid droplet contact if the patient coughs.
4. Instruct the patient to tilt back the head and open the mouth wide.	Allows adequate evaluation of the collection site and ease in specimen collection.
5. Direct light onto the back of the throat using a small flashlight or other light source.	Illuminates areas of inflammation, ulceration, exudation, or capsule formation.
6. Depress the tongue with a tongue depressor and ask the patient to say "ah."	Depressing the tongue helps avoid touching other areas of the mouth and contaminating the sample during collection. Saying "ah" raises the uvula (soft tissue hanging from the back of the throat) out of the way.

---

[c] Stat is an abbreviation of the Latin word "statim," meaning "immediately."

Step	Rationale
7. Swab both tonsils, tonsilar crypts (crevasses), the back of the throat, and any areas of ulceration, exudation, or inflammation, being careful not to touch the swab to the lips, tongue, or uvula.	Standard protocol that ensures sampling of the problem area. Touching other areas of the mouth can contaminate the swab with microbes from the oral cavity and not the throat. Touching the uvula can cause a gag reflex.
8. Maintain tongue depressor position while removing the swab and then discard it.	Keeping the tongue depressor in place until the swab is removed prevents the tongue from contaminating the swab.
9. Place the swab back in the transport tube, embed in medium, and secure cover. (Follow instructions to crush ampule and release medium first if applicable.)	The transport medium keeps the microbes alive until they can be cultured in the laboratory.
10. Label specimen.	Prompt labeling is essential to ensure correct specimen identification.
11. Remove gloves and sanitize hands.	Proper glove removal and hand decontamination prevents the spread of infection.
12. Arrange transport or deliver to the laboratory as soon as possible.	Timely processing is necessary to prevent overgrowth of normal flora.

From McCall RE, Tankersley CM. *Phlebotomy Essentials*. 5th ed. Philadelphia, PA: Lippincott Williams & Wilkins; 2012.

Wound Specimens

Whenever possible, a wound specimen should be an aspirate (i.e., pus that has been collected using a small needle and syringe assembly), rather than a swab specimen. Specimens collected by swab are frequently contaminated with indigenous skin microbes and often dry out before they can be processed in the CML. The person collecting the specimen should always indicate the type of wound infection (e.g., dog bite, surgical site, or burn wound infection) on the laboratory test requisition and the anatomical site from which the specimen was obtained. This provides valuable information that will enable CML personnel to inoculate appropriate types of media and be on the lookout for specific organisms. For example, *Pasteurella multocida* is frequently isolated from dog bite wound infections, but this Gram-negative

> The laboratory test requisition that accompanies a wound specimen must indicate the type of wound and its anatomical location.

bacillus is rarely encountered in other types of specimens. Merely stating "wound" on the laboratory test requisition is insufficient.

GC Cultures

The initials GC represent an abbreviation for *gonococci*, a term referring to *N. gonorrhoeae*. As mentioned earlier, *N. gonorrhoeae* is a fastidious bacterium that is microaerophilic and capnophilic. Only Dacron, calcium alginate, or nontoxic cotton swabs should be used to collect GC specimens. Ordinary cotton swabs contain fatty acids, which can be toxic to *N. gonorrhoeae*. When attempting to diagnose gonorrhea, swabs (vaginal, cervical, urethral, throat, and rectal) should be inoculated immediately onto Thayer–Martin or Martin-Lewis medium and incubated in a carbon dioxide (CO_2) environment.

> When attempting to culture *N. gonorrhoeae*, one should remember that it is a fastidious ("fussy"), microaerophilic, and capnophilic organism.

Alternatively, they should be inoculated into a tube or bottle (e.g., Transgrow) that contains an appropriate culture medium and an atmosphere containing 5% to 10% CO_2 (Fig. 13-8). To prevent loss of the CO_2, the bottle should be held in an upright position while inoculating. Otherwise, the CO_2 spills out and is displaced by room air. These cultures should be incubated at 37°C overnight and then shipped to a microbiology laboratory for positive identification of *N. gonorrhoeae*. If it is necessary to transport a swab specimen, the swab should be placed into a transport medium for shipment. Never refrigerate GC swabs because the low temperature might kill the *N. gonorrhoeae*.

Fecal Specimens

Ideally, fecal specimens (stool specimens) should be collected at the laboratory and processed immediately to prevent a decrease in temperature, which allows the pH to

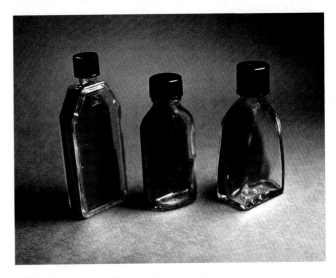

Figure 13-8. Transgrow bottles used in gonococcal cultures. (Available from Remel Products, Lenexa, KS.) (Courtesy of Dr. A. Schroeter and the CDC.)

drop, causing the death of many *Shigella* and *Salmonella* species. Alternatively, the specimen may be placed in a container with a preservative that maintains a pH of 7.0.

Because the colon is anaerobic, fecal bacteria are obligate, aerotolerant, and facultative anaerobes. However, fecal specimens are cultured anaerobically only when *Clostridium difficile*–associated disease is suspected or to diagnose clostridial food poisoning. In gastrointestinal infections, the pathogens frequently overwhelm the indigenous intestinal microbiota, so that they are the predominant organisms seen in smears and cultures. A combination of direct microscopic examination, culture, biochemical tests, and immunologic tests may be performed to identify Gram-negative and Gram-positive bacteria (e.g., enteropathogenic *Escherichia coli*, *Salmonella* spp., *Shigella* spp., *Clostridium perfringens*, *C. difficile*, *Vibrio cholerae*, *Campylobacter* spp., and *Staphylococcus* spp.), fungi (*Candida*), intestinal protozoa (*Giardia*, *Entamoeba*), and intestinal helminths.

> In gastrointestinal infections, the pathogens frequently overwhelm the indigenous intestinal microbes, so that they are the predominant organisms seen in smears and cultures.

The Pathology Department ("The Lab")

The clinical specimens just described are submitted to the CML. Within a hospital setting, the CML is an integral part of the Pathology Department (which is frequently referred to simply as "the lab"). Because virtually all healthcare personnel will interact in some way(s) with the Pathology Department, they should understand how it is organized and the types of laboratory tests that are performed there.

> Within a hospital, the CML is an integral part of the Pathology Department.

The Pathology Department is under the direction of a *pathologist* (a physician who has had extensive, specialized training in *pathology*—the study of the structural and functional manifestations of disease). As shown in Figure 13-9, the Pathology Department consists of two major divisions: Anatomical Pathology and Clinical Pathology.

Anatomical Pathology

Most pathologists work in Anatomical Pathology, where they perform autopsies in the morgue and examine diseased organs, stained tissue sections, and cytology specimens. Other healthcare professionals employed in

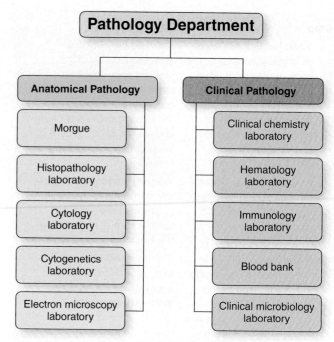

Figure 13-9. Organization of a typical Pathology Department.

Anatomical Pathology include cytogenetic technologists, cytotechnologists, histologic technicians, histotechnologists, and pathologist's assistants.

In addition to the morgue, Anatomical Pathology houses the Histopathology Laboratory, the Cytology Laboratory, and the Cytogenetics Laboratory. In some Pathology Departments, the Electron Microscopy Laboratory is also located in Anatomical Pathology.

Clinical Pathology

In addition to the CML, Clinical Pathology consists of several other laboratories: the Clinical Chemistry Laboratory (or Clinical Chemistry/Urinalysis Laboratory), the Hematology Laboratory (or Hematology/Coagulation Laboratory), the Blood Bank (or Immunohematology Laboratory), and the Immunology Laboratory (described in Chapter 16). In smaller hospitals, immunodiagnostic procedures are performed in the Immunology Section (or Serology Section) of the CML.

Personnel working in Clinical Pathology include pathologists; specialized scientists such as chemists and microbiologists, who have graduate degrees in their specialty areas; **medical laboratory scientists** (also known as *medical technologists* or *MTs*), who have 4-year baccalaureate degrees; and **medical laboratory technicians** (also known as *medical laboratory technicians* or *MLTs*), who have 2-year associate degrees.

> The CML is located in the Clinical Pathology division of the Pathology Department.

SPOTLIGHTING
Medical Laboratory Professionals

Medical laboratory professionals are important members of the highly skilled medical team who work together to collect clinical data and diagnose diseases. Medical laboratory professionals include pathologists, medical laboratory scientists (MLSs; also known as medical technologists, MTs), MLTs, histologic technicians, cytotechnologists, blood bank technologists, phlebotomy technicians, pathologist assistants, and cytogeneticists. Practice settings for these professionals include hospital laboratories; clinics; nursing homes; city, state, and federal public health facilities (e.g., the Centers for Disease Control and Prevention [CDC]); molecular diagnostic and biotechnology laboratories; research laboratories; educational institutions; and commercial companies (e.g., pharmaceutical companies and food service industries).

MLSs (or MTs) and MLTs work in all areas of the clinical laboratory, including blood bank, chemistry, hematology, immunology, urinalysis, and microbiology. They perform a wide variety of laboratory tests used in the detection, diagnosis, and treatment of many diseases. MLSs have many responsibilities and are held accountable for accurate and reliable test results.

Education and training in Clinical Laboratory Science not only prepare the individual for a rewarding career in the profession, but also serve as a foundation for jobs in other fields (e.g., medicine, medical research, forensics, biotechnology). Individuals interested in pursuing a career in Clinical Laboratory Science should have a strong background in the high school and college sciences (i.e., biology and chemistry), as well as math and computer science.

There are two levels of Medical Laboratory Science training available. The minimum formal education requirements for an MLT are a 2-year associate degree and completion of an accredited MLT program. MLTs perform routine tests in all areas of the laboratory under the supervision of an MLS. The MLS requires a 4-year baccalaureate degree and clinical experience in an accredited Medical Laboratory Science program. MLSs are able to correlate results with disease states, establish and monitor quality control, and operate complex electronic equipment and computers. MLSs must be able to work in stressful situations and they must be reliable, self-sufficient, precise, and thorough. Clinical education programs for MLSs may be located in hospitals or university settings and include instruction in microbiology, chemistry, hematology, immunology, blood banking, virology, phlebotomy, urinalysis, management, and education. To ensure competency, graduates of both MLS and MLT clinical education programs must be certified by one or both of the two national credentialing agencies: the American Society for Clinical Pathology (ASCP), or the National Credentialing Agency (NCA). Additional information concerning these professions, including educational programs, certification, and salaries can be found at the following web sites:

- American Medical Association (http://www .ama-assn.org)
- American Society for Clinical Laboratory Science (http://www.ascls.org)
- American Society for Clinical Pathology (http:// www.ascp.org)
- National Accrediting Agency for Clinical Laboratory Sciences (http://www.naacls.org)
- National Credentialing Agency (http://www .nca-info.org)

The Clinical Microbiology Laboratory

Organization

Depending on the size of the hospital, the CML may be under the direction of a pathologist, a microbiologist (having either a master or doctor of clinical microbiology degree), or, in smaller hospitals, an MT who has had many years of experience working in microbiology. Most of the actual bench work that is performed in the CML is performed by MLSs and MLTs.

As shown in Figure 13-10, the CML is divided into various sections, which, to a large degree, correspond to the various categories of microbes. With the exception of the Immunology Section, the responsibilities of the specific sections of the CML are described in this chapter. Procedures performed in the Immunology Section are described in Chapter 16.

Responsibilities

The primary mission of the CML is to assist clinicians in the diagnosis and treatment of infectious diseases. To accomplish this mission, the four major, day-to-day responsibilities of the CML are to:

> The four major responsibilities of the CML are to (a) process clinical specimens, (b) isolate pathogens, (c) identify (speciate) pathogens, and (d) perform antimicrobial susceptibility testing when appropriate to do so.

1. Process the various clinical specimens that are submitted to the CML (described previously)
2. Isolate pathogens from those specimens
3. Identify (speciate) the pathogens
4. Perform antimicrobial susceptibility testing when appropriate to do so

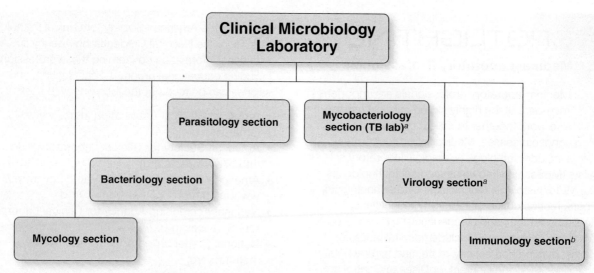

Figure 13-10. Organization of a typical Clinical Microbiology Laboratory. [a]Virology and Mycobacteriology Sections are usually found only in larger hospitals and medical centers. Lacking these sections, most of the smaller hospitals would instead send virology and mycobacteriology specimens to a reference laboratory. [b]Only smaller hospitals would have Immunology Sections, where some immunodiagnostic procedures would be performed. Larger hospitals and medical centers would have an Immunology Laboratory, which would perform a much wider variety of immunologic procedures and would operate independently of the CML.

> In general, the processing of clinical specimens in the CML includes (a) examining the specimen macroscopically, (b) examining the specimen microscopically, and (c) inoculating the specimen to appropriate culture media.

The exact steps in the processing of clinical specimens vary from one specimen type to another and also depend on the specific section of the CML to which the specimen is submitted. In general, processing includes the following steps:

- Examining the specimen macroscopically and recording pertinent observations (e.g., cloudiness or the presence of blood, mucus, or an unusual odor)
- Examining the specimen microscopically and recording pertinent observations (e.g., the presence of WBCs or microorganisms)
- Inoculating the specimen to appropriate culture media in an attempt to isolate the pathogen(s) from the specimen and get them growing in pure culture in the laboratory

such is usually *not* the case with CML procedures. CML procedures frequently require a pure culture of the suspected pathogen, which often takes a minimum of 24 hours to obtain. Once a pure culture is available, an additional 24 hours or more are often required to obtain a species identification and antimicrobial susceptibility test results. **Therefore, individuals who submit specimens to the CML should expect a 1- or 2-day delay between submission of the specimens and receipt of CML results.** Fortunately, some of the newer techniques (such as molecular and immunodiagnostic procedures) do provide same day results.

The CML is sometimes called on to assume an additional responsibility, namely the processing of environmental samples (i.e., samples collected from within the hospital environment). Such samples are processed by the CML whenever there is an outbreak or epidemic within the hospital, in an attempt to locate the source of the pathogen involved. Environmental samples include those collected from appropriate hospital sites (e.g., floors, sink drains, showerheads, whirlpool baths, respiratory therapy equipment) and employees (e.g., nasal swabs, material from open wounds).

> A less frequent responsibility of the CML is to process environmental samples whenever there is an outbreak or epidemic within the hospital.

Frequently, CML personnel are the first people to recognize that an outbreak is occurring within the hospital. For example, CML personnel might note an unusually

SOMETHING TO THINK ABOUT

Although the results of some laboratory procedures (such as certain of the automated procedures performed in the Chemistry Section) are often available within hours after arrival of the specimens in the laboratory, high number of isolates of a particular pathogen from specimens submitted from a particular ward. The CML would notify the Hospital Infection Control Committee (described in Chapter 12) of the unusually high number of isolates, and the committee would then be responsible for collecting appropriate environmental samples and submitting them to the CML for processing.

Isolation and Identification (Speciation) of Pathogens

In an effort to isolate bacteria (including mycobacteria) and fungi (yeasts and moulds) from clinical specimens, the specimens are inoculated into liquid culture media or onto solid culture media. The goal is to get any pathogens

> To isolate bacteria and fungi from clinical specimens, specimens are inoculated into liquid culture media or onto solid culture media.

that are present in the specimen growing in pure culture (by themselves), and in large number, so that there will be a sufficient quantity of the organism to inoculate appropriate identification and antimicrobial susceptibility testing systems. Specific types of media were discussed in Chapter 8. The manner in which pathogens are identified depends on the particular section of the CML to which the specimen was submitted. (Note: As previously mentioned, throughout this book, the term "to identify an organism" means to learn the organism's name; i.e., to speciate it.)

Bacteriology Section

The overall responsibility of the Bacteriology Section of the CML is to assist clinicians in the diagnosis of bacterial diseases. In the Bacteriology Section, various types of

> The overall responsibility of the Bacteriology Section of the CML is to assist clinicians in the diagnosis of bacterial diseases.

> CML professionals gather "clues" (phenotypic characteristics) about a pathogen until they have sufficient information to identify (speciate) it.

clinical specimens are processed, bacterial pathogens are isolated from the specimens, tests are performed to identify the bacterial pathogens, and antimicrobial susceptibility testing is performed whenever it is appropriate to do so (Fig. 13-11). Once they are isolated from clinical specimens, bacterial pathogens are identified by gathering clues (phenotypic characteristics). Thus, CML professionals are very much like detectives and crime scene investigators (Fig. 13-12), gathering "clues" about a pathogen until they are have sufficient clues to identify it.

The various phenotypic characteristics (clues) useful in identifying bacteria include the following:

- Gram reaction (i.e., Gram-positive or Gram-negative)
- Cell shape (e.g., cocci, bacilli, curved, spiral-shaped, filamentous, branching)

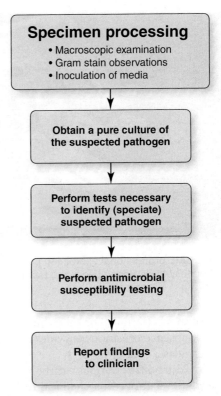

Specimen processing
- Macroscopic examination
- Gram stain observations
- Inoculation of media

↓

Obtain a pure culture of the suspected pathogen

↓

Perform tests necessary to identify (speciate) suspected pathogen

↓

Perform antimicrobial susceptibility testing

↓

Report findings to clinician

Figure 13-11. Flowchart illustrating the sequence of events that occur within the Bacteriology Section of the Clinical Microbiology Laboratory.

- Morphologic arrangement of cells (e.g., pairs, tetrads, chains, clusters)
- Growth or no growth on various types of plated media
- Colony morphology (e.g., color, general shape, elevation, margin) (Fig. 13-13)
- Presence or absence of a capsule
- Motility
- Number and location of flagella
- Ability to sporulate

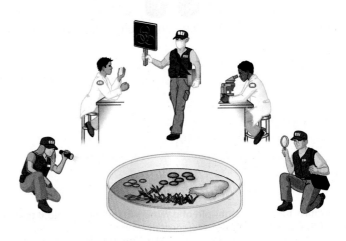

Figure 13-12. Clinical Microbiology Laboratory professionals are very much like detectives and crime scene investigators. They gather "clues" about a pathogen until they have enough information to identify (speciate) the culprit.

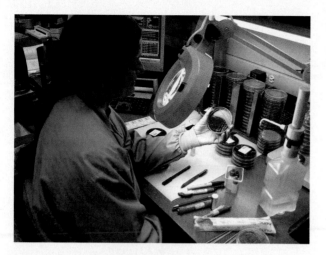

Figure 13-13. CML professional examining bacterial colonies. (Courtesy of Dr. Robert Fader and Biomed Ed, Round Rock, TX.)

- Location of spores (terminal or subterminal)
- Presence or absence of various enzymes (e.g., catalase, coagulase, oxidase, urease)
- Ability to catabolize various carbohydrates and amino acids (miniaturized biochemical test systems—"minisystems"—are often used for this purpose; see Fig. 13-14)
- Ability to reduce nitrate
- Ability to produce indole from tryptophan
- Atmospheric requirements
- Type of hemolysis produced (Fig. 13-15)

Mycology Section

The overall responsibility of the Mycology Section of the CML is to assist clinicians in the diagnosis of fungal infections (mycoses). In the Mycology Section, various types of clinical specimens are processed, fungal pathogens are isolated, and tests are performed to identify the fungal pathogens. In general, the specimens processed in the Mycology Section are the same types of specimens that are processed in the Bacteriology Section. However, three types are specimens are much more commonly submitted to the Mycology Section than to the Bacteriology Section: hair clippings, nail clippings, and skin scrapings.

> The overall responsibility of the Mycology Section of the CML is to assist clinicians in the diagnosis of fungal infections (mycoses).

A potassium hydroxide preparation (KOH prep) is performed on hair clippings, nail clippings, and skin scrapings. (See Appendix 5 on thePoint for details of the KOH preparation.) The KOH acts as a clearing agent by dissolving keratin in the specimens. This enables the technologist to see into the specimens when they are examined microscopically, and to determine whether any fungal elements (e.g., yeasts or hyphae) are present in the specimen. Stained tissue specimens are also examined for the presence of hyphae (Fig. 13-16).

Specimens will also be inoculated onto Sabouraud dextrose agar, a selective medium for fungi. Bacteria do not grow on this medium because of the low pH (pH 5.6), but most fungi grow quite well.

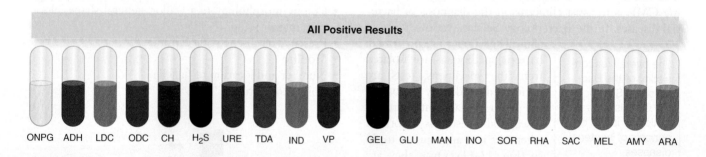

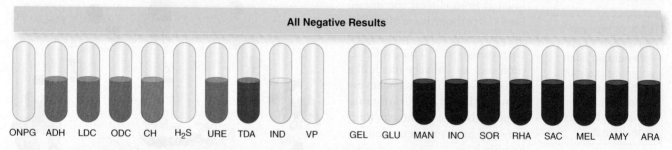

Figure 13-14. An example of a miniaturized biochemical test system (minisystem). The minisystem illustrated here, called the API-20E, is primarily used for identification of *E. coli* and other members in the bacterial family Enterobacteriaceae. It is manufactured by bioMerieux, Hazelwood, MO. The API-20E consists of a plastic strip and 20 plastic cupules. Each cupule contains a different substrate. The lower strip shows the color of each cupule immediately after inoculation. Following 18 to 20 hours of incubation, the colors in the compartments are interpreted as either positive or negative results. (Negative reactions are illustrated in the lower strip, and positive reactions are illustrated in the upper strip.) Based on the pattern of positive and negative reactions, a seven-digit biotype number is calculated. In most cases, the number is specific for a particular bacterial species. (Redrawn from Harvey RA et al. *Lippincott's Illustrated Reviews: Microbiology.* 3rd ed. Philadelphia, PA: Lippincott Williams & Wilkins; 2013.)

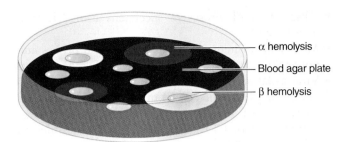

Figure 13-15. Diagram illustrating the three types of hemolysis that can be observed on a blood agar plate. α-hemolysis is a green zone around the bacterial colony. α-hemolytic bacteria produce an enzyme that causes a partial breakdown of hemoglobin in the RBCs in the medium, resulting in a green color. β-hemolysis is a clear zone around the bacterial colony. β-hemolytic bacteria produce an enzyme that completely destroys (lyses) the RBCs, thus producing a clear zone. γ-hemolysis is no hemolysis at all (neither a green nor a clear zone around the bacterial colony). γ-hemolytic bacteria (also referred to as nonhemolytic bacteria) produce neither of these enzymes and, therefore, cause no change in the RBCs.

> When isolated from clinical specimens, yeasts are identified using various biochemical tests, primarily based on their ability to catabolize various carbohydrates.

When isolated from clinical specimens, yeasts are identified by using various biochemical tests, primarily by their ability to catabolize various carbohydrates. Moulds are identified using a combination of rate of growth and macroscopic and microscopic observations, *not* by performing biochemical tests. Macroscopic observations are things that you can learn about the mycelium by looking at it with the naked eye—like color, texture, and topography (see Figs. 13-17 and 13-18).

To examine a mould microscopically, a tease mount is prepared. A drop of stain is placed on a glass microscope slide. A small piece of the mycelium is placed into the drop. Teasing needles (also known as dissecting needles) are used

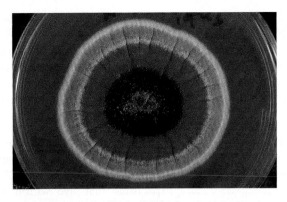

Figure 13-17. A colony (mycelium) of an *Aspergillus* species. Moulds in the genus *Aspergillus* can cause sinusitis, lower respiratory infections, and infections of the eyes, heart, kidneys, skin, and other organs, most commonly in immunosuppressed patients. (From Winn WC Jr, et al. *Koneman's Color Atlas and Textbook of Diagnostic Microbiology*. 6th ed. Philadelphia, PA: Lippincott Williams & Wilkins; 2006.)

to gently pull (tease) the piece of mycelium apart, enabling the CML professional to see various identifying characteristics of the mould. A glass coverslip is added, and the tease mount preparation is examined under the microscope. The stain that is used in the tease mount is lactophenol cotton blue, containing lactic acid, phenol, and cotton blue. The lactic acid preserves morphology. The phenol kills the organisms, so they will not be infectious. The cotton blue stains the mycelial structures blue.

> When isolated from clinical specimens, moulds are identified using a combination of rate of growth and macroscopic and microscopic observations.

When the tease mount preparation is examined microscopically, the first thing to determine is whether the mould has septate or aseptate hyphae (described in Chapter 5). Next, the technologist will look for spores and the structures on or within which the spores are produced. The appearance of these structures further

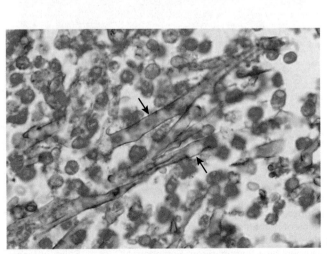

Figure 13-16. Fungal hyphae (*arrows*) in a stained heart valve specimen from a patient with zygomycosis. (Courtesy of Dr. Libero Ajello and the CDC.)

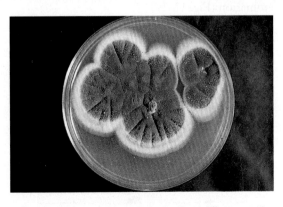

Figure 13-18. Colonies (mycelia) of a *Penicillium* species. Although penicillin is derived from *Penicillium*, various species in this genus can also cause lung, liver, and skin infections in immunosuppressed patients. (From Winn WC Jr, et al. *Koneman's Color Atlas and Textbook of Diagnostic Microbiology*. 6th ed. Philadelphia, PA: Lippincott Williams & Wilkins; 2006.)

enables the technologist to identify the mould (refer back to Fig. 5-10 in Chapter 5).

Susceptibility testing of fungi is not currently performed in most CMLs; however, because of the ever-growing problem of drug resistance in fungi, it is likely that such testing will become routine in the near future.

Parasitology Section

The overall responsibility of the Parasitology Section of the CML is to assist clinicians in the diagnosis of parasitic diseases—specifically, infections caused by endoparasites (parasites that live within the body), such as parasitic protozoa and helminths (parasitic worms). In general, parasitic infections are diagnosed by observing and recognizing various parasite life cycle stages (e.g., trophozoites and cysts of protozoa; microfilariae, eggs, and larvae of helminths) in clinical specimens. Parasites are identified primarily by the characteristic appearance (e.g., size, shape, internal details) of the various life cycle stages that are seen in clinical specimens. Sometimes, whole worms or segments of worms are observed in fecal specimens. Parasites are described in detail in Chapter 21.

> The overall responsibility of the Parasitology Section of the CML is to assist clinicians in the diagnosis of parasitic diseases. Parasites are identified primarily by their characteristic appearance.

Virology Section

The overall responsibility of the Virology Section of the CML is to assist clinicians in the diagnosis of viral diseases. Many viral diseases are diagnosed using immunodiagnostic procedures (described in Chapter 16). Other techniques used to identify viral pathogens are:

> The overall responsibility of the Virology Section of the CML is to assist clinicians in the diagnosis of viral diseases.

- Observation of intracytoplasmic or intranuclear viral inclusion bodies in specimens by cytologic or histologic examination (Fig. 13-19)

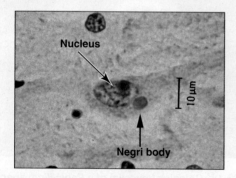

Nucleus

Negri body

10 µm

Figure 13-19. Intracytoplasmic inclusion body (called a Negri body) in a brain cell from a patient with rabies. (From Harvey RA et al. *Lippincott's Illustrated Reviews: Microbiology.* 3rd ed. Philadelphia, PA: Lippincott Williams & Wilkins; 2013.)

- Observation of viruses in specimens using electron microscopy
- Molecular techniques such as nucleic acid probes and polymerase chain reaction assays (described on thePoint)
- Virus isolation by use of cell cultures; viruses are identified primarily by the type(s) of cell lines that they are able to infect and the physical changes (called cytopathic effect or CPE) that they cause in the infected cells (Fig. 13-20).

Mycobacteriology Section

The primary responsibility of the Mycobacteriology Section (or "TB Lab," as it is often called) of the CML is to assist clinicians in the diagnosis of tuberculosis. In the Mycobacteriology Section, various types of specimens (primarily sputum specimens) are processed, acid-fast staining is performed, mycobacteria are isolated and identified, and susceptibility testing is performed. *Mycobacterium* spp. are identified using a combination of growth characteristics (e.g., growth rate, colony pigmentation,

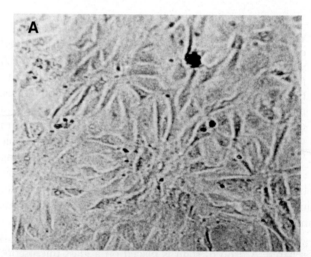

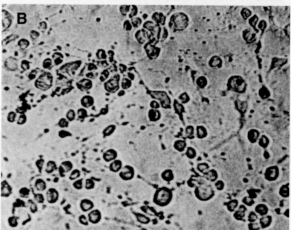

Figure 13-20. Cytopathic effect (CPE). A. Normal appearance of human diploid fibroblasts. **B.** The appearance of the same cells, 48 hours after being inoculated with herpes simplex type 2 virus. (From Engleberg NC, et al. *Schaechter's Mechanisms of Microbial Disease.* 4th ed. Philadelphia, PA: Lippincott Williams & Wilkins; 2007.)

photoreactivity, and morphology) and various biochemical tests. *Mycobacterium tuberculosis*, the primary cause of human tuberculosis, is a very slow-growing organism. Fortunately, the acid-fast stain (described in Chapter 4) enables rapid presumptive diagnosis of tuberculosis.

Additional information pertaining to the CML, including molecular diagnostic procedures, antimicrobial susceptibility testing, quality assurance and quality control in the CML, and safety in the CML, can be found in Appendix 4 on thePoint: ("Responsibilities of the Clinical Microbiology Laboratory").

SOMETHING TO THINK ABOUT

"In addition to diagnosing infections caused by well-established pathogens, clinical microbiologists uncover new pathogens, acting as sentinels for possible epidemics. They also provide statistical and clinical information regarding pathogens on the scene and spur demands on research to create novel diagnostic tools. In fact, development of such tools is taking place so swiftly that, in not too many years, the practice of clinical microbiology may well become unrecognizable. Not only is the use of nucleic acid-based techniques expected to expand, but other sophisticated techniques such as mass spectrometry will make microbiological diagnoses ever more rapid and accurate."

Schaechter E. The excitement of clinical microbiology. *Microbe*. 2013;8:11–14.

ON thePoint

- Terms Introduced in This Chapter
- Review of Key Points
- A Closer Look:
  - Specimen Quality and Clinical Relevance
  - The Polymerase Chain Reaction
- Increase Your Knowledge
- Critical Thinking
- Additional Self-Assessment Exercises

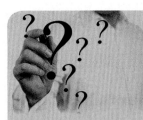

Self-Assessment Exercises

After studying this chapter, answer the following multiple-choice questions.

1. Assuming that a CCMS urine was processed in the CML, which of the following colony counts is (are) indicative of a UTI?
   a. 10,000 CFU/mL
   b. 100,000 CFU/mL
   c. >100,000 CFU/mL
   d. both b and c

2. Which of the following statements about blood is false?
   a. As it circulates throughout the human body, blood is usually sterile.
   b. Following centrifugation, the layer of leukocytes and platelets is referred to as the buffy coat.
   c. Bacteremia and septicemia are synonyms.
   d. Plasma constitutes about 55% of whole blood.

3. Which of the following statements about CSF specimens is false?
   a. They are collected only by clinicians.
   b. They are treated as STAT (emergency) specimens in the laboratory.
   c. They should always be refrigerated.
   d. They should be rushed to the laboratory after collection.

4. All clinical specimens submitted to the CML must be:
   a. properly and carefully collected
   b. properly labeled
   c. properly transported to the laboratory
   d. all of the above

5. Which of the following is *not* one of the three parts of a urine culture?
   a. isolation and identification of the pathogen
   b. performing a colony count
   c. performing a microscopic observation of the urine specimen
   d. performing antimicrobial susceptibility testing

6. Which of the following matches is false?

   a. CPE.. Virology Section
   b. KOH preparation.. Mycology Section
   c. Tease mount.. Bacteriology Section
   d. Type of hemolysis.. Bacteriology Section

7. Who is primarily responsible for the quality of specimens submitted to the CML?

   a. microbiologist who is in charge of the CML
   b. pathologist who is in charge of "the lab"
   c. person who collects the specimen
   d. person who transports the specimen to the CML

8. Which of the following is not one of the four major day-to-day responsibilities of the CML?

   a. identify (speciate) pathogens
   b. isolate pathogens from clinical specimens
   c. perform antimicrobial susceptibility testing when appropriate
   d. process environmental samples

9. Which of the following sections is *least* likely to be found in the CML of a small hospital?

   a. Bacteriology Section
   b. Mycology Section
   c. Parasitology Section
   d. Virology Section

10. In the Mycology Section of the CML, moulds are identified by _____.

    a. biochemical test results
    b. macroscopic observations
    c. microscopic observations
    d. a combination of b and c

14

Pathogenesis of Infectious Diseases

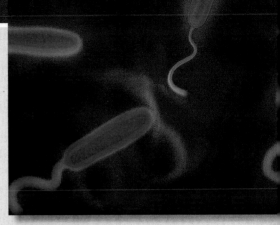

Artist rendering of pathogenic bacteria emitting virulence factors such as toxins and destructive enzymes.

CHAPTER OUTLINE

Introduction

Infection versus Infectious Disease

Why Infection Does Not Always Occur

Four Periods or Phases in the Course of an Infectious Disease

Localized versus Systemic Infections

Acute, Subacute, and Chronic Diseases

Symptoms of a Disease versus Signs of a Disease

Latent Infections

Primary versus Secondary Infections

Steps in the Pathogenesis of Infectious Diseases

Virulence

Virulence Factors
Attachment
    Receptors and Adhesins
    Bacterial Fimbriae (Pili)
Obligate Intracellular Pathogens
Facultative Intracellular Pathogens
    Intracellular Survival Mechanisms
Capsules
Flagella
Exoenzymes
    Necrotizing Enzymes
    Coagulase
    Kinases
    Hyaluronidase
    Collagenase
    Hemolysins
    Lecithinase

Toxins
    Endotoxin
    Exotoxins
Mechanisms by Which Pathogens Escape Immune Responses
    Antigenic Variation
    Camouflage and Molecular Mimicry
    Destruction of Antibodies

LEARNING OBJECTIVES

After studying this chapter, you should be able to:

- Cite four reasons why an individual might not develop an infectious disease after exposure to a pathogen
- Discuss the four periods or phases in the course of an infectious disease
- Differentiate between localized and systemic infections
- Explain how acute diseases differ from subacute and chronic diseases
- Differentiate between "symptoms" of a disease and "signs" of a disease and cite several examples of each
- Cite several examples of latent infections
- Differentiate between primary and secondary infections
- List six steps in the pathogenesis of an infectious disease
- Define virulence and virulence factors
- List three bacterial structures that serve as virulence factors
- List six bacterial exoenzymes that serve as virulence factors
- Differentiate between endotoxins and exotoxins
- List six bacterial exotoxins and the diseases they cause
- Describe three mechanisms by which pathogens escape the immune response

Introduction

By definition, microbes are too small to be seen with the unaided eye. How is it possible for such tiny organisms and infectious particles to cause disease in plants and animals, which are gigantic in comparison to microbes? This chapter will attempt to answer that question, with emphasis on disease in humans.

> Words containing the prefix "path-" or "patho-" pertain to disease.

The prefix *path-* comes from the Greek word "pathos," meaning disease. Examples of words containing this prefix are *pathogen* (a microbe capable of causing disease), *pathology* (the study of the structural and functional manifestations of disease), *pathologist* (a physician who has specialized in pathology), *pathogenicity* (the ability to cause disease), and *pathogenesis* (the steps or mechanisms involved in the development of a disease).

Infection versus Infectious Disease

As discussed previously in this book, an infectious disease is a disease caused by a microbe, and the microbes that cause infectious diseases are collectively referred to as pathogens. The word *infection* tends to be confusing because the term is used in different ways. Most commonly, infection is used as a synonym for infectious disease. For example, saying that "the patient has an ear infection" is the same thing as saying that "the patient has an infectious disease of the ear." Because this is how the word infection is used by physicians, nurses, other healthcare professionals, the mass media, and most other people, this is how infection is used in this book.

> In general usage, the terms *infection* and *infectious disease* are synonyms.

Many microbiologists, however, reserve use of the word infection to mean colonization by a pathogen (i.e., when a pathogen lands on or enters a person's body and establishes residence there, then the person is infected with that pathogen). That pathogen may or may not go on to cause disease in the person. In other words, it is possible for a person to be infected with a certain pathogen, but *not* have the infectious disease caused by that pathogen (recall the discussion of carriers in Chapter 11).

Why Infection Does Not Always Occur

Many people who are exposed to pathogens do not get sick. Listed here are some possible explanations:

- The microbe may land at an anatomic site where it is unable to multiply. For example, when a respiratory pathogen lands on the skin, it may be unable to grow there because the skin lacks the necessary warmth, moisture, and nutrients required for growth of that particular microbe. Additionally, the low pH and presence of fatty acids make the skin a hostile environment for certain organisms.

> Many factors influence whether or not exposure to a pathogen results in disease, including a person's immune, nutritional, and overall health status.

- Many pathogens must attach to specific receptor sites (described later) before they are able to multiply and cause damage. If they land at a site where such receptors are absent, they are unable to cause disease.
- Antibacterial factors that destroy or inhibit the growth of bacteria (e.g., the lysozyme that is present in tears, saliva, and perspiration) may be present at the site where a pathogen lands.
- The indigenous microbiota of that site (e.g., mouth, vagina, intestine) may inhibit growth of the foreign microbe by occupying space and using up available nutrients. This is a type of *microbial antagonism*, in which one microbe or group of microbes wards off another.
- The indigenous microbiota at the site may produce antibacterial factors (proteins called **bacteriocins**) that destroy the newly arrived pathogen. This is also a type of microbial antagonism.
- The individual's nutritional and overall health status often influences the outcome of the pathogen–host encounter. A person who is in good health, with no underlying medical problems, would be less likely to become infected than a person who is malnourished or in poor health.
- The person may be immune to that particular pathogen, perhaps as a result of prior infection with that pathogen or having been vaccinated against that pathogen. Immunity and vaccination are discussed in Chapter 16.
- Phagocytic white blood cells (phagocytes) present in the blood and other tissues may engulf and destroy the pathogen before it has an opportunity to multiply, invade, and cause disease. Phagocytosis is discussed in Chapter 15.

Four Periods or Phases in the Course of an Infectious Disease

Once a pathogen has gained entrance to the body, the course of an infectious disease has four periods or phases (Fig. 14-1):

1. **The incubation period** is the time that elapses between arrival of the pathogen and the onset of symptoms. The length of the incubation period is influenced by many factors, including the overall health and nutritional status of the host, the immune status

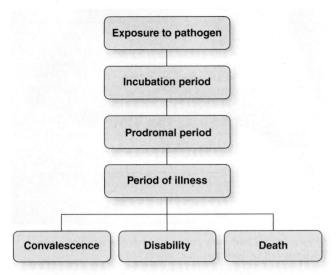

Figure 14-1. Periods in the course of an infectious disease.

of the host (i.e., whether the host is immunocompetent or immunosuppressed), the virulence of the pathogen, and the number of pathogens that enter the body.

> The four periods or phases of an infectious disease are the (a) incubation period, (b) prodromal period, (c) period of illness, and (d) convalescent period.

2. **The prodromal period** is the time during which the patient feels "out of sorts" but does not yet experience actual symptoms of the disease. Patients may feel like they are "coming down with something" but are not yet sure what it is.

3. **The period of illness** is the time during which the patient experiences the typical symptoms associated with that particular disease (e.g., sore throat, headache, sinus congestion). Communicable diseases are most easily transmitted during this third period.

4. **The convalescent period** is the time during which the patient recovers. For certain infectious diseases, especially viral respiratory diseases, the convalescent period can be quite long. Although the patient may recover from the illness itself, permanent damage may be caused by destruction of tissues in the affected area. For example, brain damage may follow encephalitis or meningitis, paralysis may follow poliomyelitis, and deafness may follow ear infections.

Localized versus Systemic Infections

Once an infectious process is initiated, the disease may remain localized to one site or it may spread. Pimples, boils, and abscesses are examples of **localized infections**.

If the pathogens are not contained at the original site of infection, they may be carried to other parts of the body by way of lymph, blood, or, in some cases, phagocytes. When the infection has spread throughout the body, it is referred to as either a **systemic infection** or a *generalized infection*. For example, the bacterium that causes tuberculosis—*Mycobacterium tuberculosis*—may spread to many internal organs, a condition known as miliary (disseminated) tuberculosis.

> An infection may remain localized or it may spread, becoming a systemic or generalized infection.

Acute, Subacute, and Chronic Diseases

A disease may be described as being acute, subacute, or chronic. An **acute disease** has a rapid onset, usually followed by a relatively rapid recovery; measles, mumps, and influenza are examples. A **chronic disease** has an insidious (slow) onset and lasts a long time; examples are tuberculosis, leprosy (Hansen disease), and syphilis. Sometimes, a disease having a sudden onset can develop into a long-lasting disease. Some diseases, such as bacterial endocarditis, come on more suddenly than a chronic disease, but less suddenly than an acute disease; they are referred to as **subacute diseases**. An example of a subacute disease is subacute bacterial endocarditis, often referred to merely as SBE.

> A disease may be acute, subacute, or chronic, depending on the length of its incubation period and duration.

Symptoms of a Disease versus Signs of a Disease

A **symptom of a disease** is defined as some evidence of a disease that is experienced or perceived by the patient—something that is subjective. Examples of symptoms include any type of ache or pain, a ringing in the ears (tinnitus), blurred vision, nausea, dizziness, itching, and chills. Diseases, including infectious diseases, may be either symptomatic or asymptomatic. A **symptomatic disease** (or clinical disease) is a disease in which the patient is experiencing symptoms. An **asymptomatic disease** (or subclinical disease) is a disease that the patient is unaware of because he or she is not experiencing any symptoms.

> Symptoms of a disease are subjective, in that they are perceived by the patient.

In its early stages, gonorrhea (caused by the bacterium, *Neisseria gonorrhoeae*) is usually symptomatic in male patients (who develop a urethral discharge and experience pain while urinating), but asymptomatic in female patients. Only after several months, during which the organism may have caused extensive damage to her reproductive organs, pain is experienced by the infected woman. In trichomoniasis (caused by the protozoan, *Trichomonas vaginalis*), the situation is reversed. Infected women are usually symptomatic (experiencing vaginitis), whereas infected men are usually asymptomatic. These two sexually transmitted diseases are especially difficult to control because people are often unaware that they are infected and unknowingly transmit the pathogens to others during sexual activities.

A **sign of a disease** is defined as some type of objective evidence of a disease. For example, while palpating a patient, a physician might discover a lump or an enlarged liver (hepatomegaly) or spleen (splenomegaly). Other signs of disease include abnormal heart or breath sounds, blood pressure, pulse rate, and laboratory results as well as abnormalities that appear on radiographs, ultrasound studies, or computed tomography scans.

> Signs of a disease are objective findings, such as laboratory test results, which are not perceived by the patient.

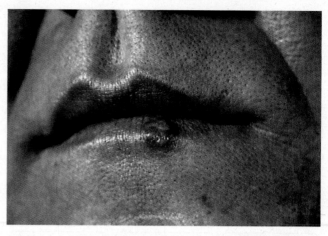

Figure 14-2. Cold sore caused by herpes simplex virus. (Courtesy of Dr. Hermann and the CDC.)

fever, and mucous membrane lesions. These symptoms disappear within weeks to 12 months, and the disease enters a latent stage, which may last for weeks to years (sometimes for a lifetime). During the latent stage, the patient has few or no symptoms. In tertiary syphilis, the spirochetes cause destruction of the organs in

> If not successfully treated, syphilis can progress through several stages, including a latent stage.

Latent Infections

An infectious disease may go from being symptomatic to asymptomatic and then, sometime later, go back to being symptomatic. Such diseases are referred to as **latent infections**, from the Greek word "latens," meaning to lie hidden. Herpes virus infections, such as cold sores (fever blisters), genital herpes infections, and shingles, are examples of latent infections. Cold sores occur intermittently, but the patient continues to harbor the herpes virus between cold sore episodes (Fig. 14-2). The virus remains dormant within cells of the nervous system until some type of stress acts as a trigger. The stressful trigger may be a fever, sunburn, extreme cold, or emotional stress. A person who had chickenpox as a child may harbor the virus throughout his or her lifetime and then, later in life, as the immune system weakens, that person may develop shingles. Shingles, a painful infection of the nerves, is considered a latent manifestation of chickenpox.

> A latent disease is a disease that is lying dormant, not currently manifesting itself.

If not successfully treated, syphilis progresses through primary, secondary, latent, and tertiary stages (Fig. 14-3). During the primary stage, the patient has an open lesion called a chancre, which contains the spirochete *Treponema pallidum* (Fig. 14-4). Four to six weeks after the spirochete enters the bloodstream, the chancre disappears, and the symptoms of the secondary stage arise, including rash,

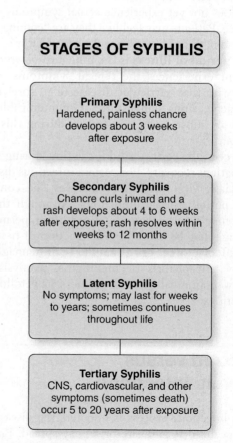

STAGES OF SYPHILIS

Primary Syphilis
Hardened, painless chancre develops about 3 weeks after exposure

Secondary Syphilis
Chancre curls inward and a rash develops about 4 to 6 weeks after exposure; rash resolves within weeks to 12 months

Latent Syphilis
No symptoms; may last for weeks to years; sometimes continues throughout life

Tertiary Syphilis
CNS, cardiovascular, and other symptoms (sometimes death) occur 5 to 20 years after exposure

Figure 14-3. Stages of syphilis.

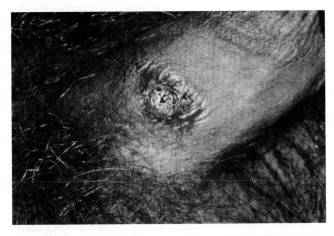

Figure 14-4. Syphilis chancre on penile shaft. (Courtesy of Dr. Gavin Hart, Dr. NJ Fiumara, and the CDC.)

which they have been hiding—the brain, heart, and bone tissue—sometimes leading to death.

Primary versus Secondary Infections

One infectious disease may commonly follow another, in which case the first disease is referred to as a **primary infection** and the second disease is referred to as a **secondary infection**. For example, serious cases of bacterial pneumonia frequently follow relatively mild viral respiratory infections. During the primary infection, the virus causes damage to the ciliated epithelial cells that line the respiratory tract. The function of these cells is to move foreign materials up and out of the respiratory tract and into the throat where they can be swallowed. While coughing, the patient may inhale some saliva, containing an opportunistic bacterial pathogen, such as *Streptococcus pneumoniae* or *Haemophilus influenzae*. Because the ciliated epithelial cells were damaged by the virus, they are unable to clear the bacteria from the lungs. The bacteria then multiply and cause pneumonia. In this example, the viral infection is the primary infection and bacterial pneumonia is the secondary infection.

> A primary infection caused by one pathogen can be followed by a secondary infection caused by a different pathogen.

Steps in the Pathogenesis of Infectious Diseases

In general, the pathogenesis of infectious diseases often follows the following sequence (Fig. 14-5):

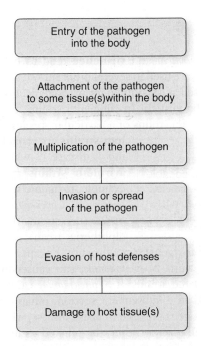

Figure 14-5. Steps in the pathogenesis of infectious diseases. Not all infectious diseases involve *all* of the steps shown. For example, once ingested, some exotoxin-producing intestinal pathogens are capable of causing disease without adhering to the intestinal wall or invading tissue.

1. **Entry** of the pathogen into the body. Portals of entry include penetration of skin or mucous membranes by the pathogen, inoculation of the pathogen into bodily tissues by an arthropod, inhalation (into the respiratory tract), ingestion (into the gastrointestinal tract), introduction of the pathogen into the genitourinary tract, or introduction of the pathogen directly into the blood (e.g., through blood transfusion or the use of shared needles by intravenous drug abusers).
2. **Attachment** of the pathogen to some tissue(s) within the body.
3. **Multiplication** of the pathogen. The pathogen may multiply in one location of the body, resulting in a localized infection (e.g., abscess), or it may multiply throughout the body (a systemic infection).
4. **Invasion or spread** of the pathogen.
5. **Evasion** of host defenses.
6. **Damage to host tissue(s).** The damage may be so extensive as to cause the death of the patient.

> An infection may follow the sequence of entry, attachment, multiplication, invasion, evasion of host defenses, and damage to host tissues.

It is important to understand that not all infectious diseases involve *all* these steps. For example, once ingested, some exotoxin-producing intestinal pathogens are capable of causing disease without adhering to the intestinal wall or invading tissue.

Virulence

The terms *virulent* and **virulence** tend to be confusing because they are used in several different ways. Sometimes virulent is used as a synonym for pathogenic. For example, there may be virulent (pathogenic) strains and *avirulent* (nonpathogenic) strains of a particular species. The **virulent strains** are capable of causing disease, whereas the **avirulent strains** are not. For example, toxigenic strains of the bacterium, *Corynebacterium diphtheriae* (i.e., strains that produce diphtheria toxin) are virulent, whereas nontoxigenic strains are not. Encapsulated strains of the bacterium, *S. pneumoniae*, can cause disease, but nonencapsulated strains of *S. pneumoniae* cannot. As will be discussed in a subsequent section, piliated strains of certain pathogens are able to cause disease, whereas nonpiliated strains are not; thus, the piliated strains are virulent, but the nonpiliated strains are avirulent.

> Virulent strains of a microbe are capable of causing disease, whereas avirulent strains are not.

Sometimes virulence is used to express a measure or degree of pathogenicity. Although all pathogens cause disease, some are more virulent than others (i.e., they are better able to cause disease). In bacterial diarrhea, for example, it only takes about 10 *Shigella* cells to cause shigellosis, but it takes between 100 and 1,000 *Salmonella* cells to cause salmonellosis. Thus, *Shigella* is considered to be more virulent than *Salmonella*. In some cases, certain strains

> Some strains of a given pathogen can be more virulent than other strains.

of a particular species are more virulent than others. For example, the "flesh-eating" strains of the bacterium, *Streptococcus pyogenes*, are more virulent than other strains of *S. pyogenes* because they produce certain necrotizing enzymes that are not produced by the other strains. Similarly, only certain strains of *S. pyogenes* produce **erythrogenic toxin** (the cause of scarlet fever); these strains are considered more virulent than the strains of *S. pyogenes* that do not produce erythrogenic toxin. Strains of the bacterium *Staphylococcus aureus* that produces toxic shock syndrome toxin 1 (TSST-1) are considered more virulent than those that do not produce this toxin.

Sometimes virulence is used in reference to the severity of the infectious diseases that are caused by the pathogens. Used in this manner, one pathogen is more virulent than another if it causes a more serious disease.

Virulence Factors

The physical attributes or properties of pathogens that enable them to escape various host defense mechanisms and cause disease are called **virulence factors**. Virulence factors are phenotypic characteristics that, like all phenotypic characteristics, are dictated by the organism's genotype. Toxins are obvious virulence factors, but other virulence factors are not so obvious. Some virulence factors are shown in Figure 14-6.

> Virulence factors are phenotypic characteristics that enable microbes to be virulent (to cause disease).

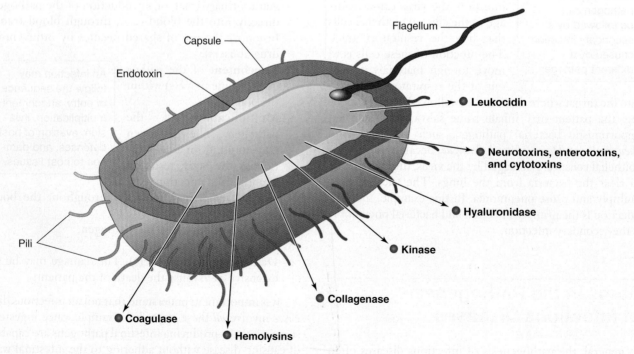

Figure 14-6. Bacterial virulence factors. See text for details.

Flagellum

Capsule

Endotoxin

Leukocidin

Neurotoxins, enterotoxins, and cytotoxins

Hyaluronidase

Kinase

Pili

Collagenase

Coagulase

Hemolysins

Attachment

Perhaps you have noticed that certain pathogens infect dogs but not humans, whereas others infect humans but not dogs. Perhaps you have wondered why certain pathogens cause respiratory infections, whereas others cause gastrointestinal infections. Part of the explanation has to do with the type or types of cells to which the pathogen is able to attach. To cause disease, some pathogens must be able to anchor themselves to cells after they have gained access to the body.

Receptors and Adhesins

The general terms *receptor* and *integrin* are used to describe the molecule on the surface of a host cell that a particular pathogen is able to recognize and attach to (Fig. 14-7). Often, these receptors are glycoprotein molecules. A particular pathogen can only attach to cells bearing the appropriate receptor. Thus, certain viruses cause respiratory infections because they are able to recognize and attach to certain receptors that are present on cells that line the respiratory tract. Because those particular receptors are not present on cells lining the gastrointestinal tract, that virus is unable to cause gastrointestinal infections. Similarly, certain viruses cause infections in dogs, but not in humans, because dog cells possess a receptor that human cells lack.

> Molecules on a host cell's surface that pathogens are able to recognize and attach to are called receptors or integrins.

S. pyogenes cells have an adhesin (called protein F) on their surfaces that enables this pathogen to adhere to a protein—fibronectin—that is found on many host cell surfaces. Human immunodeficiency virus (HIV; the virus that causes acquired immunodeficiency syndrome [AIDS]) is able to attach to cells bearing a surface receptor called CD4. Such cells are known as CD4$^+$ cells. A category of lymphocytes called T-helper cells (the primary target cells for HIV) are examples of CD4$^+$ cells.

The general terms *adhesin* and *ligand* are used to describe the molecule on the surface of a pathogen that is able to recognize and bind to a particular receptor (Fig. 14-7). For example, the adhesin on the envelope of HIV that recognizes and binds to the CD4 receptor is a glycoprotein molecule designated *gp*120. (Entry of HIV into a host cell is a rather complex event, requiring several adhesins and several co-receptors.)

> Molecules on a pathogen's surface that recognize and attach to receptors on a host cell's surface are called adhesins or ligands.

Because adhesins enable pathogens to attach to host cells, they are considered virulence factors. In some cases, antibodies directed against such adhesins prevent the pathogen from attaching and, thus, prevent

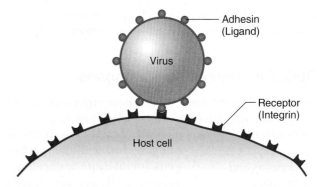

Figure 14-7. Adhesins and receptors. See text for details.

infection by that pathogen. (As will be discussed in Chapter 16, antibodies are proteins that our immune systems produce to protect us from pathogens and infectious diseases.)

Bacterial Fimbriae (Pili)

Bacterial fimbriae (pili) are long, thin, hairlike, flexible projections composed primarily of an array of proteins called pilin (refer back to Fig. 3-13). Fimbriae are considered to be virulence factors because they enable bacteria to attach to surfaces, including various tissues within the human body. Fimbriated (piliated) strains of *N. gonorrhoeae* are able to anchor themselves to the inner walls of the urethra and cause urethritis. Should nonfimbriated (nonpiliated)

> Bacterial fimbriae (pili) are virulence factors, in that they enable fimbriated (piliated) bacteria to adhere to cells and tissues within the human body.

strains of *N. gonorrhoeae* gain access to the urethra, they are flushed out by urination and are thus unable to cause urethritis. Therefore, with respect to urethritis, fimbriated strains of *N. gonorrhoeae* are virulent and nonfimbriated strains are avirulent.

Similarly, fimbriated strains of *Escherichia coli* that gain access to the urinary bladder are able to anchor themselves to the inner walls of the bladder and cause cystitis; thus, with respect to cystitis, fimbriated strains of *E. coli* are virulent. Should nonfimbriated strains of *E. coli* gain access to the urinary bladder, they are flushed out by urination and are unable to cause cystitis; thus, nonfimbriated strains are avirulent.

The fimbriae of group A, β-hemolytic streptococci (*S. pyogenes*) contain molecules of M-protein. M-protein serves as a virulence factor in two ways: (a) it enables the bacteria to adhere to pharyngeal cells; and (b) it protects the cells from being phagocytized by white blood cells (i.e., the M-protein serves an antiphagocytic function).

Other bacterial pathogens possessing fimbriae are *Vibrio cholerae*, *Salmonella* spp., *Shigella* spp., *Pseudomonas aeruginosa*, and *Neisseria meningitidis*. Because bacterial fimbriae enable bacteria to colonize surfaces, they are sometimes referred to as colonization factors.

Obligate Intracellular Pathogens

Certain pathogens, such as Gram-negative bacteria in the genera *Rickettsia* and *Chlamydia* must live within host cells to survive and multiply; they are referred to as **obligate intracellular pathogens** (or obligate intracellular parasites). Rickettsias invade and live within endothelial cells and vascular smooth muscle cells. Rickettsias are capable of

> Rickettsias and chlamydias are obligate intracellular pathogens.

synthesizing proteins, nucleic acids, and adenosine triphosphate (ATP), but are thought to require an intracellular environment because they possess an unusual membrane transport system; they are said to have leaky membranes.

The different species and serotypes of chlamydias invade different types of cells, including conjunctival epithelial cells and cells of the respiratory and genital tracts. Although chlamydias produce ATP molecules, they preferentially use ATP molecules produced by host cells; this has earned them the title of "energy parasites." In the laboratory, obligate intracellular pathogens are propagated using cell cultures, laboratory animals, or embryonated chicken eggs.

Ehrlichia spp. and *Anaplasma phagocytophilum* are Gram-negative bacteria that closely resemble *Rickettsia* spp. They are **intraleukocytic pathogens**. *Ehrlichia* spp. live within monocytes, causing a disease known as human monocytic ehrlichiosis. *A. phagocytophilum* lives within granulocytes, causing a condition known as human anaplasmosis (formerly called human granulocytic ehrlichiosis). Certain sporozoan

> *Ehrlichia* and *Anaplasma* spp. are intraleukocytic pathogens, whereas *Plasmodium* and *Babesia* spp. are intraerythrocytic pathogens.

protozoa, such as the *Plasmodium* spp. that cause human malaria and the *Babesia* spp. that cause human babesiosis, are **intraerythrocytic pathogens** (i.e., they live within erythrocytes).

Facultative Intracellular Pathogens

Some pathogens, referred to as **facultative intracellular pathogens** (or facultative intracellular parasites), are capable of both an intracellular and extracellular existence. Many facultative intracellular pathogens that

> Pathogens that can live both within and outside of host cells are called facultative intracellular pathogens.

can be grown in the laboratory on artificial culture media are also able to survive *within* phagocytes. How facultative

intracellular pathogens are able to survive within phagocytes is discussed in the next section. Phagocytosis is discussed in greater detail in Chapter 15.

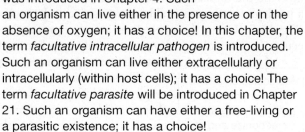

STUDY AID
The Word Facultative

Wherever the word *facultative* appears in this book, it implies a choice. For example, the term *facultative anaerobe* was introduced in Chapter 4. Such an organism can live either in the presence or in the absence of oxygen; it has a choice! In this chapter, the term *facultative intracellular pathogen* is introduced. Such an organism can live either extracellularly or intracellularly (within host cells); it has a choice! The term *facultative parasite* will be introduced in Chapter 21. Such an organism can have either a free-living or a parasitic existence; it has a choice!

Intracellular Survival Mechanisms

As will be discussed in Chapter 15, phagocytes play an important role in our defenses against pathogens. The two most important categories of phagocytes in the human body (referred to as "professional phagocytes") are macrophages and neutrophils. Once phagocytized, most pathogens are destroyed within the phagocytes by hydrolytic enzymes (e.g., lysozyme, proteases, lipases, DNase, RNase, myelo-

> The two most important categories of phagocytes in the human body—referred to as "professional phagocytes"—are macrophages and neutrophils.

peroxidase), hydrogen peroxide, superoxide anions, and other mechanisms. However, certain pathogens are able to survive and multiply within phagocytes after being ingested (Table 14-1).

Some pathogens (such as the bacterium, *M. tuberculosis*) have a cell wall composition that resists digestion. Mycobacterial cell walls contain waxes, and it is thought that these waxes protect the organisms from digestion. Other pathogens (such as the protozoan, *Toxoplasma gondii*) prevent the fusion of lysosomes

> Many bacteria, including *M. tuberculosis*, are facultative intracellular pathogens.

(vesicles that contain digestive enzymes) with the phagocytic vacuole (phagosome). Other pathogens, such as the bacterium, *Rickettsia rickettsii*, produce phospholipases that destroy the phagosome membrane, thus preventing

Table 14-1 Pathogens That Routinely Remain Virulent and Multiply within Macrophages

Category of Pathogens	Examples	Disease(s)
Viruses	Herpes viruses	Genital herpes, herpes labialis (cold sores or fever blisters)
	HIV	AIDS
	Rubeola virus	Measles
	Poxviruses	Smallpox, monkeypox
Rickettsias	R. rickettsii	Rocky Mountain spotted fever
	Rickettsia prowazeki	Epidemic (louseborne) typhus
Other bacteria	Brucella spp.	Brucellosis
	L. pneumophila	Legionellosis
	L. monocytogenes	Listeriosis
	Mycobacterium leprae	Hansen disease (leprosy)
	M. tuberculosis	Tuberculosis
Protozoa	Leishmania spp.	Leishmaniasis
	T. gondii	Toxoplasmosis
	Trypanosoma cruzi	Chagas disease (American trypanosomiasis)
Fungi	C. neoformans	Cryptococcosis

lysosome–phagosome fusion. Other pathogens (such as the bacteria, *Brucella abortus, Francisella tularensis, Legionella pneumophila, Listeria monocytogenes, Salmonella* spp., and *Yersinia pestis*) are able to survive by means of mechanisms that are not yet understood.

Capsules

Bacterial capsules (refer back to Fig. 3-10) are considered to be virulence factors because they serve an antiphagocytic function (i.e., they protect encapsulated bacteria from being phagocytized by phagocytic white blood cells). Phagocytes are unable to attach to encapsulated bacteria because they lack surface receptors for the polysaccharide material of which the capsule is made. If they cannot adhere to the bacteria, they cannot ingest them. Because encapsulated bacteria that gain access to the bloodstream or tissues are protected from phagocytosis, they are able to multiply, invade, and cause disease. Nonencapsulated bacteria, on the other

> Bacterial capsules serve an antiphagocytic function (i.e., they protect encapsulated bacteria from being phagocytized).

hand, are phagocytized and killed. Encapsulated bacteria include *S. pneumoniae, Klebsiella pneumoniae, H. influenzae,* and *N. meningitidis.* The capsule of the yeast, *Cryptococcus neoformans,* is also considered to be a virulence factor (refer back to Fig. 5-12).

Flagella

Bacterial *flagella* are considered virulence factors because flagella enable flagellated (motile) bacteria to invade aqueous areas of the body that nonflagellated (nonmotile) bacteria are unable to reach. Perhaps flagella also enable bacteria to avoid phagocytosis—it is more difficult for phagocytes to catch a moving target.

> Flagella are considered to be virulence factors because they enable flagellated bacteria to invade areas of the body that nonflagellated bacteria cannot reach.

Exoenzymes

Although pili, capsules, and flagella are considered virulence factors, they really do not explain how bacteria and other pathogens actually *cause* disease. **The major mechanisms by which pathogens cause disease are certain exoenzymes or toxins that they produce.** Some pathogens (e.g., certain strains of *S. pyogenes*) produce *both* exoenzymes and toxins.

> The most important virulence factors are certain exoenzymes and toxins that pathogens produce.

Some pathogens release enzymes (called **exoenzymes**) that enable them to evade host defense mechanisms, invade, or cause damage to body tissues.[a] These exoenzymes include necrotizing enzymes, coagulase, kinases, hyaluronidase, collagenase, hemolysins, and lecithinase.

Necrotizing Enzymes

Many pathogens produce exoenzymes that destroy tissues; these are collectively referred to as necrotizing enzymes. Notorious examples are the flesh-eating strains of *S. pyogenes,* which produce proteases and other enzymes that cause very rapid destruction of soft tissue, leading to a disease called necrotizing fasciitis

> Necrotizing enzymes are exoenzymes that cause destruction of cells and tissues.

(Fig. 14-8). The various *Clostridium* species that cause gas gangrene (myonecrosis) produce a variety of necrotizing enzymes, including proteases and lipases.

[a]Enzymes that are produced within cells and remain within those cells to catalyze intracellular reactions are called endoenzymes.

① **Day 0:** Right lower leg was edematous with an erythematous area below the knee.

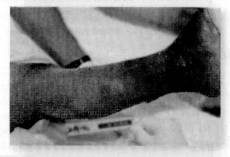

② **Day 2:** Initial debridement revealed necrotic tissue with many layers of thrombosed blood vessels.

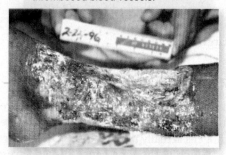

③ **Day 6:** Radical debridement was performed because the infectious process was progressing toward the knee. Subsequent skin grafts (not shown) took well and the wound healed without complications.

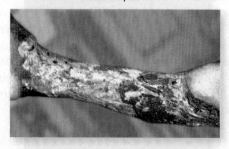

Figure 14-8. Progress of the disease known as necrotizing fasciitis. Edematous means swollen, erythematous means reddened, debridement refers to removal of damaged tissue, and thrombosed means clotted. (From Harvey RA, et al. *Lippincott's Illustrated Reviews: Microbiology.* 3rd ed. Philadelphia, PA: Lippincott Williams & Wilkins; 2013.)

Coagulase

An important identifying feature of *S. aureus* in the laboratory is its ability to produce a protein called **coagulase**. Coagulase binds to prothrombin, forming a complex called staphylothrombin. The protease activity of thrombin is activated in this complex, causing the

> Coagulase is a virulence factor that causes clotting.

conversion of fibrinogen to fibrin. In the body, coagulase may enable *S. aureus* to clot plasma and thereby to form a sticky coat of fibrin around themselves for protection from phagocytes, antibodies, and other host defense mechanisms.

Kinases

Kinases (also known as fibrinolysins) have the opposite effect of coagulase. Sometimes the host will cause a fibrin clot to form around pathogens in an attempt to wall them off and prevent them from invading deeper into body tissues. Kinases are enzymes that lyse (dissolve) clots; therefore, pathogens that produce kinases are able to escape from clots. **Streptokinase** is the name of a

> Kinases are exoenzymes that dissolve clots.

kinase produced by streptococci, and **staphylokinase** is the name of a kinase produced by staphylococci. Streptokinase has been used to treat patients with coronary thrombosis. Because *S. aureus* produces both coagulase and staphylokinase, it can not only cause the formation of clots, but also dissolve them.

Hyaluronidase

The "spreading factor," as **hyaluronidase** is sometimes called, enables pathogens to spread through connective tissue by breaking down **hyaluronic acid**, the polysaccharide "cement" that holds tissue cells together. Hyaluronidase is secreted by several pathogenic species of *Staphylococcus, Streptococcus*, and *Clostridium*.

> Hyaluronidase and collagenase are virulence factors that dissolve hyaluronic acid and collagen, respectively, enabling pathogens to invade deeper into tissues.

Collagenase

The enzyme **collagenase**, produced by certain pathogens, breaks down collagen (the supportive protein found in tendons, cartilage, and bones). This enables the pathogens to invade tissues. *Clostridium perfringens*, a major cause of gas gangrene, spreads deeply within the body by secreting both collagenase and hyaluronidase.

Hemolysins

Hemolysins are enzymes that cause damage to the host's red blood cells (erythrocytes). The lysis (bursting or destruction) of red blood cells not only harms the host but also provides the pathogens with a source

> Hemolysins are enzymes that damage red blood cells.

of iron. In the laboratory, the effect an organism has on the red blood cells in blood agar enables differentiation between α-hemolytic and β-hemolytic bacteria. The hemolysins produced by α-hemolytic bacteria cause a partial breakdown of hemoglobin in the red blood cells, resulting in a green zone around the colonies of α-hemolytic bacteria. The hemolysins produced by β-hemolytic bacteria cause complete lysis of the red blood cells, resulting in a clear zone around the colonies of β-hemolytic bacteria (refer back to Fig. 13-15). Hemolysins are produced by many pathogenic bacteria, but the type of hemolysis produced by an organism is of most importance when attempting to speciate a *Streptococcus* in the laboratory. Some *Streptococcus* spp. are α-hemolytic, some are β-hemolytic, and some are γ-hemolytic (nonhemolytic).

Lecithinase

C. perfringens, the major cause of gas gangrene, is able to rapidly destroy extensive areas of tissue, especially muscle tissue. One of the enzymes produced by *C. perfringens*, called **lecithinase**, breaks down phospholipids that are collectively referred to as **lecithin**. This enzyme is destructive to cell membranes of red blood cells and other tissues.

> Lecithinase is an exoenzyme that causes destruction of host cell membranes.

Toxins

The ability of pathogens to damage host tissues and cause disease may depend on the production and release of various types of poisonous substances, referred to as toxins. The two major categories of toxins are endotoxins and exotoxins. **Endotoxins**, which are integral parts of the cell walls of Gram-negative bacteria, can cause a number of adverse physiologic effects. **Exotoxins**, on the other hand, are toxins that are produced within cells and then released from the cells.

> The two major categories of toxins are endotoxins and exotoxins.

Endotoxin

Septicemia (often referred to as *sepsis*) is a very serious disease consisting of chills, fever, prostration (extreme exhaustion), and the presence of bacteria or their toxins in the bloodstream. Septicemia caused by Gram-negative bacteria, sometimes referred to as Gram-negative sepsis, is an especially serious type of septicemia. The cell walls of Gram-negative bacteria contain lipopolysaccharide, the lipid portion of which is called lipid-A or endotoxin. Endotoxin can cause serious, adverse, physiologic effects such as fever and shock. Substances that cause fever are known as **pyrogens**.

> Endotoxin is a component of the cell walls of Gram-negative bacteria. It can cause fever and shock.

Shock is a life-threatening condition resulting from very low blood pressure and an inadequate blood supply to body tissues and organs, especially the kidneys and brain. The type of shock that results from Gram-negative sepsis is known as **septic shock**. Symptoms include reduced mental alertness, confusion, rapid breathing, chills, fever, and warm, flushed skin. As shock worsens, several organs

begin to fail, including the kidneys, the lungs, and the heart. Blood clots may form within blood vessels. More than 500,000 cases of sepsis occur annually in the United States; approximately half of these are caused by Gram-negative bacteria. There is a 30% to 35% mortality rate associated with Gram-negative sepsis.

Exotoxins

Exotoxins are poisonous proteins that are secreted by a variety of pathogens; they are often named for the target organs that they affect. Examples include neurotoxins, enterotoxins, cytotoxins, exfoliative toxin, erythrogenic toxin, and diphtheria toxin.

> Exotoxins are poisonous proteins that are secreted by a variety of pathogens.

The most potent exotoxins are **neurotoxins**, which affect the central nervous system (CNS). The neurotoxins produced by *Clostridium tetani* and *Clostridium botulinum*—tetanospasmin and botulinal toxin—cause tetanus and botulism, respectively. Tetanospasmin affects control of nerve transmission, leading to a spastic, rigid type of paralysis in which the patient's muscles are contracted (Fig. 14-9). Botulinal toxin also blocks nerve impulses but by a different mechanism, leading to a generalized, flaccid type of paralysis in which the patient's muscles are relaxed. Both diseases are often fatal. See thePoint for "A Closer Look at Botulinal Toxin."

> Neurotoxins are exotoxins that adversely affect the CNS.

Other types of exotoxins, called **enterotoxins**, are toxins that affect the gastrointestinal tract, often causing diarrhea and sometimes vomiting. Examples of bacterial pathogens that produce enterotoxins are *Bacillus cereus*, certain serotypes of *E. coli*, *Clostridium difficile*, *C. perfringens*, *Salmonella* spp., *Shigella* spp., *Vibrio cholerae*, and some strains of *S. aureus*. In addition to releasing an enterotoxin (called toxin A), *C. difficile* also produces a cytotoxin (called toxin B) that damages the lining of the colon, leading to a condition known as pseudomembranous colitis.

> Enterotoxins are exotoxins that adversely affect the gastrointestinal tract.

Symptoms of toxic shock syndrome are caused by exotoxins secreted by certain strains of *S. aureus* and, less commonly, *S. pyogenes*. Staphylococcal TSST-1 primarily affects the integrity of capillary walls. **Exfoliative toxin** (or epidermolytic toxin) of *S. aureus* causes the epidermal layers of skin to slough away, leading to a disease known as scalded skin syndrome. *S. aureus* also produces a variety of toxins that destroy cell membranes.

> Erythrogenic toxin, produced by some strains of *S. pyogenes*, causes scarlet fever.

Erythrogenic toxin, produced by some strains of *S. pyogenes*, causes scarlet fever. **Leukocidins** are toxins that destroy white blood cells (leukocytes). Thus, leukocidins

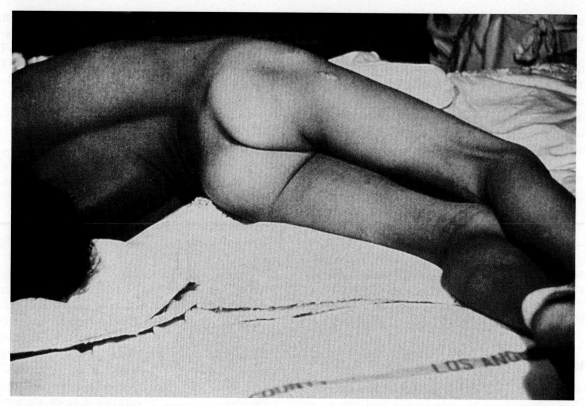

Figure 14-9. Tetanus patient displaying the bodily posture known as opisthotonos. This condition of abnormal posturing involves rigidity and severe arching of the back, with the head thrown backward. If a patient displaying opisthotonos was placed on their back, only the back of their head and their heels would touch the supporting surface. (Courtesy of the CDC.)

(which are produced by some staphylococci, streptococci, and clostridia) cause destruction of the very cells that the body sends to the site of infection to ingest and destroy pathogens.

Diphtheria toxin, produced by toxigenic strains of *C. diphtheriae*, inhibits protein synthesis. It kills mucosal epithelial cells and phagocytes and adversely affects the heart and nervous system. The toxin is actually coded for by a bacteriophage gene. Thus, only *C. diphtheriae* cells that are "infected" with that particular bacteriophage are able to produce diphtheria toxin. Other exotoxins that inhibit protein synthesis are *Pseudomonas aeruginosa* exotoxin A, Shiga toxin (produced by *Shigella* spp.), and Shiga-like toxins produced by certain serotypes of *E. coli*.

> Diphtheria toxin is produced by some strains of *C. diphtheriae*, referred to as toxigenic strains.

Table 14-2 provides a recap of bacterial virulence factors described so far.

Mechanisms by Which Pathogens Escape Immune Responses

Immunology, the study of the immune system, is discussed in detail in Chapter 16. A primary role of the immune system is to recognize and destroy pathogens that invade our bodies. However, there are many ways in which pathogens avoid being destroyed by immune responses. Several mechanisms will be mentioned here; others are beyond the scope of this book.

Antigenic Variation

As discussed in Chapter 16, antigens are foreign molecules that evoke an immune response—often stimulating the immune system to produce antibodies. Some pathogens are able to periodically change their surface antigens, a phenomenon known as **antigenic variation**. About the time that the host has produced antibodies in response to the pathogen's surface antigens, those antigens are shed and new ones appear in their place. This renders the antibodies worthless, because they have nothing to adhere to. Examples of pathogens capable of antigenic variation are influenza viruses, HIV, *Borrelia recurrentis* (the causative agent of relapsing fever), *N. gonorrhoeae*, and the parasitic trypanosomes that cause African trypanosomiasis. Trypanosomes can keep up their antigenic variation for 20 years, never presenting the same surface antigens twice.

> Some pathogens periodically change their surface antigens, a phenomenon known as antigenic variation.

Camouflage and Molecular Mimicry

Adult schistosome worms (trematodes that cause schistosomiasis) are able to conceal their foreign nature by coating themselves with host proteins—a sort of

Table 14-2 Recap of Bacterial Virulence Factors

Virulence Factor	Comments
Bacterial structures	
Flagella	Enable bacteria to gain access to anatomic areas that nonmotile bacteria cannot reach; may enable bacteria to "escape" from phagocytes
Capsules	Serve an antiphagocytic function
Pili	Enable bacteria to attach to surfaces
Enzymes	
Coagulase	Enables bacteria to produce clots within which to "hide"
Kinases	Enable bacteria to dissolve clots
Hyaluronidase	Dissolves hyaluronic acid, enabling bacteria to penetrate deeper into tissues
Lecithinase	Destroys cell membranes
Necrotizing enzymes	Cause massive destruction of tissues
Toxins	
Endotoxin	Released from the cell walls of Gram-negative bacteria; causes fever and septic shock
Exotoxins	Produced within the cell, but then released from the cell
Neurotoxins	Cause damage to the CNS; tetanospasmin and botulinal toxin are examples
Enterotoxins	Cause gastrointestinal disease
C. difficile toxin B	The cytotoxin that causes pseudomembranous colitis
S. aureus TSST-1	The toxin that causes most cases of toxic shock syndrome
Exfoliative toxin	Produced by some strains of *S. aureus*; causes scalded skin syndrome
Erythrogenic toxin	Produced by some strains of *S. pyogenes*; causes scarlet fever
Diphtheria toxin	Produced by toxigenic strains of *C. diphtheriae*; causes diphtheria
Leukocidins	Cause the destruction of leukocytes

subdued immune response against the pathogens, it is known that the hyaluronic acid capsule of streptococci is almost identical to the hyaluronic acid component of human connective tissue. It is also interesting that in mycoplasmal pneumonia, antibodies produced by the host against antigens of *Mycoplasma pneumoniae* can cause damage to the host's heart, lung, brain, and red blood cells.

Destruction of Antibodies
Several bacterial pathogens, including *H. influenzae*, *N. gonorrhoeae*, and streptococci, produce an enzyme (IgA protease) that destroys IgA antibodies. Thus, these pathogens are capable of destroying some of the antibodies that the host's immune system has produced in an attempt to destroy them.

ON thePoint

- Terms Introduced in This Chapter
- Review of Key Points
- A Closer Look at Botulinal Toxin
- Increase Your Knowledge
- Critical Thinking
- Additional Self-Assessment Exercises

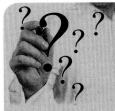

Self-Assessment Exercises

After studying this chapter, answer the following multiple-choice questions.

1. Which of the following virulence factors enable(s) bacteria to attach to tissues?
   a. capsules
   b. endotoxin
   c. flagella
   d. pili

2. Neurotoxins are produced by:
   a. *Clostridium botulinum* and *Clostridium tetani*
   b. *Clostridium difficile* and *Clostridium perfringens*
   c. *Pseudomonas aeruginosa* and *Mycobacterium tuberculosis*
   d. *Staphylococcus aureus* and *Streptococcus pyogenes*

camouflage. In molecular mimicry, the pathogen's surface antigens closely resemble host antigens and are therefore not recognized as being foreign. Although there is little evidence to prove that molecular mimicry leads to a

In molecular mimicry, pathogens cover their surface antigens with host proteins, so the pathogens will not be recognized as being foreign.

3. Which of the following pathogens produce enterotoxins?

a. *Bacillus cereus* and certain serotypes of *Escherichia coli*
b. *C. difficile* and *C. perfringens*
c. *Salmonella* spp. and *Shigella* spp.
d. all of the above

4. A bloodstream infection with _____ could result in the release of endotoxin into the bloodstream.

a. *C. difficile* or *C. perfringens*
b. *Neisseria gonorrhoeae* or *E. coli*
c. *S. aureus* or *M. tuberculosis*
d. *S. aureus* or *S. pyogenes*

5. Communicable diseases are most easily transmitted during the:

a. incubation period
b. period of convalescence
c. period of illness
d. prodromal period

6. Enterotoxins affect cells in the:

a. central nervous system
b. gastrointestinal tract
c. genitourinary tract
d. respiratory tract

7. Which of the following bacteria is *least* likely to be the cause of septic shock?

a. *E. coli*
b. *Haemophilus influenzae*
c. *Mycoplasma pneumoniae*
d. *Neisseria meningitidis*

8. Which of the following produces both a cytotoxin and an enterotoxin?

a. *C. botulinum*
b. *C. difficile*
c. *C. tetani*
d. *Corynebacterium diphtheriae*

9. Which of the following virulence factors enable(s) bacteria to avoid phagocytosis by white blood cells?

a. capsule
b. cell membrane
c. cell wall
d. pili

10. Which of the following can cause toxic shock syndrome?

a. *C. difficile* and *C. perfringens*
b. *M. pneumoniae* and *M. tuberculosis*
c. *N. gonorrhoeae* and *E. coli*
d. *S. aureus* and *S. pyogenes*

15

Nonspecific Host Defense Mechanisms

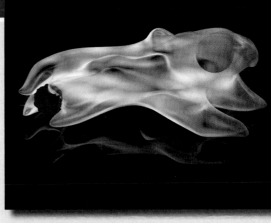

Artist rendering of a phagocytic white blood cell phagocytizing an object.

 CHAPTER OUTLINE

Introduction

Nonspecific Host Defense Mechanisms

First Line of Defense

Skin and Mucous Membranes as Physical Barriers
Cellular and Chemical Factors
Microbial Antagonism

Second Line of Defense

Transferrin
Fever
Interferons
The Complement System
Acute-Phase Proteins
Cytokines
Inflammation
Phagocytosis
    Chemotaxis
    Attachment
    Ingestion
    Digestion
Mechanisms by Which Pathogens Escape Destruction
   by Phagocytes
Disorders and Conditions That Adversely Affect
   Phagocytic and Inflammatory Processes
    Leukopenia
    Disorders and Conditions Affecting Leukocyte Motility
     and Chemotaxis
    Disorders and Conditions Affecting Intracellular Killing
     by Phagocytes
    Additional Factors

 LEARNING OBJECTIVES

After studying this chapter, you should be able to:

- Define the following terms: host defense mechanisms, antibody, antigen, lysozyme, microbial antagonism, colicin, bacteriocins, superinfection, pyrogen, interferon, complement cascade, complement, opsonization, inflammation, vasodilation, phagocytosis, and chemotaxis
- Briefly describe the three lines of defense used by the body to combat pathogens and give one example of each
- Explain what is meant by "nonspecific host defense mechanisms" and how they differ from "specific host defense mechanisms"
- Identify three ways by which the digestive system is protected from pathogens
- Describe how interferons function as host defense mechanisms
- Name three cellular and chemical responses to microbial invasion
- Describe the major benefits of complement activation
- List the four main signs and symptoms associated with inflammation
- Discuss the four primary purposes of the inflammatory response
- Describe the four steps in phagocytosis
- Identify the three major categories of leukocytes and the three categories of granulocytes
- State four ways in which pathogens escape destruction by phagocytes
- Categorize the disorders and conditions that affect the body's nonspecific host mechanisms

Introduction

In Chapter 14, you discovered the ways in which pathogens cause infectious diseases. In this chapter and the next, you will learn how our bodies combat pathogens in an attempt to prevent the infectious diseases that they cause.

Humans and animals have survived on Earth for hundreds of thousands of years because they have many built-in or naturally occurring mechanisms of defense against pathogens and the infectious diseases that they cause. The ability of any animal to resist these invaders and recover from disease is attributable to many complex interacting functions within the body.

Host defense mechanisms—ways in which the body protects itself from pathogens—can be thought of as an army consisting of three lines of defense (Fig. 15-1).

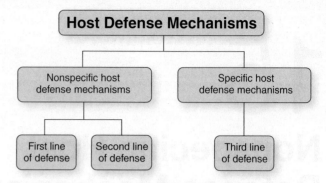

Figure 15-2. **Categories of host defense mechanisms.**

If the enemy (the pathogen) breaks through the first line of defense, it will encounter and, hopefully, be stopped by the second line of defense. If the enemy manages to break through and escape the first two lines of defense, there is a third line of defense ready to attack it.

The first two lines of defense are nonspecific; these are ways in which the body attempts to destroy *all* types of substances that are foreign to it, including pathogens. The third line of defense, the immune response, is very specific. In the third line of defense (or *specific host defense mechanisms*), special proteins called *antibodies* are usually produced in the body in response to the presence of foreign substances. These foreign substances are called **antigens** because they stimulate the production of specific antibodies; they are "**anti**body-**gen**erating" substances. The antibodies that are produced are very specific,

> The first two lines of defense are nonspecific, in the sense that they are directed against *any* foreign substances that enter our bodies. The third line of defense, on the other hand, is very specific.

in that they usually can only recognize and attach to the antigen that stimulated their production. Immune responses are discussed in greater detail in Chapter 16. The various categories of host defense mechanisms are summarized in Figure 15-2.[a]

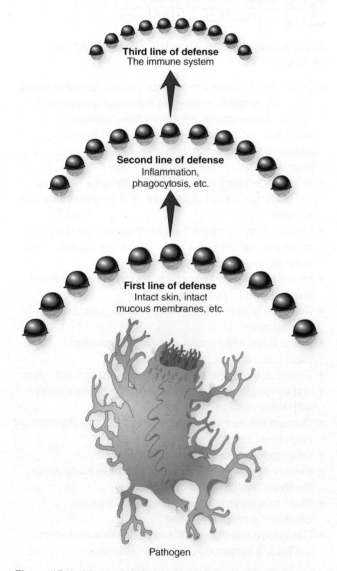

Figure 15-1. **Lines of defense.** Host defense mechanisms—ways in which the body protects itself from pathogens—can be thought of as an entrenched army consisting of three lines of defense. (See text for details.)

Nonspecific Host Defense Mechanisms

Nonspecific host defense mechanisms are general and serve to protect the body against many harmful substances. One of the nonspecific host defenses is the

---

[a]Some immunologists consider both the second and third lines of defense as parts of the immune system. They refer to the second line of defense as *innate immune responses* (those not requiring immunologic memory) and the third line of defense as *acquired immune responses*.

innate, or inborn, resistance observed among some species of animals and some persons who have a natural resistance to certain diseases. Innate or inherited characteristics make these people and animals more resistant to some diseases than to others. The exact factors that produce this innate resistance are not well understood, but are probably related to chemical, physiologic, and temperature differences between the species as well as the general state of physical and emotional health of the person and environmental factors that affect certain races, but not others.

Although we are usually unaware of it, our bodies are constantly in the process of defending us against microbial invaders. We encounter pathogens and potential pathogens many times per day, every day of our lives. Usually, our bodies successfully ward off or destroy the invading microbes. Nonspecific host defense mechanisms discussed in this chapter include mechanical and physical barriers to invasion, chemical factors, microbial antagonism by our indigenous microbiota, fever, the inflammatory response (inflammation), and phagocytic white blood cells (phagocytes).

First Line of Defense

Skin and Mucous Membranes as Physical Barriers

The intact, unbroken skin that covers our bodies represents a nonspecific host defense mechanism, in that it serves as a physical or mechanical barrier to pathogens. Very few pathogens are able to penetrate intact skin. Although certain helminth infections (e.g., hookworm infection, schistosomiasis) are acquired by penetration of the skin by parasites, it is unlikely that many, if any, bacteria are capable of penetrating intact skin. In most cases, it is only when the skin is cut, abraded (scratched), or burned that pathogens gain entrance or when they are injected through the skin (e.g., by arthropods or the sharing of needles by intravenous drug abusers). Even the tiniest of cuts (a paper cut, for example) can serve as a portal of entry for pathogens.

Although they are composed of only a single layer of cells, mucous membranes also serve as a physical or mechanical barrier to pathogens. Most pathogens can only pass through when these membranes are cut or scratched. As is true for skin, even the tiniest of cuts can serve as portals of entry for pathogens. The sticky mucus that is produced by goblet cells within the mucous membranes serves to entrap invaders; thus, it is considered part of the first line of defense.

> Intact skin and mucous membranes act as nonspecific host defense mechanisms by serving as physical or mechanical barriers to pathogens.

Cellular and Chemical Factors

Not only does skin provide a physical barrier, but there are several additional factors that account for the skin's ability to resist pathogens. The dryness of most areas of skin inhibits colonization by many pathogens. Also, the acidity (pH ~5.0) and temperature ($<37°C$) of the skin inhibit the growth of pathogens. The oily sebum that is produced by sebaceous glands in the skin contains fatty acids, which are toxic to some pathogens. Perspiration serves as a nonspecific host defense mechanism by flushing organisms from pores and the surface of the skin. Perspiration also contains the enzyme, *lysozyme*, which degrades peptidoglycan in bacterial cell walls (especially Gram-positive bacteria). Even the sloughing off of dead skin cells removes potential pathogens from the skin.

> The dryness, acidity, and temperature of the skin inhibit colonization and growth of pathogens; perspiration flushes them away.

In addition to being sticky, the mucus produced at mucous membranes contains a variety of substances (e.g., lysozyme, lactoferrin, lactoperoxidase) that can kill bacteria or inhibit their growth. As previously mentioned, lysozyme destroys bacterial cell walls by degrading peptidoglycan. *Lactoferrin* is a protein that binds iron, a mineral that is required by all pathogens. Because they are unable to compete with lactoferrin for free iron, the pathogens are deprived of this essential nutrient. *Lactoperoxidase* is an enzyme that produces superoxide radicals, highly reactive forms of oxygen, which are toxic to bacteria.

> Sticky mucus serves as a nonspecific host defense mechanism by trapping pathogens. It also contains toxic substances, such as lysozyme, lactoferrin, and lactoperoxidase.

Because mucosal cells are among the most rapidly dividing cells in the body, they are constantly being produced and released from mucous membranes. Bacteria that are adhering to the cells are often expelled along with the cells to which they are attached.

The respiratory system would be particularly accessible to invaders that could ride in on dust or other particles inhaled with each breath were it not for the hair, mucous membranes, and irregular chambers of the nose that serve to trap much of the inhaled debris. Also, the cilia (mucociliary covering) present on epithelial cells of the posterior nasal membranes, nasal sinuses, bronchi, and trachea sweep the trapped dust and microbes upward toward the throat, where they are swallowed or expelled by sneezing and coughing. Damage

> The mucociliary covering on epithelial cells in the respiratory tract moves trapped dust and microbes upward toward the throat, where they are swallowed or expelled.

to these ciliated epithelial cells (e.g., damage caused by smoking, other pollutants, bacterial or viral respiratory infections) can increase a person's susceptibility to bacterial respiratory infections. Phagocytes in the mucous membranes may also be involved in this mucociliary clearance mechanism.

Lysozyme and other enzymes that lyse or destroy bacteria are present in nasal secretions, saliva, and tears. Even the swallowing of saliva can be thought of as a nonspecific host defense mechanism because thousands of bacteria are removed from the oral cavity every time we swallow. Humans swallow approximately 1 L of saliva per day.

To a certain extent, the following factors protect the gastrointestinal (GI) tract from bacterial colonization and are therefore considered to be nonspecific host defense mechanisms:

- Digestive enzymes
- Acidity of the stomach (pH ~1.5)
- Alkalinity of the intestines

> Pathogens entering the GI tract are often killed by digestive enzymes or the acidity or alkalinity of different anatomical regions.

Bile, which is secreted from the liver into the small intestine, lowers the surface tension and causes chemical changes in bacterial cell walls and membranes that make bacteria easier to digest. As a result of the combination of stomach acid, bile salts, and the rapid flow of its contents, the small intestine is relatively free of bacteria. Many invading microbes are trapped in the sticky, mucous lining of the digestive tract, where they may be destroyed by bactericidal enzymes and phagocytes. Peristalsis and the expulsion of feces serve to remove bacteria from the intestine. Bacteria make up about 50% of feces.

> Peristalsis and urination serve to remove pathogens from the GI tract and urinary tract, respectively.

The urinary tract is usually sterile in healthy persons, with the exception of indigenous microbes that colonize the distal urethra (that part of the urethra furthest from the urinary bladder). Microbes are continually flushed from the urethra by frequent urination and expulsion of mucus secretions. Many urinary bladder infections result from infrequent urination, including the failure to urinate after sexual intercourse. Conditions that obstruct urine flow (e.g., benign prostatic hyperplasia) also increase the chances of developing cystitis. The low pH of vaginal fluid usually inhibits colonization of the vagina by pathogens. However, women who are taking certain oral contraceptives are particularly susceptible to some infections because the contraceptives increase the pH of the vagina.

> The acidity of vaginal fluid usually inhibits colonization of the vagina by pathogens.

Microbial Antagonism

As mentioned in Chapter 10, when resident microbes of the indigenous microbiota prevent colonization by new arrivals to a particular anatomical site, it is known as *microbial antagonism*. This is another example of a nonspecific host defense mechanism. The inhibitory capability of the indigenous microbiota has been attributed to the following factors:

- Competition for colonization sites
- Competition for nutrients
- Production of substances that kill other bacteria

> When indigenous microbiota prevent the establishment of arriving pathogens, it is known as microbial antagonism.

It is thought that the indigenous microbiota of the skin, oral cavity, upper respiratory tract, and colon play a major role as a nonspecific host defense mechanism by preventing pathogens and potential pathogens from colonizing these sites. The effectiveness of microbial antagonism is frequently decreased after prolonged administration of broad-spectrum antibiotics. The antibiotics reduce or eliminate certain members of the indigenous microbiota (e.g., the vaginal and GI microbes), leading to overgrowth by bacteria or fungi that are resistant to the antibiotic(s) being administered. This overgrowth or "population explosion" of organisms is called a *superinfection*. A superinfection of *Candida albicans* yeasts in the vagina may lead to the condition known as yeast vaginitis. A superinfection of *Clostridium difficile* bacteria in the colon may lead to *C. difficile*–associated diseases known as antibiotic-associated diarrhea (AAD) and pseudomembranous colitis (PMC).

> A decrease in the number of indigenous microbiota at a particular anatomical site can lead to an overgrowth of pathogens or opportunistic pathogens present at the site; this is referred to as a *superinfection*.

Some bacteria produce proteins that kill other bacteria; collectively, these antibacterial substances are known as *bacteriocins*. An example is *colicin*, which is produced by certain strains of *Escherichia coli*. Similar antibacterial substances are produced by some strains of *Pseudomonas* and *Bacillus* species as well as by certain other bacteria. Bacteriocins have a narrower range of activity than do antibiotics, but they are more potent than antibiotics.

> Colicin and other bacteriocins are proteins produced by some bacteria that kill other bacteria.

Second Line of Defense

Pathogens able to penetrate the first line of defense are usually destroyed by nonspecific cellular and chemical responses, collectively referred to as the second line of

> Transferrin, fever, interferons, the complement system, inflammation, and phagocytosis are all part of the second line of defense.

defense. A complex sequence of events develops involving production of fever, production of interferons, activation of the complement system, inflammation, chemotaxis, and phagocytosis. Each of these responses is discussed in this chapter.

Transferrin

Transferrin, a glycoprotein synthesized in the liver, has a high affinity for iron. Its normal function is to store and deliver iron to host cells. Like lactoferrin (mentioned earlier), transferrin serves as a nonspecific host defense mechanism by sequestering iron and depriving pathogens of this essential nutrient. Studies have shown that transferrin levels in the blood increase dramatically in response to systemic bacterial infections.

> Transferrin serves as a host defense mechanism by depriving pathogens of iron.

Fever

Normal body temperature fluctuates between 36.2° and 37.5°C (97.2° and 99.5°F), with an average of about 37°C (98.6°F). A body temperature greater than 37.8°C (100°F) is generally considered to be a fever. Substances that stimulate the production of fever are called *pyrogens* or *pyrogenic substances*. Pyrogens may originate either outside or inside the body. Those from outside the body include pathogens and various pyrogenic substances that they produce or release (e.g., endotoxin). Interleukin 1 (IL-1), a cytokine that is produced by certain white blood cells, is an example of an endogenous pyrogen (i.e., one that originates within the body). The resulting increased body temperature (fever) is considered to be a nonspecific host defense mechanism.

> Substances that stimulate the production of fever are called pyrogens or pyrogenic substances.

Fever augments the host's defenses in the following ways:

- By stimulating white blood cells (leukocytes) to deploy and destroy invaders
- By reducing available free plasma iron, which limits the growth of pathogens that require iron for replication and synthesis of toxins
- By inducing the production of IL-1, which causes the proliferation, maturation, and activation of lymphocytes in the immunologic response

> A fever can slow down the growth rate of certain pathogens and can even kill some especially fastidious ones.

Elevated body temperatures also slow down the growth rate of certain pathogens and can even kill some especially fastidious pathogens.

The following scenario illustrates one way in which fever develops during an infectious disease:

1. A patient has septicemia caused by Gram-negative bacteria (referred to as *Gram-negative sepsis*). Recall from Chapter 13 that septicemia is a serious disease characterized by chills, fever, prostration, and the presence of bacteria or their toxins in the bloodstream.
2. The bacteria release endotoxin into the patient's bloodstream. (Endotoxin is part of the cell wall structure of Gram-negative bacteria; it is the lipid component of lipopolysaccharide.)
3. Phagocytes ingest (phagocytize) the endotoxin.
4. The ingested endotoxin stimulates the phagocytes to produce IL-1, an endogenous pyrogen. IL-1 is produced primarily by macrophages.
5. IL-1 stimulates the hypothalamus (a part of the brain referred to as the body's thermostat) to produce prostaglandins.
6. Once metabolized, the prostaglandins cause the hypothalamic thermostat to be set at a higher level.
7. The increased thermostatic reading sends out signals to the nerves surrounding peripheral blood vessels. This causes the vessels to contract, thus conserving heat.
8. The increased body heat, resulting from vasoconstriction, continues until the temperature of the blood supplying the hypothalamus matches the elevated thermostat reading. The thermostat can be reset to the normal body temperature when the concentration of endogenous pyrogen decreases.

There are, of course, detrimental aspects of fever—especially prolonged high fevers. These include increased heart rate, increased metabolic rate, increased caloric demand, and mild to severe dehydration.

Interferons

Interferons are small, antiviral proteins produced by virus-infected cells. They are called interferons because they "interfere" with viral replication. The three known

STUDY AID

Beware of Similar Sounding Terms

A **pyogen** is a pus-producing microbe (i.e., a pyogenic microbe). A **pyrogen** is a fever-producing substance (i.e., a pyrogenic substance).

> Interferons are small, antiviral proteins produced by virus-infected cells. They interfere with viral replication.

types of interferon, referred to as alpha (α), beta (β), and gamma (γ) interferons, are induced by different stimuli, including viruses, tumors, bacteria, and other foreign cells. The different types of interferons are produced by different types of cells. α-Interferon is produced by B lymphocytes (B cells), monocytes, and macrophages; β-interferon, by fibroblasts and other virus-infected cells; and γ-interferon, by activated T lymphocytes (T cells) and natural killer cells (NK cells).[b]

The interferons produced by a virus-infected cell are unable to save that cell from destruction, but once they are released from that cell, they attach to the membranes of surrounding cells and prevent viral replication from occurring in those cells. Thus, the spread of the infection is inhibited, allowing other body defenses to fight the disease more effectively. In this way, many viral diseases (e.g., colds, influenza, and measles) are limited in duration. Similarly, the acute phase of herpes simplex cold sores is of limited duration. The herpes virus then enters a latent phase and hides in nerve ganglion cells where it is protected until the person's defenses are down; the cycle of disease and latency is repeated over and over.

Interferons are not virus-specific, meaning that they are effective against a variety of viruses, not just the particular type of virus that stimulated their production. Interferons are species-specific, however, meaning that they are effective only in the species of animal that produced them. Thus, rabbit interferons are only effective in rabbits and could not be used to treat viral infections in humans. Human interferons are industrially produced by genetically engineered bacteria (bacteria into which human interferon genes have been inserted) and are used experimentally to treat certain viral infections (e.g.,

> Interferons are not virus-specific, but they are host-specific.

warts, herpes simplex, hepatitis B and C) and cancers (e.g., leukemias, lymphomas, Kaposi sarcoma in patients with acquired immune deficiency syndrome or acquired immunodeficiency syndrome [AIDS]). In addition to interfering with viral multiplication, interferons also activate certain lymphocytes (NK cells) to kill virus-infected cells.

In addition to the beneficial aspects of the interferons that are produced in response to certain viral infections, they actually cause the nonspecific flulike symptoms (malaise, myalgia, chills, fever) that are associated with many viral infections.

The Complement System

Complement is not a single entity, but rather a group of approximately 30 different proteins (including nine proteins designated as C1 through C9) that

are found in normal blood plasma. These proteins make up what is called "the complement system"—so named because it is complementary to the action of the immune system. The proteins of the complement system, sometimes collectively referred to as complement components, interact with each other in a stepwise manner, known as the **complement cascade**. A discussion of the somewhat complex steps in the complement cascade is beyond the scope of this book. What is of primary importance is that activation of the complement system is considered a nonspecific host defense mechanism; it assists in the destruction of many different pathogens.

> The proteins of the complement system (collectively referred to as complement components) interact with each other in a stepwise manner, known as the complement cascade—a nonspecific host defense mechanism that assists in the destruction of many different pathogens.

The major consequences of complement activation are listed here:

• Initiation and amplification of inflammation
• Attraction of phagocytes to sites where they are needed (chemotaxis; to be discussed later)
• Activation of leukocytes
• Lysis of bacteria and other foreign cells
• Increased phagocytosis by phagocytic cells (opsonization)

See thePoint for "A Closer Look at the Complement System."

Opsonization is a process by which phagocytosis is facilitated by the deposition of **opsonins**, such as antibodies or certain complement fragments, onto the surface of particles or cells. In some cases, phagocytes are unable to ingest certain particles or cells (e.g., encapsulated bacteria) until opsonization occurs. One of the products formed during the complement cascade, called C3b, is an opsonin. It is deposited on the surface of microbes. Neutrophils and macrophages possess surface molecules (receptors) that can recognize and bind to C3b.

> Opsonization is a process by which phagocytosis is facilitated by the deposition of opsonins (e.g., antibodies or certain complement fragments) onto the surface of particles or cells.

Complement fragments C3a, C4a, and C5a cause mast cells to degranulate and release histamine, leading to increased vascular permeability and smooth muscle contraction. (Mast cells are discussed in Chapter 16.) C5a also acts as a chemoattractant (chemotactic agent) for neutrophils and macrophages. Chemoattractants are discussed later in the chapter.

There are a variety of hereditary complement deficiencies that interfere with activities of the complement system. Some of these inherited deficiencies are associated

---

[b]B cells, T cells, and NK cells are discussed in Chapter 16.

with defects in activation of the classical pathway.[c] A deficiency of C3 leads to a defect in activation of both the classical and alternative pathways. Defects of properdin impair activation of the alternative pathway.[d] Any of these defects leads to increased susceptibility to pyogenic (pus-producing) staphylococcal and streptococcal infections.

Acute-Phase Proteins

Plasma levels of molecules collectively referred to as *acute-phase proteins* increase rapidly in response to infection, inflammation, and tissue injury. They serve as host defense mechanisms by enhancing resistance to infection and promoting the repair of damaged tissue. Acute-phase proteins include C-reactive protein (which is used as a laboratory marker for, or indication of, inflammation), serum amyloid A protein, protease inhibitors, and coagulation proteins.

Cytokines

Cytokines are chemical mediators that are released from many different types of cells in the human body. They enable cells to communicate with each other. They act as chemical messengers both within the immune system (discussed in Chapter 16) and between the immune system and other systems of the body. A cell is able to "sense" the presence of a cytokine if it possesses appropriate surface receptors that can recognize the cytokine. The cytokine mediates (causes) some type of response in a cell that is able to sense its presence. Some cytokines are chemoattractants (to be discussed later), recruiting phagocytes to locations where they are needed. Others, like interferons (previously discussed), have a direct role in host defense.

> Cytokines are chemical mediators that are released from many different types of cells in the human body. They act as chemical messengers, enabling cells to communicate with each other.

Inflammation

The body normally responds to any local injury, irritation, microbial invasion, or bacterial toxin by a complex series of events collectively referred to as **inflammation** or the *inflammatory response* (Fig. 15-3). The three major events in acute inflammation are as follows:

- An increase in the diameter of capillaries (**vasodilation**), which increases blood flow to the site
- Increased permeability of the capillaries, allowing the escape of plasma and plasma proteins
- Escape of leukocytes from the capillaries and their accumulation at the site of injury

The primary purposes of the inflammatory response (Fig. 15-4) are to:

- Localize an infection
- Prevent the spread of microbial invaders
- Neutralize any toxins being produced at the site
- Aid in the repair of damaged tissue

> The three major events in acute inflammation are vasodilation, increased permeability of the capillaries, and escape of leukocytes from the capillaries.

> The primary purposes of the inflammatory response are to localize an infection, prevent the spread of microbial invaders, neutralize toxins, and aid in the repair of damaged tissue.

During the inflammatory process, many nonspecific host defense mechanisms come into play. These interrelated physiologic reactions result in the four cardinal (main) signs and symptoms of inflammation: redness, heat, swelling (**edema**), and pain.[e] There is often pus formation, and occasionally a loss of function of the damaged area (e.g., an inflamed elbow might prevent bending of the arm).

A complex series of physiologic events occurs immediately after the initial damage to the tissue. One of the initial events is vasodilation at the site of injury, mediated by vasoactive agents (e.g., histamine and prostaglandins) released from damaged cells. Vasodilation allows more blood to flow to the site, bringing redness and heat. Additional heat results from increased metabolic activities in the tissue cells at the site. Vasodilation causes the endothelial cells that line the capillaries to stretch and separate, resulting in increased permeability. Plasma escapes from the capillaries into the surrounding area, causing the site to become **edematous** (swollen). Sometimes the swelling is severe enough to interfere with the bending of a particular joint (e.g., knuckle, elbow, knee, ankle), leading to a loss of function.

> The four cardinal or main signs and symptoms of inflammation are redness, heat, swelling (edema), and pain.

> Vasodilation— an increase in the diameter of capillaries—leads to redness, heat, and edema.

A variety of chemotactic agents (to be discussed later) are produced at the site of inflammation, leading to an influx of phagocytes. The pain or tenderness that accompanies inflammation may result from actual damage of the nerve fibers because of the injury, irritation by microbial toxins or other cellular secretions (such as prostaglandins), or increased pressure on nerve endings because of the edema.

---

[c]As explained on thePoint, the complement system can be activated by any of the three pathways: the classical (or classic) pathway, the alternative pathway, and the lectin pathway.

[d]Properdin (also known as factor P) is a nonimmunoglobulin γ-globulin component of the alternative pathway of complement activation.

[e]In his written work, *De Medicina* (On Medicine), Aulus Cornelius Celsus, a Roman encyclopedist who lived and died before the time of Christ, described the cardinal signs of inflammation using the Latin terms *rubor* (redness), *calor* (warmth), *dolor* (pain), and *tumor* (swelling). These Latin terms are sometimes taught in Physiology courses.

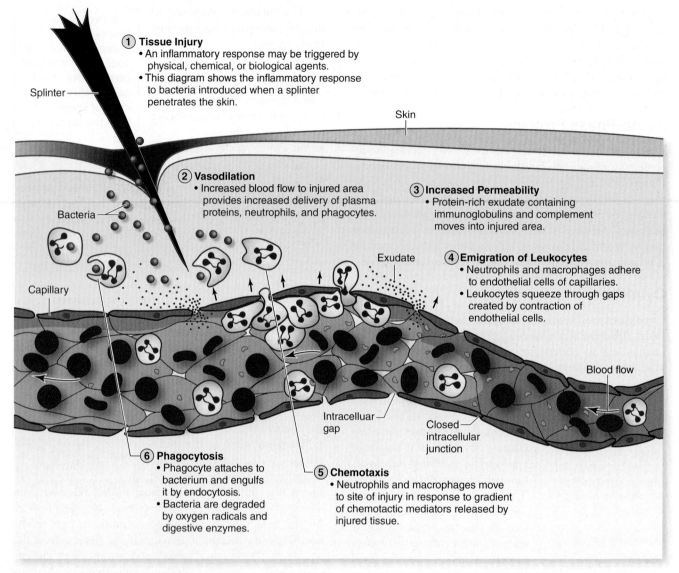

Figure 15-3. Sequence of events in inflammation. (Redrawn from Harvey RA, Champe RA, eds. *Lippincott Illustrated Reviews: Microbiology*. Philadelphia, PA: Lippincott Williams & Wilkins; 2001.) (An animated version of this figure can be found on thePoint.)

The accumulation of fluid, cells, and cellular debris at the inflammation site is referred to as an **inflammatory exudate**. If the exudate is thick and greenish yellow, containing many live and dead leukocytes, it is known as a **purulent exudate** or *pus*. However, in many inflammatory responses, such as arthritis or pancreatitis, there is no exudate and are no invading microbes. When **pyogenic microbes** (pus-producing microbes), such as staphylococci and streptococci, are present, additional pus is produced as a result of the killing effect of bacterial toxins on phagocytes and tissue cells. Although most pus is greenish yellow, the exudate is often bluish green in infections caused by *Pseudomonas aeruginosa*. This is caused by the bluish green pigment (called *pyocyanin*) produced by this organism.

> A purulent inflammatory exudate is often referred to as pus.

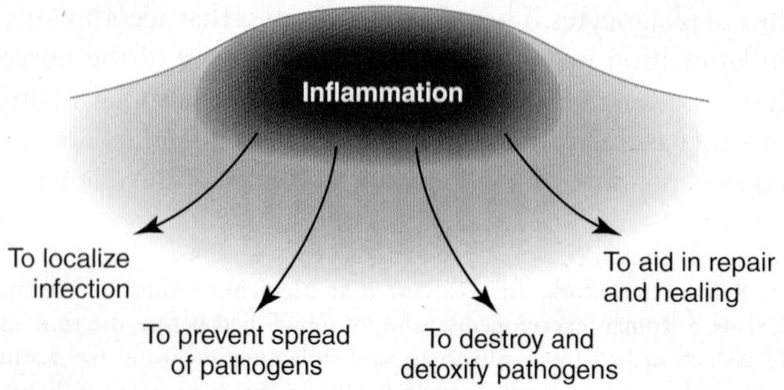

When the inflammatory response is over and the body has won the battle, phagocytes clean up the area and help to restore order. The cells and tissues can then repair the damage and begin to function normally again in a homeostatic (equilibrated) state, although some permanent damage and scarring may result.

The lymphatic system—including lymph (the fluid component of the lymphatic system), lymphatic vessels, lymph nodes, and lymphatic organs (tonsils, spleen, and

Inflammation

To localize infection

To prevent spread of pathogens

To destroy and detoxify pathogens

To aid in repair and healing

Figure 15-4. The purposes of inflammation.

The primary functions of the lymphatic system include draining and circulating intercellular fluids from tissues, transporting digested fats from the digestive system to the blood, removing foreign matter and microbes from the lymph, and producing antibodies and other factors to aid in the destruction and detoxification of any invading microbes.

thymus gland)—also plays an important role in defending the body against invaders. The primary functions of this system include draining and circulating intercellular fluids from the tissues and transporting digested fats from the digestive system to the blood. Also, macrophages, B cells, and T cells in the lymph nodes serve to filter the lymph by removing foreign matter and microbes, and by producing antibodies and other factors to aid in the destruction and detoxification of any invading microbes.

The body continually wages war against damage, injury, malfunction, and microbial invasion. The outcome of each battle depends on the person's age, hormonal balance, genetic resistance, and overall state of physical and mental health, as well as the virulence of the pathogens involved.

Phagocytosis

The cellular elements of blood are shown in Figure 15-5. Recall from Chapter 13 that the three major categories of leukocytes found in blood are monocytes, lymphocytes, and granulocytes. The three types of granulocytes are neutrophils, eosinophils, and basophils.

The three major categories of leukocytes found in blood are monocytes, lymphocytes, and granulocytes.

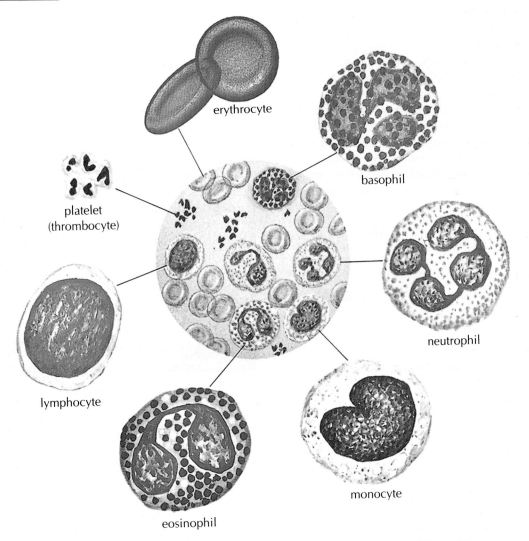

Figure 15-5. Cellular elements of the blood, as seen in a Wright's-stained peripheral blood smear. Wright's stain contains two dyes: eosin (a reddish orange acidic dye, which stains basic substances) and methylene blue (a dark blue dye, which stains acidic substances). Eosinophil granules stain reddish orange because their contents are basic and, therefore, attract the acidic dye. Basophil granules stain dark blue because their contents are acidic and, therefore, attract the basic dye. The contents of neutrophil granules are neutral (neither basic nor acidic) and therefore attract neither the acidic dye nor the basic dye. (From McCall RE, Tankersley CM. *Phlebotomy Essentials*. 2nd ed. Philadelphia, PA: Lippincott-Raven Publishers; 1998.)

Phagocytic white blood cells are called **phagocytes**, and the process by which phagocytes surround and engulf (ingest) foreign material is called **phagocytosis**. The two most important groups of phagocytes in the human body are macrophages and neutrophils; they are sometimes called "professional phagocytes," because phagocytosis is their major function.[f] Macrophages serve as a "clean-up crew" to rid the body of unwanted and often harmful substances, such as dead cells, unused cellular secretions, debris, and microbes.

> The two most important groups of phagocytes in the human body—sometimes referred to as "professional phagocytes"—are macrophages and neutrophils.

Granulocytes are named for the prominent cytoplasmic granules that they possess. Phagocytic granulocytes include **neutrophils** and **eosinophils**. Neutrophils (also known as polymorphonuclear cells, polys, and PMNs) are much more efficient at phagocytosis than eosinophils. An abnormally high number of eosinophils in the peripheral bloodstream is known as **eosinophilia**. Examples of conditions that cause eosinophilia are allergies and helminth infections. **Basophils**, a third type of granulocyte, are also involved in allergic and inflammatory reactions, although they are not phagocytes. Basophil granules contain histamine and other chemical mediators. Basophils are further discussed in Chapter 16.

> Granulocytes include basophils, eosinophils, and neutrophils.

Macrophages develop from a type of leukocyte called **monocytes** during the inflammatory response to infections. Those that leave the bloodstream and migrate to infected areas are called **wandering macrophages**. **Fixed macrophages** (also known as *histocytes* or *histiocytes*) remain within tissues and organs and serve to trap foreign debris. Macrophages are extremely efficient phagocytes. They are found in tissues of the **reticulo-endothelial system** (RES). This nonspecific defensive system includes cells in the liver (Kupffer cells), spleen, lymph nodes, and bone marrow as well as the lungs (alveolar or dust cells), blood vessels, intestines, and brain (microglia). The principal function of the entire RES is the engulfment and removal of foreign and useless particles, living or dead, such as excess cellular secretions, dead and dying leukocytes, erythrocytes, and tissue cells as well as foreign debris and microbes that gain entrance to the body.

> Wandering macrophages leave the bloodstream and migrate to sites of infection and other areas where they are needed. Fixed macrophages remain within tissues and organs.

The four steps in phagocytosis are chemotaxis, attachment, ingestion, and digestion. They are discussed next and are summarized in Table 15-1.

Chemotaxis

Phagocytosis begins when phagocytes move to the site where they are needed. This directed migration is called **chemotaxis** and is the result of chemical attractants referred to as **chemotactic agents** (also called chemotactic factors, chemotactic substances, and chemoattractants). Chemotactic agents that are produced by various cells of the human body are called **chemokines**.[g] Chemotactic agents are produced during the complement cascade and inflammation. The phagocytes move along a concentration gradient, meaning that they move from

Table 15-1	Four Steps in Phagocytosis
Step	**Brief Description**
1. Chemotaxis	Phagocytes are attracted by chemotactic agents to the site where they are needed
2. Attachment	A phagocyte attaches to an object
3. Ingestion	Pseudopodia surround the object, and it is taken into the cell
4. Digestion	The object is broken down and dissolved by digestive enzymes and other mechanisms

[f]Macrophages and neutrophils are not the only body cells capable of phagocytosis, but they are the most important phagocytic cells.

[g]Various types of cells within the human body, including cells of the immune system, communicate with each other. They do so by means of chemical messages—proteins known as cytokines. If the cytokines are chemotactic agents, attracting leukocytes to areas where they are needed, they are referred to as chemokines.

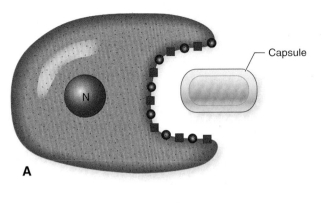

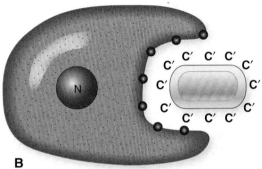

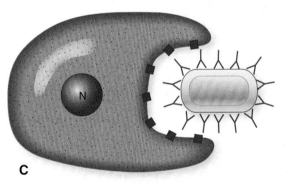

> The directed migration of phagocytes is called chemotaxis. It is caused by chemicals referred to as chemotactic agents.

areas of low concentrations of chemotactic agents to the area of highest concentration. The area of highest concentration is the site where the chemotactic agents are being produced or released—often the site of inflammation. Thus, the phagocytes are attracted to the site where they are needed. Different types of chemotactic agents attract different types of leukocytes; some attract monocytes, others neutrophils, and still others eosinophils.

Attachment

The next step in phagocytosis is attachment of the phagocyte to the object (e.g., a yeast or bacterial cell) to be ingested. Phagocytes can only ingest objects to which they can attach. As previously mentioned, opsonization is sometimes necessary to enable phagocytes to attach to certain particles (e.g., encapsulated bacteria). In opsonization, the particle becomes coated with opsonins (either complement fragments or anti-

> In opsonization, a particle becomes coated with opsonins—either complement fragments or antibodies.

bodies). Because the phagocyte possesses surface molecules (receptors) for complement fragments and antibodies, the phagocyte can now attach to the particle (Fig. 15-6).

Ingestion

The phagocyte then surrounds the object with pseudopodia, which fuse together, and the object is ingested (is

> During ingestion, the particle becomes surrounded by a membrane. The membrane-bound vesicle is called a phagosome.

phagocytized or phagocytosed) (Fig. 15-7). Phagocytosis is one type of endocytosis, the process of ingesting material from outside a cell. Within the cytoplasm of the phagocyte, the object is contained within a membrane-bound vesicle called a **phagosome**.

Digestion

The phagosome next fuses with a nearby lysosome to form a digestive vacuole (**phagolysosome**), within which killing and digestion occur (Fig. 15-8). Recall from Chapter 3 that lysosomes are membrane-bound vesicles containing digestive en-

> The fusion of a lysosome and a phagosome results in a phagolysosome, within which the ingested particle is digested.

zymes. Digestive enzymes found within lysosomes include lysozyme, β-lysin, lipases, proteases, peptidases, DNAses, and RNases, which degrade carbohydrates, lipids, proteins, and nucleic acids.

Other mechanisms also participate in the destruction of phagocytized microbes. In neutrophils, for example, a membrane-bound enzyme called nicotinamide adenine

Figure 15-6. Opsonization. A. The phagocyte shown here is unable to attach to the encapsulated bacterium because there are no molecules (receptors) on the surface of the phagocyte that can recognize or attach to the polysaccharide capsule. **B.** Complement fragments (represented by the symbol C') have been deposited onto the surface of the capsule. (In this example, the opsonins are complement fragments.) Now the phagocyte can attach to the bacterium because there are receptors (represented by red circles) on the phagocyte's surface that can recognize and bind to complement fragments. **C.** Antibodies (the Y-shaped molecules) have attached to the capsule. (In this example, the opsonins are antibodies.) Now the phagocyte can attach to the bacterium because there are receptors (represented by green squares) on the phagocyte's surface that can recognize and bind to the F_c region of antibody molecules. (See text for additional details.) N, nucleus.

dinucleotide phosphate (NADPH) oxidase reduces oxygen to very destructive products such as superoxide anions, hydroxyl radicals, hydrogen peroxide, and singlet oxygen. These highly reactive reduction products assist in the destruction of the ingested microbes. Another killing mechanism involves the enzyme myeloperoxidase. After

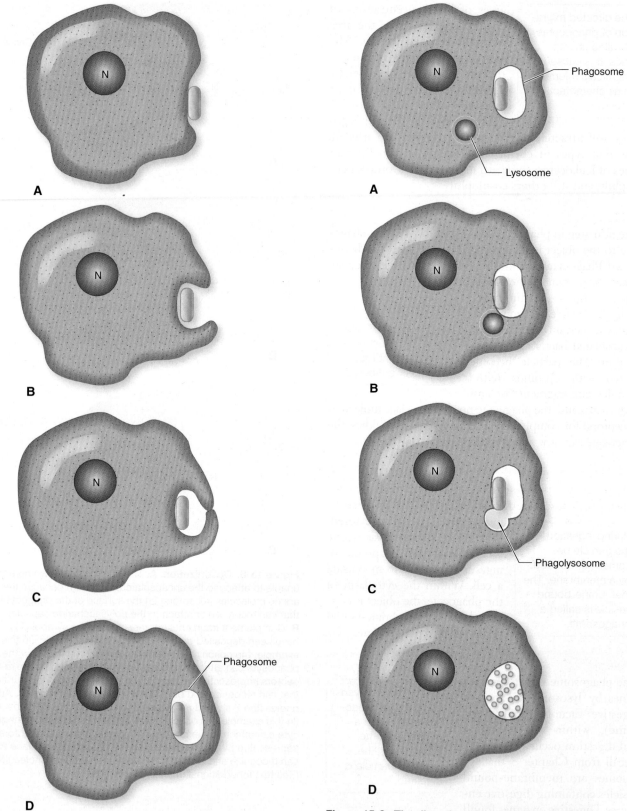

Figure 15-7. The ingestion phase of phagocytosis.
A. A phagocyte has attached to a bacterial cell. **B.** Pseudo-podia extend around the bacterial cell. **C.** The pseudopodia meet and fuse together. **D.** The bacterial cell, surrounded by a membrane, is now inside the phagocyte. The membrane-bound structure, containing the ingested bacterial cell, is called a phagosome. N, nucleus. (An animated version of Figures 15-7 and 15-8 can be found on thePoint.)

Figure 15-8. The digestion phase of phagocytosis.
A. A lysosome, containing digestive enzymes, approaches a phagosome. **B.** The lysosome membrane fuses with the phagosome membrane. **C.** The lysosome and phagosome become a single membrane-bound vesicle, known as a phagolysosome. The phagolysosome contains the ingested bacterial cell plus digestive enzymes. **D.** The bacterial cell is digested within the phagolysosome. N, nucleus.

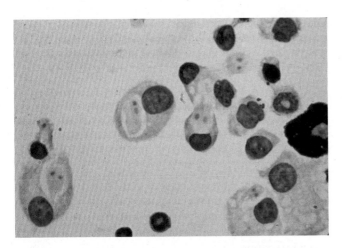

Figure 15-9. Photomicrograph of rat leukocytes, some of which contain phagocytized *Giardia* trophozoites. The phagocytosis occurred under experimental conditions in a research laboratory. Each *Giardia* trophozoite contains two darkly-stained nuclei, giving the appearance of eyes. (Courtesy of Biomed Ed, Round Rock, TX.)

lysosome fusion, myeloperoxidase is released, which, in the presence of hydrogen peroxide and chloride ion, produces a potent microbicidal agent called hypochlorous acid.

Figures 15-9 and 15-10 depict *Giardia lamblia* trophozoites being phagocytized by rat leukocytes. *G. lamblia* (also known as *Giardia intestinalis*) is a flagellated protozoan parasite that causes a diarrheal disease known as giardiasis. These photomicrographs and electron micrographs were taken during a laboratory research project involving opsonization of *Giardia* trophozoites.

Mechanisms by Which Pathogens Escape Destruction by Phagocytes

During the initial phases of infection, capsules serve an antiphagocytic function, protecting encapsulated bacteria from being phagocytized. Some bacteria produce an exoenzyme (referred to as a toxin by some scientists) called *leukocidin*, which kills phagocytes. As mentioned in Chapter 14, not all bacteria engulfed by phagocytes are destroyed within phagolysosomes. For example, waxes in the cell wall of *Mycobacterium tuberculosis* protect the organism from digestion. The bacteria are even able to multiply within the phagocytes and are transported within them to other parts of the body. Other pathogens that are able to survive within phagocytes include bacteria such as *Rickettsia rickettsii, Legionella pneumophila, Brucella abortus, Coxiella burnetii, Listeria monocytogenes,* and *Salmonella* spp., as well as protozoan parasites such as *Toxoplasma gondii, Trypanosoma cruzi,* and *Leishmania* spp. The mechanism by which each pathogen evades digestion by lysosomal enzymes differs from one pathogen to another; in some cases, the mechanism is not yet understood. These pathogens may remain dormant within phagocytes for months or years before they escape to cause disease. Thus, these types of virulent pathogens usually win the battle with phagocytes. Unless antibodies or complement fragments are present to aid in the destruction of these pathogens, the infection may progress unchecked.

> Some bacteria and protozoa are able to survive within phagocytes.

Ehrlichia and *Anaplasma* spp., closely related to rickettsias, are obligate, intracellular, Gram-negative bacteria that live within leukocytes (i.e., they are *intraleukocytic pathogens*). These organisms cause two endemic, tick-borne diseases in the United States. *Ehrlichia* spp. cause human monocytic ehrlichiosis, a condition in which the bacteria infect monocytic phagocytes. *Anaplasma* spp. cause human anaplasmosis (or human granulocytic ehrlichiosis, as it is sometimes called), a condition in which the bacteria infect granulocytes. The bacteria are somehow able to prevent the fusion of lysosomes with phagosomes.

> *Ehrlichia* and *Anaplasma* spp. are intraleukocytic bacteria, which are able to live and multiply within leukocytes.

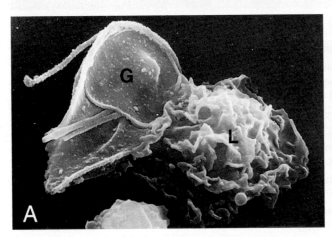
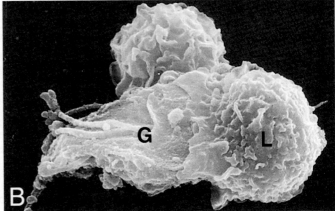

Figure 15-10. Scanning electron micrographs (A, B) illustrating the phagocytosis of *Giardia* trophozoites (G) by rat leukocytes (L). The phagocytosis occurred under experimental conditions in a research laboratory. (Courtesy of Dr. Stanley Erlandsen and Biomed Ed, Round Rock, TX.)

Disorders and Conditions That Adversely Affect Phagocytic and Inflammatory Processes

Leukopenia

Some patients have an abnormally low number of circulating leukocytes—a condition known as **leukopenia**. (Although the terms *leukopenia* and *neutropenia* are often used synonymously, they are not really synonyms. Technically, neutropenia is an abnormally low number of circulating neutrophils; neutropenia = neutrophilic leukopenia.) Leukopenia may result from bone marrow injury as a result of ionizing radiation or drugs, nutritional deficiencies, or congenital stem cell defects.

> Leukopenia—an abnormally low number of circulating leukocytes. Neutropenia—an abnormally low number of circulating neutrophils.

STUDY AID

Beware of Similar Sounding Words

When a patient has an abnormally low number of circulating leukocytes, the condition is known as **leukopenia**. When a patient has an abnormally high number of circulating leukocytes, the condition is known as **leukocytosis** (which is usually the result of an infection). **Leukemia** is a type of cancer in which there is a proliferation of abnormal leukocytes in the blood. Actually, there are several different types of leukemia, classified by the dominant type of leukocyte.

Disorders and Conditions Affecting Leukocyte Motility and Chemotaxis

The inability of leukocytes to migrate in response to chemotactic agents may be related to a defect in the production of actin, a structural protein associated with motility. Some drugs (e.g., corticosteroids) can also inhibit the chemotactic activity of leukocytes. Decreased neutrophil chemotaxis also occurs in the inherited childhood disease known as Chediak–Higashi syndrome (CHS). In addition, the PMNs of individuals with CHS contain abnormal lysosomes that do not readily fuse with phagosomes, resulting in decreased bactericidal activity. CHS is characterized by symptoms such as albinism, central nervous system abnormalities, and recurrent bacterial infections.

Disorders and Conditions Affecting Intracellular Killing by Phagocytes

The phagocytes of some individuals are capable of ingesting bacteria, but are incapable of killing certain species. This is usually the result of deficiencies in myeloperoxidase or an inability to generate superoxide anion, hydrogen peroxide, or hypochlorite. Chronic granulomatous disease (CGD) is an often fatal genetic disorder that is characterized by repeated bacterial infections. The PMNs of individuals with CGD can ingest bacteria but cannot kill certain species. In one form of CGD, the person's PMNs are unable to produce hydrogen peroxide. In another hereditary disorder, the individual's PMNs completely lack myeloperoxidase. Their PMNs do possess other microbicidal mechanisms, however, so these individuals usually do not experience recurrent infections.

Additional Factors

Table 15-2 lists some additional factors that can impair host defense mechanisms.

Table 15-2   Additional Factors That Can Impair Host Defense Mechanisms

Factor	Comments
Nutritional status	Malnutrition is accompanied by decreased resistance to infections
Increased iron levels	High concentrations of iron make it easier for bacteria to satisfy their iron requirements; high concentrations of iron reduce the chemotactic and phagocytic activities of phagocytes; increased iron levels may result from a variety of conditions or habits
Stress	People living under stressful conditions are more susceptible to infections than people living under less stressful conditions
Age	Newborn infants lack a fully developed immune system; the efficiency of the immune system and other host defenses declines after age 50
Cancer and cancer chemotherapy	Cancer chemotherapeutic agents kill healthy cells and malignant ones
AIDS	Destruction of the AIDS patient's T_H cells decreases the patient's ability to produce antibodies to certain pathogens (discussed in Chapter 16)
Drugs	Steroids and alcohol, for example
Various genetic defects	B-cell and T-cell deficiencies, for example

ON thePoint

- Terms Introduced in This Chapter
- Review of Key Points
- A Closer Look at the Complement System
- Increase Your Knowledge
- Critical Thinking
- Additional Self-Assessment Exercises

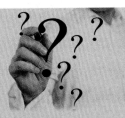

Self-Assessment Exercises

After studying this chapter, answer the following multiple-choice questions.

1. Host defense mechanisms—ways in which the body protects itself from pathogens—can be thought of as an army consisting of how many lines of defense?

   a. two
   b. three
   c. four
   d. five

2. Which of the following is not part of the body's first line of defense?

   a. fever
   b. intact skin
   c. mucus
   d. pH of the stomach contents

3. Each of the following is considered a part of the body's second line of defense except:

   a. fever
   b. inflammation
   c. interferons
   d. lysozyme

4. Which of the following is *not* a consequence of activation of the complement system?

   a. attraction and activation of leukocytes
   b. increased phagocytosis by phagocytic cells (opsonization)
   c. lysis of bacteria and other foreign cells
   d. repair of damaged tissue

5. Each of the following is a primary purpose of the inflammatory response except:

   a. to localize the infection
   b. to neutralize any toxins being produced at the site
   c. to prevent the spread of microbial invaders
   d. to stimulate the production of opsonins

6. Which of the following cells is a granulocyte?

   a. eosinophil
   b. lymphocyte
   c. macrophage
   d. monocyte

7. All the following would be considered an aspect of microbial antagonism except:

   a. competition for nutrients
   b. competition for space
   c. production of bacteriocins
   d. production of lysozyme

8. Which of the following function as opsonins?

   a. antibodies
   b. antigens
   c. complement fragments
   d. both a and c

9. Which of the following statements about interferons is false?

   a. Interferons are virus-specific
   b. Interferons have been used to treat hepatitis C and certain types of cancer
   c. Interferons produced by a virus-infected cell will not save that cell from destruction
   d. Interferons produced by virus-infected rabbit cells cannot be used to treat viral diseases in humans

10. Which of the following is not one of the four cardinal signs or symptoms of inflammation?

    a. edema
    b. heat
    c. loss of function
    d. redness

16

Specific Host Defense Mechanisms: An Introduction to Immunology

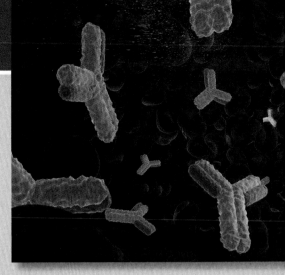

Artist rendering of antibody molecules in the bloodstream.

 CHAPTER OUTLINE

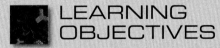 LEARNING OBJECTIVES

After studying this chapter, you should be able to:

- Define the following terms: immunology, immunity, antigenic determinant, immunoglobulins, primary

response, secondary response, agammaglobulinemia, hypogammaglobulinemia, T cell, B cell, plasma cell, and immunosuppression
- Differentiate between humoral immunity and cell-mediated immunity
- Distinguish between active acquired immunity and passive acquired immunity
- Differentiate between natural active acquired immunity and artificial active acquired immunity and cite an example of each
- Distinguish between natural passive acquired immunity and artificial passive acquired immunity and cite an example of each
- Outline the steps involved in the processing of T-independent antigens and T-dependent antigens
- Identify the two primary functions of the immune system
- Construct a diagram of a monomeric antibody molecule
- Identify and describe the five immunoglobulin classes (isotypes)
- List the types of cells that are killed by natural killer (NK) cells
- Name the four types of hypersensitivity reactions
- Outline the steps involved in allergic reactions, starting with the initial sensitization to an allergen and ending with the typical symptoms of an allergic reaction
- Cite six examples of allergens
- List five possible explanations for a positive tuberculosis (TB) skin test

Introduction

Immunology is the scientific study of the immune system and immune responses. Scientists who study various aspects of the immune system are called immunologists.

> The immune system is considered to be a specific host defense mechanism and the third line of defense.

The immune system is considered to be the third line of defense. It is considered a *specific* host defense mechanism because it springs into action to defend against a specific pathogen (or other foreign object) that has gained entrance to the body.

since its inception. The roots of medical laboratory immunology are found in clinical microbiology—the very first immunologic procedures were designed to diagnose infectious diseases. In some medical facilities (primarily small ones), immunologic procedures are still performed in microbiology laboratories. In larger hospitals and medical centers, immunologic procedures are performed in an immunology laboratory, which is separate from the microbiology laboratory.

Immune responses involve complex interactions among many different types of body cells and cellular secretions. Only certain basic fundamentals of immunology and immune responses are presented in this chapter. Topics briefly discussed here include active and passive acquired immunity to infectious agents, vaccines, antigens and antibodies, processes involved in antibody production, cell-mediated immune responses, allergies and other types of hypersensitivity reactions, autoimmune diseases, immunosuppression, and immunodiagnostic procedures (IDPs).

The Key to Understanding Immunology

An understanding of immunology boils down to an understanding of two terms: *antigens* and *antibodies*. For the moment, think of antigens as molecules (usually proteins) that stimulate a person's immune system to produce antibodies. Think of antibodies as protein molecules that a person's immune system produces in response to antigens. Later in the chapter, antigens and antibodies will be discussed in more detail. As you study this chapter, keep in mind that if you understand antigens and antibodies, you are well on your way to understanding immunology.

> Antigens are molecules that stimulate the immune system to produce antibodies. Antibodies are proteins produced by the immune system in response to antigens.

Primary Functions of the Immune System

According to accepted doctrine, the primary functions of the immune system are to:

> The primary functions of the immune system are to differentiate between "self" and "nonself" (something foreign), and destroy that which is nonself.

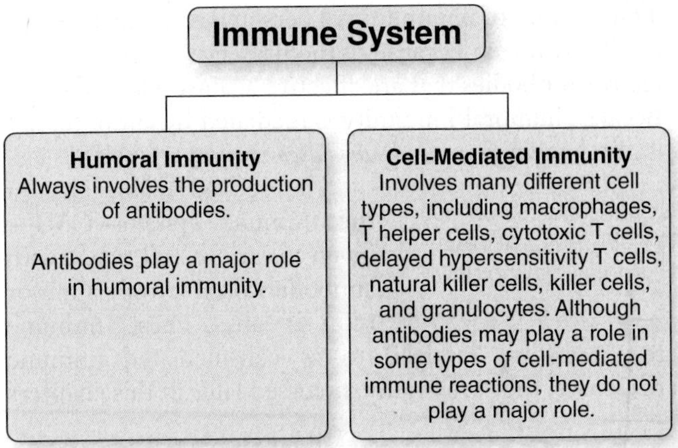

Figure 16-1. **The two major arms of the immune system.**

- Differentiate between "self" and "nonself" (something foreign), and
- Destroy that which is nonself.[a]

Major Arms of the Immune System

There are two major arms of the immune system: humoral immunity and cell-mediated immunity (CMI) (Fig. 16-1).

Humoral immunity always involves the production of antibodies in response to antigens. After their production, these humoral (circulating) antibodies remain in blood plasma, lymph, and other body secretions where they protect against the specific pathogens that stimulated their production.

> Antibodies play a major role in humoral immunity, but play only a minor role, if any, in CMI.

---

[a]An Alternative Viewpoint. For more than 50 years, immunologists have relied on the self/nonself theory of immunity, which states that the immune system reacts to, or "does battle with," nonself (foreign molecules), but does not react to self (molecules that are part of the human body). However, there are certain immunologic events that are seemingly at odds with this theory. An alternative model of immunity has been proposed, called the Danger Model. This model "suggests that the immune system is more concerned with [tissue] damage than with foreignness, and is called into action by [danger or] alarm signals [emitted] from injured tissues, rather than by the recognition of non-self.... When distressed, [the tissues] stimulate immunity, and... they may also determine the [specific type] of [immune] response." The immune response "is tailored to the tissue in which the response occurs, rather than being tailored by the targeted pathogen." Thus, "immunity is controlled by an internal conversation between tissues and the cells of the immune system." (From Matzinger P. The danger model: a renewed sense of self. *Science* 2002;296:301–305.) It should be noted that the Danger Model has not won universal acceptance. Many immunologists believe that the immune response is mainly fueled by receptors that recognize patterns expressed by bacteria and other microbes and do not see cell death in the absence of pathogens as a primary driver of immune response. These ideas, however, do not explain how the immune system rejects transplants or tumors, or induces autoimmune diseases. (en. Wikipedia.org.)

Thus, in humoral immunity, a person is immune to a particular pathogen because of the presence of specific protective antibodies that are effective against that pathogen. Because humoral immunity is mediated by antibodies, it is also known as *antibody-mediated immunity* (AMI).

> CMI involves various cell types, with antibodies playing only a minor role, if any.

The second major arm of the immune system—**CMI**—involves various cell types, with antibodies playing only a minor role, if any. These immune responses are referred to as cell-mediated immune responses; they are briefly discussed later in this chapter.

Immunity

A significant result of immune responses is to make a person resistant to certain infectious diseases. When one is resistant to a certain disease, he/she is said to be immune. The condition of being immune is usually referred to as **immunity**. Humans are immune to certain infectious diseases simply because they are humans. For example, humans are not infected with some of the pathogens that infect their pets. One explanation for this is that human cells do not possess the appropriate cell surface receptors for some of the pathogens that cause diseases of pets. Other reasons for this natural or innate resistance are far more complex and, in some cases, not fully understood, and will not be addressed here.

STUDY AID

Different Uses of the Term Resistant

As you have learned in previous chapters, bacteria can become resistant to certain antibiotics, meaning that they are no longer killed by those antibiotics. Such bacteria are said to be drug resistant. Humans do not become resistant to antibiotics. Humans can become resistant (immune) to certain infectious diseases, however, in ways that are discussed in this chapter.

What will be discussed in this section are the various types of immunities that humans acquire as life progresses, from conception onward—these types of immunity are collectively referred to as *acquired immunity*. Such immunity is often the result of the presence of protective antibodies that are directed against various pathogens.

Acquired Immunity

Immunity that results from the active production or receipt of protective antibodies during one's lifetime is called **acquired immunity**. If the antibodies are actually produced within the person's body, the immunity is called **active acquired immunity**; such protection is usually long lasting. In **passive acquired immunity**, the person receives antibodies that were produced by another person or by more than one person, or, in some cases, by an animal; such protection is usually only temporary. In either case, active or passive, the immunity may result from either a natural or an artificial event. The four categories of acquired immunity are summarized in Table 16-1.

> Immunity that results from the active production or receipt of protective antibodies during one's lifetime is called acquired immunity.

Active Acquired Immunity

There are two types of active acquired immunity:

1. Natural (or naturally occurring) active acquired immunity, which, as the name implies, occurs naturally.
2. Artificial (or artificially occurring) active acquired immunity, which does not occur naturally; rather, it is artificially induced.

> Acquired immunity may be the result of a natural or artificial event.

People who have had a specific infection usually have developed some resistance to reinfection by the causative pathogen because of the presence of antibodies and stimulated lymphocytes. This is called **natural active acquired immunity**. Symptoms of the disease may or

Table 16-1 Types of Acquired Immunity	
Active acquired immunity	
Natural active acquired immunity	Immunity that is acquired in response to the entry of a live pathogen into the body (i.e., in response to an actual infection)
Artificial active acquired immunity	Immunity that is acquired in response to vaccines
Passive acquired immunity	
Natural passive acquired immunity	Immunity that is acquired by a fetus when it receives maternal antibodies in utero or by an infant when it receives maternal antibodies contained in colostrum
Artificial passive acquired immunity	Immunity that is acquired when a person receives antibodies contained in antisera or gamma globulin

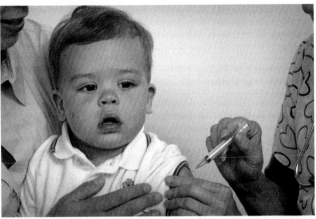

Figure 16-2. Child receiving a vaccine. (Courtesy of Judy Schmidt, James Gathany, and the CDC.)

may not be present when these antibodies are formed. Such resistance to reinfection may be permanent, lasting for a person's entire lifetime, or it may only be temporary. Antibodies that protect us from infection or reinfection are called **protective antibodies**. Sometimes, there is no immunity to reinfection after recovery from certain infectious diseases, even though antibodies are produced against the pathogens that cause these diseases. This is because the antibodies that are produced are *not* protective antibodies.

> Antibodies that protect us from infection or reinfection are called protective antibodies.

Artificial active acquired immunity is the second type of active acquired immunity. This type of immunity results when a person receives a vaccine. The administration of a vaccine (Fig. 16-2) stimulates a person's immune system to produce specific protective antibodies—antibodies that will protect the person should he or she become colonized with that particular pathogen in the future. Vaccines are discussed more fully in the following section.

> Immunity that results from receipt of a vaccine is called artificial active immunity.

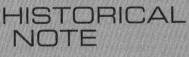

HISTORICAL NOTE

Vaccination

Since the time of the ancient Greeks, it has been observed that people who have recovered from certain infectious diseases, such as plague, smallpox, and yellow fever, rarely contract the same diseases again. The use of vaccines to prevent diseases may date as far back as the 11th century, when the Chinese used a powder prepared from dried smallpox scabs to immunize people, either by introducing the powder into a person's skin or by having him/her inhale the powder. This method of preventing smallpox—using actual smallpox scabs—was known as the *Chinese method*. One of those immunized in this manner was Edward Jenner, a British physician. Some years later, Jenner investigated the widespread belief that milkmaids, who usually had clear, unblemished skin, never developed smallpox. He hypothesized that having had cowpox (a much milder disease than smallpox and one that leaves no scars) protected the milkmaids from getting smallpox. He prepared a smallpox vaccine, using material obtained from cowpox lesions. People injected with Jenner's vaccine were protected from smallpox. The words "vaccine" and "vaccination" come from *vacca*, the Latin word for cow. Because Jenner was the first person to publish (in 1798) the successful results of vaccination, he is generally given credit for originating the concept. During the late 19th century, Louis Pasteur developed successful vaccines to prevent cholera in chickens, anthrax in sheep and cattle, and rabies in dogs and humans. It was actually Pasteur who first used the terms *vaccine* and *vaccination*.

Vaccines. The mere mention of the names of certain infectious diseases struck fear into the hearts of our ancestors. Today, thanks to childhood vaccines, residents of the United States rarely hear of those diseases, let alone live in fear of them. Here is what the Centers for Disease Control and Prevention (CDC) has stated: "It's true, some diseases (like polio and diphtheria) are becoming very rare in the U.S. Of course, they are becoming rare largely because we have been vaccinating against them. But it is still reasonable to ask whether it's really worthwhile to keep vaccinating. It's much like bailing out a boat with a slow leak. When we started bailing, the boat was filled with water. But we have been bailing fast and hard, and now it is almost dry. We could say, 'Good. The boat is dry now, so we can throw away the bucket and relax.' But the leak hasn't stopped. Before long we'd notice a little water seeping in, and soon it might be back up to the same level as when we started. Unless we 'stop the leak' (eliminate the disease), it is important to keep immunizing. Even if there are only a few cases of disease today, if we take away the protection given by vaccination, more and more people will be infected and will spread disease to others. Soon we will undo the progress we have made over the years. If we stop vaccinating, diseases that are almost unknown would stage a comeback. Before long we would see epidemics of diseases that are nearly under control today. More children would get sick and more would die. We don't vaccinate just to protect our children.

We also vaccinate to protect our grandchildren and their grandchildren. If we keep vaccinating now, parents in the future may be able to trust that diseases like polio and meningitis won't infect, cripple, or kill children" (http://www.cdc.gov/vaccines).

A **vaccine** is defined as material that can artificially induce immunity to an infectious disease, usually after injection or, in some cases, ingestion of the material (e.g., oral polio vaccine). A person is deliberately exposed to a harmless version of a pathogen (or toxin), which will stimulate his/her immune system to produce protective antibodies and memory cells (described later in the chapter), but will not cause disease in him/her. In this manner, the person's immune system is primed to mount a strong protective response should the actual pathogen (or toxin) be encountered in the future.

> Vaccination deliberately exposes a person to a harmless version of a pathogen (or toxin), to stimulate his/her immune system to produce protective antibodies and memory cells.

An ideal vaccine is one that:

- contains enough antigenic determinants to stimulate the immune system to produce protective antibodies (i.e., antibodies that will protect individuals from infection by the pathogen)
- contains antigenic determinants from all the strains of the pathogen that cause that disease (e.g., the three strains of virus that cause polio); such vaccines are referred to as multivalent or polyvalent vaccines
- has few (preferably, no) side effects
- does not cause disease in the vaccinated person

Types of Vaccines. Various materials are used in vaccines (Table 16-2). Most vaccines are made from living or dead (inactivated) pathogens or from certain toxins they produce. The use of such vaccines illustrates a very important and practical

> Some vaccines contain weakened (attenuated) pathogens, whereas others contain dead (inactivated) pathogens.

Table 16-2   Types of Available Vaccines

Type of Vaccine	Examples
Attenuated vaccines. The process of weakening pathogens is called attenuation, and the vaccines are referred to as *attenuated vaccines*. Most live vaccines are avirulent (nonpathogenic) mutant strains of pathogens that have been derived from the virulent (pathogenic) organisms; this is accomplished by growing them for many generations under various conditions or by exposing them to mutagenic chemicals or radiation. Attenuated vaccines should not be administered to immunosuppressed individuals, because even weakened pathogens could cause disease in these persons.	**Attenuated viral vaccines:** adenovirus, chicken pox (varicella), measles (rubeola), mumps, German measles (rubella), polio (oral Sabin vaccine), rotavirus, smallpox, yellow fever **Attenuated bacterial vaccines:** BCG (for protection against TB), cholera, tularemia, typhoid fever (oral vaccine)
Inactivated vaccines. Vaccines made from pathogens that have been killed by heat or chemicals—called *inactivated vaccines*—can be produced faster and more easily, but they are less effective than live vaccines. This is because the antigens on the dead cells are usually less effective and produce a shorter period of immunity.	***Inactivated viruses or viral antigens:*** hepatitis A, influenza, Japanese encephalitis, other (EEE, WEE, Russian) encephalitis vaccines, polio (subcutaneous Salk vaccine), rabies ***Inactivated bacterial vaccines:*** anthrax, cholera, pertussis, plague, typhoid fever (subcutaneous vaccine), Q fever
Subunit vaccines. A *subunit vaccine* (or *acellular vaccine*) is one that uses antigenic (antibody-stimulating) portions of a pathogen, rather than using the whole pathogen. For example, a vaccine containing pili of *Neisseria gonorrhoeae* could theoretically stimulate the body to produce antibodies that would attach to *N. gonorrhoeae* pili, thus preventing the bacteria from adhering to cells. If *N. gonorrhoeae* cells cannot adhere to cells that line the urethra, they cannot cause urethritis. The material that is used to protect healthcare workers and others from hepatitis caused by hepatitis B virus (HBV) is being produced by genetically engineered yeasts. The genes that code for hepatitis B surface protein were introduced into yeast cells, which then produced large quantities of that protein. The proteins are then injected into people. Antibodies against the protein are produced in their bodies, and these antibodies serve to protect the people from HBV hepatitis.	Anthrax, hepatitis B, Lyme disease, whooping cough

Table 16-2 Types of Available Vaccines (*Continued*)	
Type of Vaccine	**Examples**
Conjugate vaccines. Successful conjugate vaccines have been made by conjugating bacterial capsular antigens (which by themselves are not very antigenic) to molecules that stimulate the immune system to produce antibodies against the less antigenic capsular antigens.	Hib (for protection against *H. influenzae* type b), meningococcal meningitis (*Neisseria meningitidis* serogroup C), pneumococcal pneumonia
Toxoid vaccines. A **toxoid** is an exotoxin that has been inactivated (made nontoxic) by heat or chemicals. Toxoids can be injected safely to stimulate the production of antibodies that are capable of neutralizing the exotoxins of pathogens, such as those that cause tetanus, botulism, and diphtheria. Antibodies that neutralize toxins are called **antitoxins**, and a serum containing such antitoxins is referred to as an **antiserum**.	Diphtheria, tetanus. Commercial antisera containing antitoxins are used to treat diseases such as tetanus and botulism. Such antisera are also used in certain types of laboratory tests, known as IDPs.
DNA vaccines. Currently, *DNA vaccines* or *gene vaccines* are only experimental. A particular gene from a pathogen is inserted into plasmids, and the plasmids are then injected into skin or muscle tissue. Inside host cells, the genes direct the synthesis of a particular microbial protein (antigen). Once the cells start churning out copies of the protein, the body then produces antibodies directed against the protein, and these antibodies protect the person from infection with the pathogen.	Laboratory animals have been successfully protected using this technique, and reports of the induction of cellular immune responses in humans to a malarial parasite antigen, using DNA vaccines, have been published.
Autogenous vaccines. An autogenous vaccine is one that has been prepared from bacteria isolated from a localized infection, such as a staphylococcal boil. The pathogens are killed and then injected into the same person to induce production of more antibodies.	

application of the principles of microbiology and immunology. In general, vaccines made from living organisms are most effective, but they must be prepared from harmless organisms that are antigenically closely related to the pathogens or from weakened (attenuated) pathogens that have been genetically changed so that they are no longer pathogenic.

As microbiologists made further studies of the characteristics of vaccines, they found that it was practical to vaccinate against several diseases by combining specific vaccines in a single injection. For example, the diphtheria–tetanus–pertussis (DTaP) vaccine contains toxoids to prevent diphtheria and tetanus and antigenic portions of killed bacteria (*Bordetella pertussis*) to prevent whooping cough (pertussis). Another example is the measles–mumps–rubella (MMR) vaccine.

According to the CDC, American children should receive the following vaccines between birth and entry into school (http://www.cdc.gov/vaccines):

- Hepatitis B (Hep B) vaccine
- Rotavirus vaccine
- Diphtheria toxoid–tetanus toxoid–acellular pertussis (DTaP) vaccine
- *Haemophilus influenzae* type b (Hib) conjugate vaccine
- Inactivated poliovirus vaccine
- MMR vaccine
- Varicella (chickenpox) vaccine
- Influenza vaccine (yearly)
- Pneumococcal vaccine
- Hepatitis A vaccine
- Meningococcal vaccine

Many additional vaccines are available for use when needed. They include vaccines for protection against anthrax, cervical cancer, human papillomavirus, H1N1 flu, Japanese encephalitis, Lyme disease, monkeypox, rabies, smallpox, TB, typhoid fever, and yellow fever. A successful vaccine for colds has not been developed, because so many different types of viruses cause colds. Maintaining a successful vaccine for influenza is difficult because influenza viruses frequently change their surface antigens—a phenomenon known as **antigenic variation**.

SOMETHING TO THINK ABOUT

"In some surprising ways, we are in danger of becoming the victims of our own success. As our collective memory of infectious diseases like whooping cough and polio fades, the rare complications from vaccination loom large. Because of concerns about such complications, some parents are choosing not to have their children appropriately immunized. This poses a significant threat to the public health, because the microbes that cause the diseases are still very much with us. With the appearance of a large number of susceptible people again, we can expect to see the return of diseases we thought conquered." (From Needham C, et al. *Intimate Strangers: Unseen Life on Earth*. Washington, DC: ASM Press; 2000.) The quote is as true today as when it was published.

How Vaccines Work. Vaccines stimulate the recipient's immune system to produce protective antibodies. The protective antibodies and/or memory cells produced in response to the vaccine then remain in the recipient's body to "do battle with" a particular pathogen, should that pathogen enter the recipient's body at some time in the future.

For example, when a person receives tetanus toxoid (an altered form of the toxin, tetanospasmin), protective antibodies referred to as antitoxins are produced. The antitoxins remain in the person's body. Should *Clostridium tetani* enter the person's body at some time in the future, and start to produce tetanospasmin, the antitoxins are there to attach to and neutralize the toxin.

Some vaccines stimulate the body to produce protective antibodies that are directed against surface antigens. When the pathogen enters the person's body, the antibodies attach to the surface antigens. This prevents the pathogen from adhering to host cells. In the case of viruses, if they are unable to attach, they are unable to enter the cell and are thus unable to multiply and cause cell destruction. Antibodies produced in response to molecules on the surface of bacterial pili would adhere to the pili, preventing the bacteria from attaching to tissues and, thus, preventing the bacteria from causing disease.

In some cases, protective antibodies attached to pathogens' surface antigens act as opsonins (discussed in Chapter 15), enabling phagocytes to attach to the pathogens. Once attached to a pathogen, the phagocyte can ingest and digest it. In other cases, attachment of protective antibodies to surface antigens activates the complement cascade, with the end result being lysis of the pathogen.

Passive Acquired Immunity

Passive acquired immunity differs from active acquired immunity, in that antibodies formed in one person are transferred to another to protect the latter from infection. Thus, in passive

> In passive acquired immunity, a person *receives* antibodies, rather than producing them. This can occur naturally or artificially.

acquired immunity, a person *receives* antibodies, rather than producing them. Because the person receiving the antibodies did not actively produce them, the immunity is temporary, lasting only about 3 to 6 weeks. The antibodies of passive acquired immunity may be transferred naturally or artificially.

In **natural passive acquired immunity**, small antibodies (such as immunoglobulin G [IgG], which is described later in this chapter) present in the mother's blood cross the placenta to reach the fetus while it is in the uterus (in utero). Also, colostrum, the thin, milky fluid secreted by mammary glands a few days before and after delivery, contains maternal antibodies to protect the infant during the first months of life.

> A fetus receiving maternal antibodies in utero and an infant receiving maternal antibodies in colostrum are examples of natural passive acquired immunity.

Artificial passive acquired immunity is accomplished by transferring antibodies from an immune person to a susceptible person. After a patient has been exposed to a disease, the length of the incubation period usually does not allow sufficient time for postexposure vaccination to be an effective preventive measure. This is because a span of about 2 weeks is needed before sufficient antibodies are formed to protect the exposed person. To provide temporary protection in these situations, the patient is given human gamma globulin or "pooled" immune serum globulin (ISG), that is, antibodies taken from the blood of many immune people. In this manner, the patient receives some antibodies

> Receiving a shot of gamma globulin is an example of artificial passive acquired immunity.

to all of the diseases to which the donors are immune. The ISG may be given to provide temporary protection against measles, mumps, polio, diphtheria, and hepatitis in people, especially infants, who are not immune and have been exposed to these diseases.

Hyperimmune serum globulin (or specific immune globulin) has been prepared from the serum of persons with high antibody levels (titer) against certain diseases. For example, hepatitis B immune globulin (HBIG) is given to protect those who have been, or are apt to be, exposed to hepatitis B virus; tetanus immune globulin is used to prevent tetanus in nonimmunized patients with deep, dirty wounds; and rabies immune globulin may be given to prevent rabies after a person is bitten by a rabid animal. Other examples include chickenpox immune globulin, measles immune globulin, pertussis immune globulin, poliomyelitis immune globulin, and zoster immune globulin. In potentially lethal cases of botulism, antitoxin antibodies are used to neutralize the toxic effects of the botulinal toxin. Remember that passive acquired immunity is always temporary because the antibodies are not actively produced by the B cells of the protected person.

Cells of the Immune System

As stated earlier, the immune system involves very complex interactions among many different types of cells and cellular secretions. The major cell types that participate in immune responses are:

- T lymphocytes (T cells)
- B lymphocytes (B cells)
- NK cells (a category of lymphocytes)
- Macrophages

The cells involved in immune responses originate in bone marrow, from which most blood cells develop. Three lines of lymphocytes—B lymphocytes (B cells), T lymphocytes (T cells), and NK cells—are derived from lymphoid stem cells of bone marrow.

There are two major categories of T cells: helper T cells and cytotoxic T cells. Helper T cells are also known as T-helper cells, T_H cells, and $CD4^+$ cells. The term $CD4^+$ cells refers to the fact that these cells possess on their surface an antigen designated as CD4. The primary function of helper T cells is secretion of cytokines. T_H1 cells and T_H2 cells are subcategories of helper T cells. Cytokines secreted by T_H1 cells (referred to as type 1 cytokines) support cell-mediated immune responses (described later in the chapter), involving macrophages, cytotoxic T cells, and NK cells. Cytokines secreted by T_H2 cells (referred to as type 2 cytokines) support humoral immune responses (described later in the chapter) by inducing B-cell activation and differentiation of activated B cells into plasma cells.

> The two major types of T cells are helper T cells and cytotoxic T cells.

Cytotoxic T cells are also known as T cytotoxic cells, T_C cells, and $CD8^+$ cells. The term $CD8^+$ cells refers to the fact that these cells possess on their surface an antigen designated as CD8. The primary function of cytotoxic T cells is to destroy virally infected host cells, foreign cells, and tumor cells. (An animated overview of the immune response can be found on thePoint.)

STUDY AID

Sorting Out the -Kines

Various types of cells within the human body, including cells of the immune system, communicate with each other. They do so by means of chemical messages—proteins known as **cytokines**. If the cytokines are chemotactic agents, attracting leukocytes to areas where they are needed, they are referred to as **chemokines**.

Where Do Immune Responses Occur?

Although it encompasses the whole body, the lymphatic system is the site and source of most immune activity. Immune responses to antigens in the blood are usually initiated in the spleen, whereas responses to microbes and other antigens in tissues are generated in lymph nodes located near the affected area. Antigens entering the body through mucosal surfaces (e.g., after inhalation or ingestion) activate immune responses in mucosa-associated lymphoid tissues. For example, immune responses to intranasal and inhaled antigens occur in the tonsils and adenoids. Ingested antigens enter specialized epithelial cells called microfold or M cells, which then transport the antigens to Peyer patches in the intestinal mucosa, where the immune responses are initiated. All of the various types of cells (macrophages, B cells, T cells, etc.) that collaborate to produce immune responses are present at these sites (spleen, lymph nodes, tonsils, adenoids, Peyer patches).

> Immune responses occur at many body sites, including the spleen, lymph nodes, tonsils, and adenoids.

Humoral Immunity

In **humoral immunity**, special glycoproteins (molecules composed of carbohydrate and protein) called antibodies are produced by B cells in response to antigens. In many cases, these antibodies are capable of recognizing, binding to, and inactivating or destroying specific pathogens.

A Closer Look at Antigens

Most **antigens** are foreign organic substances that are large enough to stimulate the production of antibodies; in other words, an antigen generates antibody production—it is an *anti*body-*gen*erating substance. Substances capable of stimulating the production of antibodies are said to be **antigenic** or **immunogenic**. Antigens may be proteins of more than 10,000 daltons[b] (Da) molecular weight, polysaccharides larger than 60,000 Da, large molecules of DNA or RNA, or any combination of biochemical molecules (e.g., glycoproteins, lipoproteins, and nucleoproteins) that are cellular components of either microorganisms or macroorganisms (e.g., helminths). Foreign proteins are the best antigens.

> Antigens stimulate the immune system to produce antibodies.

A bacterial cell has many molecules on its surface capable of stimulating the production of antibodies; these

---

[b]The term dalton is a unit of mass equal to 1/12 the mass of a carbon-12 (^{12}C) atom. A dalton is equal to 1 in the atomic mass scale. Daltons are used to express molecular weight.

individual molecules or antigenic sites are known as **antigenic determinants** (or *epitopes*). A bacterial cell could be described as a mosaic of antigenic determinants. The important point is that, in most cases, antigens must be *foreign* materials that the human body does not recognize as *self* antigens. Certainly, all invading microbes fall into this category. Some small molecules called **haptens** may act as antigens only if they are coupled with a large carrier molecule such as a protein. Then the antibodies formed against the antigenic determinant(s) of the hapten may combine with the hapten molecules when they are not coupled with the carrier protein. As an example, penicillin and other low–molecular-weight chemical molecules may act as haptens, causing some people to become allergic (or hypersensitive) to them.

> Individual molecules that stimulate the production of antibodies are referred to as antigenic determinants or epitopes.

Processing of Antigens in the Body

For antibodies to be produced within the body, a complex series of events must occur, some of which are not completely understood. It is known that macrophages, T cells, and B cells often are involved in a cooperative effort. (The processing of antigens within the body is actually far more complex than the abbreviated explanation that follows.)

> The processing of T-dependent antigens requires the participation of helper T cells, as well as macrophages and B cells.

T-dependent antigens. The majority of antigens are referred to as *T-dependent antigens*, because T cells (specifically, T_H cells) are involved in their processing. In other words, processing of these antigens is *dependent* on T cells. The processing of T-dependent antigens also involves macrophages and B cells.

T-independent antigens. Other antigens are known as *T-independent antigens*, the processing of which requires only B cells. In other words, the processing occurs independently of T cells (see Fig. 16-3). T-independent antigens are large polymeric molecules (usually polysaccharides) containing repeating antigenic determinants; examples include the lipopolysaccharide (LPS) found in the cell walls of Gram-negative bacteria, bacterial flagella, and bacterial capsules.

> Helper T cells are not involved in the processing of T-independent antigens; only B cells are required.

> The cells that secrete antibodies are called plasma cells; they are derived from B cells.

Table 16-3 summarizes the processing of T-independent and T-dependent antigens. Note that the processing of either

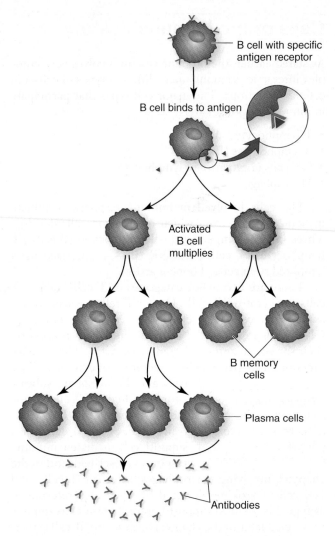

Figure 16-3. Processing of T-independent antigens. See Table 16-3 for details. (Redrawn from Cohen BJ. *Memmler's The Human Body in Health and Disease.* 11th ed. Philadelphia, PA: Lippincott Williams & Wilkins; 2009.)

category of antigen—T-independent or T-dependent—results in B cells developing into **plasma cells** that are capable of secreting antibodies.

The initial immune response to a particular antigen is called the **primary response**. In the primary response to an antigen, it takes about 10 to 14 days for antibodies to be produced. When the antigen is used up, the number of antibodies in the blood declines as the plasma cells die. Other antigen-stimulated B cells become memory cells, which are small lymphocytes that can be stimulated to rapidly produce large quantities of antibodies when later exposed to the same antigens. This increased production of antibodies after the second exposure to the antigen (e.g., a booster shot) is called the **secondary response**, *anamnestic*

> The initial response to an antigen is called the primary response, whereas a subsequent response to the same antigen is referred to as the secondary, anamnestic, or memory response.

Labels in figure:
- B cell with specific antigen receptor
- B cell binds to antigen
- Activated B cell multiplies
- B memory cells
- Plasma cells
- Antibodies

Table 16-3 Mechanisms by Which T-Dependent and T-Independent Antigens Are Processed by the Immune System

T-Independent Antigen	T-Dependent Antigen
Processing of T-independent antigens is initiated when an appropriate B cell makes physical contact with the free antigenic determinant (i.e., an antigenic determinant not bound to a major histocompatibility complex [MHC] molecule[a]).	After invasion of the body, an antigen (e.g., a bacterial cell) is ingested and digested by a macrophage.
↓	↓
The activated B cell next undergoes extensive cell division, producing a clone of identical B cells.	Within the macrophage, antigenic determinants of the bacterial cell (referred to as antigenic peptides or APs) attach to molecules called MHC molecules.
↓	↓
Some of the members of the newly formed clone mature into antibody-producing plasma cells, whereas others become memory cells (Fig. 16-3).	The combined AP–MHC molecules are then displayed on the surface of the macrophage; at this point, the macrophage is referred to as an **antigen-presenting cell** (APC).
	↓
	A T$_H$ cell attaches to one of the AP-MHC molecules, divides, and "sends out" (secretes) chemical signals (cytokines). (Note that T$_H$ cells assist in the production of antibodies, but do not manufacture antibodies themselves.)
	↓
	When the chemical signals reach a B cell that is capable of recognizing that particular signal, the activated B cell divides, producing a clone of identical B cells.
	↓
	Some of the members of the newly formed clone mature into antibody-producing plasma cells. Antibodies are expelled rapidly for several days until the plasma cell dies. Each plasma cell makes only one type of antibody; one that will bind with the antigenic determinant that activated the B cell and stimulated production of that antibody. Members of the clone that do not become plasma cells, and some of the activated T cells, remain in the body as memory cells, able to respond very quickly should the antigen enter the body again at a later date.

[a]MHC molecules are cell surface molecules that play roles in antigen presentation and rejection of foreign tissue transplants.

response, or *memory response*. A second booster shot of antigen many months later causes the antibody concentration to exceed the level of the secondary response. This is the reason why booster shots are given to protect against certain pathogens that one might encounter throughout life, such as the bacterium, *C. tetani* (the cause of tetanus). In addition to memory B cells, memory T cells also contribute to immunologic memory.

A Closer Look at Antibodies

Humoral immunity (or AMI) involves the production of antibodies, as opposed to CMI (discussed later in this chapter), which does not involve antibody production. *Antibodies* are proteins produced by lymphocytes in response to the presence of an antigen. (As previously described, the antibody-producing cells are a specific type of lymphocyte called B lymphocytes [or B cells],

STUDY AID

Immunologic Memory

During the processing of both T-dependent and T-independent antigens, memory cells are produced, in addition to antibody-secreting plasma cells. Memory cells are B cells and T cells that are primed to respond to a given antigen the *next time* that the antigen enters the body. This response is referred to as the secondary, anamnestic, or memory response. It occurs very rapidly and results in the production of large quantities of IgG antibodies directed against the antigen. Booster shots are given to trigger the secondary response.

which usually work in coordination with T lymphocytes [T cells] and macrophages.) A bacterial cell has numerous antigenic determinants on its cell membrane, cell wall, capsule, and flagella that stimulate the production of many different antibodies. Usually, an antibody is specific in that it will recognize and bind to only the antigenic determinant that stimulated its production. **Example:** Antibodies produced against molecules located on bacterial pili can recognize and bind to only those particular molecules. Occasionally, however, an antibody will bind to an antigenic determinant that is similar, but not identical, in structure to the antigenic determinant that stimulated its production; in this case, it is referred to as a *cross-reacting antibody*.

> Antibodies are usually very specific, binding only with the antigenic determinant that stimulated their production.

All antibodies are in a category of proteins called **immunoglobulins**—globular glycoproteins in the blood that participate in immune reactions. The term *antibodies* is used to refer to immunoglobulins with particular specificity for an antigen. In addition to being found in blood, immunoglobulins are found in lymph, tears, saliva, and colostrum (Fig. 16-4). Antibodies found in the blood are called humoral or circulating antibodies. As previously mentioned, antibodies that provide protection against infectious diseases are called protective antibodies.

> An antibody is an immunoglobulin having particular specificity for an antigen.

The amount and type of antibodies produced by a given antigenic stimulation depend on the nature of the antigen, the site of antigenic stimulus, the amount of antigen, and the number of times the person is exposed to the antigen. After the initial exposure to an antigen (such as a vaccine), there is a delayed primary response in the production of antibodies. During this lag phase, the antigen is processed by cells of the immune system. As previously mentioned, it takes about 10 to 14 days for antibodies to be produced.

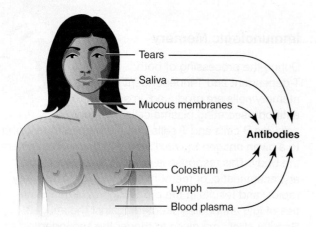

Figure 16-4. Body fluids and sites where antibodies are found.

- Tears
- Saliva
- Mucous membranes
- **Antibodies**
- Colostrum
- Lymph
- Blood plasma

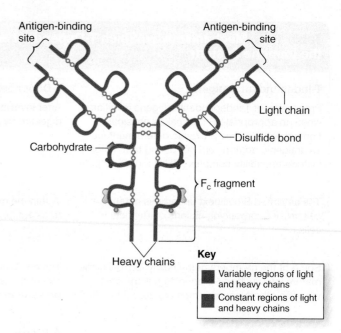

Figure 16-5. Basic structure of a monomeric immunoglobulin molecule. This molecule contains two light chains, two heavy chains, an F_C region, and two antigen-binding sites.

Labels in figure: Antigen-binding site; Antigen-binding site; Light chain; Disulfide bond; Carbohydrate; F_C fragment; Heavy chains

Key
- Variable regions of light and heavy chains
- Constant regions of light and heavy chains

Antibody Structure

As previously stated, antibodies belong to a category of glycoproteins called immunoglobulins. All antibodies are immunoglobulins, but not all immunoglobulins are antibodies. (However, to avoid any confusion, the terms are used synonymously in this book.) Antibodies are produced by plasma cells in response to stimulation of B cells by foreign antigens.

The basic structure of an immunoglobulin molecule resembles the letter Y (Fig. 16-5). It consists of two identical light polypeptide chains (located at the top of the Y), two identical heavy polypeptide chains, two antigen-binding sites (located at the very top of the Y), and a fragment crystallizable (F_C) region (located at the base of the Y). In this basic form, the molecule is referred to as a **monomer**. The light chains, which contain fewer amino acids than the heavy chains, are shorter and lighter in weight than the heavy chains. The chains are connected to each other by disulfide (—S—S—) bonds. The monomer is bivalent in the

> A monomer resembles the letter Y. It consists of two heavy chains, two light chains, two antigen-binding sites, and an F_C region.

sense that it has two sites (called *antigen-binding sites*) that can bind specifically to the antigenic determinant that stimulated production of that antibody.[c] The amino acid sequence within the variable regions of heavy and light chains enables the antibody molecule to bind to a particular antigenic determinant. The F_C region enables the

---

[c]It is important to note that the two antigen-binding sites can attach only to copies of the antigenic determinant that stimulated production of that antibody.

molecule to bind to cells (e.g., neutrophils, macrophages, basophils, mast cells) that possess surface receptors able to recognize various sites on the F$_C$ region.

> The five immuno-globulin classes are IgA, IgD, IgE, IgG, and IgM.

Studies of the gamma globulin component of human blood have revealed that five classes (or *isotypes*) of immunoglobulins exist, designated IgA, IgD, IgE, IgG, and IgM. (Ig stands for immunoglobulin.) IgA and IgG have subclasses. The amino acid sequence within the constant regions of heavy and light chains varies from one immunoglobulin class to another. Information about the various classes of immunoglobulins is presented in Table 16-4 and Figure 16-6.

Antigen–Antibody Complexes

When an antibody combines with an antigen, an **antigen–antibody complex** (or Ag–Ab complex, or *immune complex*) is formed. Antigen–antibody complexes are capable of activating the complement cascade (by the classical pathway), resulting in, among other effects, the

Table 16-4 Immunoglobulin Classes

IG Class	Molecular Weight (Da)	% of Total Ig in Serum (Approximate)	Functions
IgA	160,000–385,000; can exist as a monomer or as a dimer (two monomers held together by a short protein chain called a J-chain ["J" for joining])	10–20	The predominant immunoglobulin class in saliva, tears, seminal fluid, colostrum, breast milk, and mucous secretions of the nose, lungs, and gastrointestinal tract. In secretions, IgA is primarily present as secretory IgA (sIgA), a dimer that contains an additional protein called the secretory component. The secretory component apparently facilitates the transport of sIgA into secretions and may serve to protect the IgA molecule from enzymatic damage within the gastrointestinal tract. Protects external openings and mucous membranes from the attachment, colonization, and invasion of pathogens. IgA in colostrum and breast milk helps protect nursing newborns. In the intestine, IgA attaches to viruses, bacteria, and protozoal parasites, such as *Entamoeba histolytica*, and prevents the pathogens from adhering to mucosal surfaces, thus preventing invasion
IgD	180,000–184,000 (a monomer)	<1	Found in large quantities on the surface of B cells. Its function is unknown, but it is possible that the IgD molecules on the B cell's surface serve as antigen receptors and determine which specific antigen that particular B cell is able to respond to.
IgE	188,000–200,000 (a monomer)	<1	In atopic individuals, IgE is produced in response to allergens. Found on the surfaces of basophils and mast cells. Plays a major role in allergic responses. (Basophils are granulocytes that circulate in the blood. Mast cells are morphologically very similar to basophils, but they are found in tissues—especially tissues that surround the eyes, nose, respiratory tract, and gastrointestinal tract.)
IgG	146,000–170,000 (a monomer; the lightest of the immunoglobulins)	70–85 (the most abundant immunoglobulin type in serum)	The only class of immunoglobulin that can cross the placenta. Maternal IgG antibodies that cross the placenta help protect the newborn during its first months of life. Antigen-bound IgG can bind to and activate complement, a process known as "complement fixation." IgG molecules can bind to a wide range of cellular receptors to promote phagocytosis and antibody-dependent cytotoxicity. As a result of memory cells, high levels of IgG are produced very rapidly (within 1–3 days) during the secondary response to antigens (described earlier). IgG antibodies are long-lived, sometimes persisting for the lifetime of the individual.
IgM	900,000–970,000 (a pentamer, consisting of five monomers held together by a J-chain; the largest of the immunoglobulins)	10	Because a pentamer has 10 antigen-binding sites, IgM can potentially bind to 10 identical antigenic determinants. Theoretically, an IgM molecule could bind to 10 separate virus particles, thus preventing the viruses from attaching to target cells. IgM antibodies are the first antibodies formed in the primary response to antigens (including pathogens), although IgG antibodies later become the most prevalent class. IgM antibodies are relatively short-lived, remaining in the bloodstream for only a few months. Because of its large size, IgM does not cross the placenta. Provides protection in the earliest stages of infection. Bactericidal to Gram-negative bacteria. IgM is the most efficient complement-fixing (complement-binding) immunoglobulin.

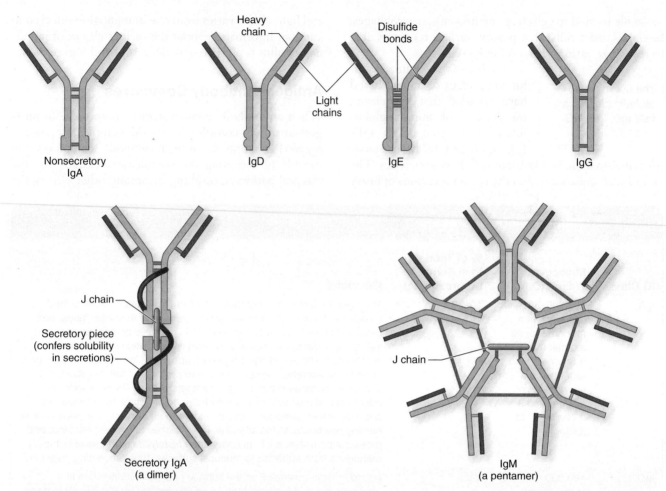

Figure 16-6. Structures of the different classes of antibodies. IgG, IgD, IgE, and nonsecretory IgA are monomers. Secretory IgA is a dimer (composed of two monomers), and IgM is a pentamer (composed of five monomers). J chains ("J" for joining) are short protein chains that bind monomers together. The secretory piece (or component) protects IgA molecules from proteolytic (protein-splitting) enzymes and facilitates transport of IgA molecules through membranes.

> The combination of an antibody and an antigen is called an antigen–antibody complex, Ag–Ab complex, or immune complex.

activation of leukocytes, lysis of bacterial cells, and increased phagocytosis as a result of opsonization. Thus, acute extracellular bacterial infections are controlled almost entirely by AMI. There is also a "dark side" to immune complexes, which will be discussed in a later section ("Type III Hypersensitivity Reactions").

How Antibodies Protect Us from Pathogens and Infectious Diseases

As previously mentioned, once they are produced, antibodies are very specific. Usually, a given antibody can recognize and bind to only the antigenic determinant that stimulated its production. Table 16-5 illustrates several of the ways in which antigen–antibody interactions protect us from pathogens and infectious diseases. Some examples are given here:

Example 1. A pathogen has entered a person's body and has started producing a toxin. That person's immune system responds by producing antibodies against the toxin; such antibodies are called **antitoxins**. Once produced, the antitoxins recognize, bind to, and neutralize the toxin molecules, so that they can no longer cause harm (i.e., they are no longer toxic).

Example 2. Recall from Chapter 14 that viruses can bind only to the host cells that bear the appropriate receptor on their surface. The molecule on the virus that recognizes and binds to the receptor is called an adhesin. A person has received a vaccine containing an attenuated virus (a virus that is no longer infectious). The vaccine stimulates that person's immune system to produce antibodies against the adhesin molecules. At some later date, should that same virus enter the person's body, those antibodies will adhere to the adhesin molecules, making it impossible for the virus to bind to host cells. If the virus is unable to bind to the appropriate host cell, it is unable to enter the cell, and the person is protected from infection with that virus.

Table 16-5 Antigen–Antibody Interactions and Their Effects

Interaction	Effects
Prevention of attachment	A pathogen coated with antibody is prevented from attaching to a cell.
Clumping of antigen	Antibodies link antigens together, forming a cluster that phagocytes can ingest.
Neutralization of toxins	Antibodies bind to toxin molecules to prevent them from damaging cells.
Help with phagocytosis	Phagocytes can attach more easily to antigens that are coated with antibody.
Activation of complement	When complement attaches to antibody on a cell surface, a series of reactions begins that activates complement to destroy cells.
Activation of NK cells	NK cells respond to antibody adhering to a cell surface and attack the cell.

Courtesy of Cohen BJ. *Memmler's The Human Body in Health and Disease*. 11th ed. Philadelphia, PA: Lippincott Williams & Wilkins; 2009.

Example 3. A person is infected with a piliated bacterium. (Recall that pili enable bacteria to attach to host cells, which, with certain bacterial pathogens, is necessary for the bacteria to cause disease.) That person's immune system responds by producing antibodies against the pili. The antibodies bind to the pili, making it impossible for the bacterial cells to bind to tissue. If the bacteria are unable to attach to tissue, they are unable to cause disease.

Example 4. A person is infected with an encapsulated bacterium. (Recall that bacterial capsules serve an antiphagocytic function, meaning that phagocytic white blood cells are unable to phagocytize encapsulated bacteria. The reason for this is that the phagocytes have no receptors on their surface that recognize the polysaccharide molecules. If the phagocyte is unable to attach to the encapsulated bacterium, it is unable to phagocytize it.) That person's immune system responds by producing antibodies against the capsular polysaccharide molecules. The antibodies attach to the capsule. This makes it possible for the phagocytes to bind to the encapsulated bacteria. Why? Because the phagocytes have receptors on their surface that can recognize and bind to antibody molecules.

> Among other functions, antibodies can neutralize toxins, prevent attachment of pathogens to host cells, and promote phagocytosis.

Monoclonal Antibodies

Purified antibodies that are directed against specific antigens have been produced in laboratories by an innovative technique in which a single plasma cell that produces only one specific type of antibody is fused with a rapidly dividing tumor cell. The new long-lived, antibody-producing cell is called a **hybridoma**. These hybridomas are capable of producing large amounts of specific antibodies called **monoclonal antibodies**. The first monoclonal antibodies were produced in 1975; since then, many uses have been found for them. They are commonly used in **IDPs**—immunologic procedures used in laboratories to diagnose diseases. The first diagnostic kit containing monoclonal antibodies was approved for use in the United States in 1981. Many other monoclonal antibody-based IDPs have been developed during the past 30+ years. Monoclonal antibodies are also being evaluated for possible use in fighting diseases, killing tumor cells, boosting the immune system, and preventing organ rejection.

> Monoclonal antibodies are produced by long-lived cells called hybridomas.

Cell-Mediated Immunity

Antibodies are unable to enter cells, including cells containing intracellular pathogens. Fortunately, there is an arm of the immune system capable of controlling chronic infections by intracellular pathogens (e.g., bacteria, protozoa, fungi, viruses). It is called CMI—a complex system of interactions among many types of cells and cellular secretions (cytokines). (Only a brief overview of CMI can be provided here.) Included among the various cells that participate in CMI are macrophages, T_H cells, T_C cells, NK cells, and granulocytes. Although CMI does not involve the production of antibodies, antibodies produced during humoral immunity can play a minor role in some cell-mediated responses.

> Cell-mediated immune responses involve many types of cells and cytokines; antibodies are rarely, if ever, involved.

A typical cell-mediated cytotoxic response would involve the following steps:

Step 1. A macrophage engulfs and partially digests a pathogen. Fragments (antigenic determinants) of the pathogen are then displayed on the surface of the macrophage (i.e., the macrophage acts as an antigen-presenting cell).

Step 2. A T_H cell binds to one of the antigenic determinants being displayed on the macrophage surface. The T_H cell produces cytokines, which reach an effector cell of the immune system (e.g., a T_C cell or NK cell).

Step 3. The effector cell binds to a target cell (i.e., a pathogen-infected host cell displaying the same antigenic determinant on its surface).

Step 4. Vesicular contents of the effector cell are discharged. These include perforin and other proteins and enzymes, which literally punch holes in the target cell membrane. Other cytokines released by effector cells are tumor necrosis factor and NK cytotoxic factor.

Step 5. Toxins produced by the effector cells enter the target cell, causing disruption of DNA and organelles. The target cell dies.

Both humoral and cell-mediated immune responses play a role in the body's defense against viral infections. In cytolytic viral infections (e.g., herpes infections), the viruses can be neutralized and destroyed by antibodies and the complement system when they move in body fluids from a lysed cell to an intact cell. When the virus is established within body cells, the cell-mediated immune response can destroy the virus-infected cells, preventing viral multiplication. If the virus is not completely destroyed, however, it may become latent in nerve ganglion cells, as in herpes infections (e.g., shingles).

T_C cells and NK cells kill infected host cells when pathogens are established inside the cells. Thus, infected liver cells are destroyed in hepatitis infections during the body's battle against the disease. The acquired immunodeficiency syndrome (AIDS) virus (human immunodeficiency virus [HIV]) that targets T_H cells is particularly destructive because it destroys the very cells that would have helped fight the infection. The lack of T_H cells impairs both humoral immunity and CMI, making AIDS patients very susceptible to many opportunistic infections and malignancies.

Natural Killer Cells

NK cells are in a subpopulation of lymphocytes called large granular lymphocytes. Although they morphologically resemble lymphocytes, NK cells lack typical T- or B-cell surface markers. They also differ from T and B cells in other ways. For example, they do not proliferate in response to antigen and appear not to be involved in antigen-specific recognition. As the name implies, NK cells kill target cells, including foreign cells, host cells infected with viruses or bacteria, and tumor cells. Although NK cell activity is not dependent on antibodies, NK cells have receptors on their surface for the F_C region of IgG antibodies. These receptors enable the cells to attach to and kill antibody-coated target cells; this is known as antibody-dependent cellular cytotoxicity. Once attached to an antibody-coated target cell, the NK cell inserts a molecule called perforin into the cell membrane of the target cell, creating an opening (pore), through which cytotoxic granules called granzymes are injected. Although firm evidence is lacking

> Cytotoxic T cells and NK cells kill foreign cells, host cells infected with viruses or bacteria, and tumor cells.

for an immune surveillance system within our bodies that monitors for and destroys malignant cells, NK cells may participate in such a system.

Hypersensitivity and Hypersensitivity Reactions

The term *hypersensitivity* refers to an overly sensitive or overly reactive immune system. In such situations, the immune system, in an attempt to protect the person, causes irritation or damage to certain cells and tissues in the body.

> Hypersensitivity can be thought of as an overly sensitive immune system.

There are several different types of **hypersensitivity reactions**. Some types involve antibodies, whereas others do not. All types depend on the presence of antigen and T cells that are sensitized to that antigen. Hypersensitivity reactions are divided into two general categories—immediate-type and delayed-type—depending on the nature of the immune reaction and the time required for an observable reaction to occur (Table 16-6). **Immediate-type hypersensitivity reactions** occur from within a few minutes to 24 hours after contact with a particular antigen. There are three categories of immediate-type hypersensitivity reactions, referred to

> Immediate-type hypersensitivity reactions occur within 24 hours of exposure to an antigen, whereas DTH reactions take longer than 24 hours to manifest themselves.

Table 16-6 Types of Hypersensitivity Reactions	
Immediate-type hypersensitivity reactions (occur from within a few minutes to 24 hours after contact with a particular antigen):	
Type I hypersensitivity reactions	Anaphylactic reactions (allergic reactions)
Type II hypersensitivity reactions	Cytotoxic reactions (involve damage to or death of body cells)
Type III hypersensitivity reactions	Immune complex reactions (damage to tissues and organs is initiated by antigen–antibody complexes)
DTH reactions (usually take 24 to 48 hours or longer to manifest themselves):	
Type IV hypersensitivity reactions	Also known as cell-mediated reactions; antibodies play only a minor role, if any; an example is a positive TB skin test

as type I, type II, and type III hypersensitivity reactions. A **delayed-type hypersensitivity (DTH) reaction** usually takes more than 24 hours to manifest itself. DTH reactions are also known as type IV hypersensitivity reactions and cell-mediated reactions.

Type I Hypersensitivity Reactions

> Classic allergic responses such as hay fever and food allergies are examples of type I hypersensitivity reactions, which are immediate-type hypersensitivity reactions.

Type I hypersensitivity reactions (also known as *anaphylactic reactions*) include classic allergic responses such as hay fever symptoms, asthma, hives, and gastrointestinal symptoms that result from food allergies; allergic responses to insect stings and drugs; and anaphylactic shock. These reactions all involve IgE antibodies and the release of chemical mediators (especially histamine) from mast cells and basophils.

The Allergic Response

Type I immediate hypersensitivity is probably the most commonly observed one, because more than half the American population is allergic to something. People who are prone to allergies (**atopic persons**) produce IgE (sometimes called reagin) antibodies when they are exposed to **allergens** (antigens that cause allergic reactions). The IgE molecules bind to the surface of basophils and mast cells by their F_C regions. The type and severity of an allergic reaction depend on a combination of factors, including the nature of the antigen, the amount of antigen entering the body, the route by which it enters, the length of time between exposures to the antigen, the person's ability to produce IgE antibodies, and the site of IgE attachment (Fig. 16-7).

> People who are prone to allergies are described as being atopic. They produce IgE antibodies when they are exposed to allergens (antigens that cause allergic reactions).

The allergic reaction results from the presence of IgE antibodies bound to basophils in the blood or to mast cells[d] in connective tissues—IgE antibodies that were produced in response to the person's first exposure to the allergen. When the allergen binds to cell-bound IgE during a subsequent exposure to the allergen, the sensitized cells respond by degranulation—the discharge and outpouring of granules and their irritating and damaging contents (chemical mediators) (Figs. 16-8 to 16-10). These mediators of the allergic responses include histamine, prostaglandins, serotonin, bradykinin, slow-reacting substance of anaphylaxis (SRS-A), leukotrienes, and chemicals that attract eosinophils (eosinophilotactic agents).

> Following their production, IgE antibodies bind to the surface of basophils and mast cells. Degranulation of the basophils and mast cells occurs when allergen later binds to these IgE antibodies.

STUDY AID

Examples of Allergens

Animal dander (e.g., cat dander)	Insect venom
Drugs (e.g., penicillin)	Latex
Foods (e.g., peanuts, shellfish, dairy products)	Mold spores
House dust (dust–mite feces)	Pollens

Localized Anaphylaxis

Type I hypersensitivity reactions (**anaphylactic reactions**) may be localized or systemic. Localized reactions usually involve mast cell degranulation, whereas systemic reactions usually involve basophil degranulation. Hay fever, asthma, and hives are examples of localized anaphylaxis. The symptoms depend on how the allergen enters the body and the sites of IgE attachment. If the allergen (e.g., pollens, dust, fungal spores) is inhaled and deposits on the mucous membranes of the respiratory tract, the IgE antibodies that are produced attach to mast cells in

> Type I hypersensitivity reactions (anaphylactic reactions) may be either localized or systemic. Systemic reactions tend to be more severe than localized reactions.

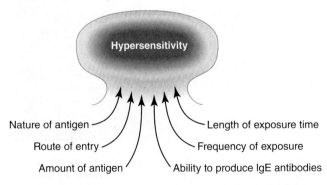

Figure 16-7. Factors in the development of type I hypersensitivity (allergies).

---

[d]Mast cells can be thought of as basophils that reside in tissues other than blood. They are most plentiful in the tissues that surround the eyes, respiratory tract, and gastrointestinal tract.

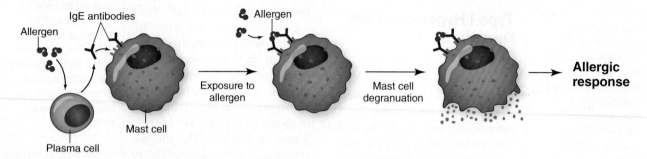

① Mast Cell Sensitization

First exposure to antigen causes plasma cell to produce specific IgE antibodies, which attach to the surface of tissue mast cells and blood basophils.

② Binding of Allergen

Receptor-bound IgE molecules are cross-linked by antigen (allergen).

③ Mast Cell Degranulation

The sensitized mast cells are stimulated to release granules containing histamine, leukotrienes, prostaglandins, and other potent chemical mediators.

Figure 16-8. Events that occur in type I hypersensitivity reactions. (Redrawn from Harvey RA, Champe PA, eds. *Lippincott Illustrated Reviews: Microbiology*. Philadelphia, PA: Lippincott Williams & Wilkins; 2001.)

that area. Subsequent exposure to those inhaled allergens allows them to bind to the attached IgE, causing mast cell degranulation. The released histamine initiates the classic symptoms of hay fever. Antihistamines function by binding to and, thus, blocking the sites where histamine binds. However, antihistamines are not as effective in treating asthma, because the mediators of this lower respiratory allergy include chemical mediators in addition to histamine. Allergens (e.g., food and drugs) entering through the digestive tract can also sensitize the host, and subsequent exposure may result in the symptoms of food allergies (hives, vomiting, and diarrhea).

Systemic Anaphylaxis

Systemic **anaphylaxis** results from the release of chemical mediators from basophils in the bloodstream. It occurs throughout the body and thus tends to be a more serious condition than localized anaphylaxis. It may lead to a severe, potentially fatal condition known as **anaphylactic shock**. Most often, the allergens involved in systemic anaphylaxis are drugs or insect venom to which the host has been sensitized. Penicillin is an example of a hapten—a substance that must first bind to a host blood protein (a carrier protein) before IgE antibodies are produced. The IgE antibodies then bind to circulating basophils. Subsequent injections of penicillin into the sensitized host may cause degranulation of the basophils and release of large amounts of histamine and other chemical mediators into the circulatory system.

> Systemic anaphylactic reactions can lead to anaphylactic shock, which, if not treated quickly and properly, can lead to death.

The shock reaction usually occurs immediately (within 20 minutes) after re-exposure to the allergen. The first

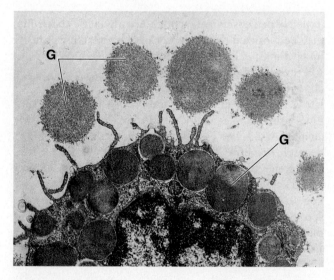

Figure 16-9. Transmission electron micrograph showing degranulation of a rat mast cell. The degranulation occurred under experimental conditions in a research laboratory. G, granule. (Courtesy of Biomed Ed, Round Rock, TX.)

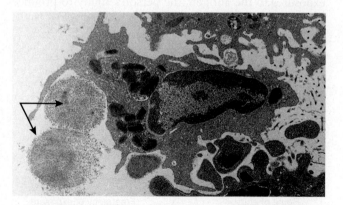

Figure 16-10. Transmission electron micrograph showing phagocytosis of rat mast cell granules (*arrows*) by a rat eosinophil. The phagocytosis occurred under experimental conditions in a research laboratory. (Courtesy of Biomed Ed, Round Rock, TX.)

symptoms are flushing of the skin with itching, headache, facial swelling, and difficulty breathing; this is followed by falling blood pressure, nausea, vomiting, abdominal cramps, and urination (caused by smooth muscle contractions). In many cases, acute respiratory distress, unconsciousness, and death may follow shortly. Swift treatment with epinephrine (adrenaline) and antihistamine usually stops the reaction.

Healthcare professionals must take particular care to ask patients whether they have any allergies or sensitivities before administering drugs. In particular, those people with allergies to penicillin and other drugs and to insect stings should wear MedicAlert jewelry, so that they do not receive improper treatment during a medical crisis.

Latex Allergy

Healthcare workers frequently come in contact with latex by wearing latex gloves and using other products containing latex. The National Institute for Occupational Safety and Health (NIOSH) has stated that "for some workers, exposures to latex may result in skin rashes; hives; flushing; itching; nasal, eye, or sinus symptoms; and (rarely) shock" (http://www.cdc.gov/niosh/docs/97-135). "Reports indicate that from 1% to 6% of the general population and about 8% to 12% of regularly exposed healthcare workers are sensitized to latex." Latex can trigger any of the following three types of reactions:

- **Irritant contact dermatitis.** This is the most common reaction to latex products. The affected individual experiences dry, itchy, irritated areas on the skin, usually the hands. This is not a true allergy because the immune system is not involved.
- **Allergic contact dermatitis.** This results from exposure to chemicals added to latex during harvesting, processing, or manufacturing. These chemicals can cause skin reactions similar to those caused by poison ivy. This is a type of delayed hypersensitivity or type IV allergy.
- **Latex allergy.** This is an immediate-type hypersensitivity that can be a more serious reaction to latex than irritant contact dermatitis or allergic contact dermatitis. Certain products in latex may cause sensitization. Subsequent exposure to latex can then trigger mild to severe reactions. Mild reactions include skin redness, hives, or itching. More severe reactions include respiratory symptoms (runny nose, sneezing), itchy eyes, scratchy throat, and asthma. Rarely, shock may occur. Latex allergy is a systemic type I, IgE-mediated reaction.

Latex allergy can be diagnosed using antibody detection procedures and skin testing. Once an individual becomes allergic to latex, special precautions are needed to prevent exposures. Certain medications may reduce the allergy symptoms,

> Many healthcare workers develop latex allergy, necessitating measures to avoid contact with latex-containing products.

but complete latex avoidance, although quite difficult, is the most effective approach. Many healthcare facilities maintain latex-safe areas for affected patients and workers. Additional information about the diagnosis and treatment of latex allergy can be found at the NIOSH web site.

Allergy Skin Testing and Allergy Shots

Anaphylactic reactions can be prevented by avoiding known allergens. In some cases, skin tests (scratch tests or intradermal injections of allergens) are used to identify the offending allergens. A skin test is considered positive if **cutaneous anaphylaxis** (i.e., swelling and redness at the scratch or injection site) occurs; this is often referred to as a "wheal and flare" reaction.

> A positive skin test result is swelling and redness (wheal and flare) at the site that the allergen was introduced into the skin.

Once the offending allergen is identified, immunotherapy may be accomplished by injecting small doses of allergen, repeatedly, several days apart. In hyposensitization, circulating IgG antibodies are produced rather than IgE antibodies. In theory, when the patient is later exposed in a natural manner to the allergen, the circulating IgG antibodies should bind with the allergen and block its attachment to the basophil- or mast cell–bound IgE. Such circulating IgG molecules, produced in response to allergy shots, are called **blocking antibodies.** Immunotherapy has been used in patients allergic to plant allergens, insect venoms, cat dander, and fire ant venom.

> Allergy shots result in the production of IgG blocking antibodies, which prevent the allergen from attaching to basophil- or mast cell–bound IgE.

Type II Hypersensitivity Reactions

Type II hypersensitivity reactions are cytotoxic reactions, meaning that body cells are destroyed during these reactions. These include the cytotoxic reactions that occur in incompatible blood transfusions, Rh incompatibility reactions, and myasthenia gravis; all of these reactions involve IgG or IgM antibodies and complement. A typical type II hypersensitivity reaction might follow this sequence:

> Type II hypersensitivity reactions are cytotoxic reactions.

Step 1. A particular drug binds to the surface of a body cell.
Step 2. Antidrug antibodies then bind to the drug.
Step 3. This initiates complement activation on the cell surface.
Step 4. The complement cascade leads to lysis of the body cell.

Type III Hypersensitivity Reactions

Recall that immune complexes are the result of binding of an antibody with the antigen that stimulated its produc-

> Type III hypersensitivity reactions are immune complex reactions.

tion. Earlier in the chapter, it was stated that immune complexes have a "dark side." The dark side is that immune complexes can result in *type III hypersensitivity reactions* (also known as immune complex reactions). Examples of type III hypersensitivity reactions are serum sickness and certain autoimmune diseases (e.g., systemic lupus erythematosus [SLE] and rheumatoid arthritis). These reactions involve IgG or IgM antibodies, complement, and neutrophils. Serum sickness is a cross-reacting antibody immune reaction in which antibodies formed to globular proteins in horse serum may also bind with similar proteins in the patient's blood. The formation of these immune complexes (antigen + antibody + complement) causes the symptoms of hives, fever, kidney malfunction, and joint lesions of serum sickness. Horse serum containing antitoxins is used to treat botulism. About 10% of patients receiving this antiserum develop serum sickness.

Certain complications (sequelae) of untreated or inadequately treated strep throat and other *Streptococcus pyogenes* infections are the result of type III hypersensitivity reactions. IgG and IgM antibodies produced in response

> Immune complications of *Streptococcus pyogenes* infections include rheumatic heart, arthritis, and glomerulonephritis.

to *S. pyogenes* infection may bind with streptococcal antigens (e.g., M-protein). The resultant immune complexes become deposited in heart tissue, joints, or the glomeruli of the kidney. This causes inflammation at the site, leading to scarring and, in some cases, abnormalities in or loss of function. Deposition of immune complexes in heart tissue leads to rheumatic heart, in joints leads to arthritis, and in kidneys leads to glomerulonephritis.

Type IV Hypersensitivity Reactions

Type IV hypersensitivity reactions are referred to as *delayed-type hypersensitivity* or cell-mediated immune reactions,

> Type IV hypersensitivity reactions are also known as delayed-type hypersensitivity reactions or cell-mediated immune reactions. They typically take 24 to 48 hours to manifest themselves.

and are part of CMI. (Recall that the two major arms of the immune system are humoral immunity and CMI.) Type IV hypersensitivity reactions are called DTH reactions because they are usually observed 24 to 48 hours or longer after exposure or contact. They occur in tuberculin and fungal skin tests, contact dermatitis, and transplantation rejection. DTH is

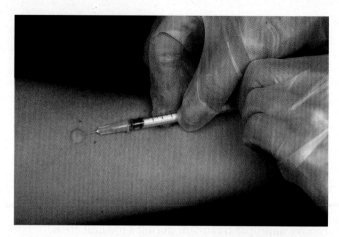

Figure 16-11. Mantoux skin test. This test is performed by injecting 0.1 mL of tuberculin or PPD intradermally and observing the results 48 to 72 hours later. If the person has been exposed to mycobacteria in the past, redness and swelling will occur at the injection site; this constitutes a positive TB skin test result. The diameter of induration (the palpable raised hardened area)—not the area of redness—is measured and the results are interpreted using standardized criteria. (Courtesy of Gabrielle Benenson, Greg Knobloch, and the CDC.)

the prime mode of defense against *intracellular* bacteria and fungi. DTH involves various cell types, including macrophages, cytotoxic T cells, and NK cells, but antibodies do not play a major role.

A classic example of a DTH reaction is a positive TB skin test (also called the Mantoux skin test).[e] Either tuberculin or purified protein derivative (PPD), protein extracts prepared from *Mycobacterium tuberculosis* cultures, is injected intradermally into a person (Fig. 16-11). If an "immunologic memory" of the *M. tuberculosis* proteins exists in the person's body, a DTH reaction will occur, producing the typical swelling and redness (wheal and flare) associated with a positive test result.

The following events occur to produce the positive reaction:

Step 1. Within 2 to 3 hours after injection of the PPD, there is an influx of polymorphonuclear cells (PMNs) into the site.

Step 2. This is followed by an influx of lymphocytes and macrophages while the PMNs disperse.

Step 3. Within 12 to 18 hours, the area becomes red (*erythematous*) and swollen (*edematous*).

Step 4. The *erythema* (redness) and *edema* (swelling) reach maximum intensity between 24 and 48 hours.

Step 5. With time, as the swelling and redness disappear, the lymphocytes and macrophages disperse.

A positive TB skin test result does not necessarily mean that a person has TB, although that is one possibility.

---

[e]The Mantoux skin test is named after Charles Mantoux, the French physician who introduced this test in 1908.

Actually, a positive TB skin test result may indicate any of the following five possibilities:

> A positive TB skin test indicates that an individual has been exposed to mycobacterial antigens. That individual may or may not have active TB.

1. The person has active TB (in which case, a chest radiograph will reveal the disease, the person will probably be coughing, and his/her sputum will contain acid-fast bacilli).
2. The person had TB at some time in the past and recovered (in this case, the person should remember having had TB or his/her medical records will contain this information).
3. The person was infected with *M. tuberculosis* at some time in the past, but the organisms were killed by his/her host defense mechanisms (even though this person currently harbors no live *M. tuberculosis* cells, he or she will receive a 6-month course of isoniazid, because there is no way to differentiate possibility 3 from possibility 4).
4. The person currently harbors live *M. tuberculosis* organisms but does not actually have TB (in this case, a 6-month course of isoniazid will be initiated in an attempt to kill any *M. tuberculosis* cells in his/her body).
5. The person had received Bacillus Calmette–Guérin (BCG) vaccine at some time in the past (he/she should remember having received BCG vaccine or he or she is from a country where BCG vaccine is routinely administered).

Many countries (excluding the United States) routinely immunize their citizens against TB using BCG vaccine. BCG vaccine is prepared from an attenuated strain of *Mycobacterium bovis*.[f] Although this vaccine is only about 50% effective in preventing TB, it does cause recipients to have positive TB skin test results for variable periods after immunization.

A reaction that is similar to the positive TB skin test occurs in contact dermatitis (contact hypersensitivity), after contact with certain metals, the catechols of poison ivy, cosmetics, and topical medications. The rejection of transplanted tissues containing foreign histologic (tissue) antigens appears to occur in a similar manner, except that cytokines and antibodies cause the rejection of the transplant.

Autoimmune Diseases

An **autoimmune disease** results when a person's immune system no longer recognizes certain body tissues as self and attempts to destroy those tissues as if they were

nonself or foreign. This may occur with certain tissues that are not exposed to the immune system during fetal development, so that they are not recognized as self. Such tissues may include the lens of the eye, the brain and spinal cord, and sperm. Subsequent exposure to this tissue (by surgery or injury) may allow antibodies (IgG or IgM) to be formed, which together with complement could cause destruction of these tissues, resulting in blindness, allergic encephalitis, or sterility. It is believed that certain drugs and viruses may alter the antigens on host cells, thus inducing the formation of autoantibodies or sensitized T cells to react against these altered tissue cells.

> An autoimmune disease results when a person's immune system attacks his/her body tissues as if they were nonself or foreign.

There are more than 80 recognized autoimmune diseases. It has been estimated that more than 10 million people in the United States suffer from these diseases.

Autoimmune diseases can be classified as organ-specific and non–organ-specific. Examples of organ-specific autoimmune diseases are Hashimoto thyroiditis, Graves disease, and primary myxoedema thyrotoxicosis (all three of which affect the thyroid); pernicious anemia affects the gastric mucosa; Addison disease affects the adrenal glands; and insulin-dependent diabetes mellitus, also known as type 1 diabetes, affects the pancreas. Non–organ-specific autoimmune diseases involve the skin, kidneys, joints, and muscles; examples include myasthenia gravis (affects muscle), dermatomyositis (affects skin), systemic lupus erythematosis (SLE; affects kidneys, lungs, skin, and brain), scleroderma (affects skin, lungs, kidneys, and the gastrointestinal tract), and rheumatoid arthritis (affects joints). Autoimmune diseases are the result of type II, III, or IV hypersensitivity reactions. For example, myasthenia gravis is the result of type II hypersensitivity, whereas rheumatoid arthritis and SLE are the result of type III hypersensitivity.

Immunosuppression

If a person's immune system is functioning properly, he/she is said to be an **immunocompetent person**. If a person's immune system is not functioning properly, he/she is said to be **immunosuppressed**, *immunodepressed*, or *immunocompromised*. The most common cause of immune deficiency worldwide is malnutrition. In addition, there are acquired and inherited immunodeficiencies.

> If a person's immune system is not functioning properly, he/she is said to be immunosuppressed, immunodepressed, or immunocompromised.

Acquired immunodeficiencies may be caused by drugs (e.g., cancer chemotherapeutic agents and drugs given to transplant

> Immunodeficiencies may be either inherited or acquired.

---

[f]BCG vaccine is named for Albert Calmette and Camille Guérin, French bacteriologists who developed this vaccine. The vaccine was first tested in 1921.

patients), irradiation, or certain infectious diseases (e.g., HIV infection). HIV infection leads to a decrease in T_H cells, which in turn prevents the production of antibodies against T-dependent antigens and, consequently, results in an inability to fight off certain pathogens. These pathogens overwhelm the patient's host defenses, eventually causing death. Persons with AIDS usually die of various devastating infectious diseases, including viral, bacterial, fungal, and parasitic diseases. Immune responsiveness and the ability to produce antibodies also decline as the normal body ages, perhaps the result of a declining ability of T cells to regulate the immune response. This, in turn, results in greater susceptibility of the elderly to serious infectious diseases.

Inherited immunodeficiency diseases can be the result of deficiencies in antibody production, complement activity, phagocytic function, or NK cell function. Several inherited immunodeficiency diseases have already been mentioned: chronic granulomatous disease, and Chediak–Higashi syndrome. Others include severe combined immune deficiency (SCID), DiGeorge syndrome, and Wiskott–Aldrich syndrome. SCID patients have deficiencies of B cells or T cells or both, resulting in severe recurrent infections.

In DiGeorge syndrome, there is a congenital absence of the thymus and parathyroid glands; patients suffer frequent infections and delayed development. Wiskott–Aldrich syndrome patients have deficiencies in B cells, T cells, monocytes, and platelets; effects on the patient include bleeding, recurrent infections, and eczema. Bone marrow transplantation and gene therapy may be valuable in treating certain immunodeficiency diseases.

It is hoped that the increased knowledge of genetics that is being gained as a result of the Human Genome Project will lead to an increased understanding of these diseases and various new methods by which they may be treated.

Some people are born lacking the ability to produce protective antibodies. Because they are unable to produce antibodies, they have no gamma globulins in their blood. This abnormality is called **agammaglobulinemia**. These persons are very susceptible to infections by even the least virulent microbes in their environment. One treatment for agammaglobulinemia that is often successful consists of a bone marrow transplant, which involves the transfer of precursor white blood cells from a closely related person. Some of these cells become lymphocytes. These lymphocytes may be implanted in the lymph nodes and become immunocompetent (i.e., capable of being stimulated by antigens to produce antibodies).

Persons who produce an insufficient amount of antibodies are said to have **hypogammaglobulinemia**.

> A person lacking the ability to produce antibodies is said to have agammaglobulinemia, whereas a person who produces too few antibodies is said to have hypogammaglobulinemia.

Their resistance to infection is lower than normal, so they usually do not recover from infectious diseases as readily as most other persons. One type, called Bruton hypogammaglobulinemia, is a hereditary disease in which the numbers of circulating B cells are profoundly low or totally absent.

The Immunology Laboratory

As mentioned in Chapter 13, immunologic procedures may be performed in an Immunology Laboratory that is separate from the Clinical Microbiology Laboratory (CML), or within the Immunology Section of the CML, depending on the size of the medical facility. Immunologic procedures include tests to diagnose infectious diseases and immune system disorders, determine tissue compatibility for organ and tissue transplants, and detect and measure various serum components (immunochemical procedures). Only a few of these procedures are discussed here.

Immunodiagnostic Procedures

Historically, the amount of time it takes to get laboratory results has been the most common criticism of the CML. Sometimes days or even weeks are necessary to isolate pathogens from clinical specimens, to get them growing in pure culture and large numbers, and to perform the tests necessary to identify them. With certain infectious diseases, it is impossible to isolate the pathogens, because they are either obligate intracellular pathogens or extremely fastidious.

One solution to these problems has been the development of IDPs—laboratory procedures that help to diagnose infectious diseases by detecting either antigens or antibodies in clinical specimens. The results of such procedures are often available on the same day that the clinical specimen is collected from the patient. IDPs performed on serum specimens are sometimes referred to as **serologic procedures**.

> Immunodiagnostic procedures are laboratory procedures that use principles of immunology to diagnose diseases.

Some IDPs are designed to detect antigens, whereas others detect antibodies (Fig. 16-12). Detection of antigens in a clinical specimen is an indication that a particular pathogen is present in the patient, thus providing direct evidence that the patient is infected with that pathogen. Detection of antibodies directed against a particular pathogen is indirect evidence of infection with that pathogen. In reality,

> Detecting antibodies to a particular pathogen in a clinical specimen may represent present infection, past infection, or prior vaccination against that pathogen.

Immunodiagnostic Procedures

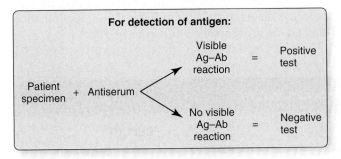

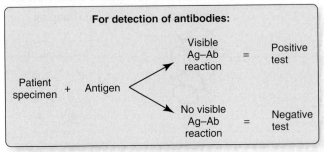

Figure 16-12. Principles of antigen and antibody detection procedures. Depending on the type of IDP being performed, the visible antigen–antibody (Ag–Ab) reaction might be agglutination (clumping) of cells or latex particles, formation of a precipitin line or band, fluorescence, or production of a color (as in enzyme immunoassays).

there are four possible explanations for the presence of antibodies to a particular pathogen:

- Present infection (i.e., the person is currently infected with the pathogen).
- Past infection (i.e., the person was infected with the pathogen in the past, and antibodies are still present in his/her body).
- Vaccination (i.e., the antibodies are the result of the person having been vaccinated against that particular pathogen at some time in the past; for example, a person's serum may contain antibodies against influenza viruses because he/she received a flu shot last year).
- Although we consider antibodies to be very specific, there are instances where antibodies can react with epitopes that are molecularly similar to, but not identical to, the epitope that stimulated production of the antibodies.[g] This is known as **cross-reactivity** or a **cross reaction**. Fortunately, in most IDPs, cross-reactivity is not a common event.

Because several explanations are possible for the presence of antibodies in a clinical specimen, the presence of antigens provides the best proof of current infection. Unfortunately, antigen detection procedures are not available for many infectious diseases. Another problem with antibody detection procedures is that it takes a person approximately 10 to 14 days to produce detectable antibodies; thus, even if the person is infected with a particular pathogen, antibodies will not be detectable for about 2 weeks.

Two ways to increase the value of antibody detection procedures to diagnose present infection are (a) to specifically test for IgM antibodies and (b) to use paired sera. Because IgM antibodies are the first antibodies to be produced during the initial exposure to an antigen (the primary response) and are relatively short-lived, the presence of IgM antibodies directed against a particular pathogen is evidence that the pathogen is currently infecting the individual.

To test paired sera, one serum specimen (called the *acute serum*) is collected during the acute stage of the disease and another (called the *convalescent serum*) is collected 2 weeks later. A significant rise in antibody titer (concentration) between the acute and convalescent sera is evidence that the patient was actively producing antibodies against that pathogen during the 2-week period and, therefore, that pathogen is the cause of the patient's current infection. The use of paired sera is useful for epidemiologic purposes (e.g., to determine the prevalent strain of influenza virus during a seasonal flu epidemic).

> The value of antibody detection procedures can be improved by specific detection of IgM antibodies or via the use of paired sera (i.e., acute and convalescent sera).

Laboratories purchase the reagents used to detect either antigens or antibodies from commercial companies. The reagent used to detect antigens contains antibodies and is called an antiserum. An antiserum is usually prepared by inoculating a laboratory animal with the pathogen (usually dead pathogens are used), and then collecting blood from the animal several weeks later. The blood is allowed to clot, and the serum is drawn off. The reagent used to detect antibodies contains antigens. This is usually a suspension of the dead pathogen.

A variety of different laboratory tests have been designed so that a visible reaction will be

> The reagent used to detect antigens contains antibodies and is called an antiserum. The reagent used to detect antibodies contains antigens.

> Tests used to determine that an antigen–antibody reaction occurred include agglutination, precipitin procedures, immunofluorescence procedures, and ELISAs.

---

[g]As an example, let us consider IDPs for the detection of antibodies directed against *Treponema pallidum* (the bacterium that causes syphilis). Antibodies produced against other pathogenic treponemes (e.g., the causative agents of yaws and pinta), as well as nonpathogenic treponemes, will cross-react with antigenic determinants possessed by *T. pallidum*. Thus, a positive test result for anti-*T. pallidum* antibodies may be due to antibodies that the patient's immune system has produced against some other treponemes, resulting in a false-positive test result.

observed if an antigen–antibody reaction takes place. Such tests, which include agglutination (involving the clumping of particles such as red blood cells [RBCs] or latex beads), precipitin procedures (involving the production of a precipitate), immunofluorescence procedures, and enzyme-linked immunosorbent assays (ELISAs), are represented diagrammatically in Table 16-7. Agglutination procedures are illustrated in Figure 16-13.

Table 16-7 IDPs for Detection of Antibodies in a Patient's Serum

Reaction In Vitro	REAGENTS			RESULTS	
	Antigen	Antibody	Other	Positive	Negative
Agglutination	Red blood cells or bacteria	Patient's serum		Clumping	No clumping
Precipitin	Toxins, hormones, proteins	Patient's serum	Agar or solution	Precipitate	No precipitate
Lysis by Complement	Cells, bacteria	Patient's serum	Complement	Lysis	No lysis
Fluorescent Antibody Technique	Pathogen	Patient's serum	Fluorescein-tagged rabbit antihuman antiserum	Fluorescent pathogen	No fluorescence
Capsular Swelling (Quellung Reaction)	Encapsulated bacteria	Patient's serum		Capsule appears to swell	No appearance of swelling
Enzyme-linked assay	Test microbe	Patient's serum	Enzyme-linked antibody +Substrate	Color change	No color change

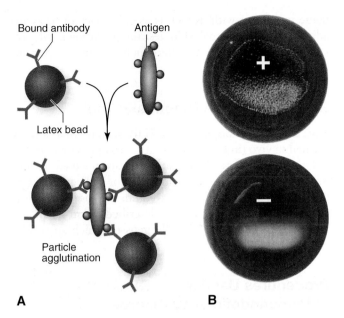

Bound antibody Antigen

Latex bead

Particle agglutination

A   B

Table 16-8	Blood Typing		
A Person Is Considered This Blood Type …	**IF THESE ANTIGENS ARE PRESENT ON THE SURFACE OF THEIR RBCS:**		
	A Antigen	**B Antigen**	**Rh Antigen**
Type A+	Present	Absent	Present
Type A–	Present	Absent	Absent
Type B+	Absent	Present	Present
Type B–	Absent	Present	Absent
Type AB+	Present	Present	Present
Type AB–	Present	Present	Absent
Type O+	Absent	Absent	Present
Type O–	Absent	Absent	Absent

Figure 16-13. Agglutination procedure. A. Schematic representation illustrating how antigen can agglutinate antibody-bound latex beads. This results in clumping of the latex beads. **B.** Actual latex agglutination test illustrating positive results (clumping of latex beads) and negative results (no clumping of latex beads). (A was redrawn from Harvey RA, et al. *Lippincott's Illustrated Reviews: Microbiology*. 3rd ed. Philadelphia, PA: Lippincott Williams & Wilkins; 2013.)

Antigen Detection Procedures

For detection of antigen, the clinical specimen is mixed with a particular antiserum (see Fig. 16-12). A visible reaction is the result of the formation of antigen–antibody complexes and indicates that the antigen is present in the clinical specimen; in such a case, the test result is considered positive. If the visible reaction is not observed, then the antigen is not present in the specimen and the test result is negative. **Example:** A drop of cerebrospinal fluid (CSF) from a patient with meningitis is mixed with a drop of antiserum containing antibodies against *H. influenzae*. A visible antigen–antibody reaction is evidence that the patient's CSF contained *H. influenzae* antigens, and the patient's condition is diagnosed as meningitis caused by *H. influenzae*.

Blood Typing

Agglutination tests are used in the Blood Bank to learn a person's blood type, which is determined by the types of antigens present on the surface of his/her RBCs. Three reagents are used for ABO and Rh typing:

Anti-A antiserum (a serum containing antibodies against A antigen)

Anti-B antiserum (a serum containing antibodies against B antigen)

Anti-Rh antiserum (a serum containing antibodies against Rh antigen)[h]

In three separate tests, each antiserum is mixed together with the person's RBCs. In each test, agglutination (clumping) of the RBCs will occur if that particular antigen is present on the RBCs (see Table 16-8). Reactions with anti-A and anti-B antisera are depicted in Figure 16-14.

Example 1: A person is said to be A positive (A+) if his/her RBCs have A antigen and Rh antigen on their surface, but lack B antigen.

Example 2: A person is said to be O negative (O–) if his/her RBCs lack A antigen, B antigen, and Rh antigen.

It is important to remember that, in addition to the antigens that determine a person's ABO blood type and Rh status, the surface of RBCs contains many other antigens.

Antibody Detection Procedures

For detection of antibodies, the clinical specimen is mixed with a suspension of a particular antigen (see Fig. 16-12). A visible reaction indicates that antibodies against that pathogen are present in the clinical specimen, and the test result is positive. If the visible reaction is not observed, then antibodies against that pathogen are not

[h]The Rhesus blood group system is based on another important group of RBC antigens. "Rh" stands for "Rhesus factor." In reality, the Rh blood group system consists of 50 defined blood group antigens. "Rh factor" strictly refers only to the most immunogenic of these antigens-called *D antigen*. A person either has or does not have Rh factor on the surface of his/her RBCs. If Rh factor is present, he/she is considered Rh positive; if not, he/she is considered Rh negative. The original antiserum used to detect this antigen was produced in the 1940s by injecting rabbits with RBCs from a rhesus monkey; the term "Rhesus" is still in use.

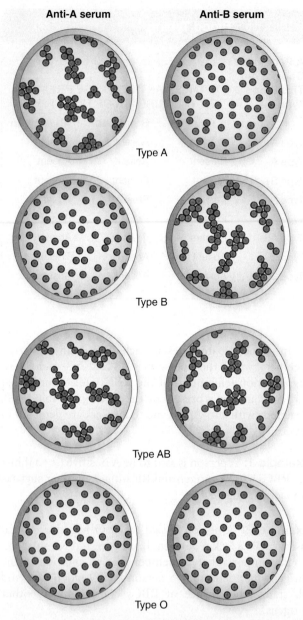

Figure 16-14. Agglutination procedure used for ABO blood typing. Clumping of the person's RBCs with either anti-A antiserum or anti-B antiserum signifies that A antigen and/or B antigen is present on his/her RBCs. (From Cohen BJ. *Memmler's The Human Body in Health and Disease.* 11th ed. Philadelphia, PA: Lippincott Williams & Wilkins; 2009.)

present in the specimen and the test result is negative. **Example:** A drop of serum from a patient suspected of having Lyme disease is mixed with a suspension of *Borrelia burgdorferi* (the bacterium that causes Lyme disease). A visible antigen–antibody reaction is evidence that the patient's serum contained antibodies against *B. burgdorferi*, and the patient's condition is diagnosed as Lyme disease.

The radioallergosorbent test (RAST) is used to detect and measure circulating IgE antibodies produced against allergens that individuals inhale, ingest, or otherwise come in contact with. RAST is used in place of or as an adjunct to intradermal skin testing (traditional allergy testing) to determine the allergen(s) to which a person is allergic.

Skin Testing as a Diagnostic Tool

Skin testing is another type of IDP, but one that is performed in vivo (in the patient) rather than in vitro (in the laboratory). In skin testing, antigens are injected within or beneath the skin (intradermally or subcutaneously, respectively). An example of a commonly used skin test is the TB skin test (previously described). Skin testing is also used to determine the allergens to which an atopic individual is allergic.

Procedures Used in the Diagnosis of Immunodeficiency Disorders

In addition to IDPs, tests are performed in the Immunology Laboratory that enable the assessment of a patient's immune status and evaluation of immunodeficiency disorders. These include tests to diagnose B-cell deficiency states (humoral immunodeficiencies), cell-mediated immunodeficiencies, combined humoral and cell-mediated immunodeficiencies, phagocytic deficiency states, and complement deficiencies.

ON **the Point**

- Terms Introduced in This Chapter
- Review of Key Points
- Increase Your Knowledge
- Critical Thinking
- Additional Self-Assessment Exercises

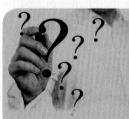

Self-Assessment Exercises

After studying this chapter, answer the following multiple-choice questions.

1. Of the following, which is the *least* likely to be involved in CMI?
   a. antibodies
   b. cytokines
   c. macrophages
   d. T cells

2. Antibodies are secreted by:
   a. basophils
   b. macrophages
   c. plasma cells
   d. T cells

3. Humoral immunity involves all the following except:
   a. antibodies
   b. antigens
   c. NK cells
   d. plasma cells

4. Immunity that develops as a result of an actual infection is called:
   a. artificial active acquired immunity
   b. artificial passive acquired immunity
   c. natural active acquired immunity
   d. natural passive acquired immunity

5. Artificial passive acquired immunity would result from:
   a. having the measles
   b. ingesting colostrum
   c. receiving a gamma globulin injection
   d. receiving a vaccine

6. The vaccines that are used to protect people from diphtheria and tetanus are:
   a. antitoxins
   b. attenuated vaccines
   c. inactivated vaccines
   d. toxoids

7. Natural passive acquired immunity would result from:
   a. having the measles
   b. ingesting colostrum
   c. receiving a gamma globulin injection
   d. receiving a vaccine

8. Which of the following statements about IgM is *false*?
   a. IgM contains a J-chain
   b. IgM has a total of 10 antigen-binding sites
   c. IgM is a pentamer
   d. IgM is a long-lived molecule

9. Which of the following could be an effect of type III hypersensitivity?
   a. glomerulonephritis
   b. rheumatoid arthritis
   c. SLE
   d. all of the above

10. Most likely, immunology got its start in 1890 when these scientists discovered antibodies while developing a diphtheria antitoxin.
    a. Edward Jenner and Louis Pasteur
    b. Elie Metchnikoff and Robert Koch
    c. Emil Behring and Kitasato Shibasaburo
    d. Jonas Salk and Albert Sabin

17

Overview of Human Infectious Diseases

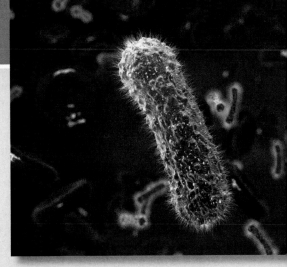

Artist rendering of a bacterial bloodstream infection.

 CHAPTER OUTLINE

 LEARNING OBJECTIVES

After studying this chapter, you should be able to:

- Define the terms and abbreviations introduced in this chapter
- Categorize various infectious diseases by body system (e.g., cystitis is an infection of the urinary bladder, which is part of the genitourinary [GU] system; myelitis is an infection of the brain and spinal cord)

Introduction

Human diseases fall into many different categories, including:

- Degenerative diseases
- Immune disorders
- Infectious diseases
- Metabolic disorders
- Neoplasms (cancers and other types of tumors)
- Nutritional disorders
- Psychiatric disorders

Of these disease categories, only infectious diseases are caused by microbes.[a] Recall from Chapter 1 that pathogens actually cause two general categories of diseases: microbial intoxications and infectious diseases. **Microbial intoxications**, which follow ingestion of a toxin produced outside the body (in vitro) by a pathogen, are discussed in Appendix 1 on thePoint. **Infectious diseases (or infections)**, on the other hand, follow colonization

---

[a]Some types of cancer are also known to be caused by viruses, but these are only briefly discussed in Chapter 4.

> Infectious diseases are diseases that are caused by pathogens, following colonization of some body site by the pathogen.

of some body site by a pathogen. This chapter provides an overview of the major infectious diseases of humans. Chapters 18 through 21 provide detailed information about specific infectious diseases.

This chapter is divided into sections that describe infectious diseases of various anatomical sites, including skin, ears, eyes, respiratory system, the oral region, gastrointestinal (GI) tract, GU system, circulatory system, and central nervous system (CNS). Although a particular disease may be described within one particular section of this chapter (e.g., in the section describing infectious diseases of the respiratory system), readers should keep in mind that some infectious diseases involve several body systems simultaneously, and that the pathogen(s) causing a particular infection may move from one body site to another during the course of that disease.

> Some infectious diseases affect more than one anatomical site, and some pathogens move from one body site to another during the course of a disease.

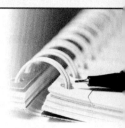

STUDY AID

What to Learn?

After studying Chapter 17, students should be able to define the terms and abbreviations introduced in this chapter and categorize various infectious diseases by body system (e.g., that myocarditis is an inflammation of the muscular walls of the heart—the myocardium; that encephalitis is an inflammation of the brain).

Infectious Diseases of the Skin

As mentioned in Chapter 15, intact skin is a type of nonspecific host defense mechanism, serving as a physical barrier (Fig. 17-1). It is part of the body's first line of defense. Very few pathogens can penetrate intact skin.

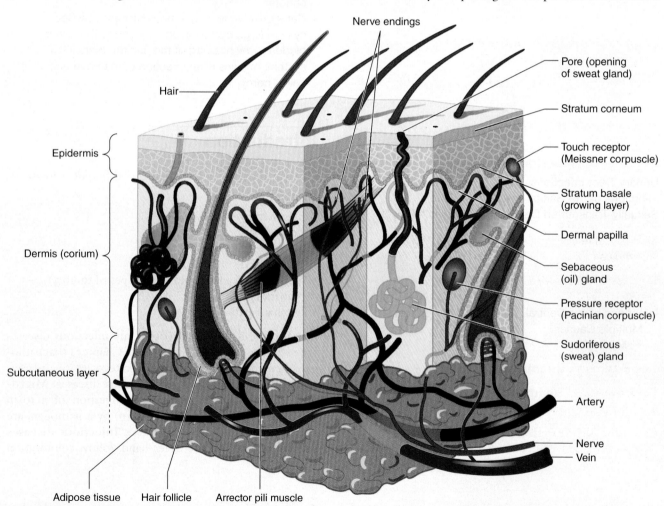

Figure 17-1. Cross section of the skin. (From Cohen BJ. *Memmler's The Human Body in Health and Disease*. 11th ed. Philadelphia, PA: Lippincott Williams & Wilkins; 2009.)

The indigenous microbiota of the skin, a low pH, and the presence of chemical substances such as lysozyme and sebum also serve to prevent colonization of the skin by pathogens. Nonetheless, skin infections do occur. Listed here are some terms relating to skin and infectious diseases of the skin:

- **Epidermis.** The superficial portion of the skin.
- **Dermis.** The inner layer of skin, containing blood and lymphatic vessels, nerves, nerve endings, glands, and hair follicles.
- **Dermatitis.** Inflammation of the skin.
- **Sebaceous glands.** Glands in the dermis that usually open into hair follicles and secrete an oily substance known as **sebum**.
- **Folliculitis.** Inflammation of a hair follicle, the sac that contains a hair shaft.
- **Sty (or stye).** Inflammation of a sebaceous gland that opens into a follicle of an eyelash.
- **Furuncle.** A localized pyogenic (pus-producing) infection of the skin, usually resulting from folliculitis; also known as a **boil**.
- **Carbuncle.** A deep-seated pyogenic infection of the skin, usually arising from a coalescence of furuncles.
- **Macule.** A surface lesion that is neither raised nor depressed, such as the lesions of measles.
- **Papule.** A surface lesion that is firm and raised, such as the lesions of chickenpox.
- **Vesicle.** A blister or small fluid-filled sac, such as is seen in chickenpox and shingles.
- **Pustule.** A pus-filled surface lesion.

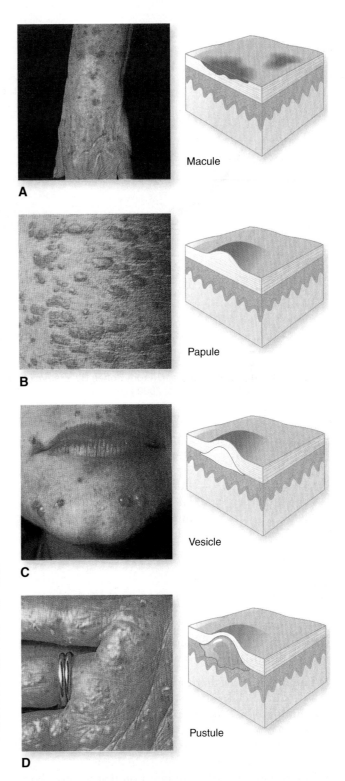

Figure 17-2. Types of surface lesions. A. Macules, **(B)** papules, **(C)** vesicles, and **(D)** pustules. (From Cohen BJ. *Memmler's The Human Body in Health and Disease.* 11th ed. Philadelphia, PA: Lippincott Williams & Wilkins; 2009.)

> ## STUDY AID
>
> ### The Suffix "itis"
>
> Words ending in "itis" refer to an inflammation of a particular anatomical region. For example, *meningitis* means an inflammation of the meninges (the membranes that surround the brain and the spinal column). Although inflammation is often the result of an infection, it can be caused by other factors (e.g., toxins and chemicals).

Various types of surface lesions are shown in Figure 17-2.

Infectious Diseases of the Ears

The anatomy of the ear is shown in Figure 17-3. There are three pathways for pathogens to enter the ear: (a) through the eustachian (auditory) tube, from the throat and nasopharynx; (b) from the external ear; and (c) via the blood or lymph. Usually, bacteria are trapped in the middle ear when a bacterial infection in the throat and nasopharynx causes the eustachian tube to close. The result is an anaerobic condition in the middle ear, allowing obligate and facultative anaerobes to proliferate and cause pressure on the tympanic membrane (eardrum). Swollen

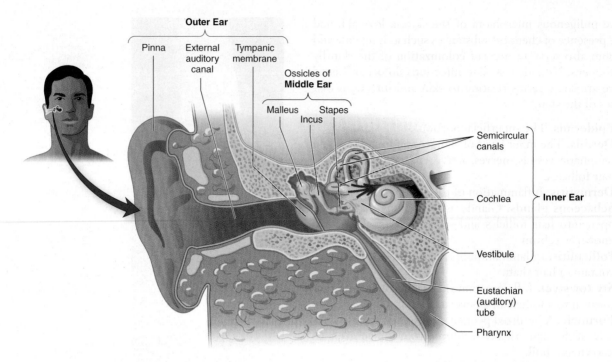

Figure 17-3. Anatomy of the ear. (From Cohen BJ. *Memmler's The Human Body in Health and Disease.* 11th ed. Philadelphia, PA: Lippincott Williams & Wilkins; 2009.)

> Infection of the middle ear is known as otitis media, whereas infection of the outer ear canal is known as otitis externa.

lymphoid (adenoid) tissues, viral infections, and allergies may also close the eustachian tube, especially in young children. Infection of the middle ear is known as **otitis media**, whereas infection of the outer ear canal is known as **otitis externa**.

Infectious Diseases of the Eyes

The anatomy of the eye is shown in Figure 17-4. Terms relating to the eye and infectious diseases of the eye include the following:

- **Conjunctiva.** The thin, tough lining that covers the inner wall of the eyelid and the sclera (the white of the eye).
- **Conjunctivitis.** An infection or inflammation of the conjunctiva.
- **Keratitis.** An infection or inflammation of the cornea—the domed covering over the iris and lens.
- **Keratoconjunctivitis.** An infection that involves both the cornea and conjunctiva.

Infectious Diseases of the Respiratory System

For practical purposes, the discussion of the respiratory system is divided into the upper respiratory tract (URT) and the lower respiratory tract (LRT). The URT

includes the paranasal sinuses, nasopharynx, oropharynx, epiglottis, and larynx ("voice box"). The LRT includes the trachea ("windpipe"), bronchial tubes, and alveoli of the lungs. The respiratory system is depicted in Figure 17-5.

Indigenous microbiota of the URT may cause opportunistic infections of the respiratory system. Infectious diseases of the URT (e.g., colds and sore throats) are more common than infectious diseases of the LRT. They may predispose the patient to more serious infections, such as sinusitis, otitis media, bronchitis, and pneumonia. LRT infections are the most common cause of death from infectious diseases.

> LRT infections are the most common cause of death from infectious diseases.

Terms relating to infectious diseases of the respiratory system include the following:

- **Bronchitis.** Inflammation of the mucous membrane lining of the bronchial tubes; most commonly caused by respiratory viruses.
- **Bronchopneumonia.** Combination of bronchitis and pneumonia.
- **Epiglottitis.** Inflammation of the epiglottis (the mouth of the windpipe); may cause respiratory obstruction, especially in children; frequently caused by *Haemophilus influenzae* type b (Hib).
- **Laryngitis.** Inflammation of the mucous membrane of the larynx (voice box).
- **Pharyngitis.** Inflammation of the mucous membrane and underlying tissue of the pharynx; commonly referred to as **sore throat**. "Strep throat" is pharyngitis

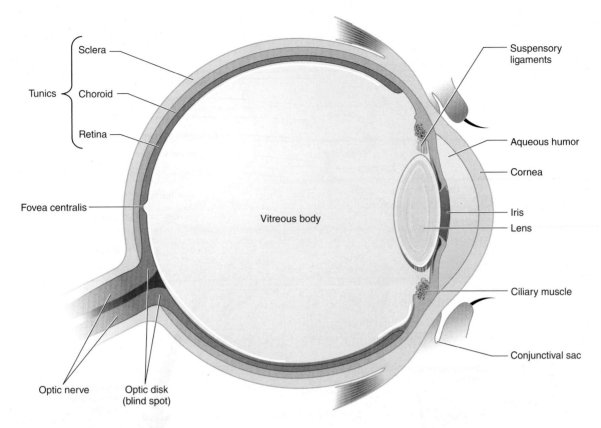

Figure 17-4. Anatomy of the eye. (From Cohen BJ. *Memmler's The Human Body in Health and Disease.* 11th ed. Philadelphia, PA: Lippincott Williams & Wilkins; 2009.)

caused by *Streptococcus pyogenes*. Even though *S. pyogenes* is the most "publicized" cause of pharyngitis, most cases of pharyngitis are caused by viruses.

- **Pneumonia.** Inflammation of one or both lungs. Alveolar sacs become filled with exudate, inflammatory cells, and fibrin. Most cases of pneumonia are caused by bacteria or viruses, but it can also be caused by fungi and protozoa.
- **Sinusitis.** Inflammation of the lining of one or more of the paranasal sinuses. The most common causes are the bacteria, *Streptococcus pneumoniae* and *H. influenzae*. Less common causes are the bacteria, *S. pyogenes*, *Moraxella catarrhalis*, and *Staphylococcus aureus*.

> Even though *S. pyogenes* is the most widely "publicized" cause of pharyngitis, viruses cause most cases of pharyngitis.

nausea, diarrhea, and vomiting. X-ray abnormalities are proportional to the physical symptoms. Common causes of typical pneumonia are the bacteria, *S. pneumoniae*, *H. influenzae*, and *S. aureus*, and viruses such as influenza virus types A and B, parainfluenza viruses, and respiratory syncytial virus (RSV). Other causes are *Legionella pneumophila*, *Mycoplasma pneumoniae*, *Chlamydophila pneumoniae*, and other Gram-negative bacilli. **Atypical pneumonia** has a more insidious (slower) onset than typical pneumonia. Patients present with headache, fever, cough with little sputum, and myalgia. X-ray abnormalities are usually greater than the physical symptoms would predict. Common causes of atypical pneumonia are the bacteria, *M. pneumoniae*, *C. pneumoniae*, and *L. pneumophila*, and viruses such as influenza viruses, RSV, and adenoviruses. Other causes are *Chlamydophila psittaci* (a bacterium), *Pneumocystis jiroveci* (a fungus), varicella-zoster virus, and parainfluenza viruses. Note that some pathogens can produce either typical or atypical pneumonia.

STUDY AID

Typical versus Atypical Pneumonia

Patients with **typical pneumonia** experience chest pain, dyspnea (shortness of breath), fever, chills, and a productive cough (one that produces purulent sputum). Less common symptoms include anorexia, headache,

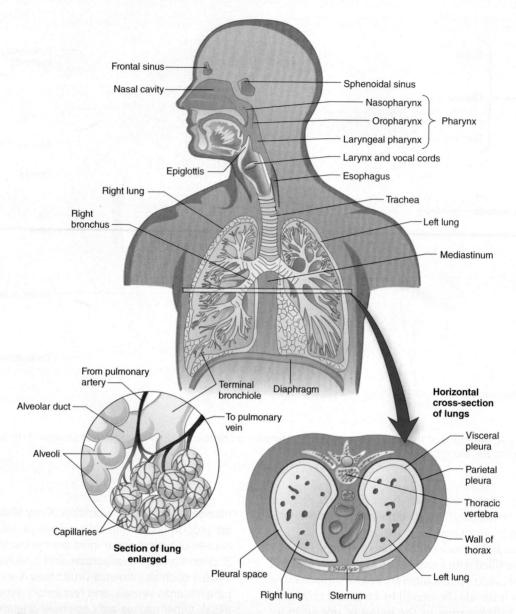

Figure 17-5. Anatomy of the respiratory system. (From Cohen BJ. *Memmler's The Human Body in Health and Disease.* 11th ed. Philadelphia, PA: Lippincott Williams & Wilkins; 2009.)

SPOTLIGHTING

Respiratory Therapists

As stated in the American Medical Association's (AMA) Health Care Careers Directory (available under "Education," Health Service Careers Directory at http://www.ama-assn.org), "Respiratory therapists work in a wide variety of settings to evaluate, treat, and manage patients of all ages with respiratory illnesses and cardiopulmonary disorders. Entry-level respiratory therapists perform general respiratory care procedures. They may assume clinical responsibility for specified respiratory care modalities involving the application of therapeutic

techniques under the supervision of an advanced-level therapist and/or a physician. The advanced-level respiratory therapist participates in clinical decision-making and patient education, develops and implements respiratory care plans, applies patient-driven protocols, utilizes evidence-based clinical practice guidelines, and participates in health promotion, disease prevention, and disease management. The advanced-level respiratory therapist may be required to exercise considerable independent judgment, under the supervision of a physician, in the respiratory care of patients." Information concerning educational requirements and programs, certification, and salary can be found on the AMA Web site.

Infectious Diseases of the Oral Region

As discussed in Chapter 10, the oral cavity (mouth) is a complex ecosystem suitable for growth and interrelationships of many types of microorganisms (Fig. 17-6). Although the actual indigenous microbiota of the mouth varies greatly from one person to the next, studies have shown that it includes about 300 identified species of bacteria, both aerobes and anaerobes. Many additional, as yet unclassified bacteria also live there. Some members of the oral microbiota are beneficial in that they produce secretions that are antagonistic to other bacteria. Although several bacterial species, such as *Streptococcus* (*Streptococcus salivarius*, *Streptococcus mitis*, *Streptococcus sanguis*, and *Streptococcus mutans*) and *Actinomyces* spp., often interact to protect the oral surfaces, in other circumstances, they are involved in oral disease.

> Most infections of the oral cavity are caused by members of the indigenous oral microbiota, sometimes one member acting independently and other times several members acting together.

In the healthy mouth, saliva secreted by salivary glands helps control the growth of opportunistic oral microbes. Saliva contains enzymes (including lysozyme), immunoglobulins (IgA), and buffers to control the near-neutral pH and continually flushes microbes and food particles through the mouth. Other antimicrobial secretions and phagocytes are found in the mucus that coats the oral surfaces. The hard, complex, calcium tooth enamel, bathed in protective saliva, usually resists damage by oral microbes. However, if the ecological balance is upset or is not properly maintained, oral disease may result. The following terms relate to infectious diseases of the oral cavity:

- **Dental caries**. Tooth decay or cavities. Dental caries start when the external surface (the enamel) of a tooth is dissolved by organic acids produced by masses of microorganisms attached to the tooth (dental plaque). This is followed by enzymatic destruction of the protein matrix, cavitation, and bacterial invasion. The most common cause of tooth decay is *S. mutans*, which produces lactic acid as an end product in the fermentation of glucose.
- **Gingivitis**. Inflammation of the gingiva (gums).
- **Periodontitis**. Inflammation of the periodontium (tissues that surround and support the teeth, including the gingiva and supporting bone); in severe cases, teeth loosen and fall out.

> The most common cause of tooth decay is *S. mutans*.

Oral infections result from a combination of the unique microbial population, reduced host defenses, improper diet, and poor dental hygiene. These diseases are the consequence of at least four microbial activities, including (a) formation of dextran (a polysaccharide) from sugars by streptococci, (b) acid production by lactic acid–producing bacteria, (c) deposition of calculus by *Actinomyces*, and (d) secretion of inflammatory substances (endotoxin) by *Bacteroides* species. This combination of circumstances damages the teeth, soft tissues (gingiva), alveolar bone, and the periodontal fibers that attach teeth to bone. Oral diseases such as gingivitis, periodontitis, and trench mouth are collectively known as **periodontal diseases**.

> Oral diseases such as gingivitis, periodontitis, and trench mouth are collectively known as periodontal diseases.

Periodontal diseases can be prevented by maintaining good health, proper oral hygiene (tooth brushing, using tartar-control toothpaste, and flossing), an adequate diet without sugars, and regular fluoride treatments to help control the microbial population and to prevent damaging bacterial interactions. Severe gingivitis and periodontitis require professional care by a specially trained dentist called a periodontist. Using techniques known as scaling and planing, periodontists remove tartar that has accumulated on tooth surfaces up to one fifth of an inch below the gum line—areas where tooth brushing and flossing cannot reach. After dental surgery, periodontists often prescribe a chlorhexidine mouth rinse as a temporary substitute for brushing and flossing.

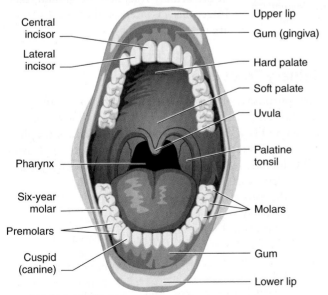

Central incisor
Lateral incisor
Pharynx
Six-year molar
Premolars
Cuspid (canine)
Upper lip
Gum (gingiva)
Hard palate
Soft palate
Uvula
Palatine tonsil
Molars
Gum
Lower lip

Figure 17-6. Anatomy of the mouth. (From Cohen BJ. *Memmler's The Human Body in Health and Disease.* 11th ed. Philadelphia, PA: Lippincott Williams & Wilkins; 2009.)

Infectious Diseases of the Gastrointestinal Tract

The GI tract consists of a long tube with many expanded areas designed for digestion of food, absorption of nutrients, and elimination of undigested materials (Fig. 17-7). Transient and resident microbes continuously enter and leave the GI tract. Most of the microorganisms ingested with food are destroyed in the stomach and duodenum by

- **Gastritis.** Inflammation of the mucosal lining of the stomach.
- **Gastroenteritis.** Inflammation of the mucosal linings of the stomach and intestines.
- **Hepatitis.** Inflammation of the liver; usually the result of viral infection, but can be caused by toxic agents.

Diarrhea is a symptom in a wide variety of conditions and diseases. It can be caused by certain foods or drugs, or it may be the result of an infectious disease. If diarrhea results from an infectious disease, the pathogen may be a virus, a bacterium, a protozoan, or a helminth. Dysentery may also be caused by various pathogens, including bacteria (e.g., *Shigella* spp. cause bacillary dysentery) and protozoa (e.g., amebiasis and balantidiasis, which are described in Chapter 21).

> Diarrhea is a symptom in a wide variety of conditions and diseases. It can be caused by certain foods or drugs, or it may be the result of an infectious disease.

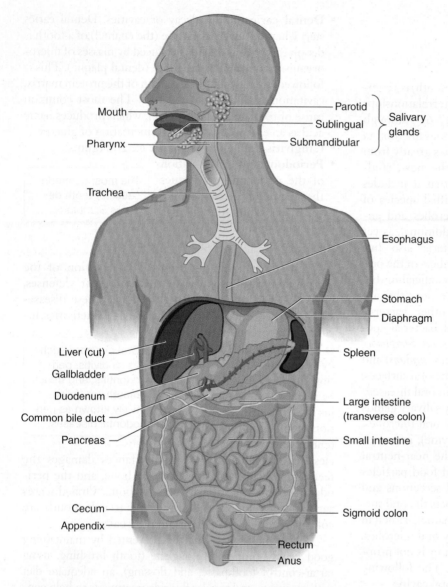

Figure 17-7. Anatomy of the gastrointestinal tract. (From Cohen BJ. *Memmler's The Human Body in Health and Disease.* 11th ed. Philadelphia, PA: Lippincott Williams & Wilkins; 2009.)

Labels in figure: Mouth, Pharynx, Trachea, Parotid, Sublingual, Submandibular, Salivary glands, Esophagus, Stomach, Diaphragm, Liver (cut), Gallbladder, Duodenum, Common bile duct, Pancreas, Spleen, Large intestine (transverse colon), Small intestine, Cecum, Appendix, Sigmoid colon, Rectum, Anus

the low pH (gastric contents have a pH of approximately 1.5) and are inhibited from growing in the lower intestines by the resident microbiota (microbial antagonism). They are then flushed from the colon during defecation, along with large numbers of indigenous microbes. The indigenous microbiota of the GI tract were discussed in Chapter 10. Terms relating to infectious diseases of the GI tract include the following:

- **Colitis.** Inflammation of the colon (the large intestine).
- **Diarrhea.** An abnormally frequent discharge of semisolid or fluid fecal matter. Some laboratory workers define diarrheal specimens as "stool specimens that conform to the shape of the container."
- **Dysentery.** Frequent watery stools, accompanied by abdominal pain, fever, and dehydration. The stool specimens may contain blood or mucus.
- **Enteritis.** Inflammation of the intestines, usually referring to the small intestine.

Infectious Diseases of the Genitourinary System

The GU or urogenital system consists of the urinary tract and the genital tract. Infectious diseases of the urinary tract are described first.

Urinary Tract Infections

For purposes of discussion, urinary tract infections (UTIs) can be divided into upper UTIs and lower UTIs. Upper UTIs include infections of the kidneys (nephritis or **pyelonephritis**) and ureters (ureteritis). Lower UTIs include infections of the urinary bladder (cystitis), the urethra (urethritis), and, in men, the prostate (prostatitis). The anatomy of the urinary tract is shown in Figure 17-8.

UTIs may be caused by any of various microorganisms, introduced by poor personal hygiene, sexual intercourse, the insertion of catheters, and other means. The urinary tract is usually protected from pathogens

> UTIs may be caused by any of a variety of microorganisms, introduced by poor personal hygiene, sexual intercourse, the insertion of catheters, and some other means.

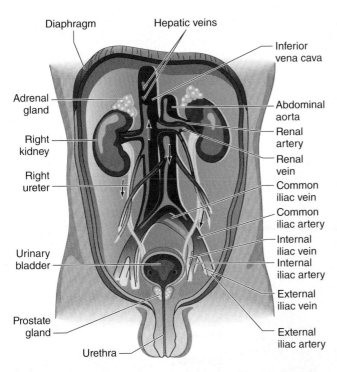

Diaphragm
Hepatic veins
Inferior vena cava
Adrenal gland
Abdominal aorta
Renal artery
Right kidney
Renal vein
Right ureter
Common iliac vein
Common iliac artery
Internal iliac vein
Urinary bladder
Internal iliac artery
External iliac vein
Prostate gland
External iliac artery
Urethra

Figure 17-8. Anatomy of the urinary tract. (From Cohen BJ. *Memmler's The Human Body in Health and Disease.* 11th ed. Philadelphia, PA: Lippincott Williams & Wilkins; 2009.)

by the frequent flushing action of urination. The acidity of normal urine also discourages growth of many microorganisms. Indigenous microbiota are found at and near the outer opening (meatus) of the urethra of both men and women.

Terms relating to infectious diseases of the urinary tract include the following:

- **Cystitis.** Inflammation of the urinary bladder; the most common type of UTI. The most common cause of cystitis is *Escherichia coli.* Other common causes of cystitis are species of *Klebsiella, Proteus, Enterobacter, Pseudomonas,* and *Enterococcus* as well as *Staphylococcus saprophyticus, Staphylococcus epidermidis,* and *Candida albicans.*
- **Nephritis.** General term referring to inflammation of the kidneys. *Pyelonephritis* is inflammation of the renal parenchyma. *E. coli* is the most common cause of nephritis and pyelonephritis. Most often, nephritis is preceded by cystitis; the bacteria migrate up the ureters, from the urinary bladder to the kidneys. Bacteria may also gain access to the kidneys via the bloodstream.
- **Ureteritis.** Inflammation of one or both ureters. Usually caused by the spreading of infection upward from the urinary bladder or downward from the kidneys.
- **Urethritis.** Inflammation of the urethra. Pathogens are usually transmitted sexually. The most common cause of urethritis is the bacterium, *Chlamydia trachomatis,* but *Neisseria gonorrhoeae,* ureaplasmas, and mycoplasmas can also be the cause. Urethritis that is *not* caused by *N. gonorrhoeae* is often referred to as nonspecific urethritis or nongonococcal urethritis.

- **Prostatitis.** Inflammation of the prostate gland. Most often, prostatitis is not an infectious disease. If it is caused by a pathogen, the pathogen may be a bacterium, a virus, a fungus, or a protozoan.

> The most common cause of cystitis, nephritis, and pyelonephritis is *E. coli,* whereas the most common cause of urethritis is the bacterium, *Chlamydia trachomatis.*

Infections of the Genital Tract

As previously mentioned, indigenous microbiota are found at and near the outer opening of the urethra and within the distal urethra[b] of both men and women. Additionally, the female genital region supports the growth of many other microorganisms. The adult vaginal microbiota contains many species of *Lactobacillus, Staphylococcus, Streptococcus, Enterococcus, Neisseria, Clostridium, Actinomyces, Prevotella,* diphtheroids, enteric bacilli, and *Candida.* The balance among these microbes depends on the estrogen levels and pH of the site. For example, should something (e.g., antibiotic use) kill the resident lactobacilli, an overgrowth (superinfection) of *C. albicans* can occur, leading to the condition known as yeast vaginitis. Should any of these or other microorganisms invade further into the GU system, various nonspecific infections may occur. The male and female reproductive systems are shown in Figure 17-9.

> Destruction of some members of the vaginal microbiota can lead to an overgrowth (superinfection) of other members.

Genital infections can be caused by a wide variety of microbes. Terms relating to infectious diseases of the genital tract are as follows:

- **Bartholinitis.** Inflammation of the Bartholin ducts in women.
- **Cervicitis.** Inflammation of the cervix (that part of the uterus that opens into the vagina).
- **Endometritis.** Inflammation of the endometrium (the inner layer of the uterine wall).
- **Epididymitis.** Inflammation of the epididymis (an elongated structure connected to the testis).
- **Pelvic inflammatory disease.** Inflammation of the fallopian tubes; also known as **salpingitis**.
- **Vaginitis.** Inflammation of the vagina. The three most common causes of vaginitis in the United States, each causing about one-third of the cases, are *C. albicans* (a yeast), *Trichomonas vaginalis* (a protozoan), and a mixture of bacteria (including bacteria in the genera

> The three most common causes of vaginitis in the United States are *C. albicans* (a yeast), *T. vaginalis* (a protozoan), and a mixture of bacteria.

[b]The distal urethra is that section of the urethra farthest from the urinary bladder and closest to the external opening.

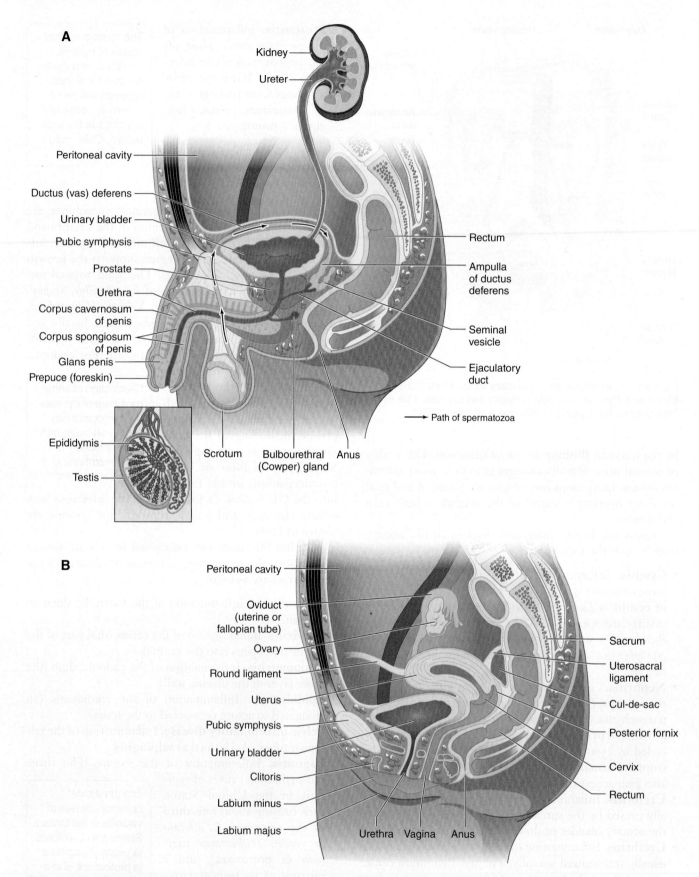

Figure 17-9. Anatomy of the reproductive system. A. Male. **B.** Female. (From Cohen BJ. *Memmler's The Human Body in Health and Disease.* 11th ed. Philadelphia, PA: Lippincott Williams & Wilkins; 2009.)

Mobiluncus and *Gardnerella*). When caused by a mixture of bacteria, the infection is referred to as *bacterial vaginosis*. In general, infections that result from the actions of two or more bacteria are called synergistic or polymicrobial infections. A saline wet mount preparation is usually used to diagnose vaginitis (see Appendix 5 on thePoint).

- **Vulvovaginitis.** Inflammation of the vulva (the external genitalia of women) and the vagina.

Sexually Transmitted Diseases of the Genital Tract

The term sexually transmitted disease (STD), formerly called venereal disease (VD), includes any of the infections transmitted by sexual activities. It is important to understand that STDs affect not

> STDs affect not only the genital tract, but also the skin, mucous membranes, blood, lymphatic and digestive systems, and many other anatomic sites.

only the genital tract, but also the skin, mucous membranes, blood, lymphatic and digestive systems, and many other body areas. Epidemic STDs include acquired immunodeficiency syndrome (AIDS), chlamydial and herpes infections, gonorrhea, and syphilis. The AIDS virus (human immunodeficiency virus [HIV]) primarily causes damage to helper T cells and thus inhibits antibody production; it is discussed in Chapter 18 in the section entitled "Viral Diseases of the Circulatory System." Diseases such as hepatitis B, amebiasis, and giardiasis can also be transmitted by sexual activities, as can many other diseases. The Centers for Disease Control and Prevention (CDC) estimates that 20 million cases of STDs occur annually in the United States.

Infectious Diseases of the Circulatory System

The circulatory system consists of the cardiovascular system and the lymphatic system. The cardiovascular (*cardio* for heart, and *vascular* for the various types of blood vessels) system includes the heart, arteries, capillaries, veins, and blood. Blood is composed of plasma (the liquid portion) plus the various cellular elements. (The cellular elements of blood are discussed in Chapters 13 and 15.) Terms relating to infectious diseases of the cardiovascular system are as follows:

- **Endocarditis.** Inflammation of the endocardium—the endothelial membrane that lines the cavities of the heart (Fig. 17-10).
- **Myocarditis.** Inflammation of the myocardium—the muscular walls of the heart.
- **Pericarditis.** Inflammation of the pericardium—the membranous sac around the heart.

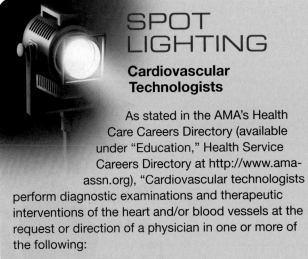

SPOT LIGHTING

Cardiovascular Technologists

As stated in the AMA's Health Care Careers Directory (available under "Education," Health Service Careers Directory at http://www.ama-assn.org), "Cardiovascular technologists perform diagnostic examinations and therapeutic interventions of the heart and/or blood vessels at the request or direction of a physician in one or more of the following:

- Invasive cardiovascular laboratories—cardiac catheterization, blood gas, and electrophysiology laboratories
- Noninvasive cardiovascular laboratories—echocardiology, exercise stress test, and electrocardiology laboratories
- Noninvasive peripheral vascular studies laboratories—Doppler ultrasound and thermography laboratories

Through subjective sampling and/or recording, the cardiovascular technologist creates an easily definable foundation of data from which a correct anatomic and physiologic diagnosis may be established for each patient."

"The cardiovascular technologist is qualified by specific didactic, laboratory, and clinical technological education to perform various cardiovascular/peripheral vascular diagnostic and therapeutic procedures. The role of the cardiovascular technologist may include but is not limited to:

- Reviewing and/or recoding pertinent patient history and supporting clinical data
- Performing appropriate clinical procedures and obtaining a record of anatomical, pathological, and/or physiological data for interpretation by a physician
- Exercising discretion and judgment in the performance of cardiovascular diagnostic and therapeutic services."

Information concerning educational requirements and programs, certification, and salary can be found on the AMA Web site.

Normally, blood is sterile; it contains no resident microbiota. The presence of bacteria in the bloodstream is known as **bacteremia**, which can be, but is not always, a sign of disease. **Transient bacteremia** (the temporary

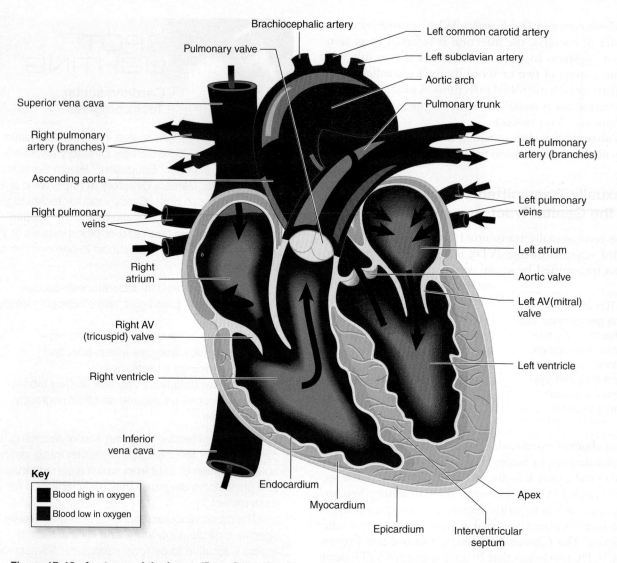

Brachiocephalic artery
Pulmonary valve
Left common carotid artery
Left subclavian artery
Aortic arch
Pulmonary trunk
Superior vena cava
Right pulmonary artery (branches)
Left pulmonary artery (branches)
Ascending aorta
Left pulmonary veins
Right pulmonary veins
Left atrium
Aortic valve
Right atrium
Left AV (mitral) valve
Right AV (tricuspid) valve
Left ventricle
Right ventricle
Inferior vena cava
Endocardium
Myocardium
Apex
Epicardium
Interventricular septum

Key
Blood high in oxygen
Blood low in oxygen

Figure 17-10. Anatomy of the heart. (From Cohen BJ. *Memmler's The Human Body in Health and Disease*. 11th ed. Philadelphia, PA: Lippincott Williams & Wilkins; 2009.)

> The presence of bacteria in a person's bloodstream is known as bacteremia. It may or may not be a sign of disease.

> Septicemia is a disease in which the patient experiences chills, fever, and prostration (extreme exhaustion) and has bacteria and/or their toxins in their bloodstream.

presence of bacteria in the blood) often results from dental extractions, wounds, bites, and damage to the intestinal, respiratory, or reproductive tract mucosa. Even aggressive tooth brushing, which causes bleeding of the gums, can lead to transient bacteremia.

However, when pathogenic organisms are capable of resisting or overwhelming the phagocytes and other body defenses—or when an individual is immunosuppressed or is otherwise more susceptible than normal—a systemic disease called *septicemia* may occur.

A patient with septicemia experiences chills, fever, and prostration (extreme exhaustion) and has bacteria and/or their toxins in the bloodstream.

Although dozens of infectious diseases can be transmitted by donated blood, only the following tests are routinely performed on donor blood in the United States:

- *Treponema pallidum* antigen (*T. pallidum* is the cause of syphilis)
- HIV-1 antibody
- HIV-2 antibody
- HTLV-I and HTLV-II antibody (human T-cell lymphotropic virus type 1 has been associated with several kinds of diseases, including demyelinating diseases, leukemia, and lymphoma; HTLV-II has not been clearly linked to any specific disease, but has been associated with several neurological disorders)
- Hepatitis B (HBV) surface antigen
- Hepatitis B (HBV) core antibody
- Hepatitis C (HCV) antibody
- Nucleic acid amplification testing for HIV-1, HCV, and West Nile Virus
- Antibody test for *Trypanosoma cruzi*, the cause of Chagas disease

The lymphatic system consists of lymphatic vessels, lymphoid tissue (including lymph nodes, tonsils, thymus, and spleen), and lymph (the liquid that circulates through the lymphatic system). Lymph occasionally picks up microorganisms from the intestine, lungs, and other areas, but these transient organisms are usually quickly engulfed by phagocytic cells in the liver and lymph nodes. The lymphatic system contains many lymphocytes (discussed in Chapter 16). Terms relating to infectious diseases of the lymphatic system include:

- **Lymphadenitis.** Inflamed and swollen lymph nodes.
- **Lymphadenopathy.** Diseased lymph nodes.
- **Lymphangitis.** Inflamed lymphatic vessels.

Infectious Diseases of the Central Nervous System

The nervous system is composed of the CNS and the peripheral nervous system (Fig. 17-11). The CNS consists

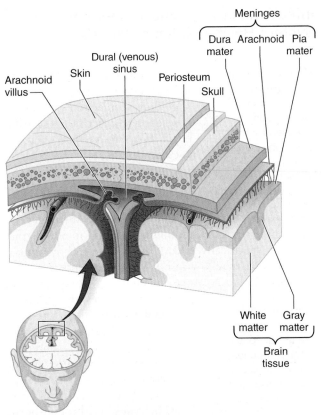

Figure 17-12. **Section of the top of the head showing the meninges and related structures.** (From Cohen BJ. *Memmler's The Human Body in Health and Disease*. 11th ed. Philadelphia, PA: Lippincott Williams & Wilkins; 2009.)

of the brain, the spinal cord, and the three membranes (or **meninges** [sing., **meninx**]) that cover the brain and spinal cord (Fig. 17-12). The CNS is well protected and remarkably resistant to infection; it is encased in bone, bathed and cushioned in cerebrospinal fluid (CSF), and nourished by capillaries. These capillaries make up the blood–brain barrier, supplying nutrients but not allowing larger particles, such as macromolecules (e.g., antibodies and most antibiotics), cells of the immune system, and microorganisms, to pass from the blood into the brain. The peripheral nervous system consists of nerves that branch from the brain and spinal cord.

There are no indigenous microbiota of the nervous system. Microbes gain access to the CNS through trauma (fracture or medical procedure), via the blood and lymph to the CSF, or along the peripheral nerves. Terms relating to infectious diseases of the CNS include the following:

- **Encephalitis.** Inflammation of the brain.
- **Encephalomyelitis.** Inflammation of the brain and spinal cord.
- **Meningitis.** Inflammation of the membranes (meninges) that surround the brain and spinal cord.
- **Meningoencephalitis.** Inflammation of the brain and meninges.
- **Myelitis.** Inflammation of the spinal cord.

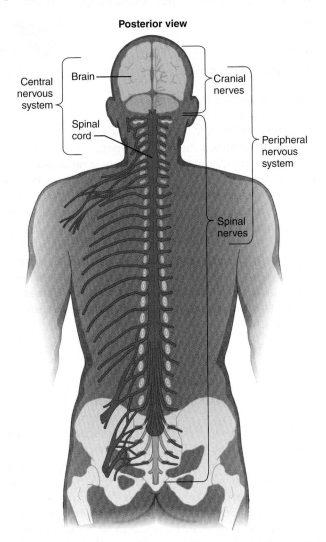

Figure 17-11. **Anatomy of the central nervous system.** (From Cohen BJ. *Memmler's The Human Body in Health and Disease*. 11th ed. Philadelphia, PA: Lippincott Williams & Wilkins; 2009.)

Infections of the Central Nervous System Having Multiple Causes

Meningitis

Meningitis—inflammation of the meninges—can have many causes, including the ingestion of poisons, the in-

> Meningitis can be caused by the ingestion of poisons, the ingestion or injection of drugs, a reaction to a vaccine, or a pathogen.

gestion or injection of drugs, a reaction to a vaccine, or a pathogen. If caused by a pathogen, the culprit might be a virus, a bacterium, a fungus, or a protozoan.

Viral meningitis may be caused by a virus that specifically infects the meninges, or may be the result of an immune reaction to a virus that does not specifically infect the brain (e.g., chickenpox, measles, and rubella viruses). Viral meningitis is sometimes referred to as "aseptic meningitis," because in about

> Viral meningitis is sometimes referred to as "aseptic meningitis" because in about 50% of the cases, the pathogen cannot be identified.

50% of the cases, the pathogen cannot be identified. The various types of viruses that cause meningitis include enteroviruses (the major cause in the United States), coxsackieviruses, echoviruses, mumps virus, **arboviruses** (arthropod-borne viruses), poliovirus, adenoviruses, measles virus, herpes simplex, and varicella virus. Viral meningitis tends to be less serious than bacterial meningitis.

Historically, the three major causes of bacterial meningitis have been *H. influenzae* (the primary cause in children), *Neisseria meningitidis* (the

> Historically, the three major causes of bacterial meningitis have been *H. influenzae*, *N. meningitidis*, and *S. pneumoniae*.

primary cause in adolescents), and *S. pneumoniae* (the primary cause in the elderly). Vaccination of children with the Hib vaccine[c] has drastically reduced the incidence of *H. influenzae* meningitis in children in the United States. Less common causes of bacterial meningitis are *S. aureus*, *Pseudomonas aeruginosa*, *Salmonella*, and *Klebsiella*.

The major causes of bacterial meningitis in neonates are *Streptococcus agalactiae* (Group B, β-hemolytic streptococci), *E. coli* and other members of the family Enterobacteriaceae, and *Listeria monocytogenes*.

Early symptoms of bacterial meningitis include fever, headache, stiff neck, sore throat, and vomiting. Then neurologic symptoms of dizziness, convulsions, minor paralysis, and coma occur; death may result within a few hours. Meningitis is a medical emergency and steps must be taken immediately to determine the cause. Diagnosis is usually made by a combination of patient symptoms,

physical examination, and Gram staining and culture of the CSF.

Free-living amebas that may cause *meningoencephalitis* are in the genera *Naegleria* and *Acanthamoeba*. Other protozoa that may invade the meninges are *Toxoplasma* and *Trypanosoma*. Occasionally, fungal pathogens,

> Parasites that can cause CNS diseases include free-living amebas and *Toxoplasma* and *Trypanosoma* spp.

especially *Cryptococcus neoformans* (an encapsulated yeast), cause meningitis.

Toxins. Several CNS diseases are caused by toxins. Examples of bacterial neurotoxins are botulinal toxin (the exotoxin that causes botulism) and **tetanospasmin** (the cause of tetanus). Diseases caused by fungal toxins (mycotoxins) include ergot from grain moulds and mushroom poisoning. *Gonyaulax*, an alga found in algal "blooms," produces neurotoxins, which may concentrate in bivalve shell fish and cause paralytic symptoms following ingestion of the contaminated shellfish. A variety of other algae also produce neurotoxins (see Appendix 1 on thePoint).

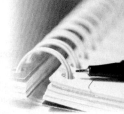

STUDY AID

Aseptic Meningitis

The term *aseptic meningitis* implies meningitis that is not caused by a pathogen. Although it is true that some cases of meningitis result from events unrelated to pathogens (e.g., the ingestion of poisons or certain drugs), many cases of aseptic meningitis are actually the result of infections. The term probably originated from meningitis cases where no organisms were recovered on routine bacteriological culture. However, many cases of meningitis are caused by microbes that will not grow on standard bacteriological culture media. Examples of such pathogens are viruses (many different types), fungi, leptospira, and *T. pallidum*. Cases of meningitis caused by these types of organisms are collectively referred to as aseptic meningitis.

Opportunistic Infections

Recall from Chapter 1 that certain microbes are referred to as "opportunistic pathogens" or "opportunists." These are microbes that usually do not cause disease, but have the potential to cause disease under certain conditions. The term **opportunistic infections** (OIs), refers to infections that normally would not occur in healthy, immunocompetent individuals or would, at most, cause only mild infections. On the other hand, OIs are relatively common in immunosuppressed individuals, and often contribute

---

[c]The Hib in Hib vaccine stands for *Haemophilus influenzae* type b, the capsular type of *H. influenzae* that, prior to use of Hib vaccine, was the major cause of meningitis in children.

to their death. Immunosuppressed individuals present an "opportunity" for the pathogens to cause disease.

Listed here are some of the most common OIs:

- **Aspergillosis and other mould infections** (including bread mould infections); can become a systemic infection in immunosuppressed individuals
- **Candidiasis**. A yeast infection of the mouth (thrush), throat, or vagina; can become a systemic infection in immunosuppressed individuals
- **Cytomegalovirus infection**. Can cause eye disease that can lead to blindness
- **Herpes simplex virus infections**. The cause of oral herpes (cold sores) and genital herpes, which can occur in immunocompetent individuals, but are more frequent and more severe in immunosuppressed individuals
- **Malaria**. A parasitic infection that occurs in immunocompetent individuals, but is more common and more severe in immunosuppressed individuals
- *Mycobacterium avium* **complex**. A bacterial infection that can cause recurring fevers, problems with digestion, and serious weight loss
- *Pneumocystis* **pneumonia**. A fungal infection that can cause a fatal pneumonia; prior to newer and more aggressive treatments was once the major killer of AIDS patients
- **Toxoplasmosis ("toxo")**. A protozoal infection of the eyes and brain
- **Tuberculosis (TB)**. A bacterial lower respiratory infection; can cause meningitis; occurs in immunocompetent individuals, but is more common and more severe in immunosuppressed individuals

Emerging and Reemerging Infectious Diseases

It was not so many years ago that scientists believed that they had infectious diseases "on the run."[d] They were confident that a combination of surveillance, quarantine, vaccines, antibiotics, and other antimicrobial agents marked the beginning of the end for pathogen-caused diseases. They were wrong!

Not only do "new" (previously unknown) infectious diseases continue to emerge, but other infectious diseases, once thought to be contained or eradicated, continue to reemerge. Causes of emerging diseases include changes in human demographics and behavior; ecological changes

such as dams, deforestation, and climate change; increased international travel; increased exposure to exotic animals; misuse of antibiotics and other antimicrobial agents; and breakdown of public health measures. Listed here are some of the infectious diseases that have emerged in the last 30 years:

Avian influenza ("bird flu")
Cryptosporidiosis
E. Coli O157 infections (including hemolytic uremic syndrome)
Ebola hemorrhagic fever
Hantavirus pulmonary syndrome (HPS)
Hendra virus infection
HIV infection and AIDS
Human monkeypox
Lassa fever
Legionellosis
Lyme disease
Marburg hemorrhagic fever
Nipah virus encephalitis
Severe acute respiratory syndrome (SARS)
Variant Creutzfeldt–Jakob disease
West Nile virus encephalitis

Causes of reemerging infectious diseases include pathogen mutations and genetic recombinations, acquired drug resistance, decreased compliance with vaccination policies and other breakdowns in public health measures, population shifts, war and civil conflicts, famine, floods, droughts, and bioterrorism. Infectious diseases that have reemerged or shown up in new geographic areas in recent years include cholera, dengue fever, diphtheria, malaria, Rift Valley fever, TB, yellow fever, and infections caused by methicillin-resistant *S. aureus* and other "superbugs."

The journal, *Emerging Infectious Diseases*, published monthly by the Centers for Disease Control and Prevention (CDC), is available at no cost at http://www.cdc.gov/ncidod/EID/index.htm.

---

[d]In the late 1960s, based on progress that had been made reducing the incidence of such infectious diseases as smallpox, polio, and rheumatic fever, the Surgeon General of the United States, William H. Stewart, declared that it was time to close the book on infectious diseases and, to instead, pay closer attention to chronic ailments such as cancer and heart disease.

SOMETHING TO THINK ABOUT

"Climatic factors influence the emergence and reemergence of infectious diseases, in addition to multiple human, biological, and ecological determinants. Climatologists have identified upward trends in global temperatures and now estimate an unprecedented rise of 2.0°C by the year 2100. Of major concern is that these changes can affect the introduction and dissemination of many serious infectious diseases."

"The incidence of mosquito-borne diseases, including malaria, dengue, and viral encephalitides, are among those diseases most sensitive to climate. Climate change would directly affect disease transmission by shifting the vector's geographic range and increasing reproductive and biting rates and by shortening the pathogen incubation period. Climate-related increases in sea surface temperature and sea level can lead to higher incidence of water-borne infectious and toxin-related illnesses, such as cholera and shellfish poisoning. Human migration and damage to health infrastructures from the projected increase in climate variability could indirectly contribute to disease transmission. Human susceptibility to infections might be further compounded by malnutrition due to climate stress on agriculture and potential alterations in the human immune system caused by increased flux of ultraviolet radiation."

(Patz JA, et al. Global climate change and emerging infections. *JAMA* 1996;275:217–223.)

Possible Relationships between Disease States and Our Microbiome

"We tend to think that we are exclusively a product of our own cells, upwards of ten trillion of them. But the microbes we harbor add another 100 trillion cells into the mix… And while our 21,000 or so human genes help make us who we are, our resident microbes possess another eight million or so genes, many of which collaborate behind the scenes handling food, tinkering with the immune system, turning human genes on and off, and otherwise helping us function… Microbes inhabit almost every corner of the body,…all told more than 10,000 species… But the real news is that the microbial community makes a significant difference in how we live and even how we think and feel." Unfortunately, our microbiome has been under attack ever since the dawn of the antibiotic era. Whenever we receive antibiotics, "good" bacteria are killed, along with the "bad" bacteria. In addition to antibiotics, our microbiome has been altered as a result of our obsession with cleanliness and antibacterial soaps, lotions, household cleaners, and other products. "Recent studies have linked changes in the microbiome to some of the most pressing medical problems of our time, including obesity, allergies, diabetes, bowel disorders, and even psychiatric problems like autism, schizophrenia, and depression… Researchers generally can't say for sure if changes in the microbiome cause certain conditions, or merely occur as a consequence of those conditions." Additional research into possible relationships between us and our microbiome is obviously needed, and we must come to realize that we and our microbes are intimate partners that clearly influence our daily lives. (Quoted material is from Coniff R. Microbes: the trillions of creatures governing your health. Smithsonianmag.com. May 2013.)

ON thePoint

- Terms Introduced in This Chapter
- Review of Key Points
- Increase Your Knowledge
- Additional Self-Assessment Exercises

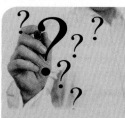

Self-Assessment Exercises

After studying this chapter, answer the following multiple-choice questions.

1. Otitis media is an inflammation or infection of the:
   a. ear
   b. eye
   c. brain
   d. urinary bladder

2. Keratitis is an inflammation or infection of the:
   a. conjunctiva
   b. cornea
   c. kidney
   d. skin

3. Which of the following is/are the most common cause of pharyngitis?
   a. *Escherichia coli*
   b. *Staphylococcus aureus*
   c. *Streptococcus pyogenes*
   d. viruses

4. Which of the following is the most common cause of tooth decay?
   a. *S. aureus*
   b. *Streptococcus agalactiae*
   c. *Streptococcus mutans*
   d. *S. pyogenes*

5. An infection of the urinary bladder is known as:
    a. cystitis
    b. pyelonephritis
    c. ureteritis
    d. urethritis

6. The most common cause of cystitis is:
    a. *Candida albicans*
    b. *E. coli*
    c. *Staphylococcus epidermidis*
    d. *Staphylococcus saprophyticus*

7. The most common cause of urethritis is:
    a. *Chlamydia trachomatis*
    b. *E. coli*
    c. *Mycoplasma pneumoniae*
    d. *S. aureus*

8. Which of the following terms means swollen lymph glands?
    a. lymphadenitis
    b. lymphadenopathy
    c. lymphangitis
    d. lymphitis

9. Inflammation or infection of the brain is called:
    a. encephalitis
    b. meningitis
    c. myelitis
    d. otitis externa

10. Which of the following is not one of the three most common causes of bacterial meningitis?
    a. *E. coli*
    b. *Haemophilus influenzae*
    c. *Neisseria meningitidis*
    d. *Streptococcus pneumoniae*

18

Viral Infections of Humans

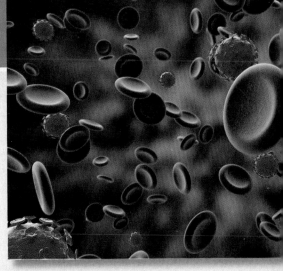

Artist rendering of a viral bloodstream infection.

CHAPTER OUTLINE

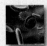

LEARNING OBJECTIVES

After studying this chapter, you should be able to:

- Correlate various viral diseases with body systems (e.g., rhinoviruses with the respiratory system)
- Correlate a particular viral disease with its major characteristics, etiologic agent, reservoir(s), mode(s) of transmission, and diagnostic laboratory procedures
- Name several nationally notifiable viral diseases
- Briefly describe how viruses cause disease
- Describe *Koplik spots* and state the disease with which they are associated
- Characterize the various hepatitis viruses as being either DNA or RNA viruses
- List several viral diseases that are sexually transmitted

Introduction

It would be impossible in a book this size to describe *all* of the human infectious diseases caused by viruses. Thus, only selected viral diseases are described in this chapter.

Certain of the viral diseases described in this chapter are nationally notifiable infectious diseases, meaning that when a patient is diagnosed with one of these diseases in the United States, the information must be reported to the Centers for Disease Control and Prevention (CDC). As of 2010, there were approximately 25 nationally notifiable viral diseases (see Table 18-1). Most of them are described in this chapter, as are some viral diseases that are not nationally notifiable.

Table 18-1 Nationally Notifiable Viral Diseases

Viral Disease	Number of New U.S. Cases Reported to the CDC in 2010[a]
Arthropod-borne viral (arboviral) diseases	
Encephalitis caused by members of the California serogroup	75
Eastern equine encephalitis	10
Powassan virus encephalitis	8
St. Louis encephalitis	10
West Nile virus encephalitis	1,021
Western equine encephalitis (WEE)	0
Dengue fever	700
Hantavirus pulmonary syndrome (HPS)	20
Hepatitis A	1,670
Hepatitis B	3,374
Hepatitis C	849
HIV diagnosis	35,741
Influenza-associated pediatric mortality	61
Measles	63
Mumps	2,612
Poliomyelitis	0
Rabies, human	2
Rubella	5
SARS	0
Smallpox	0
Varicella (chickenpox)	15,431
Viral hemorrhagic fevers	1
Yellow fever	0

Source: http://www.cdc.gov.

[a]These figures provide insight as to how frequently these diseases occur in the United States. For updated information, go to the CDC web site; click on "Morbidity & Mortality Weekly Report"; then click on "Notifiable Diseases"; then click on the most recent year that is listed.

How Do Viruses Cause Disease?

Recall from Chapter 4 that viruses can infect only the cells bearing appropriate surface receptors (i.e., surface receptors that the virus is able to recognize and bind to). Thus, viruses are specific as to the type of cell(s) that they can infect. For this reason, certain viruses cause only respiratory infections, whereas others cause only gastrointestinal (GI) infections, and so on.

Viruses multiply within host cells, and it is during their escape from those cells—by either cell lysis or budding—that the host cells are destroyed. This cell destruction leads to most of the symptoms of the viral infection, which vary depending on the location of the infection. Other symptoms are the result of immunological injury (i.e., injury that results from the immune response to the viral pathogen). In the case of the acquired immunodeficiency syndrome (AIDS) virus (human immunodeficiency virus [HIV]), the virus destroys cells of the immune system. This renders the patient unable to ward off various viral, bacterial, fungal, and parasitic pathogens. The AIDS patient's death results from overwhelming infections caused by these pathogens.

STUDY AID

What to Learn?

This chapter contains a large amount of information. Of primary importance will be your ability to later recall the name of the virus that causes a particular viral disease and the manner in which the disease is transmitted. If applicable, you should be able to state the vector that is involved in the transmission of the disease. For example, if your teacher says "dengue fever," you should be able to state the name of the virus that causes the disease (dengue virus), the manner in which dengue fever is transmitted (mosquito bite), and the vector that is involved in the transmission of dengue fever (mosquitoes in the genus *Aedes*).

Viral Infections of the Skin

Table 18-2 lists information pertaining to viral infections of the skin.

STUDY AID

Beware of Similar-Sounding Names

Do not confuse varicella, variola, and vaccinia viruses. **Varicella virus** (which is a type of herpes virus) is the cause of chickenpox. **Variola virus** is the cause of smallpox and is often referred to as smallpox virus. **Vaccinia virus** is the cause of cowpox; it is used to make the vaccine that protects against smallpox. The words *vaccine* and *vaccination* are derived from *vacca*, Latin for cow.

Table 18-2 Viral Infections of the Skin

Disease	Additional Information
Chickenpox and shingles. (a) Chickenpox (also known as varicella) is an acute, generalized viral infection, with fever and a skin rash (Fig. 18-1). Vesicles also form in mucous membranes. It is usually a mild, self-limiting disease, but can be severely damaging to a fetus. Serious complications include pneumonia, secondary bacterial infections, hemorrhagic complications, and encephalitis. Reye (pronounced "rize") syndrome (a severe encephalomyelitis with liver damage) may follow clinical chickenpox if aspirin is given to children younger than 16 years of age. Chickenpox is the leading cause of vaccine-preventable death in the United States. (b) Shingles (also known as herpes zoster) is a reactivation of the varicella virus, often the result of immunosuppression. Shingles involves inflammation of sensory ganglia of cutaneous sensory nerves, producing fluid-filled blisters, pain, and paresthesia (numbness and tingling). Shingles may occur at any age, but is most common after age 50. **Patient care.** Use Airborne and Contact Precautions for hospitalized patients until their lesions become dry and crusted.	**Pathogen.** Chickenpox and shingles are caused by varicella-zoster virus (VZV); a herpes virus (family Herpesviridae) that is also known as human herpesvirus 3; a DNA virus. **Reservoirs and mode of transmission.** Infected humans serve as reservoirs. Transmission is from person to person by direct contact or droplet or airborne spread of vesicle fluid or secretions of the respiratory system of persons with chickenpox. **Laboratory diagnosis.** Diagnosis is usually made on clinical and epidemiologic grounds. Immunodiagnostic and molecular diagnostic procedures are available, as are cell culture and electron microscopy.
German measles (rubella). German measles is a mild, febrile viral disease. A fine, pinkish, flat rash begins 1 or 2 days after the onset of symptoms (Fig. 18-2). The rash starts on the face and neck and spreads to the trunk, arms, and legs. Rubella is a milder disease than hard measles with fewer complications. If acquired during the first trimester of pregnancy, rubella may cause congenital rubella syndrome in the fetus. This can lead to intrauterine death, spontaneous abortion, or congenital malformations of major organ systems. **Patient care.** Use Droplet Precautions for hospitalized patients until 7 days after the onset of rash.	**Pathogen.** Rubella is caused by rubella virus, an RNA virus in the family Togaviridae. **Reservoirs and mode of transmission.** Infected humans serve as reservoirs. Transmission occurs by droplet spread or direct contact with nasopharyngeal secretions of infected people. **Laboratory diagnosis.** Immunodiagnostic and molecular diagnostic procedures are available for diagnosis of rubella. The virus can be propagated in cell culture.

(continued)

Table 18-2 Viral Infections of the Skin (continued)

Disease	Additional Information
Measles (hard measles, rubeola). Measles is an acute, highly communicable viral disease with fever, conjunctivitis, cough, photosensitivity (light sensitivity), Koplik spots in the mouth, and red blotchy skin rash (Fig. 18-3). Koplik spots are small red spots, in the center of which can be seen a minute bluish white speck when observed under a strong light (Fig. 18-4). The rash begins on the face between days 3 and 7 and then becomes generalized. Complications include bronchitis, pneumonia, otitis media, and encephalitis. Rarely, autoimmune, subacute, sclerosing panencephalitis (SSPE) may follow a latent period of several years. SSPE is characterized by gradual progressive psychoneurological deterioration, including personality changes, seizures, photosensitivity, ocular abnormalities, and coma. **Patient care.** Use Airborne Precautions for hospitalized patients until 4 days after the onset of rash.	**Pathogen.** Measles is caused by measles virus (also known as rubeola virus). It is an RNA virus in the family Paramyxoviridae. **Reservoirs and mode of transmission.** Infected humans serve as reservoirs. Airborne transmission occurs by droplet spread and direct contact with nasal or throat secretions of infected persons or with articles freshly soiled with nose and throat secretions. **Laboratory diagnosis.** Diagnosis of measles is usually made on clinical and epidemiologic grounds. Immunodiagnostic and molecular diagnostic procedures are available, and the virus can be isolated in cell culture.
Monkeypox. Monkeypox is a rare viral disease that causes fever, headache, muscle aches, backache, lymphadenitis, malaise (fatigue), and a rash (Fig. 18-5). A disease milder than smallpox, monkeypox occurs primarily in central and western Africa, although several people in the United States became ill in 2003 after handling infected prairie dogs. Unlike smallpox, monkeypox is rarely fatal. **Patient care.** Use Airborne and Contact Precautions for hospitalized patients; Airborne Precautions until monkeypox is confirmed and smallpox is excluded; Contact Precautions until lesions become crusted.	**Pathogen.** Monkeypox is caused by monkeypox virus, which is in the same group of viruses (orthopoxviruses) as smallpox virus (variola virus) and the virus used in the smallpox vaccine (vaccinia virus). **Reservoirs and mode of transmission.** Infected animals serve as reservoirs. Transmission occurs via animal bite or contact with an infected animal's blood, body fluids, or rash. Person-to-person transmission does occur. **Laboratory diagnosis.** Monkeypox can be diagnosed by molecular diagnostic procedures, cell culture, electron microscopy, or immunodiagnostic procedures. (See http://www.cdc.gov/ncidod/monkeypox for more information.)
Smallpox. Smallpox is a systemic viral infection with fever, malaise, headache, prostration, severe backache, a characteristic skin rash (refer back to Fig. 11-10 in Chapter 11), and occasional abdominal pain and vomiting. The rash is similar to, and must be distinguished from, the rash of chickenpox. Smallpox can become severe, with bleeding into the skin and mucous membranes, followed by death. **Patient care.** Use Airborne and Contact Precautions for hospitalized patients until all scabs have crusted and separated (3–4 weeks). Use N95 or higher respiratory protection.	**Pathogen.** Smallpox is caused by two strains of variola virus: variola minor (with a fatality rate of <1%), and variola major (with a fatality rate of 20%–40% or higher). Variola virus is a double-stranded DNA virus in the genus Orthopoxvirus, family Poxviridae. Smallpox virus is a potential biological warfare and bioterrorism agent. **Reservoirs and mode of transmission.** Before smallpox was eradicated, infected humans were the only source of the virus. There are no known animal or environmental reservoirs. Person-to-person transmission is via the respiratory tract (droplet spread) or skin inoculation. Patients are most contagious before eruption of the rash, by aerosol droplets from oropharyngeal lesions. **Laboratory diagnosis.** Because of the potential danger of the use of smallpox virus as a bioterrorism agent, physicians must become familiar with the clinical and epidemiologic features of smallpox and how to distinguish smallpox from chickenpox. Laboratory diagnosis is by cell culture, virus neutralization tests, molecular diagnostic procedures, or electron microscopy. These procedures are performed only in biosafety level 4 (BSL-4) facilities.
Warts. Warts consist of many varieties of skin and mucous membrane lesions, including common warts (verrucae vulgaris), venereal warts, and plantar warts. Most are harmless, but some can become cancerous. Venereal or genital warts are discussed in more detail later in the chapter.	**Pathogens.** Warts are caused by at least 70 types of human papillomaviruses (HPV). They are classified in the genus Papillomavirus within the family Papovaviridae. They are DNA viruses. **Reservoirs and mode of transmission.** Infected humans serve as reservoirs. Transmission usually occurs by direct contact. Genital warts are sexually transmitted. They are easily spread from one area of the body to another, but most are not very contagious from person to person (genital warts are an exception). **Laboratory diagnosis.** Diagnosis is made on clinical grounds.

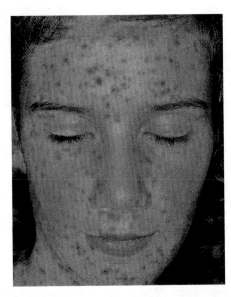

Figure 18-1. Chickenpox with lesions at all stages of development. (From Harvey RA, et al. *Lippincott's Illustrated Reviews: Microbiology*. 3rd ed. Philadelphia, PA: Lippincott Williams & Wilkins; 2013.)

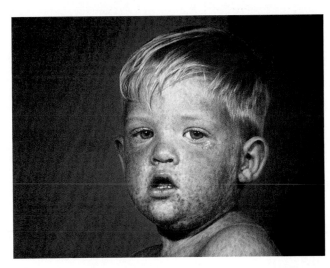

Figure 18-3. Child with measles. (Courtesy of the CDC.)

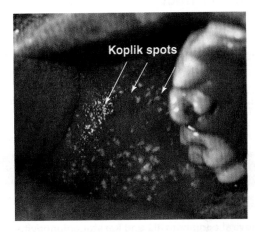

Figure 18-4. Koplik spots. Koplik spots, which appear on the inner membrane of the cheek, are an early sign of measles; they usually appear prior to the onset of skin rash. Koplik spots are irregularly shaped, bright-red spots, often having a bluish white central dot. (From Harvey RA, et al. *Lippincott's Illustrated Reviews: Microbiology*. 2nd ed. Philadelphia, PA: Lippincott Williams & Wilkins; 2007.)

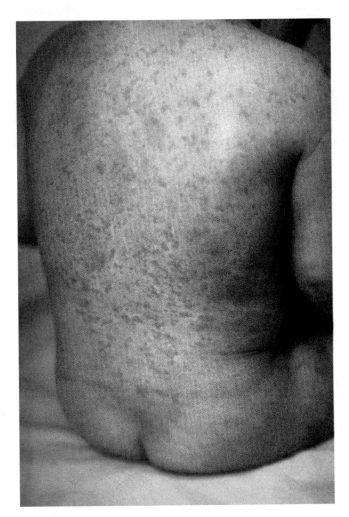

Figure 18-2. Child with rubella. The lesions are not as intensely red as those of measles. (Courtesy of the CDC.)

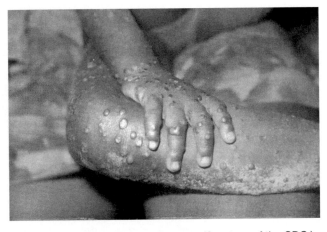

Figure 18-5. Child with monkeypox. (Courtesy of the CDC.)

Viral Infections of the Ears

Information about viral and bacterial ear infections can be found in Table 19-3 in Chapter 19.

Viral Infections of the Eyes

Table 18-3 lists information about viral infections of the eyes.

Viral Infections of the Respiratory System

Viral Infections of the Upper Respiratory Tract

The Common Cold (Acute Viral Rhinitis, Acute Coryza)

Disease. The common cold is a viral infection of the lining of the nose, sinuses, throat, and large airways. Symptoms include coryza (profuse discharge from nostrils), sneezing, runny eyes, sore throat, chills, and malaise. Additionally, laryngitis, tracheitis, or bronchitis may accompany a cold. Secondary bacterial infections, including sinusitis and otitis media, may follow. The common cold occurs most frequently in fall, winter, and spring. On average, most people have one to six colds annually. It is not a nationally notifiable disease in the United States.

Patient Care. Use Droplet Precautions for hospitalized patients.

Pathogens. Many different viruses cause colds. Rhinoviruses, of which there are more than 100 serotypes, are the major cause in adults. Other cold-causing viruses include coronaviruses, parainfluenza viruses, respiratory syncytial virus (RSV), influenza viruses, adenoviruses, and enteroviruses.

Reservoirs and Mode of Transmission. Infected humans serve as reservoirs of infection. Transmission is via respiratory secretions by way of hands and fomites or direct contact with or inhalation of airborne droplets.

Laboratory Diagnosis. Laboratory diagnosis of the common cold usually is not required, but cell culture techniques can often demonstrate the specific viral pathogen.

Table 18-3 **Viral Infections of the Eyes**

Disease	Additional Information
Adenoviral conjunctivitis and keratoconjunctivitis. These are acute viral diseases of one or both eyes, associated with inflammation of the conjunctiva, edema of the eyelids and periorbital tissue, pain, photophobia, and blurred vision. The cornea is involved in about 50% of cases, with permanent scarring of the cornea in severe cases. **Patient care.** Use Contact Precautions for hospitalized patients for the duration of the illness.	**Pathogens.** Adenoviral conjunctitivis and keratoconjunctivitis are caused by various types of adenoviruses. Herpes simplex viruses and VZVs can also cause keratoconjunctivitis. **Reservoirs and mode of transmission.** Infected humans serve as reservoirs. Transmission occurs via direct contact with eye secretions or contact with contaminated surfaces, instruments, or solutions. People with viral infections (e.g., cold sores) should wash their hands thoroughly before inserting or removing contact lenses or otherwise touching their eyes. **Laboratory diagnosis.** Diagnosis is made by cell culture or immunodiagnostic or molecular diagnostic procedures.
Hemorrhagic conjunctivitis. This viral disease has a sudden onset, with redness, swelling, and pain in one or both eyes. Small, discrete subconjunctival hemorrhages may enlarge to form confluent subconjunctival hemorrhages. One adenoviral syndrome, called pharyngoconjunctival fever, is characterized by upper respiratory disease, fever, and minor degrees of corneal epithelial inflammation. **Patient care.** Use Contact Precautions for hospitalized patients for the duration of the illness.	**Pathogens.** Hemorrhagic conjunctivitis is caused by adenoviruses and enteroviruses. **Reservoirs and mode of transmission.** Infected humans serve as reservoirs. Transmission occurs by direct or indirect contact with discharge from infected eyes. Adenovirus transmission may be associated with poorly chlorinated swimming pools; this "swimming pool conjunctivitis" can reach epidemic proportions. **Laboratory diagnosis.** Diagnosis is made by cell culture or immunodiagnostic or molecular diagnostic procedures.

The Common Cold versus the Flu

Colds and influenza are both respiratory diseases. Both are caused by viruses, but by quite different viruses. Actually, there are about 200 different viruses that can cause colds (they were mentioned earlier). Having a cold caused by one cold virus does not offer any protection from the many other cold viruses. Influenza (flu), on the other hand, is caused only by influenza viruses, but there are several kinds of influenza viruses (e.g., influenza A, influenza B, influenza C). Lifelong immunity usually follows influenza, but only against the particular strain of influenza virus that caused the infection. Symptoms of the common cold include sore throat, sneezing, a runny nose, nasal congestion, and sometimes a headache. People with a cold may experience muscle aches and fatigue. They usually do not have a fever, although they may at times feel chilled. Flu symptoms include high fever and chills, cough, headache, muscle aches (sometimes severe), and extreme fatigue. Patients may also experience a sore throat, runny nose, vomiting, and diarrhea. Although a flu vaccine is available, and should be taken annually, it does not protect against all strains of influenza virus. There is no vaccine to prevent colds.

Infections of the Lower Respiratory Tract Having Multiple Causes

Information pertaining to infections of the lower respiratory tract having multiple causes can be found in Chapter 19.

Viral Infections of the Lower Respiratory Tract

Table 18-4 lists information pertaining to viral infections of the lower respiratory tract.

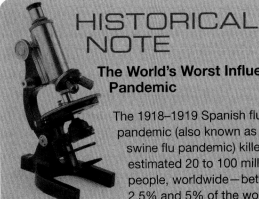

The World's Worst Influenza Pandemic

The 1918–1919 Spanish flu pandemic (also known as the swine flu pandemic) killed an estimated 20 to 100 million people, worldwide—between 2.5% and 5% of the world population. The pandemic killed between 2% and 20% of those infected compared with a mortality rate of about 0.1% for modern-day flu epidemics. Whereas most victims of modern-day flu epidemics are very young, very old, and immunosuppressed people, the 1918–1919 pandemic killed primarily healthy young adults. Scientists have recovered the virus (designated A/H1N1) that caused the pandemic from frozen tissue samples and are currently studying it. They have discovered that the virus kills by causing an overreaction of the body's immune system. This could explain why healthy young adults with strong immune systems were affected to a greater extent than those with weaker immune systems—very young, very old, and immunosuppressed individuals.

Table 18-4 Viral Infections of the Lower Respiratory Tract	
Disease	**Additional Information**
Acute, febrile, viral respiratory disease. This disease is characterized by fever and one or more of the following systemic reactions: chills, headache, general aching, malaise, anorexia, and sometimes GI disturbances in infants. The disease may include rhinitis, pharyngitis, tonsillitis, laryngitis, bronchitis, pneumonia, conjunctivitis, otitis media, and/or sinusitis. Acute, febrile, viral respiratory diseases are not nationally notifiable diseases in the United States.	**Pathogen.** Acute, febrile, viral respiratory disease can be caused by one of many viruses, including parainfluenza viruses, RSV, adenovirus, rhinoviruses, certain coronaviruses, coxsackieviruses, and echoviruses. RSV is the major viral respiratory tract pathogen of early infancy. RSV may cause pneumonia, croup, bronchitis, otitis media, and death.
Patient care. Use Standard Precautions for adult patients; add Contact Precautions for infants and young children for the duration of the illness.	**Reservoirs and mode of transmission.** Infected humans serve as reservoirs. Transmission occurs via direct oral contact or by droplets; indirectly via handkerchiefs, eating utensils, or other fomites; or for some viruses, via the fecal–oral route.
	Laboratory diagnosis. Diagnosis is made by isolation of the etiologic agent from respiratory secretions, using cell cultures. Immunodiagnostic and molecular diagnostic procedures are available.

(continued)

Table 18-4 **Viral Infections of the Lower Respiratory Tract (continued)**

Disease	Additional Information
HPS. HPS is an acute viral disease characterized by fever, myalgias (muscular pain), GI complaints, cough, difficulty breathing, and hypotension (decreased blood pressure). The Sin Nombre virus—literally, the "virus with no name"—was the cause of the epidemic that occurred in the Four Corners area of the United States in the spring and summer of 1993. Since then, sporadic cases have been reported in many states as well as in South America. **Patient care.** Use Standard Precautions for hospitalized patients.	**Pathogens.** At least five hantaviruses (Sin Nombre, Bayou, Black Creek Canal, New York-1, and Monongahela) have caused HPS in the United States. Other strains have caused HPS in South America. **Reservoirs and mode of transmission.** Rodents, including deer mice, pack rats, and chipmunks serve as reservoirs. Transmission occurs via inhalation of aerosolized rodent feces, urine, and saliva. Person-to-person transmission does not occur. **Laboratory diagnosis.** HPS can be diagnosed by immunodiagnostic and molecular procedures and by cell culture.
Influenza (flu). Influenza is an acute, viral respiratory infection with fever, chills, headache, aches, and pains throughout the body (most pronounced in the back and legs), sore throat, cough, nasal drainage. Influenza sometimes causing bronchitis, pneumonia, and death in severe cases. Nausea, vomiting, and diarrhea may occur, particularly in children. Although the term *stomach flu* is often heard, influenza viruses rarely cause GI symptoms. Stomach flu, also known as the 24-hr flu, is caused by viruses other than influenza viruses. **Patient care.** Use Droplet Precautions for hospitalized patients, usually for 5 days from onset of symptoms.	**Pathogens.** Influenza is caused by influenza viruses types A, B, and C. They are single-stranded RNA viruses in the family Orthomyxovirus. Influenza A virus cause severe symptoms and is associated with pandemics and severe disease and more localized outbreaks. Influenza C virus usually does not cause epidemics or significant disease. **Reservoirs and mode of transmission.** Infected humans are the primary reservoir; pigs and birds also serve as reservoirs. Because pig cells have receptors for both avian and human strains of influenza virus, pigs serve as "mixing bowls," resulting in new strains containing RNA segments from both avian and human strains. It is thought that the 1918 pandemic was caused by an avian influenza virus that jumped directly from birds to humans. Transmission occurs via airborne spread and direct contact. **Laboratory diagnosis.** Influenza is diagnosed by isolation of influenza virus from pharyngeal or nasal secretions or washings using cell culture techniques, antigen detection, and demonstration of a rise in antibody titer (concentration) between acute and convalescent sera (see Chapter 16), or by molecular diagnostic procedures. **Note:** Additional information about influenza can be found on thePoint.
Avian influenza (bird flu). Avian influenza, commonly referred to as bird flu, is primarily a disease of birds, but can cause human disease. In humans, the virus causes a respiratory infection with manifestations ranging from influenza-like symptoms (fever, cough, sore throat, and muscle aches) to eye infections, pneumonia, acute and severe respiratory distress, and other severe and life-threatening complications. **Patient care.** Use Droplet Precautions for hospitalized patients. (See http://www.cdc.gov/flu/avian/professional/infect-control.htm for more information.)	**Pathogens.** Bird flu is caused by avian influenza virus type A. The three prominent subtypes of the virus are designated H5, H7, and H9. The strain known as H5N1 is the most virulent strain. New strains of bird flu virus continue to emerge. **Reservoirs and mode of transmission.** Infected wild and domesticated birds serve as reservoirs. Bird-to-human transmission occurs via contact with infected poultry or surfaces that have been contaminated with excretions from infected birds. Person-to-person transmissions are relatively rare. However, influenza viruses commonly mutate, and increased instances of person-to-person transmission are likely to occur in the future. **Laboratory diagnosis.** Molecular diagnostic procedures or cell culture are the means of diagnosis. **Note:** Additional information about bird flu can be found on thePoint.
Severe acute respiratory syndrome (SARS). SARS is a viral respiratory illness with high fever, chills, headache, a general feeling of discomfort, body aches, and sometimes diarrhea. Most patients develop a dry cough followed by pneumonia. SARS was first reported in Asia in February 2003. Over the next few months, the illness spread to more than two dozen countries in Asia, Europe, South America, and North America. During the 2003 outbreak, a total of 8,098 people developed SARS, 774 of whom died. Although no cases of SARS have been reported since 2004, new strains of corona virus that cause respiratory disease in humans continue to emerge. **Patient care.** Use Standard, Airborne, Droplet, and Contact Precautions for hospitalized patients for the duration of the illness plus 10 days after resolution of fever. Use N95 or higher respiratory protection and eye protection. (See http://www.cdc.gov/ncidod/sars for more information.)	**Pathogen.** SARS is caused by SARS-associated coronavirus (SARS-CoV) (Fig. 18-6). **Reservoirs and mode of transmission.** Infected persons serve as reservoirs. It is possible that an unknown mammalian reservoir exists. Transmission occurs by respiratory droplets or by touching the mouth, nose, or eye after touching a contaminated surface or object. **Laboratory diagnosis.** Immunodiagnostic or molecular diagnostic procedures or cell culture can be used to diagnose SARS.

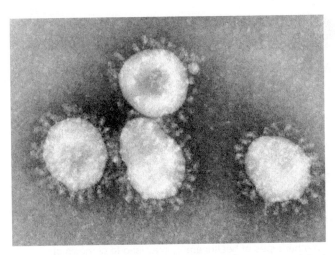

Figure 18-6. Severe acute respiratory syndrome-associated coronavirus virions. Notice the crownlike halo surrounding each virion, which gives rise to the *corona* in *coronavirus*. (Courtesy of Dr. FA Murphy and the CDC.)

Viral Infections of the Oral Region

Cold Sores (Fever Blisters, Herpes Labialis)

Cold sores are superficial clear vesicles on an erythematous (reddened) base, which may appear on the face or lips (refer back to Fig. 14-2 in Chapter 14). They crust and heal within a few days. Reactivation may be caused by trauma, fever (hence the name), physiologic changes, or disease. The infection may be severe and extensive in immunosuppressed individuals. Cold sores are usually caused by herpes simplex virus type 1 (HSV-1), although they can also be caused by herpes simplex virus type 2 (HSV-2). HSV-1 and HSV-2 are also known as human herpesvirus 1 and human herpesvirus 2, respectively. They are DNA viruses in the family Herpesviridae. Either of these viruses may also infect the genital tract, although genital herpes infections are most often caused by HSV-2.

Viral Infections of the Gastrointestinal Tract

Infections of the Gastrointestinal Tract Having Multiple Causes

Diarrhea can have many causes. It may or may not be the result of an infectious disease. When diarrhea is the result of an infectious disease, the pathogen may be a virus, a bacterium, a protozoan, or a helminth. Dysentery (a severe form of diarrhea) may also be caused by various pathogens, including bacteria (e.g., *Shigella* spp. cause bacillary dysentery) and protozoa (e.g., those that cause amebiasis and balantidiasis; see Chapter 21).

Viral Gastroenteritis (Viral Enteritis, Viral Diarrhea)

Disease. Viral gastroenteritis may be an endemic or epidemic illness in infants, children, and adults. Symptoms include nausea, vomiting, diarrhea, abdominal pain, myalgia, headache, malaise, and low-grade fever. Although most often a self-limiting disease lasting 24 to 48 hours, viral gastroenteritis (especially when caused by a rotavirus) can be fatal in an infant or young child. In developing countries, rotavirus infections are responsible for more than 800,000 diarrheal deaths per year. Although viral gastroenteritis is sometimes referred to as "stomach flu" or "24-hour flu," keep in mind that *flu* is an abbreviation of *influenza*, which is a respiratory disease. Viral gastroenteritis is not a nationally notifiable disease in the United States.

Patient Care. Use Standard Precautions for hospitalized patients. Add Contact Precautions for diapered or incontinent patients and for patients with rotavirus infections.

Pathogens. The most common viruses infecting children in their first years of life are enteric adenoviruses, astroviruses, caliciviruses (including noroviruses), and rotaviruses. Those infecting children and adults include norovirus-like viruses and rotaviruses.

Reservoirs and Mode of Transmission. Infected humans are reservoirs of these viruses; contaminated water and shellfish may also be reservoirs. Transmission is most often via the fecal–oral route. Airborne transmission and contact with contaminated fomites may cause epidemics in hospitals or cruise ships. Foodborne, waterborne, and shellfish transmission have been reported.

Laboratory Diagnosis. Diagnosis is by electron microscopic examination of stool specimens or by immunodiagnostic or molecular procedures.

Viral Hepatitis

Hepatitis, or inflammation of the liver, can have many causes, including alcohol, drugs, and viruses. Viral hepatitis refers to hepatitis caused by any one of about a dozen different viruses, including hepatitis A virus (HAV), hepatitis B virus (HBV), hepatitis C virus (HCV), hepatitis D virus (HDV), hepatitis E virus (HEV), hepatitis G virus (HGV), hepatitis GB virus A (HGBV-A), hepatitis GB virus B (HGBV-B), and hepatitis GB virus C (HGBV-C). Hepatitis can also occur as a result of viral diseases such as infectious mononucleosis, yellow fever, and cytomegalovirus infection. See Table 18-5 for information about viral types, modes of transmission, and types of disease. Use Standard Precautions for hospitalized patients; add Contact Precautions for diapered or incontinent patients. Various immunodiagnostic procedures are available for diagnosis of viral hepatitis.

Table 18-5 Common Types of Viral Hepatitis

Name of Disease	Name and Type of Virus	Mode of Transmission	Type of Disease
Type A hepatitis (also known as HAV infection, infectious hepatitis, and epidemic hepatitis)	HAV, a nonenveloped, linear ssRNA virus in the genus Hepatovirus, family Picornaviridae	Fecal–oral transmission; person-to-person; infected food handlers; fecally contaminated foods and water	Abrupt onset; varies in clinical severity from a mild illness lasting 1–2 wk to a severe, disabling disease lasting several months; no chronic infection
Type B hepatitis (also known as HBV infection and serum hepatitis)	HBV, an enveloped, circular dsDNA virus in the genus Orthohepadnavirus, family Hepadnaviridae; the only DNA virus that causes hepatitis	Sexual or household contact with an infected person; mother-to-infant before or during birth; injected drug use; tattooing; needlesticks and other types of healthcare-associated transmission	Usually has an insidious (gradual) onset; severity ranges from inapparent cases to fulminating, fatal cases; chronic infections occur; may lead to cirrhosis or hepatocellular carcinoma
Type C hepatitis (also known as HCV infection and non-A, non-B hepatitis)	HCV, an enveloped, linear ssRNA virus in the genus Hepacivirus, family Flaviviridae	Primarily parenterally transmitted (e.g., via blood transfusion); rarely sexually transmitted	Usually an insidious onset; 50%–80% of patients develop a chronic infection; may lead to cirrhosis or hepatocellular carcinoma
Type D hepatitis (also known as delta hepatitis)	HDV or delta virus, an enveloped, circular ssRNA viral satellite (a defective RNA virus) in the genus Deltavirus	Exposure to infected blood and body fluids; contaminated needles; sexual transmission; coinfection with HBV is necessary	Usually has an abrupt onset; may progress to a chronic and severe disease
Type E hepatitis	HEV, a spherical, nonenveloped, ssRNA virus in the genus Calcivirus, family Calciviridae	Fecal–oral transmission; primarily via fecally contaminated drinking water; also from person to person	Similar to type A hepatitis; no evidence of a chronic form
Type G hepatitis	HGV, a linear ssRNA virus in the genus Hepacivirus, family Flaviviridae	Parenteral	Can cause chronic hepatitis

ds, double-stranded; ss, single-stranded.

The World Health Organization (WHO) estimates that ~240 million people are chronically infected with HBV worldwide, that about 600,000 people die each year as a result of HBV infections, and that more than 2 million new acute clinical cases occur annually.

Vaccines are available for HAV and HBV. The HAV vaccine, which contains inactivated virus grown in cell culture, is recommended for people at increased risk of acquiring hepatitis A (including military personnel and others traveling to regions where HAV is endemic, homosexual and bisexual men, and users of illicit drugs). The HBV vaccine is a subunit vaccine, produced by genetically engineered *Saccharomyces cerevisiae* (common baker's yeast). At first, HBV vaccine was only recommended for persons at high risk of acquiring HBV infection (such as infants born to HBV antigen–positive mothers, household contacts of HBV carriers, homosexual and bisexual men, and users of illicit drugs), but now it is routinely administered to U.S. children. It is required for healthcare workers exposed to blood.

In addition to vaccination against HBV, healthcare personnel practice Standard Precautions (described in Chapter 12). Hepatitis B immune globulin can be given to unvaccinated people who have been exposed to HBV, perhaps by accidental needlestick injury.

Viral Infections of the Genitourinary System

Information pertaining to viral sexually transmitted diseases is listed in Table 18-6.

Viral Infections of the Circulatory System

Information pertaining to viral infections of the circulatory system is listed in Table 18-7.

Table 18-6 Viral Sexually Transmitted Diseases

Disease	Additional Information
Anogenital herpes viral infections (genital herpes). In general, herpes simplex infections are characterized by a localized primary lesion, latency, and a tendency to localized recurrence. In women, the principal sites of primary anogenital herpes virus infection are the cervix and vulva, with recurrent disease affecting the vulva, perineal skin, legs, and buttocks. In men, lesions appear on the penis (Fig. 18-7), and in the anus and rectum of those engaging in anal sex. The initial symptoms are usually itching, tingling, and soreness, followed by a small patch of redness and then a group of small, painful blisters. The blisters break and fuse to form painful, circular sores, which become crusted after a few days. The sores heal in about 10 days but may leave scars. The initial outbreak is more painful, prolonged, and widespread than subsequent outbreaks and may be associated with fever. **Patient care.** Use Standard Precautions for hospitalized patients; add Contact Precautions for severe disseminated or primary mucocutaneous herpes.	**Pathogens.** Genital herpes is usually caused by HSV-2, but is occasionally caused by HSV-1. **Reservoirs and mode of transmission.** Infected humans serve as reservoirs. Transmission occurs via direct sexual contact or oral–genital, oral–anal, or anal–genital contact during the presence of lesions. Mother-to-fetus or mother-to-neonate transmission occurs during pregnancy and birth. **Laboratory diagnosis.** Genital herpes is diagnosed by observation of characteristic cytologic changes in tissue scrapings or biopsy specimens, and the presence of multinucleated giant cells with intranuclear inclusions, and confirmation by immunodiagnostic and molecular diagnostic procedures.
Genital warts (genital papillomatosis, condyloma acuminatum). Genital warts start as tiny, soft, moist, pink or red swellings, which grow rapidly and may develop stalks. Their rough surfaces give them the appearance of small cauliflowers. Multiple warts often grow in the same area, most often on the penis in men and the vulva, vaginal wall, cervix, and skin surrounding the vaginal area in women. Genital warts also develop around the anus and in the rectum in men or women who engage in anal sex. These warts can become malignant.	**Pathogens.** Genital warts are caused by 30–40 types of HPV in the Papovaviridae family of DNA viruses (human wart viruses). HPV genotypes 16 and 18 have been associated with cervical cancer. A vaccine is available (Gardasil) which, according to the manufacturer, helps protect against two types of cancer-causing HPV and two types of HPV that cause genital warts. **Reservoirs and mode of transmission.** Infected humans serve as reservoirs. Transmission occurs via direct contact, usually sexual; through breaks in skin or mucous membranes; or from mother to neonate during birth. **Laboratory diagnosis.** Genital warts are usually diagnosed clinically. Molecular diagnostic procedures are available.

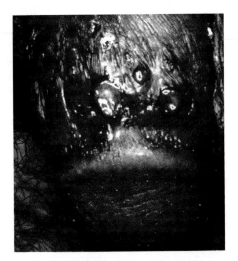

Figure 18-7. Herpes simplex lesions on a penile shaft.
(From Harvey RA, et al. *Lippincott's Illustrated Reviews: Microbiology*. 3rd ed. Philadelphia, PA: Lippincott Williams & Wilkins; 2013.)

Table 18-7 Viral Infections of the Circulatory System

Disease	Additional Information
HIV Infection and AIDS. The signs and symptoms of acute HIV infection (i.e., infection with "the AIDS virus") usually occur within several weeks to several months after infection with HIV. Initial symptoms include an acute, self-limited mononucleosis-like illness lasting 1 or 2 wk. Unfortunately, acute HIV infection is often undiagnosed or misdiagnosed, because anti-HIV antibodies are usually not present in a high enough concentration to be detected during this early phase of infection. Other signs and symptoms of acute HIV infection include fever, rash, headache, lymphadenopathy, pharyngitis, myalgia (muscle pain), arthralgia (joint pain), aseptic meningitis, retro-orbital pain, weight loss, depression, GI distress, night sweats, and oral or genital ulcers. Without appropriate anti-HIV treatment, approximately 90% of HIV-infected individuals ultimately develop AIDS. AIDS is a severe, life-threatening syndrome that represents the late clinical stage of infection with HIV. Invasion and destruction of helper T cells (see Chapter 16) leads to suppression of the patient's immune system (immunosuppression). Secondary infections caused by viruses (e.g., cytomegalovirus, herpes simplex), protozoa (e.g., *Cryptosporidium, Toxoplasma*), bacteria (e.g., mycobacteria), and/or fungi (e.g., *Candida, Cryptococcus, Pneumocystis*) become systemic and cause death. Persons with AIDS die as a result of overwhelming infections caused by a variety of pathogens, often opportunistic pathogens. Kaposi's sarcoma, a previously rare type of cancer, is a frequent complication of AIDS, thought to be caused by a type of herpes virus called human herpesvirus 8. Previously considered to be a universally fatal disease, certain combinations of drugs, referred to as cocktails, are extending the life of some HIV-positive patients. In the absence of effective anti-HIV treatment, the AIDS case–fatality rate is very high—approaching 100%. (Chapter 11 contains information about the current AIDS pandemic.) **Patient care.** Use Standard Precautions for hospitalized patients and appropriate Transmission-Based Precautions for specific infections that occur in AIDS patients.	**Pathogens.** AIDS is caused by HIV (refer back to Fig. 4-13 in Chapter 4). Two types have been identified: type 1 (HIV-1), which is the most common type, and type 2 (HIV-2). HIV viruses are single-stranded RNA viruses in the family Retroviridae (retroviruses). **Reservoirs and mode of transmission.** Infected humans serve as reservoirs. Transmission occurs via direct sexual contact (homosexual or heterosexual); sharing of contaminated needles and syringes by intravenous drug abusers; transfusion of contaminated blood and blood products; transplacental transfer from mother to child; breast-feeding by HIV-infected mothers; transplantation of HIV-infected tissues or organs; and needlestick, scalpel, and broken glass injuries (Fig. 18-8). There is no evidence of HIV transmission via biting insects. Most likely, HIV-1 first invades dendritic cells in the genital and oral mucosa. These cells then fuse with CD4+ lymphocytes (helper T cells) and spread to deeper tissues. **Laboratory diagnosis.** Immunodiagnostic procedures are available for detection of antigen and antibodies. Most HIV-infected patients develop detectable antibodies within 1–3 mo after infection. However, there may be a more prolonged interval of up to 6 mo, or even longer in some cases. The most commonly used screening test is an enzyme-linked immunosorbent assay (ELISA). If the screening test is positive, a confirmatory test such as the Western blot analysis[a] or indirect fluorescent antibody test is usually performed. Antigen detection procedures detect an HIV antigen known as p24. Molecular diagnostic procedures are also available. Quantitative assessment of viral RNA is used to monitor the effectiveness of antiviral therapy.
Infectious mononucleosis. Infectious mononucleosis (also called "mono" or the "kissing disease") is an acute viral disease that may be asymptomatic or may be characterized by fever, sore throat, lymphadenopathy (especially posterior cervical lymph nodes), **splenomegaly** (enlarged spleen), and fatigue. Infectious mononucleosis is usually a self-limited disease of 1 to several weeks' duration. It is rarely fatal. **Patient care.** Use Standard Precautions for hospitalized patients.	**Pathogen.** The etiologic agent of infectious mononucleosis is Epstein–Barr virus (EBV), which is also known as human herpesvirus 4. It is a DNA virus in the family Herpesviridae. EBV infects and transforms B cells, although it also infects other types of cells. EBV is known to be **oncogenic** (cancer causing), causing or being associated with lymphomas (e.g., Hodgkin disease and Burkitt lymphoma), carcinomas (e.g., nasopharyngeal carcinoma and gastric carcinoma), and sarcomas, among other cancers. **Reservoirs and mode of transmission.** Infected humans serve as reservoirs. Transmission occurs from person to person by direct contact with saliva. Kissing facilitates spread among adolescents. EBV can be transmitted via blood transfusion. **Laboratory diagnosis.** Patients with infectious mononucleosis usually present with a lymphocytosis (abnormally high peripheral lymphocyte count), including 10% or more abnormal lymphocyte forms, and abnormalities in liver function tests. Specific diagnosis is usually made by detection of antibodies. Molecular diagnostic procedures are also available. EBV can be cultured from the buffy coat—the layer of white blood cells that appears in centrifuged blood.

Table 18-7 Viral Infections of the Circulatory System (Continued)

Disease	Additional Information
Mumps (infectious parotitis). Mumps is an acute viral infection characterized by fever and swelling and tenderness of the salivary glands (Fig. 18-9). Complications can include **orchitis** (inflammation of the testes), **oophoritis** (inflammation of the ovaries), meningitis, encephalitis, deafness, pancreatitis, arthritis, mastitis, nephritis, thyroiditis, and pericarditis. **Patient care.** Use Droplet Precautions for hospitalized patients until 9 days after onset of swelling.	**Pathogen.** Mumps is caused by mumps virus, an RNA virus in the genus Rubulavirus, family Paramyxoviridae. **Reservoirs and mode of transmission.** Infected humans serve as reservoirs. Transmission occurs via droplet spread and direct contact with the saliva of an infected person. **Laboratory diagnosis.** Diagnosis of mumps is made using immunodiagnostic procedures or cell culture.
Viral hemorrhagic diseases. Viral hemorrhagic diseases are extremely serious, acute viral illnesses. Initial symptoms include sudden onset of fever, malaise (a feeling of general discomfort; feeling "out of sorts"), myalgia, and headache, followed by pharyngitis, vomiting, diarrhea, rash, and internal hemorrhaging. Case fatality rates for Marburg virus infection and Ebola virus infection have been 25% and 50%–90%, respectively. All known cases of both diseases occurred in or could be traced back to Africa. **Patient care.** Exercise Standard, Droplet, and Contact Precautions for hospitalized patients for the duration of the illness. Emphasize (a) use of sharps safety devices and safe work practices, (b) hand hygiene, (c) barrier protection against blood and body fluids, and (d) appropriate waste handling. Use N95 or higher respirators when performing aerosol-generating procedures.	**Pathogens.** Viral hemorrhagic fevers are caused by many different viruses, including dengue virus, yellow fever virus, Crimean-Congo hemorrhagic fever virus, Lassa virus, Ebola virus, and Marburg virus. Ebola virus and Marburg virus are filamentous viruses in the family Filoviridae. Both are extremely large viruses. Ebola virus is about 80 nm in width and up to 1 mm or longer in length. Marburg virus is about 80 nm in width and 790 nm in length. **Reservoirs and mode of transmission.** Infected humans serve as reservoirs; infected African green monkeys also serve as reservoirs of Marburg virus. Transmission is from person to person via direct contact with infected blood, secretions, internal organs, or semen, or by needlestick. The risk is highest when the patient is vomiting, having diarrhea, or hemorrhaging. Crimean-Congo hemorrhagic fever is a tickborne disease. Dengue fever and yellow fever are mosquito-borne diseases, transmitted primarily by mosquitoes in the genus *Aedes*. **Laboratory diagnosis.** Viral hemorrhagic diseases are diagnosed using immunodiagnostic and molecular procedures, cell culture, or electron microscopy. Laboratory studies of viral hemorrhagic fevers represent an extreme biohazard and should be conducted only in BSL-4 containment facilities.

[a]A Western blot analysis is a laboratory procedure in which proteins separated by electrophoresis in polyacrylamide gels are transferred (blotted) onto nitrocellulose or nylon membranes and identified by specific complexing with tagged antibodies.

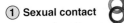
① **Sexual contact**

② **Transfusion**

③ **Contaminated needles**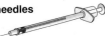

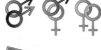
④ **Perinatal transmission**
- Transplacental
- During delivery through an infected birth canal
- As a result of ingestion of breast milk carrying virus

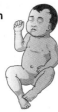

Figure 18-8. Common modes of transmission of HIV. (Redrawn from Harvey RA, et al. *Lippincott's Illustrated Reviews, Microbiology.* 3rd ed. Philadelphia, PA: Lippincott Williams & Wilkins; 2013.)

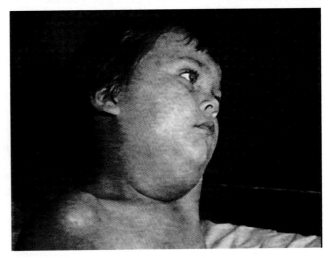

Figure 18-9. Child with mumps. (Courtesy of Barbara Rice, the National Immunization Program, and the CDC.)

STUDY AID

Viremia

The presence of viruses in the bloodstream is known as **viremia**. The viruses either may be free in the plasma, or attached to or within red blood cells or white blood cells, such as lymphocytes and monocytes. The number of viruses in the bloodstream is referred to as the **viral load**, which may be described as being heavy or light. The degree of viremia varies from one viral disease to another, and often from one stage of a particular viral infection to another.

Viral Infections of the Central Nervous System

Tables 18-8 and 18-9 list information pertaining to viral infections of the central nervous system (CNS).

Recap of Major Viral Infections of Humans

Table 18-10 provides a recap of some major viral infections of humans.

Appropriate Therapy for Viral Infections

Recommendations for the treatment of infectious diseases change frequently. The viral infections described in this chapter must be treated using appropriate antiviral drugs. For certain diseases, serum immune globulins (e.g., varicella-zoster immune globulin) are available for treatment. Additional information about antiviral agents can be found in Chapter 9 and at en.wikipedia.org/wiki/Antiviral_drug.

Table 18-8 Viral Infections of the CNS

Disease	Additional Information
Lymphocytic choriomeningitis. Lymphocytic choriomeningitis is a rodentborne viral disease that presents as aseptic meningitis, encephalitis, or meningoencephalitis. Asymptomatic or mild febrile disease also occurs. Some patients develop fever, malaise, suppressed appetite, muscle aches, headache, nausea, vomiting, sore throat, coughing, joint pain, chest pain, and salivary gland pain. Possible complications of CNS involvement include deafness and temporary or permanent neurological damage. An association between lymphocytic choriomeningitis virus infection and myocarditis has been suggested. **Patient care.** Use Standard Precautions for hospitalized patients.	**Pathogen.** Lymphocytic choriomeningitis is caused by lymphocytic choriomeningitis virus (LCMV), a member of the family Arenaviridae. **Reservoirs and mode of transmission.** Infected rodents, primarily the common house mice serve as reservoirs. Humans become infected following exposure to mouse urine, droppings, saliva, or nesting materials. The virus can enter broken skin; through nose, the eyes, or mouth; or via the bite of an infected rodent. Organ transplantation is a possible means of transmission. Person-to-person transmission does not occur. **Laboratory diagnosis.** Diagnosis is primarily by immunodiagnostic procedures and cell culture.
Poliomyelitis (polio, infantile paralysis). In most patients, poliomyelitis causes a minor illness with fever, malaise, headache, nausea, and vomiting. In about 1% of patients, the disease progresses to severe muscle pain, stiffness of the neck and back, with or without flaccid paralysis. Major illness is more likely to occur in older children and adults. Although once a major health problem in the United States, vaccines became available in the 1950s. The WHO is attempting to eradicate polio worldwide. **Patient care.** Use Contact Precautions for hospitalized patients for the duration of illness.	**Pathogens.** Poliomyelitis is caused by polioviruses, RNA viruses in the family Picornaviridae (pico = small, RNA viruses). **Reservoirs and mode of transmission.** Infected humans serve as reservoirs. Transmission is from person to person, primarily via the fecal–oral route; also by throat secretions. **Laboratory diagnosis.** Diagnosis of poliomyelitis is made by isolation of poliovirus from stool samples, cerebrospinal fluid (CSF), or oropharyngeal secretions using cell culture techniques or by immunodiagnostic or molecular diagnostic procedures.

Table 18-8 Viral Infections of the CNS (continued)

Disease	Additional Information
Rabies. Rabies is a usually fatal, acute viral encephalomyelitis of mammals, with mental depression, restlessness, headache, fever, malaise, paralysis, salivation, spasms of throat muscles induced by a slight breeze or drinking water, convulsions, and death caused by respiratory failure. The paralysis usually starts in the lower legs and moves upward through the body. Rabies is endemic in every country of the world except Antarctica and in every state except Hawaii. Worldwide, over 55,000 people die of rabies annually. **Patient care.** Use Standard Precautions for hospitalized patients.	**Pathogen.** Rabies is caused by rabies virus, a bullet-shaped, enveloped RNA virus in the family Rhabdoviridae. **Reservoirs and mode of transmission.** Reservoirs are various wild and domestic mammals, including dogs, foxes, coyotes, wolves, jackals, skunks, raccoons, mongooses, and bats. Transmission is usually via the bite of a rabid animal, which introduces virus-laden saliva. Airborne transmission from bats in caves also occurs. Person-to-person transmission is rare. **Laboratory diagnosis.** Diagnosis of rabies is made by cell culture, antibody detection in serum or CSF, antigen detection in tissue samples, molecular diagnostic procedures for brain tissue, or observation of Negri bodies in brain or other tissues. Negri bodies are viral RNA-nucleoprotein complexes found in the cytoplasm of virus-infected cells (i.e., they are intracytoplasmic inclusions).
Viral meningitis. Viral meningitis is also known as aseptic meningitis and nonbacterial or abacterial meningitis. It is a relatively common disease but, fortunately, is rarely serious. Acute illness rarely exceeds 10 days duration. Viral meningitis is characterized by sudden onset of febrile illness with the signs and symptoms of meningeal involvement. CSF findings include the presence of mononuclear white blood cells, increased protein levels, normal glucose levels, and the absence of bacteria. A rash may develop. When caused by an enterovirus, GI and respiratory symptoms may occur. **Patient care.** Use Standard Precautions for hospitalized patients. Add Contact Precautions for infants and young children.	**Pathogens.** The most common causes of viral meningitis in the United States are enteroviruses. Other causes include coxsackie viruses, arboviruses, measles virus, mumps virus, herpes simplex viruses and VZVs, lymphocytic choriomeningitis virus, and adenoviruses. Leptospirosis (a bacterial disease) can also cause aseptic meningitis. **Reservoirs and mode of transmission.** Reservoirs and modes of transmission vary with the specific etiologic agent. **Laboratory diagnosis.** During the early stages of the disease, the viral pathogen may be isolated from throat washings and stool, and occasionally from CSF and blood. Diagnosis is made by immunodiagnostic or molecular diagnostic procedures or cell culture.
Viral encephalitis (arthropod-borne viral encephalitis; Table 18-9). Arthropod-borne viral encephalitis is an acute inflammatory viral disease. A patient with this disease may be asymptomatic or have mild fever and headache. Severe infection is also possible, with headache, high fever, stupor, disorientation, coma, tremors, occasional convulsions, spastic paralysis, and death. The term *arboviruses* is sometimes used in reference to viruses that are transmitted by arthropods. **Patient care.** Exercise Standard Precautions for hospitalized patients. Transmission-Based Precautions may be necessary, depending on the etiologic agent.	**Pathogens.** See Table 18-9. Over the years, St. Louis encephalitis virus has been the most common mosquito-transmitted pathogen in the United States. The situation changed in 2002 when West Nile virus took over the number one spot. Additional information about West Nile virus can be found on thePoint. **Reservoirs and mode of transmission.** See Table 18-9. Person-to-person transmission is rare; possibly by transfusion, organ transplant, breast milk, or transplacentally. **Laboratory diagnosis.** Many of the viruses that cause encephalitis, including arboviruses, are difficult to isolate from CSF by cell culture. Appropriate containment facilities must be used when attempting to cultivate arboviruses. Viral encephalitis caused by arboviruses is usually diagnosed using immunodiagnostic or molecular diagnostic procedures, or sometimes by electron microscopy.

Table 18-9 Selected Arthropod-Borne Viral Encephalitides of the United States

Disease	Pathogen	Reservoirs	Vectors
Eastern equine encephalitis (EEE)	EEE virus, an RNA virus in the family Togaviridae	Birds, horses	*Aedes, Coquilletidia, Culex,* and *Culiseta* mosquitoes
California encephalitis	California encephalitis virus, an RNA virus in the family Bunyaviridae	Rodents, rabbits	*Aedes* and *Culex* mosquitoes
La Crosse encephalitis	La Crosse encephalitis virus, an RNA virus in the family Bunyaviridae	Chipmunks, squirrels	*Aedes* mosquitoes
St. Louis encephalitis	St. Louis encephalitis virus, an RNA virus in the family Flaviviridae	Birds	*Culex* mosquitoes
West Nile virus encephalitis	West Nile virus, an RNA virus in the family Flaviviridae	Birds, perhaps horses	*Culex* mosquitoes
WEE	WEE virus, an RNA virus in the family Togaviridae	Birds, horses	*Aedes* and *Culex* mosquitoes

Table 18-10 Recap of Some Major Viral Infections of Humans

Disease	Viral Pathogen
AIDS	HIV
Avian influenza (bird flu)	Avian influenza viruses
Chickenpox	VZV
Cold sores (fever blisters)	HSVs
Genital herpes	HSVs
HPS	Hantaviruses
Infectious mononucleosis	EBV
Influenza	Influenza viruses
Monkeypox	Monkeypox virus
Mumps	Mumps virus
Poliomyelitis	Polioviruses
Rabies	Rabies virus
Rubella (German measles)	Rubella virus
Rubeola (hard measles)	Rubeola virus
SARS	SARS-associated coronavirus
Smallpox	Variola virus
Swine flu	Swine flu viruses
Viral hepatitis	Various hepatitis viruses
Warts	Papillomaviruses
West Nile virus encephalitis	West Nile virus

ON **thePoint**

- Terms Introduced in This Chapter
- Review of Key Points
- A Closer Look:
  - Influenza Viruses, including Bird Flu and Swine Flu
  - Norovirus
  - West Nile Virus
- Increase Your Knowledge
- Critical Thinking
- Additional Self-Assessment Exercises

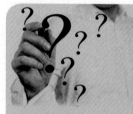

Self-Assessment Exercises

After studying this chapter, answer the following multiple-choice questions.

1. Which of the following is the cause of smallpox?
   a. Vaccinia virus
   b. Varicella virus
   c. Variola virus
   d. None of the preceding choices

2. Which of the following are considered to be oncogenic?

   a. Epstein–Barr virus and HPVs
   b. HIV and Ebola virus
   c. Rubella and rubeola viruses
   d. Variola and varicella viruses

3. Laboratory diagnosis of HIV infection is usually made by which of the following?

   a. Electron microscopy
   b. Growth of HIV in cell culture
   c. Growth of HIV in embryonated chicken eggs
   d. Immunodiagnostic procedures for the detection of antigen and antibodies

4. Which of the following is also known as infectious hepatitis?

   a. HAV
   b. HBV
   c. HCV
   d. HDV

5. Mosquitoes serve as vectors in all of the following viral diseases, except:

   a. Dengue fever
   b. Hepatitis
   c. West Nile virus disease
   d. Yellow fever

6. Which of the following viruses is/are not transmitted sexually?

   a. Hantavirus
   b. HSVs
   c. HIV
   d. Papillomaviruses

7. Which of the following is a DNA virus?

   a. HAV
   b. HBV
   c. HCV
   d. HDV

8. Which of the following is a type of herpes virus?

   a. Epstein–Barr virus
   b. Measles virus
   c. Mumps virus
   d. Rabies virus

9. Which of the following viral diseases has been acquired in the United States by handling pet prairie dogs?

   a. Chickenpox
   b. Hantavirus
   c. Monkeypox
   d. Smallpox

10. The disease known as severe acute respiratory syndrome (SARS) is caused by a type of:

   a. Coronavirus
   b. Herpes virus
   c. Papillomavirus
   d. Picornavirus

Case 1. (This case study was modified from Strohl WA, et al. *Lippincott's Illustrated Reviews: Microbiology*. Philadelphia, PA: Lippincott Williams & Wilkins; 2001. An Internet search may be required to locate answers to some of the questions.)

A 25-year-old man was admitted to the hospital in mid-June for malaise and shortness of breath of one day's duration. Three days prior to admission, he had developed sneezing and a runny and stuffy nose. Two days prior to admission he developed a nonproductive cough, a headache behind his eyes, a fever, and red blotches on his face. One day prior to admission, the rash covered most of his face and had spread to his arms and trunk. Physical examination revealed a temperature of 100°F, a relatively low total white blood cell count, labored breathing, a red face, and an erythematous maculopapular rash on the patient's trunk, palms, and extremities. Examination of his mouth revealed several salt-grain-size, raised, white spots on his buccal mucosa (the lining of his cheeks). Upon questioning, he stated that he had no known tick exposure, that his mother had told him that she thought he might have had measles as an infant, and that he had never received the measles vaccine.

A. Why do you think the patient was asked about tick exposure?

B. What disease is suggested by the combination of fever, rash, and white spots on the patient's buccal mucosa?

C. What pathogen causes this disease?

D. What are the white spots called?

E. What laboratory tests would confirm the diagnosis?

Case 2. A 27-year-old unmarried female patient presents with genital warts.

A. Which one of the following viruses is the most likely cause?

1. Herpes simplex virus
2. Epstein–Barr virus
3. Hantavirus
4. Human papillomavirus
5. Human immunodeficiency virus

B. Which one of the following diseases is this virus also associated with?

1. Syphilis
2. Gonorrhea
3. Cervical cancer
4. Nephritis
5. Urethritis

Case 3. A 54-year-old man presents with a painful, blistering skin rash on the left side of his torso, accompanied by a headache and low-grade fever. He says that he has lately been under a great deal of emotional stress.

A. Which one of the following viruses is the most likely cause?

1. Measles virus
2. Varicella-zoster virus
3. Norovirus
4. Hantavirus
5. Rubella virus

B. This condition often occurs many years after a person has had which one of the following viral diseases?

1. Measles
2. Hepatitis
3. Influenza
4. Infectious mononucleosis
5. Chickenpox

(Answers to Case Studies can be found in Appendix B.)

19

Bacterial Infections of Humans

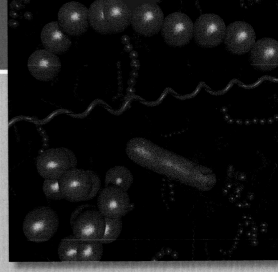

Artist rendering of a variety of bacterial pathogens.

 CHAPTER OUTLINE

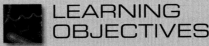 **LEARNING OBJECTIVES**

After studying this chapter, you should be able to:

- Name at least three nationally notifiable bacterial diseases
- Correlate a particular bacterial disease with its major signs and symptoms, etiologic agent, reservoir(s), mode(s) of transmission, and diagnostic laboratory procedures
- Given a particular body site (e.g., the urinary tract), state at least one example of a bacterial disease at that site
- Differentiate between gangrene and gas gangrene
- Correlate a given bacterial sexually transmitted disease (STD) with its etiologic agent
- Name at least three rickettsial or ehrlichial infections of the cardiovascular system
- Name at least three diseases caused by anaerobic bacteria
- Describe a biofilm, and name at least two human diseases thought to be associated with biofilms
- State, in general, how bacterial infections are treated

Introduction

It would be impossible in a book of this size to describe *all* of the human infectious diseases caused by bacteria. Thus, only selected bacterial diseases are described in this chapter. Although a certain disease may be described within one particular section of this chapter (e.g., in the section describing bacterial diseases of the respiratory system), readers should keep in mind that some bacterial diseases have various clinical manifestations, affecting several body systems simultaneously, and that the pathogens may move from one body site to another. Readers should also keep in mind that, although most of the bacterial diseases described in this chapter are caused by a single bacterial species, many other diseases are thought to be the result of communities of bacteria consisting of more than one species (e.g., biofilms; described in Chapter 10 and later in this chapter).

How Do Bacteria Cause Disease?

The various bacterial virulence factors, which enable pathogens to cause disease, were described in Chapter 14. Some of them are listed here:

- Adherence and colonization factors
- Factors that prevent activation of complement
- Factors that enable escape from phagocytosis by white blood cells (WBCs)
- Factors that prevent destruction within phagocytes
- Factors that suppress the host immune system (i.e., factors that cause immunosuppression)
- Endotoxin (a component of the cell walls of Gram-negative bacteria)
- Production of exotoxins (e.g., cytotoxins, enterotoxins, neurotoxins)
- Production of necrotic and other types of destructive enzymes

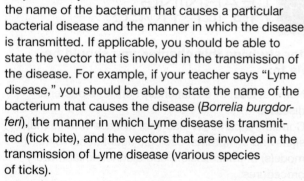

STUDY AID

What to Learn?

This chapter contains a large amount of information. Of primary importance will be your ability to later recall the name of the bacterium that causes a particular bacterial disease and the manner in which the disease is transmitted. If applicable, you should be able to state the vector that is involved in the transmission of the disease. For example, if your teacher says "Lyme disease," you should be able to state the name of the bacterium that causes the disease (*Borrelia burgdorferi*), the manner in which Lyme disease is transmitted (tick bite), and the vectors that are involved in the transmission of Lyme disease (various species of ticks).

Certain of the bacterial diseases described in this chapter are nationally notifiable infectious diseases. When a patient is diagnosed with one of these diseases in the United States, the information must be reported to the Centers for Disease Control and Prevention (CDC). As of 2010, there were approximately 35 nationally notifiable bacterial diseases (Table 19-1). Most of them are described in this chapter, as are some bacterial diseases that are not nationally notifiable (e.g., *Campylobacter* enteritis).

Bacterial Infections of the Skin

Information pertaining to bacterial infections of the skin is contained in Table 19-2.

> Gas gangrene is always caused by *Clostridium* spp.

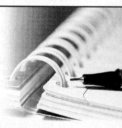

STUDY AID

Gangrene versus Gas Gangrene

The term **gangrene** refers to tissue necrosis (death) resulting from local anemia (ischemia). **Ischemia** results from an obstruction, loss, or reduction of blood supply, leading to a lack of oxygen. Gangrene may have nothing whatsoever to do with microbes. **Gas gangrene**, on the other hand, is *always* caused by microbes—specifically, *Clostridium* spp. The clostridia produce gaseous metabolic byproducts—primarily, hydrogen and nitrogen—that accumulate in the necrotic tissues. Regardless of the cause, gangrenous tissue becomes brownish black and foul smelling.

Table 19-1 Nationally Notifiable Bacterial Diseases

Bacterial Disease	Number of New U.S. Cases Reported to the CDC in 2010[a]
Anthrax	0
Botulism	112
Brucellosis	115
Chancroid	24
Chlamydia	1,307,893
Cholera	13
Diphtheria	0
Ehrlichiosis/Anaplasmosis	2,615
Gonorrhea	309,341
Haemophilus influenzae, invasive disease	3,151
Hansen disease (leprosy)	98
Hemolytic-uremic syndrome, postdiarrheal	266
Legionellosis	3,346
Listeriosis	821
Lyme disease	30,158
Meningococcal disease	833
Pertussis (whooping cough)	27,550
Plague	2
Psittacosis	4
Q fever	131
Salmonellosis	54,424
Shiga toxin-producing *Escherichia coli*	5,476
Shigellosis	14,786
Spotted fever rickettsiosis	1,985
Streptococcal disease, invasive, group A	?
Streptococcal toxic shock syndrome (TSS)	142
Streptococcus pneumoniae, invasive disease, drug-resistant, all ages	16,569
Syphilis	45,834
Tetanus	26
TSS (other than streptococcal)	82
Tuberculosis	11,182
Tularemia	124
Typhoid fever	467
Vancomycin-intermediate *S. aureus*	91
Vancomycin-resistant *S. aureus*	2

[a]These figures provide insight into how frequently these diseases occur in the United States. For updated information, go to the CDC website; click on "Morbidity & Mortality Weekly Report"; then click on "Notifiable Diseases"; then click on the most recent year that is listed.
Source: http://www.cdc.gov.

Table 19-2 Bacterial Infections of the Skin

Disease	Additional Information
Acne. Acne is a common condition in which pores become clogged with dried sebum, flaked skin, and bacteria, which leads to the formation of blackheads and whiteheads (collectively known as acne pimples) and inflamed, infected abscesses. Acne is most common among teenagers.	**Pathogens.** The etiologic agents of acne are *Propionibacterium acnes* and other *Propionibacterium* spp., all of which are anaerobic, Gram-positive bacilli. **Reservoirs and Mode of Transmission.** Infected humans serve as reservoirs, although acne is probably not transmissible. **Laboratory Diagnosis.** Diagnosis is made on clinical grounds.
Anthrax. Anthrax, also known as woolsorter's disease, can affect the skin (cutaneous anthrax), lungs (inhalation or pulmonary anthrax), or gastrointestinal tract (gastrointestinal anthrax), depending on the portal of entry of the etiologic agent. In cutaneous anthrax, depressed blackened lesions called eschars form as a result of a necrotoxin (a toxin that kills cells) (refer back to Fig. 11-9 in Chapter 11). Inhalation and gastrointestinal anthrax are often fatal, but cutaneous anthrax usually is not. Ordinarily, human cases in the United States are quite rare. However, 22 U.S. cases occurred in the fall of 2001 as a result of the mailing of letters that had purposely been contaminated with *Bacillus anthracis* spores. The 22 cases included 11 cases of inhalation anthrax (5 fatal) and 11 cases of cutaneous anthrax (nonfatal). **Patient Care.** Use Standard Precautions for hospitalized patients. Add Contact Precautions for cutaneous anthrax patients if there is a large amount of uncontained drainage. Use soap and water for handwashing; alcohol does not have sporicidal activity.	**Pathogen.** The etiologic agent of anthrax is *B. anthracis*, an encapsulated, spore-forming, Gram-positive bacillus. **Reservoirs and Mode of Transmission.** Reservoirs include anthrax-infected animals, as well as spores that may be present in soil, animal hair, wool, animal skins and hides, and products made from them. Transmission occurs via entry of endospores through breaks in skin, inhalation of spores, or ingestion of bacteria in contaminated meat. Pulmonary anthrax is not transmitted from person to person. **Laboratory Diagnosis.** Anthrax is diagnosed by isolation of *B. anthracis* from blood, lesions, or discharges, and identification using biochemical- or enzyme-based tests. Immunodiagnostic procedures are available.
Gas Gangrene (Clostridial Myonecrosis). After *Clostridium* spores enter and germinate in a wound, the vegetative pathogens produce necrotizing exoenzymes and toxins, which destroy muscle and soft tissue, allowing deeper penetration by the organisms. Gases released from the infecting pathogens cause pockets of gas to develop in the infected tissue. Tissue destruction occurs rapidly, often necessitating amputation of the infected anatomic site. In its most severe forms, gas gangrene produces massive tissue destruction, shock, and renal failure. **Patient Care.** Use Standard Precautions for hospitalized patients.	**Pathogens.** Although *Clostridium perfringens* is the most common cause of gas gangrene, other *Clostridium* spp. can also cause this condition. **Reservoirs and Mode of Transmission.** Soil is the primary reservoir. Humans become infected when soil containing clostridial spores enters an open wound. Person-to-person transmission does not occur. **Laboratory Diagnosis.** The presence of Gram-positive and/or Gram-variable bacilli in Gram-stained smears of wound specimens should lead one to suspect gas gangrene. Often, no leukocytes are observed, as they have been killed by toxins produced by the clostridia. Once isolated on culture media, the etiologic agent can be identified using various phenotypic characteristics, including reactions in biochemical- or enzyme-based tests.
Leprosy. Leprosy is today more commonly known as Hansen disease. There are two forms of leprosy: (a) lepromatous leprosy, characterized by numerous nodules in skin and possible involvement of the nasal mucosa and eyes and (b) tuberculoid leprosy, in which relatively few skin lesions occur. Peripheral nerve involvement tends to be severe, with loss of sensation. Hansen disease is named for G.A. Hansen, who, in 1873, discovered the bacillus that causes leprosy. Leprosy occurs primarily in warm, wet areas of the tropics and subtropics. The worldwide prevalence of leprosy has been estimated by the WHO to be as high as 11 million. Most U.S. cases involve people who emigrated from developing countries.	**Pathogen.** The etiologic agent of leprosy is *Mycobacterium leprae*, an acid-fast bacillus. *M. leprae* is the slowest growing of all known bacteria, with a doubling time of 13 days. (Compare that with *E. coli*, which, under ideal laboratory conditions, has a doubling time of about 20 minutes.) **Reservoirs and Mode of Transmission.** Infected humans serve as reservoirs; *M. leprae* is present in nasal discharges and is shed from cutaneous lesions. Armadillos in Texas and Louisiana have a naturally occurring disease that is identical to experimental leprosy in those animals, suggesting that transmission from armadillos to humans is possible. The exact mode of transmission has not been clearly established. The organisms may gain entrance through the respiratory system or broken skin. Leprosy does not appear to be easily transmitted from person to person. Prolonged, close contact with an infected individual appears to be necessary. The tuberculoid form of leprosy is not contagious.

Table 19-2 Bacterial Infections of the Skin (continued)

Disease	Additional Information
Patient Care. Use Standard Precautions for hospitalized patients.	**Laboratory Diagnosis.** *M. leprae* differs from all other *Mycobacterium* species in that it cannot be grown on artificial culture media. It can be cultured only in laboratory animals, such as nine-banded armadillos or mouse foot pads. Diagnosis is made by demonstration of acid-fast bacilli in skin smears or skin biopsy specimens.
Staphylococcal Skin Infections (Folliculitis, Furuncles, Carbuncles, Abscesses, Impetigo, Impetigo of the Newborn, Scalded Skin Syndrome). Virtually all infected hair follicles, boils (furuncles), carbuncles, and styes involve *Staphylococcus aureus*. The majority of common skin lesions are localized, discrete, and uncomplicated. However, seeding of the bloodstream may lead to pneumonia, lung abscess, osteomyelitis, sepsis, endocarditis, meningitis, or brain abscess. With impetigo, which occurs mainly in children, pus-filled blisters (*pustules*) may appear anywhere on the body. Impetigo of the newborn (impetigo neonatorum) and staphylococcal scalded skin syndrome (SSSS) may occur as epidemics in hospital nurseries. **Patient Care.** Use Standard Precautions for skin, burn, and wound infections if they are minor or limited, and Contact Precautions if they are major. Use Contact Precautions for patients with SSSS. Use Standard Precautions for infections caused by methicillin-resistant *S. aureus* (MRSA); add Contact Precautions if wounds cannot be contained by dressings. Use Contact Precautions for diapered or incontinent children with enterocolitis (staph food poisoning), for the duration of illness.	**Pathogen.** Most staphylococcal infections ("staph infections") are caused by *S. aureus*, a Gram-positive coccus. Impetigo may also be caused by *Streptococcus pyogenes*, which is another Gram-positive coccus. *S. aureus* spreads through skin by producing hyaluronidase (see Chapter 14). SSSS is produced by strains of *S. aureus* that produce exfoliative (or epidermolytic) toxin, which causes the top layer of skin (epidermis) to split from the rest of the skin. (See Fig. 19-1 for a summary of diseases caused by *S. aureus*.) **Reservoirs and Mode of Transmission.** Infected humans serve as reservoirs. Persons with a draining lesion or any purulent discharge are the most common sources of epidemic spread. Transmission occurs via direct contact with a person having a purulent lesion or is an asymptomatic carrier. In hospitals, staphylococcal infections can be spread by the hands of healthcare workers. **Laboratory Diagnosis.** The infecting strain must be isolated on culture media and identified using a variety of phenotypic characteristics, including reactions in biochemical- or enzyme-based tests. Susceptibility testing must be performed because many strains of *S. aureus* are multidrug resistant.
Streptococcal Skin Infections (Impetigo, Scarlet Fever, Erysipelas, Necrotizing Fasciitis). (a) Streptococcal impetigo is usually superficial but may proceed through vesicular, pustular, and encrusted stages. (b) Scarlet fever (scarlatina) includes a widespread, pink-red rash, most obvious on the abdomen, sides of the chest, and in skin folds. Severe cases may be accompanied by high fever, nausea, and vomiting. (c) Erysipelas is an acute cellulitis with fever, constitutional symptoms, and hot, tender, red eruptions (sometimes referred to as St. Anthony's fire). (d) Necrotizing fasciitis is the name of the disease caused by the so-called flesh-eating bacteria. **Fasciitis** is inflammation of the *fascia* (fibrous tissue that envelops the body beneath the skin and also encloses muscles and groups of muscles). The most common cause of necrotizing fasciitis is *Streptococcus pyogenes*. **Patient Care.** Use Standard Precautions for skin, burn, and wound infections if they are minor or limited, and Contact or Droplet Precautions if they are major. Use Droplet Precautions for infants and young children with strep throat or scarlet fever, and all patients with pneumonia or serious invasive disease. Outbreaks of serious invasive disease have occurred secondary to transmission among patients and healthcare personnel.	**Pathogen.** These infections are caused by *Streptococcus pyogenes*, a Gram-positive coccus, that is also known as group A β-hemolytic streptococcus, GAS, and "Strep A." Scarlet fever is caused by erythrogenic toxin, produced by some strains of *S. pyogenes*. Scarlet fever can be a complication (sequela) of untreated strep throat (streptococcal pharyngitis). Figure 19-2 provides a summary of diseases caused by *S. pyogenes*. **Reservoirs and Mode of Transmission.** Infected humans serve as reservoirs. Transmission occurs from person to person via large respiratory droplets or direct contact with patients or carriers. Transmission rarely occurs by indirect contact through objects. **Laboratory Diagnosis.** The infecting strain must be isolated on culture media and identified using various phenotypic characteristics, including biochemical- or enzyme-based tests. Immunodiagnostic procedures are available, some of which are referred to as "rapid strep tests." Currently, susceptibility testing is not routinely performed because *S. pyogenes* has not yet developed resistance to penicillin. Some strains have become resistant to other antimicrobial agents, however.

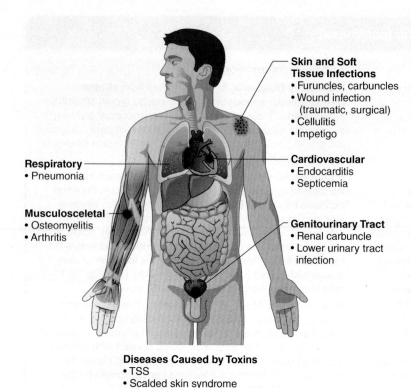

Figure 19-1. Diseases caused by *Staphylococcus aureus*. (Redrawn from Harvey RA, et al. *Lippincott's Illustrated Reviews*. 3rd ed. Philadelphia, PA: Lippincott Williams & Wilkins; 2013.)

Labels from figure 19-1:

Skin and Soft Tissue Infections
• Furuncles, carbuncles
• Wound infection (traumatic, surgical)
• Cellulitis
• Impetigo

Respiratory
• Pneumonia

Cardiovascular
• Endocarditis
• Septicemia

Musculoscleletal
• Osteomyelitis
• Arthritis

Genitourinary Tract
• Renal carbuncle
• Lower urinary tract infection

Diseases Caused by Toxins
• TSS
• Scalded skin syndrome
• Food poisoning (gastroenteritis)

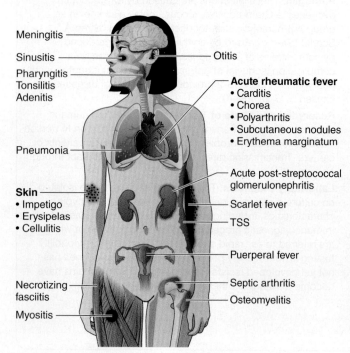

Figure 19-2. Diseases caused by *Streptococcus pyogenes*. (Redrawn from Engleberg NC, et al. *Schaechter's Mechanisms of Microbial Disease*. 5th ed. Philadelphia, PA: Lippincott Williams & Wilkins; 2013.)

Labels from figure 19-2:

Meningitis
Sinusitis
Pharyngitis
Tonsilitis
Adenitis
Pneumonia

Skin
• Impetigo
• Erysipelas
• Cellulitis

Necrotizing fasciitis
Myositis

Otitis

Acute rheumatic fever
• Carditis
• Chorea
• Polyarthritis
• Subcutaneous nodules
• Erythema marginatum

Acute post-streptococcal glomerulonephritis
Scarlet fever
TSS
Puerperal fever
Septic arthritis
Osteomyelitis

Wound Infections

When the protective skin barrier is broken as a result of burns, puncture wounds, surgical procedures, or bites, opportunistic indigenous microbiota and environmental bacteria can invade and cause local or deep tissue infections. The pathogens may spread via blood or lymph, causing serious systemic infections.

Bacterial Infections of the Ears

Information pertaining to viral and bacterial ear infections is contained in Table 19-3.

> The three most common causes of otitis media are *Streptococcus pneumoniae*, *Haemophilus influenzae*, and *Moraxella catarrhalis*.

Bacterial Infections of the Eyes

Table 19-4 contains information pertaining to bacterial infections of the eyes.

Bacterial Infections of the Respiratory System

Bacterial Infections of the Upper Respiratory Tract

Table 19-5 contains information pertaining to bacterial infections of the upper respiratory tract.

> Although we hear more about *Streptococcus pyogenes* as a cause of pharyngitis (sore throat), most cases of pharyngitis are actually caused by viruses.

Infections of the Lower Respiratory Tract Having Multiple Causes

Pneumonia

Disease. Pneumonia is an acute nonspecific infection of the small air sacs (alveoli) and tissues of the lung, with fever, productive cough (meaning that sputum is coughed up), acute chest pain, chills, and shortness of breath. It is clinically diagnosed by abnormal chest sounds and chest radiographs. Pneumonia

> Worldwide, pneumonia is the number one killer of children under five years of age.

is often a secondary infection that follows a primary viral respiratory infection. In developing countries, pneumonia

Table 19-3 Viral and Bacterial Ear Infections

Disease	Additional Information
Otitis Externa (External Otitis, Ear Canal Infection, Swimmer's Ear). Otitis externa is an infection of the outer ear canal with itching, pain, a malodorous discharge, tenderness, redness, swelling, and impaired hearing. Otitis externa is most common during the summer swimming season; trapped water in the external ear canal can lead to wet, softened skin, which is more easily infected by bacteria or fungi. Otitis externa is referred to as "swimmer's ear" because it often results from swimming in water contaminated with *Pseudomonas aeruginosa*.	**Pathogens.** The usual causes of otitis externa are the bacteria *Escherichia coli*, *P. aeruginosa*, *Proteus vulgaris*, and *Staphylococcus aureus*. Fungi, such as *Aspergillus* spp. are less common causes of otitis externa. **Reservoirs and Mode of Transmission.** Reservoirs include contaminated swimming pool water, sometimes indigenous microbiota, or articles inserted into the ear canal for cleaning out debris and wax. **Laboratory Diagnosis.** Material from the infected ear canal should be sent to the microbiology laboratory for culture and susceptibility (C&S). Most strains of *P. aeruginosa* are multidrug resistant.
Otitis Media (Middle Ear Infection). Otitis media often develops as a complication of the common cold. Manifestations can include persistent and severe earache, temporary hearing loss, pressure in the middle ear, and bulging of the eardrum (tympanic membrane). Nausea, vomiting, diarrhea, and fever may be present in young children. Otitis media may lead to rupture of the eardrum, bloody discharge, and pus. Severe complications, including bone infection, permanent hearing loss, and meningitis, may occur. Otitis media is most common in young children, particularly those between 3 months and 3 years of age.	**Pathogens.** Otitis media may be caused by bacteria or viruses. The three most common bacterial causes are *Streptococcus pneumoniae* (a Gram-positive diplococcus), *Haemophilus influenzae* (a Gram-negative bacillus; **see** Fig. 19-3), and *Moraxella catarrhalis* (a Gram-negative diplococcus). Less common bacterial causes include *Streptococcus pyogenes* and *S. aureus*. Viral causes include measles virus, parainfluenza virus, and RSV. **Reservoirs and Mode of Transmission.** Otitis media is probably not communicable. **Laboratory Diagnosis.** If present, a sample of discharge from the ear should be sent to the microbiology laboratory for C&S. β-Lactamase testing should be performed on isolates of *H. influenzae* and *S. pneumoniae*.

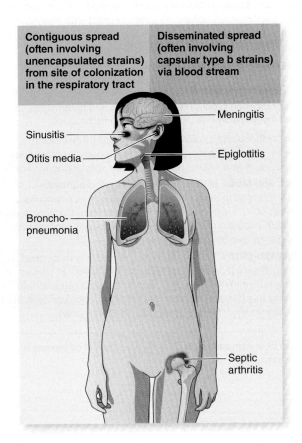

◄ **Figure 19-3. Infections caused by *Haemophilus influenzae*.**
(Redrawn from Harvey RA, et al. *Lippincott's Illustrated Reviews*. 3rd ed. Philadelphia, PA: Lippincott Williams & Wilkins; 2013.)

Table 19-4 Bacterial Infections of the Eyes

Disease	Additional Information
Bacterial Conjunctivitis ("Pinkeye"). Bacterial conjunctivitis involves irritation and reddening of conjunctiva, edema of eyelids, mucopurulent discharge, and sensitivity to light. The disease is highly contagious. **Patient Care.** Use Standard Precautions for hospitalized patients.	**Pathogens.** The most common etiologic agents of pinkeye are *Haemophilus influenzae* subsp. *aegyptius* and *Streptococcus pneumoniae*, although many other bacteria can cause these diseases. **Reservoirs and Mode of Transmission.** Infected humans serve as reservoirs. Human-to-human transmission occurs via contact with eye and respiratory discharges, contaminated fingers, facial tissues, clothing, eye makeup, eye medications, ophthalmic instruments, and contact lens-wetting and lens-cleaning agents. **Laboratory Diagnosis.** Infections of the eye caused by bacteria (including chlamydias) and viruses should be differentiated from allergic manifestations and irritation by microscopic examination of the *exudate* (oozing pus), culture of pathogens, and/or immunodiagnostic procedures.
Chlamydial Conjunctivitis (Inclusion Conjunctivitis, Paratrachoma). In neonates, acute chlamydial conjunctivitis with mucopurulent discharge may result in mild scarring of conjunctivae and cornea. It may be concurrent with chlamydial nasopharyngitis or pneumonia. In adults, chlamydial conjunctivitis may be concurrent with nongonococcal urethritis or cervicitis. **Patient Care.** Use Standard Precautions for hospitalized patients.	**Pathogens.** The etiologic agents of chlamydial conjunctivitis are certain serotypes (serovars[a]) of *Chlamydia trachomatis*, a Gram-negative bacterium and obligate intracellular pathogen. **Reservoirs and Mode of Transmission.** Infected humans serve as reservoirs. Transmission occurs via contact with genital discharges of infected people, contaminated fingers to eye, infection in newborns via an infected birth canal, or nonchlorinated swimming pools ("swimming pool conjunctivitis"). **Laboratory Diagnosis.** Chlamydias do not grow on artificial media. Diagnosis is made by cell culture and/or immunodiagnostic procedures.
Trachoma (Chlamydia Keratoconjunctivitis). Trachoma is a highly contagious, acute, or chronic conjunctival inflammation, resulting in scarring of cornea and conjunctiva, deformation of eyelids, and blindness. Trachoma is most common in poverty-stricken areas of the hot, dry Mediterranean countries and the Far East. It is the leading cause of blindness in the world. Trachoma occurs only rarely in the United States. **Patient Care.** Use Standard Precautions for hospitalized patients.	**Pathogens.** Trachoma is caused by certain serotypes (serovars) of *C. trachomatis*. **Reservoirs and Mode of Transmission.** Infected humans serve as reservoirs. Transmission occurs via direct contact with infectious ocular or nasal secretions or contaminated articles. The disease is also spread by flies serving as mechanical vectors. **Laboratory Diagnosis.** Trachoma is diagnosed by microscopic observation of intracellular chlamydial elementary bodies in epithelial cells of Giemsa-stained conjunctival scrapings or by an immunofluorescence procedure. Alternatively, the chlamydias can be isolated from specimens using cell culture techniques.
Gonococcal Conjunctivitis (Gonorrheal Ophthalmia Neonatorum). Gonococcal conjunctivitis is associated with an acute redness and swelling of conjunctiva and purulent discharge (Fig. 19-4). Corneal ulcers, perforation, and blindness may occur if the disease is untreated. **Patient Care.** Use Standard Precautions for hospitalized patient.	**Pathogen.** Gonococcal conjunctivitis is caused by *Neisseria gonorrhoeae*, a kidney bean–shaped, Gram-negative diplococcus. *N. gonorrhoeae* is also known as gonococcus (pl., gonococci) or GC. **Reservoirs and Mode of Transmission.** Infected humans—specifically, infected maternal birth canals—serve as reservoirs. Transmission occurs via contact with the infected birth canal during delivery. Adult infection can result from finger-to-eye contact with infectious genital secretions. **Laboratory Diagnosis.** Gonococcal conjunctivitis is diagnosed by microscopic observation of Gram-negative diplococci in smears of purulent material and isolation of *N. gonorrhoeae* on appropriate culture media (e.g., chocolate agar or modified chocolate agar, such as Thayer-Martin agar, Martin-Lewis agar, or Transgrow).

[a]The terms serotypes and serovars are synonyms. Serovars of a particular species differ from each other primarily as a result of differences in surface antigens. Sometimes, different serovars of a particular species cause different diseases.

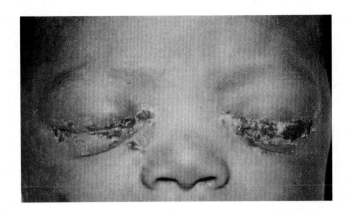

Figure 19-4. ▶ Gonococcal ophthalmia neonatorum.
(Courtesy of J. Pledger and the CDC.)

Table 19-5 Bacterial Infections of the Upper Respiratory Tract

Disease	Additional Information
Diphtheria. Diphtheria is a potentially serious upper respiratory tract disease. This acute, contagious bacterial disease primarily involves the tonsils, pharynx, larynx, and nose, and occasionally involves other mucous membranes, skin, conjunctivae, and the vagina. The characteristic lesion is a tough, asymmetrical, adherent gray-white membrane in the throat, with surrounding inflammation. Sore throat, swollen and tender cervical lymph nodes, tonsillitis, and swelling of the neck are common. The membrane may cause airway obstruction. There is also a cutaneous form of diphtheria, which is more common in the tropics. At one time, diphtheria was a major killer of children in the United States. However, as a result of widespread vaccination with diphtheria toxoid (an altered form of diphtheria toxin), diphtheria rarely occurs in the United States. Unfortunately, diphtheria continues to be a major killer of children in developing countries, where epidemics occur. **Patient Care.** Use Droplet Precautions for hospitalized patients with pharyngeal diphtheria and Contact Precautions for hospitalized patients with cutaneous diphtheria.	**Pathogen.** Diphtheria is caused by toxigenic (toxin- producing) strains of *Corynebacterium diphtheriae*, pleomorphic, Gram-positive bacilli that form characteristic V-, L-, and Y-shaped arrangements of bacilli. Only strains infected with a particular corynebacteriophage are toxigenic; the exotoxin (diphtheria toxin) is coded for by a bacteriophage gene. **Reservoirs and Mode of Transmission.** Infected humans serve as reservoirs. Transmission occurs via airborne droplets, direct contact, and contaminated fomites. **Laboratory Diagnosis.** A nasopharyngeal swab and a throat swab, preferably containing a sample of the membrane, should be sent to the microbiology laboratory for culture. Special media called Loeffler serum medium and cystine-tellurite or Tinsdale medium are used for culture and identification of *C. diphtheriae*. Toxigenicity can be determined using laboratory animals (rabbits or guinea pigs).
Streptococcal Pharyngitis (Strep Throat). Strep throat is an acute bacterial infection of the throat with soreness, chills, fever, headache, a beefy red throat, white patches of pus on pharyngeal epithelium, enlarged tonsils, and enlarged and tender cervical lymph nodes. The infection may spread to the middle ear, sinuses, or the organs of hearing. Untreated strep throat can lead to complications (sequelae) such as scarlet fever (caused by erythrogenic toxin), rheumatic fever, and glomerulonephritis. The latter two conditions result from the deposition of immune complexes beneath heart and kidney tissue, respectively. Some strains produce a pyrogenic exotoxin that causes TSS and some strains (the so-called flesh-eating bacteria) can cause necrotizing fasciitis (refer back to Fig. 14-8 in Chapter 14). More than 200,000 cases occur annually in the United States, mostly among children, 3–15 years of age. Although we hear more about *S. pyogenes* as a cause of pharyngitis, most cases of pharyngitis are actually caused by viruses. **Patient Care.** Use Droplet Precautions for hospitalized infants and young children and Standard Precautions for others.	**Pathogen.** Strep throat is caused by *Streptococcus pyogenes*, a β-hemolytic, catalase-negative, Gram-positive coccus in chains. It is also known as group A streptococcus, GAS, or Strep A. **Reservoirs and Mode of Transmission.** Infected humans serve as reservoirs. Transmission occurs human to human by direct contact, usually hands; aerosol droplets; secretions from patients and nasal carriers; and contaminated dust, lint, or handkerchiefs; contaminated milk and milk products have been associated with foodborne outbreaks of streptococcal pharyngitis. **Laboratory Diagnosis.** The sole purpose of a *routine* throat culture is to determine whether a patient does or does not have strep throat. If β-hemolytic streptococci are isolated, they are tested to determine whether they are group A streptococci. Rapid strep tests (based on detection of antigen) can be performed on throat swabs, but if the test is negative, a more traditional test (such as a throat culture and bacitracin susceptibility) should be performed.

and dehydration from severe diarrhea are the leading causes of death. Worldwide, pneumonia claimed the lives of 1.3 million children in 2011. It remains the number one killer of children under five years of age. Certain specific types of pneumonia (e.g., legionellosis and psittacosis) are nationally notifiable diseases in the United States.

Patient Care. Use Standard Precautions for all hospitalized patients; Droplet and/or Contact Precautions are required in addition to Standard Precautions for pneumonia caused by certain pathogens (e.g., *Burkholderia cepacia*, *Legionella* spp., *Neisseria meningitidis*, *Mycoplasma pneumoniae*, *Streptococcus pyogenes*).

Pathogens. A variety of microbes can cause pneumonia, including Gram-positive and Gram-negative bacteria, mycoplasmas, chlamydias, viruses, fungi, and protozoa. Community-acquired bacterial pneumonia is most frequently caused by *Streptococcus pneumoniae* (pneumococcal pneumonia). *Streptococcus pneumoniae* is the most common cause of pneumonia in the world (Fig. 19-5). Other bacterial pathogens include *Haemophilus influenzae*, *Staphylococcus aureus*, *Klebsiella pneumoniae*, and occasionally other Gram-negative bacilli and anaerobic members of the oral microbiota. Atypical pathogens include *Legionella* (legionellosis), *M. pneumoniae* (mycoplasmal pneumonia; primary atypical pneumonia), and *Chlamydiophila pneumoniae* (chlamydial pneumonia). Psittacosis (ornithosis; parrot fever), a type of pneumonia caused by *Chlamydiophila psittaci*, is normally acquired by inhalation of respiratory secretions and desiccated droppings of infected birds (e.g., parrots, parakeets). Fungi such as *Histoplasma capsulatum* (histoplasmosis), *Coccidioides immitis* (coccidioidomycosis), *Candida albicans* (candidiasis), *Cryptococcus neoformans* (cryptococcosis), *Blastomyces* (blastomycosis), *Aspergillus* (aspergillosis; see Fig. 20-4 in Chapter 20), and *Pneumocystis jiroveci* (previously considered to be a protozoan) may be etiologic agents of pneumonia, especially in immunocompromised individuals. Various species of bread molds can cause pneumonia in immunosuppressed patients; a condition known as **mucormycosis (zygomycosis)**. Viral pneumonia may be caused by adenoviruses, respiratory syncytial virus (RSV), parainfluenza viruses, cytomegalovirus, measles virus, chickenpox virus, and other viruses. Healthcare-associated bacterial pneumonia is most often caused by Gram-negative bacilli, especially *Klebsiella*, *Enterobacter*, *Serratia*, and *Acinetobacter* spp. *Pseudomonas aeruginosa* and *S. aureus* are also frequent causes of healthcare-associated pneumonias. Pneumonia is the most common fatal infection acquired in hospitals.

> *Streptococcus pneumoniae* is the most common cause of pneumonia in the world.

STUDY AID

Typical Versus Atypical Pneumonia.

Patients with **typical pneumonia** experience chest pain, dyspnea (shortness of breath), fever, chills, and a productive cough (i.e., one that produces purulent sputum). Less common symptoms include anorexia, headache, nausea, diarrhea, and vomiting. Radiographic abnormalities are proportional to the physical symptoms. Common causes of typical pneumonia are *Streptococcus pneumoniae*, *Haemophilus influenzae*, *Staphylococcus aureus*, and viruses like influenza virus types A and B, parainfluenza viruses, and RSV. Other causes are *Legionella pneumophila*, *Mycoplasma pneumoniae*, *Chlamydophila pneumoniae*, and Gram-negative bacilli. **Atypical pneumonia** has a more insidious (slower) onset than typical pneumonia. Patients present with headache, fever, cough with little sputum, and myalgia. Radiographic abnormalities are usually greater than the physical symptoms would predict. Common causes of atypical pneumonia are *M. pneumoniae*, *C. pneumoniae*, *L. pneumophila*, and viruses like influenza viruses, RSV, and adenoviruses. Other causes are *Chlamydophila psittaci*, *Pneumocystis jiroveci* (a fungus), varicella-zoster virus, and parainfluenza viruses. Note that some pathogens can cause either typical or atypical pneumonia.

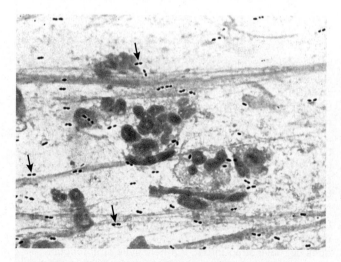

Figure 19-5. Gram-positive *Streptococcus pneumoniae* (*arrows*) in a Gram-stained smear of a purulent (pus-containing) sputum specimen from a patient with pneumococcal pneumonia. Note the typical diplococcus arrangement of this bacterium. Several larger, pink-stained polymorphonuclear neutrophils (PMNs) can also be seen. PMNs stain pink with the Gram staining procedure. (From Engleberg NC, et al. *Schaechter's Mechanisms of Microbial Disease.* 5th ed. Philadelphia, PA: Lippincott Williams & Wilkins; 2013.)

Reservoirs and Mode of Transmission. In most cases, infected humans; other reservoirs include infected psittacine birds (parrots and parakeets) in psittacosis, soil, and bird droppings in histoplasmosis and cryptococcosis. Depending on the pathogen involved, transmission is by droplet inhalation, direct oral contact, contact with contaminated hands and fomites, or inhalation of yeasts and fungal spores.

Laboratory Diagnosis. A good quality sputum specimen (coughed up from the patient's lungs) must be sent to the microbiology laboratory for culture and sensitivity (C&S). It must be sputum—*not* saliva. A laboratory workup of saliva will not provide clinically relevant information. Laboratory personnel can differentiate between saliva and sputum by preparing and examining a Gram-stained smear of the specimen. Sputum will contain numerous WBCs and few epithelial cells, whereas saliva will contain few (if any) WBCs and numerous epithelial cells.

Other Bacterial Infections of the Lower Respiratory Tract

Additional information pertaining to bacterial infections of the lower respiratory tract is contained in Table 19-6.

HISTORICAL NOTE

Tuberculosis: Captain of All These Men of Death

"[Tuberculosis] has been referred to as possibly the first born of the Mother of Pestilence and Disease and is known to have had few if any peers in causing incapacity and death of people and domestic animals. In 1913, V.A. Moore of Cornell University wrote: 'As a destroyer of man, tuberculosis has no equal; as a scourge of cattle, there is no other to compare it.'..... Reference has been made to the terrible destruction of tuberculosis in various parts of the world for many centuries and it has been given numerous names, beginning with phthisis and consumption. It was so prevalent in England in the 17th century that John Bunyan in his book, *The Life and Death of Mr. Badman* (1680), wrote of it as the 'Captain of All These Men of Death.' In 1861 Oliver Wendell Holmes named it 'The White Plague.' The name tuberculosis was coined in 1839 by K. Schoenlein..... [In 1973,] the World Health Organization referred to tuberculosis as 'The Monster.'"

(From the Preface to *Captain of All These Men of Death: Tuberculosis Historical Highlights*, by A. Arthur Myers. St. Louis, MO: Warren H. Green, Inc., 1977.)

Bacterial Infections of the Oral Region

The anaerobic environment produced by oxidation–reduction reactions of the oral microbiota allows certain genera of anaerobic bacteria (e.g., *Bacteroides*, *Porphyromonas*, *Fusobacterium*, *Prevotella*, *Actinomyces*, and *Treponema* spp.) to become involved in the production of oral diseases. The coating that forms on unclean teeth, called **dental plaque**, is a coaggregation of bacteria and their products. Many of these microbes produce a slime layer or glycocalyx that enables them to attach firmly and cause damage to the tooth enamel. Certain carbohydrates, especially sucrose, are metabolized by streptococci (especially *Streptococcus mutans*), lactobacilli, and *Actinomyces* spp., producing lactic acid, which rapidly dissolves the tooth enamel. When plaque remains on teeth for more than 72 hours, it hardens into tartar or calculus, which cannot be completely removed by brushing and flossing.

Acute Necrotizing Ulcerative Gingivitis

Acute necrotizing ulcerative gingivitis (ANUG) is also called **Vincent's angina** and **trench mouth**.

Disease. The term "trench mouth" originated in World War I, where soldiers developed the infection while fighting in trenches. It is usually the result of a combination of poor oral hygiene, physical or emotional stress, and poor diet. It involves painful, bleeding gums and tonsils, erosion of gum tissue, and swollen lymph nodes beneath the jaw. It causes extremely bad breath.

Patient Care. Use Standard Precautions for hospitalized patients.

Pathogens. Trench mouth is a synergistic (polymicrobial) infection involving two or more species of anaerobic bacteria of the indigenous oral microbiota. The most commonly involved bacteria are *Fusobacterium nucleatum* (an anaerobic, Gram-negative bacillus) and *Treponema vincentii*

> Trench mouth is a good example of a synergistic (polymicrobial) infection.

(a spirochete). Other commonly involved anaerobic Gram-negative bacilli are *Bacteroides* spp., *Prevotella intermedius*, and *Prevotella melaninogenica*.

Prevention and Control. As is true for other periodontal diseases, trench mouth can be prevented by good oral hygiene. Trench mouth is thought to be noncontagious.

Bacterial Infections of the Gastrointestinal Tract

Table 19-7 contains information pertaining to bacterial infections of the gastrointestinal (GI) tract.

Table 19-6 Bacterial Infections of the Lower Respiratory Tract

Disease	Additional Information
Legionellosis (Legionnaires' Disease, Pontiac Fever). Legionellosis is an acute bacterial pneumonia with anorexia, malaise, myalgia, headache, high fever, chills, and dry cough, followed by a productive cough, shortness of breath, diarrhea, and pleural and abdominal pain. There is about a 40% fatality rate. Pontiac fever, an influenza-like, less severe form of legionellosis, is not associated with pneumonia or death. Legionellosis was first recognized as a disease following an outbreak in a Philadelphia hotel in 1976, but evidence exists that prior epidemics and deaths were caused by *Legionella* spp. Epidemics continue to occur, often associated with hotels, cruise ships, hospitals, and supermarkets. Legionellosis usually affects elderly persons; people with preexisting respiratory disease, diabetes mellitus, renal disease, or malignancy; people who are immunocompromised; or people who smoke or drink heavily. **Patient Care.** Use Standard Precautions for hospitalized patients.	**Pathogen.** The primary etiologic agent of legionellosis is *Legionella pneumophila*, a poorly staining, Gram-negative bacillus. Other *Legionella* spp. and organisms within related genera can also cause the disease. As of 2013, 50 species of *Legionella* were known. **Reservoirs and Mode of Transmission.** Reservoirs include environmental water sources, such as ponds, lakes, and creeks; hot-water and air-conditioning systems, cooling towers, and evaporative condensers; whirlpool spas, hot tubs, shower heads, humidifiers, tap water, and water distillation systems; decorative fountains; and perhaps dust. Transmission has occurred as a result of aerosols of *Legionella* spp. that have been produced by vegetable misting devices in supermarkets. Legionellosis is not transmitted from person to person. **Laboratory Diagnosis.** Sputum and blood specimens should be sent to the microbiology laboratory for C&S. *Legionella* spp. stain poorly and require cysteine and other nutrients to grow. The recommended culture medium is buffered charcoal yeast extract agar. Immunodiagnostic procedures are available, such as antigen detection in urine.
Mycoplasmal Pneumonia (Primary Atypical Pneumonia). Mycoplasmal pneumonia has a gradual onset with headache, malaise, dry cough, sore throat, and, less often, chest discomfort. The amount of sputum the patient produces is scant at first, but may increase as the disease progresses. Illness may last from a few days to a month or more. Mycoplasmal pneumonia is most common in people 5–35 years of age. Pneumonias produced by mycoplasmas and chlamydias are the most common types of atypical pneumonias (i.e., pneumonias usually caused by organisms other than those that are the typical causes of pneumonia). **Patient Care.** Use Droplet Precautions for hospitalized patients for the duration of illness.	**Pathogen.** The etiologic agent of mycoplasmal pneumonia is *Mycoplasma pneumoniae*, a tiny, Gram-negative bacterium, lacking cell walls. **Reservoirs and Mode of Transmission.** Infected humans serve as reservoirs. Transmission occurs via droplet inhalation or direct contact with an infected person, or articles contaminated with nasal secretions or sputum from an ill, coughing patient. **Laboratory Diagnosis.** Mycoplasmal pneumonia is diagnosed by demonstration of a rise in antibody titer between acute and convalescent sera. On artificial media, *M. pneumoniae* produces tiny "fried egg" colonies, having a dense central area and a less-dense periphery (see Fig. 4-38 in Chapter 4).
Tuberculosis (TB). Tuberculosis is an acute or chronic mycobacterial infection of the lower respiratory tract with malaise, fever, night sweats, weight loss, and productive cough. Shortness of breath, chest pain, hemoptysis (coughing up blood), and hoarseness may occur in advanced stages. Widespread tuberculosis, known as military tuberculosis, involves many lesions throughout the body. (See Chapter 11 for additional information regarding the current TB pandemic.) **Patient Care.** Use Airborne Precautions for hospitalized patients with pulmonary or laryngeal disease. Use Standard Precautions for patients with extrapulmonary or meningeal TB and no draining lesions. If the patient has draining lesions, add Airborne and Contact Precautions.	**Pathogens.** Tuberculosis may be caused by any of the species in the *Mycobacterium tuberculosis* complex, but it is most often caused by *M. tuberculosis* (a slow-growing, acid-fast, Gram-positive to Gram-variable bacillus). *M. tuberculosis* is sometimes referred to as the tubercle bacillus. **Reservoirs and Mode of Transmission.** Infected humans are the primary reservoirs; rarely, primates, cattle, and other infected mammals can serve as reservoirs. Transmission occurs via airborne droplets produced by infected people during coughing, sneezing, and even talking or singing; usually following prolonged direct contact with infected individuals. Bovine tuberculosis may result from exposure to infected cattle or ingestion of unpasteurized, contaminated milk or other dairy products. **Laboratory Diagnosis.** Demonstration of acid-fast bacilli (AFB) in sputum specimens provides a rapid, presumptive diagnosis of tuberculosis. Isolation of *M. tuberculosis* on Löwenstein-Jensen or Middlebrook culture media takes about 3–6 weeks because of the organism's long generation time (about 18–24 hours). A variety of more rapid techniques are available for isolation and identification of *M. tuberculosis*, including automated and semiautomated instruments, molecular diagnostic procedures, and gas–liquid chromatography. Susceptibility testing should be performed as soon as possible, because many strains of *M. tuberculosis* are multidrug resistant. Infected patients show a positive delayed hypersensitivity skin test (the Mantoux purified protein derivative [PPD] tuberculin skin test), and pulmonary tubercles may be seen on chest radiographs. Recall from Chapter 16 that a positive TB skin test result may indicate any of five possibilities, including past infection, present infection, or receipt of Bacillus Calmette-Guérin (BCG) vaccine.

Disease	Additional Information
Whooping Cough (Pertussis). Whooping cough is a highly contagious, acute bacterial childhood (usually) infection. The first stage (the prodromal or catarrhal stage) of the disease involves mild, cold-like symptoms. The second stage (the paroxysmal stage) produces severe, uncontrollable coughing fits. The coughing often ends in a prolonged, high-pitched, deeply indrawn breath (the "whoop," from which whooping cough gets its name). The coughing fits produce a clear, tenacious mucus and vomiting. They may be so severe as to cause lung rupture, bleeding in the eyes and brain, broken ribs, rectal prolapse, or hernia. The third stage (the recovery or convalescent stage) usually begins within 4 weeks of onset. Parapertussis is a similar but milder disease. **Patient Care.** Use Droplet Precautions for hospitalized patients until 5 days after initiation of effective therapy.	**Pathogen.** Pertussis is caused by *Bordetella pertussis*, a small, encapsulated, nonmotile, Gram-negative coccobacillus that produces endotoxin and exotoxins. Parapertussis is caused by *Bordetella parapertussis*. A related organism, *Bordetella bronchiseptica*, causes respiratory infections in animals, including kennel cough in dogs. **Reservoirs and Mode of Transmission.** Infected humans serve as reservoirs. Transmission occurs via droplets produced by coughing. **Laboratory Diagnosis.** Nasopharyngeal aspirates or swabs should be sent to the microbiology laboratory. Special media, such as Bordet-Gengou agar (a potato-based medium) or Regan-Lowe agar (a charcoal/horse blood medium), are used to isolate *B. pertussis*. Molecular diagnostic and immunodiagnostic procedures are also available.

Table 19-7 Bacterial Infections of the Gastrointestinal Tract

Disease	Additional Information
Bacterial Gastritis and Gastric Ulcers. Infection with *Helicobacter pylori* can cause chronic bacterial gastritis and duodenal ulcers. Gastritis is suspected when a person has upper abdominal pain with nausea or heartburn. People with duodenal ulcers may experience gnawing, burning, aching, mild-to-moderate pain just below the breastbone, an empty feeling, and hunger. The pain usually occurs when the stomach is empty. Drinking milk, eating, or taking antacids generally relieves the pain, but it usually returns 2 or 3 hours later. Gastric ulcers and gastric adenocarcinoma are also epidemiologically associated with *H. pylori* infection. Gastric ulcers can cause swelling of the tissues leading into the small intestine, which prevents food from easily passing out of the stomach. This, in turn, can cause pain, bloating, nausea, or vomiting after eating. Gastric ulcers and duodenal ulcers are types of peptic ulcers. Complications of peptic ulcers include penetration, perforation, bleeding, and obstruction. **Patient Care.** Use Standard Precautions for hospitalized patients.	**Pathogen.** *H. pylori* is a curved, microaerophilic, capnophilic, Gram-negative bacillus that is found on the mucus-secreting epithelial cells of the stomach. No other bacteria are known to grow in the extremely acidic stomach. **Reservoirs and Mode of Transmission.** Infected humans serve as reservoirs. Transmission probably occurs via ingestion; presumed to be either oral–oral or fecal–oral transmission. **Laboratory Diagnosis.** Diagnostic techniques include staining and culturing of gastric and duodenal biopsy specimens, the urea breath test, the NH_4 excretion test, molecular diagnostic procedures, and immunodiagnostic procedures. In the urea breath test, the patient ingests radioactively labeled urea and his or her breath is analyzed 60 minutes later for radioactively labeled CO_2. The enzyme urease, produced by *H. pylori*, splits the urea into ammonia and CO_2; hence, the presence of radioactively labeled CO_2 indicates the presence of *H. pylori*. In the NH_4 excretion test, the patient consumes urea containing radioactively labeled nitrogen. The ammonia produced in the stomach by *H. pylori* is absorbed into the blood, excreted in the urine, and the amount of radioactively labeled NH_4 in the urine is measured.
***Campylobacter* enteritis.** *Campylobacter* enteritis is an acute bacterial enteric disease, ranging from asymptomatic to severe, with diarrhea, nausea, vomiting, fever, malaise, and abdominal pain. The disease is usually self-limiting, lasting 2–5 days. Stools may contain gross or occult (hidden) blood, mucus, and WBCs. *Campylobacter* spp. are the major cause of bacterial diarrhea in the United States. **Patient Care.** Use Standard Precautions for hospitalized patients. Add Contact Precautions for diapered or incontinent patients.	**Pathogens.** The etiologic agents of *Campylobacter* enteritis are *Campylobacter jejuni* and, less commonly, *Campylobacter coli*. *Campylobacter* spp. are curved, S-shaped, or spiral-shaped Gram-negative bacilli, often having a "gull-wing" morphology (a pair of curved bacilli) following cell division. They are microaerophilic and capnophilic, with an optimal growth temperature of 42°C. **Reservoirs and Mode of Transmission.** Reservoirs are animals, including poultry, cattle, sheep, swine, rodents, birds, kittens, puppies, and other pets. Most raw poultry is contaminated with *C. jejuni*, thus necessitating proper methods of cleaning and disinfecting in the kitchen. Transmission occurs via ingestion of contaminated food (e.g., chicken, pork), raw milk, or water; contact with infected pets or farm animals; or contaminated cutting boards. **Laboratory Diagnosis.** Diagnosis depends on the recovery of *Campylobacter* spp. from stool specimens, using selective medium (Campy blood agar, which contains several antimicrobial agents to suppress growth of other bacteria), a Campy gas mixture (5% O_2, 10% CO_2, 85% N_2), and 42°C incubation.

(continued)

Disease	Additional Information
Cholera. Cholera is an acute, bacterial diarrheal disease with profuse watery stools, occasional vomiting, and rapid dehydration. If untreated, circulatory collapse, renal failure, and death may occur. More than 50% of untreated people with severe cholera die. Cholera occurs worldwide, with periodic epidemics and pandemics. A cholera pandemic that started in Peru in 1991 killed more than 10,000 people. Most U.S. cases involve the ingestion of raw or undercooked seafood (e.g., oysters) from the coastal waters of Louisiana and Texas. **Patient Care.** Use Standard Precautions for hospitalized patients. Add Contact Precautions for diapered or incontinent patients.	**Pathogens.** The etiologic agents of cholera are certain biotypes of *Vibrio cholerae* serogroup 01. These are curved (comma-shaped) Gram-negative bacilli that secrete an *enterotoxin* (a toxin that adversely affects cells in the intestinal tract) called *choleragen*. Other *Vibrio* spp. (*Vibrio parahemolyticus*, *Vibrio vulnificus*) also cause diarrheal diseases. Vibrios are halophilic (salt-loving) and are thus found in marine environments. **Reservoirs and Mode of Transmission.** Reservoirs include infected humans and aquatic reservoirs (copepods and other zooplankton). Transmission occurs via the fecal–oral route, contact with feces or vomitus of infected people, ingestion of fecally contaminated water or foods (especially raw or undercooked shellfish and other seafood), or mechanical transmission by flies. **Laboratory Diagnosis.** Rectal swabs or stool specimens should be inoculated onto thiosulfate-citrate-bile-sucrose (TCBS) agar; different *Vibrio* spp. produce different reactions on this medium. Biochemical tests are used to identify the various species. Biotyping is accomplished using commercially available antisera.
Salmonellosis. Salmonellosis is gastroenteritis with sudden onset of headache, abdominal pain, diarrhea, nausea, and sometimes vomiting. Dehydration may be severe. Salmonellosis may develop into septicemia or localized infection in any tissue of the body. About 40,000 cases of salmonellosis are reported annually to the CDC. **Patient Care.** Use Standard Precautions for hospitalized patients. Add Contact Precautions for diapered or incontinent patients.	**Pathogens.** GI salmonellosis is caused by members of the family Enterobacteriaceae, currently named *Salmonella enterica* (of which there are more than 2,000 serotypes or serovars). These Gram-negative bacilli invade intestinal cells, release endotoxin, and produce cytotoxins and enterotoxins. About 200 of the *S. enterica* serotypes cause GI salmonellosis in the United States. The most commonly reported serotypes are *S. enterica* subsp. *enterica* serovar *typhimurium* (also known as *Salmonella typhimurium*) and *S. enterica* subsp. *enterica* serovar *enteritidis* (also known as *Salmonella enteritidis*). **Reservoirs and Mode of Transmission.** Reservoirs include a wide range of wild and domestic animals, such as poultry, swine, cattle, rodents, reptiles (e.g., pet iguanas and turtles), pet chicks, dogs, and cats. Infected humans (e.g., patients, carriers) are also reservoirs. Transmission occurs via ingestion of contaminated food (e.g., eggs, unpasteurized milk, meat, poultry, raw fruits and vegetables), fecal–oral transmission from person to person, food handlers, or contaminated water supplies. **Laboratory Diagnosis.** Stool specimens should be submitted to the microbiology laboratory for C&S. *Salmonella* spp. are nonlactose fermenters and thus produce colorless colonies on MacConkey agar. Biochemical tests are used for identification, and commercially available antisera are used for serotyping.
Typhoid Fever (Enteric Fever). Typhoid fever is a systemic bacterial disease with fever, severe headache, malaise, anorexia, a rash on the trunk in about 25% of patients, nonproductive cough, and constipation. Bacteremia; pneumonia; gallbladder, liver, and bone infection; endocarditis; meningitis, and other complications may occur. About 10% of untreated patients die. Worldwide, an estimated 17 million cases occur per year with approximately 600,000 deaths. **Patient Care.** Use Standard Precautions for hospitalized patients. Add Contact Precautions for diapered or incontinent patients.	**Pathogen.** Typhoid fever is caused by *Salmonella typhi* (also known as the typhoid bacillus), a Gram-negative bacillus that releases endotoxin and produces exotoxins. A similar but less severe infection is caused by *Salmonella paratyphi*. **Reservoirs and Mode of Transmission.** Infected humans serve as reservoirs for typhoid and paratyphoid; rarely, domestic animals for paratyphoid. Some people become carriers following infection, shedding the pathogens in their feces or urine. (Refer to Chapter 11 for the "Typhoid Mary" story.) Transmission occurs via the fecal–oral route; food or water contaminated by feces or urine of patients or carriers; oysters harvested from fecally contaminated waters; fecally contaminated fruits and raw vegetables; or from feces to food by mechanical transmission by flies. **Laboratory Diagnosis.** Diagnosis of typhoid fever is made by isolation of *S. typhi* from blood, urine, feces, or bone marrow, followed by identification by biochemical tests. Immunodiagnostic procedures are also available.

Table 19-7   Bacterial Infections of the Gastrointestinal Tract (continued)

Disease	Additional Information
Shigellosis (Bacillary Dysentery). Shigellosis is an acute bacterial infection of the lining of the small and large intestine, producing diarrhea (as many as 20 bowel movements a day) with blood, mucus, and pus. Other symptoms include nausea, vomiting, cramps, and fever. Sometimes *toxemia* (toxins in the blood) and convulsions (in children) occur. Other serious complications, such as hemolytic-uremic syndrome, may occur. Worldwide, shigellosis is estimated to cause approximately 600,000 deaths per year, with about two-thirds of the cases and most of the deaths occurring in children younger than 10 years. **Patient Care.** Use Standard Precautions for hospitalized patients. Add Contact Precautions for diapered or incontinent patients.	**Pathogens.** The etiologic agents of shigellosis are *Shigella dysenteriae, Shigella flexneri, Shigella boydii,* and *Shigella soneii.* They are nonmotile Gram-negative bacilli that are members of the Enterobacteriaceae family. A plasmid is associated with toxin production and virulence. Relatively few (10–100) organisms are required to cause disease. **Reservoirs and Mode of Transmission.** Infected humans serve as reservoirs. People become infected by direct or indirect fecal–oral transmission from patients or carriers; fecally contaminated hands and fingernails; or fecally contaminated food, milk, and drinking water. Flies can mechanically transfer organisms from latrines to food. **Laboratory Diagnosis.** Leukocytes will be present in stool specimens. Fresh fecal or rectal swabs should be immediately inoculated into Gram-negative (GN) enrichment broth and onto a solid medium (such as MacConkey, xylose lysine deoxycholate [XLD], or Hektoen enteric [HE] agar). *Shigella* spp. produce colorless colonies on MacConkey agar because they are nonlactose fermenters. Isolates are identified by biochemical and immunodiagnostic procedures.
***Clostridium difficile*–Associated Diseases.** *C. difficile* is the major cause of conditions known as antibiotic- associated diarrhea (AAD) and pseudomembranous colitis (PMC), which frequently occur in patients following antibiotic therapy. It does not seem to matter for what condition the patient was receiving antibiotics, which antibiotics the patient was receiving, the dosage, or the route of administration. Antibiotics that have a profound effect on colonic microbes, such as cephalosporins, ampicillin, amoxicillin, and clindamycin, are the drugs most frequently implicated. **Patient Care.** Use Contact Precautions for the duration of illness. Use soap and water for handwashing. The alcohol in waterless antiseptic hand rubs lacks sporicidal activity.	**Pathogen.** *C. difficile* (often referred to simply as "C. dif") is a spore-forming anaerobic Gram-positive bacillus. **Reservoirs and Mode of Transmission.** *C. difficile* is a member of the indigenous microbiota in about 2%–3% of healthy, nonhospitalized adults. Hospitalized patients frequently become colonized with *C. difficile* as a result of its presence in the hospital environment. It is estimated that about 20%–30% of hospitalized patients are colonized with *C. difficile.* **Laboratory Diagnosis.** *C. difficile* is identified in the laboratory using a variety of phenotypic characteristics. However, diagnosis of *C. difficile*–associated diseases is most often accomplished using some type of commercial enzyme immunoassay or cytotoxin tissue culture assay.

Enterovirulent *Escherichia coli*

Escherichia coli is a Gram-negative bacillus that is found in the GI tract of all humans. The strains and serotypes of *E. coli* that are part of the indigenous microbiota of the GI tract are opportunistic pathogens. They usually cause no harm while in the GI tract, but have the potential to cause serious infections if they gain access to the bloodstream, the urinary bladder, or a wound. *E. coli* is the major cause of septicemia, urinary tract infections (UTIs), and health-care-associated infections.

There are other strains and serotypes of *E. coli* in nature that are not indigenous microbiota of the human colon and always cause disease when they are ingested. Collectively, these strains and serotypes are referred to as enterovirulent *E. coli.* Information pertaining to two general types, the enterohemorrhagic *E. coli* and the enterotoxigenic *E. coli,* is contained in Table 19-8.

Bacterial Foodborne Intoxications (Foodborne Infections, Food Poisoning)

The term "food poisoning" is broad and may include diseases resulting from the ingestion of chemical contaminants as well as bacteria or bacterial toxins, phycotoxins, mycotoxins, viruses, or protozoa. Technically, diseases resulting from the ingestion of toxin-producing microbes are called **infectious diseases,** whereas diseases resulting from the *ingestion* of preformed microbial toxins are called **microbial intoxications.** The distinction is based on where the toxin is actually produced—in the body (in vivo) or in the food (in vitro). The incubation time (the time that elapses between ingestion and onset of symptoms) is usually shorter in microbial intoxications. If toxin-producing bacteria are ingested, the incubation time will depend on the number of bacteria ingested, their generation time, and the amount of time it takes them to produce enough toxin

Table 19-8 Enterovirulent *Escherichia coli*

Disease	Additional Information
Enterohemorrhagic *E. coli* (EHEC) Diarrhea. This disease consists of a hemorrhagic, watery diarrhea with abdominal cramping. Usually, patients have no fever or only a slight fever. About 5% of infected people (especially children younger than age 5 and the elderly) develop hemolytic-uremic syndrome (HUS), with anemia, low platelet count, and kidney failure. The first recognized outbreak of diarrhea caused by enterohemorrhagic *E. coli* (O157:H7) occurred in 1982, involving contaminated hamburger meat—hamburger meat contaminated with cattle feces. Since then, several well-publicized epidemics involving the same serotype have occurred. Not all of the outbreaks involved meat; some resulted from ingestion of unpasteurized milk or apple juice, lettuce, or other raw vegetables. It has been estimated that *E. coli* O157:H7 infection accounts for as many as 73,000 cases of illness and 60 deaths in the United States per year. **Patient Care.** Use Standard Precautions for hospitalized patients. Add Contact Precautions for diapered or incontinent patients.	**Pathogens.** *E. coli* O157:H7 (a serotype that possesses a cell wall antigen designated "O157" and a flagellar antigen designated "H7") is the most commonly involved EHEC serotype. Other EHEC serotypes include O26:H11, O111:H8, and O104:H21. These are all Gram-negative bacilli that produce potent cytotoxins called Shiga-like toxins—named for their close resemblance to Shiga toxin, produced by *Shigella dysenteriae*. **Reservoirs and Mode of Transmission.** Reservoirs include cattle and infected humans. Transmission occurs via the fecal–oral route; inadequately cooked, fecally contaminated beef; unpasteurized milk; person-to-person contact; or fecally contaminated water. **Laboratory Diagnosis.** *E. coli* O157:H7 infection should be suspected in any patient with bloody diarrhea. Stool specimens should be inoculated onto sorbitol-MacConkey (SMAC) agar. Colorless, sorbitol-negative colonies should then be assayed for O157 antigen using commercially available antiserum. Other immunodiagnostic procedures are available.
Enterotoxigenic *E. coli* (ETEC) Diarrhea (Traveler's Diarrhea). This disease consists of a watery diarrhea with or without mucus or blood, vomiting, and abdominal cramping. Dehydration and low-grade fever may occur. Enterotoxigenic strains of *E. coli* are the most common cause of traveler's diarrhea worldwide and a common cause of diarrheal disease in children in developing countries. **Patient Care.** Use Standard Precautions for hospitalized patients. Add Contact Precautions for diapered or incontinent patients.	**Pathogens.** ETEC diarrhea is caused by many different serotypes of enterotoxigenic *E. coli* that produce a heat-labile toxin, a heat-stable toxin, or both. **Reservoirs and Mode of Transmission.** Infected humans serve as reservoirs. Transmission occurs via the fecal–oral route; ingestion of fecally contaminated food or water. **Laboratory Diagnosis.** ETEC diarrhea is diagnosed by isolation of the organism from stool specimens, followed by demonstration of enterotoxin production, molecular diagnostic procedures, or immunodiagnostic procedures.

to produce symptoms. According to the CDC, approximately 76 million cases of foodborne illness occur each year in the United States, resulting in more than 5,000 deaths and 325,000 hospitalizations. Appendix 1 on thePoint contains information pertaining to microbial intoxications.

Bacterial Infections of the Genitourinary System

Urinary Tract Infections

Recall from Chapter 17 that UTIs can be divided into upper UTIs and lower UTIs. Upper UTIs include infections of the kidneys (nephritis or pyelonephritis) and ureters (ureteritis). Lower UTIs include infections of the urinary bladder (cystitis), the urethra (urethritis), and, in men, the prostate (prostatitis). Most UTIs are acquired via the ascending route, whereby the pathogen moves upward from the urethra. Far fewer UTIs occur via the descending route from the bloodstream to the kidneys.

A variety of indigenous microbes are found at and near the outer opening (meatus) of the urethra of both men and women. These microbes can ascend the urethra and gain access to the urinary bladder. UTIs may result from poor personal hygiene, sexual intercourse, the insertion of catheters, and other means. A patient with a UTI presents with dysuria (difficulty or pain on urination), lumbar pain, fever, and chills. The latter two symptoms are more common in pyelonephritis than in cystitis. The most common causes of UTIs are *E. coli* and other members of the family Enterobacteriaceae (especially *Proteus* and *Klebsiella* spp.) (Fig. 19-6). Other common causes of UTIs are *Enterococcus* spp., *Staphylococcus* spp. (especially *S. aureus*, *S. epidermidis*, and *S. saprophyticus*), and *P. aeruginosa*.

> *Escherichia coli* is the number one cause of UTIs.

UTIs may be acquired either within a healthcare setting (called healthcare-associated UTIs) or elsewhere

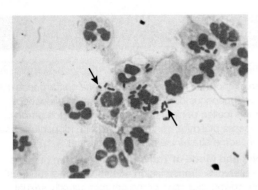

Figure 19-6. Many Gram-negative bacilli (*arrows*) and many pink-staining polymorphonuclear neutrophils can be seen in this Gram-stained urine sediment from a patient with cystitis (urinary bladder infection). (From Winn WC Jr., et al. *Koneman's Color Atlas and Textbook of Diagnostic Microbiology.* 6th ed. Philadelphia, PA: Lippincott Williams & Wilkins; 2006.)

(called community-acquired UTIs). UTIs are the most common type of healthcare-associated infection, often following urinary catheterization.

> *Chlamydia trachomatis* is the most common sexually transmitted pathogen. Genital chlamydiasis is the most commonly reported nationally notifiable disease in the United States

Infections of the Genital Tract

Common Bacterial Sexually Transmitted Diseases
Table 19-9 contains information pertaining to common bacterial STDs.

Less Common Bacterial Sexually Transmitted Diseases
Other bacterial pathogens may also be sexually transmitted. Three bacterial STDs, seen more often in parts of the world other than in the United States, are chancroid, granuloma inguinale, and lymphogranuloma venereum (LGV). Chancroid is caused by the Gram-negative bacterium *Haemophilus ducreyi*. Granuloma inguinale is a chronic infection caused by a Gram-negative bacterium named *Calymmatobacterium granulomatis* (*Donovania granulomatis*). LGV is a chlamydial infection involving the lymph nodes, rectum, and reproductive tract. It is caused by certain serotypes of *Chlamydia trachomatis*. It should be noted that many STDs are transmitted simultaneously; thus, when a patient is diagnosed with one STD, others should be sought.

Bacterial Infections of the Circulatory System

Rickettsial and Ehrlichial Infections of the Cardiovascular System

Recall that rickettsias and ehrlichias are obligate intracellular, Gram-negative bacteria. Table 19-10 contains information pertaining to rickettsial and ehrlichial diseases of the cardiovascular system.

Other Bacterial Infections of the Cardiovascular System

Infective Endocarditis
Infective (or infectious) endocarditis is usually caused by a bacterium or a fungus. It is characterized by the presence of vegetations (combinations of bacteria and blood clots) on or within the endocardium, most commonly involving a heart valve. Abnormal or damaged valves are most susceptible to infection, although valves can become contaminated during open heart surgery. The vegetations

Table 19-9 Bacterial Sexually Transmitted Diseases	
Disease	**Additional Information**
Genital Chlamydial Infections, Genital Chlamydiasis. *Chlamydia trachomatis* is considered to be the most common sexually transmitted pathogen. Different serovars of *C. trachomatis* cause different diseases. Serovars D through K are the major causes of nongonococcal urethritis (NGU) and epididymitis in men; and cervicitis, urethritis, endometritis, and salpingitis in women, causing mucopurulent urethral discharge, urethral itching, and burning on urination; may also cause infertility and proctitis in men. Most commonly causes endocervical and urethral infections, salpingitis, infertility, and chronic pelvic pain in women. Infection during pregnancy may result in premature rupture of membranes and preterm delivery as well as conjunctivitis and pneumonia in neonates. Genital chlamydial infection may be concurrent with gonorrhea. **Patient Care.** Use Standard Precautions for hospitalized patients.	**Pathogen.** Genital chlamydial infections are caused by certain serotypes of *C. trachomatis*; tiny, obligate intracellular, Gram-negative bacteria. (Less common causes of NGU are *Ureaplasma ureolyticum* [closely related to mycoplasmas], herpes simplex viruses, and *Trichomonas vaginalis*.) **Reservoirs and Mode of Transmission.** Infected humans serve as reservoirs. Transmission occurs via direct sexual contact or mother-to-neonate during birth. **Laboratory Diagnosis.** Identification of *C. trachomatis* made by cell culture, staining, and immunodiagnostic procedures.

(continued)

Table 19-9   Bacterial Sexually Transmitted Diseases (continued)

Disease	Additional Information
Gonorrhea. It is important to understand that not all clinical presentations of gonorrhea involve the genital tract. Gonorrhea may present as asymptomatic mucosal infection, ophthalmia neonatorum, urethritis, proctitis, pharyngitis, epididymitis, cervicitis, Bartholin gland infection, pelvic inflammatory disease, endometritis, salpingitis, peritonitis, and disseminated gonococcal infection. Patients with disseminated gonococcal infection have myalgia (muscular pain), arthralgia (joint pain), polyarthritis (inflammation of joints), and a characteristic dermatitis—skin lesions located primarily on the extremities. Urethral discharge and painful urination are common in infected men, usually starting 2–7 days after infection. Infected women may be asymptomatic for weeks or months, during which time severe damage to the reproductive system may occur. **Patient Care.** Use Standard Precautions for hospitalized patients.	**Pathogen.** Gonorrhea is caused by *Neisseria gonorrhoeae* (also known as gonococcus or GC), a Gram-negative diplococcus. Some strains (called penicillinase- producing *N. gonorrhoeae* or PPNG) possess plasmids containing the gene for penicillinase production; some strains are multidrug resistant. **Reservoirs and Mode of Transmission.** Infected humans serve as reservoirs. Transmission occurs via direct mucous membrane-to-mucous membrane contact, usually sexual contact; adult-to-child (may indicate sexual abuse); and mother-to-neonate during birth. **Laboratory Diagnosis.** Gonorrhea in male patients can be diagnosed by the typical appearance of Gram-stained urethral discharge specimens, with numerous WBCs and numerous intracellular and extracellular Gram-negative diplococci (Fig. 19-7). Specimens are inoculated to chocolate agar or a modified chocolate agar (such as Thayer-Martin medium, Martin-Lewis medium, or Transgrow). β-Lactamase testing of isolates is performed, followed by antimicrobial susceptibility testing if the organism is β-lactamase positive. Isolates are usually identified using biochemical tests. Immunodiagnostic procedures are also available.
Syphilis. Syphilis is a treponemal disease that occurs in four stages: (a) primary syphilis—a painless lesion known as a chancre (refer back to Fig. 14-4 in Chapter 14), which develops at the site where *Treponema pallidum* entered the genital mucosa or skin through a break in the surface; (b) secondary syphilis—a skin rash (especially on the palms and soles) about 4–6 weeks later, with fever and mucous membrane lesions, followed by (c) a long latent period (as long as 5–20 years); and then (d) tertiary syphilis—with damage to the CNS, cardiovascular system, visceral organs, bones, sense organs, and other sites. Damage to the CNS or heart is usually not reversible. **Patient Care.** Use Standard Precautions for hospitalized patients.	**Pathogen.** Syphilis is caused by *T. pallidum*, a Gram-variable, tightly coiled spirochete that is too thin to be seen with brightfield microscopy (refer back to Fig. 4-20 in Chapter 4). **Reservoirs and Mode of Transmission.** Infected humans serve as reservoirs. Transmission occurs via direct contact with lesions, body secretions, mucous membranes, blood, semen, saliva, and vaginal discharges of infected people, usually during sexual contact; blood transfusions; or transplacentally from mother to fetus. **Laboratory Diagnosis.** Primary syphilis can be diagnosed by darkfield microscopy (refer back to Fig. 2-6 in Chapter 2) of material scraped from the margin of chancres. Many immunodiagnostic procedures are available, such as the rapid plasma reagin (RPR), Venereal Disease Research Laboratory (VDRL), and fluorescent treponemal antibody absorption (FTA-Abs) tests for detecting antibodies in serum or spinal fluid specimens and fluorescent antibody procedures for detecting antigen in material obtained from lesions or lymph nodes.

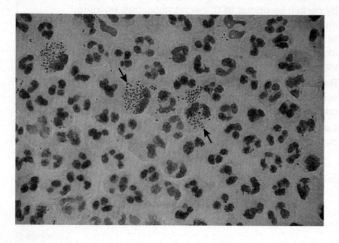

◄ **Figure 19-7. Gram-stained urethral exudate from a male patient with gonococcal urethritis.** The large pink-staining objects are polymorphonuclear neutrophils, some of which contain phagocytized Gram-negative *Neisseria gonorrhoeae* diplococci (*arrows*). (Courtesy of Joe Millar and the CDC.)

Disease	Additional Information
Spotted fever rickettsiosis (formerly called Rocky Mountain spotted fever). A tick-borne rickettsial disease characterized by sudden onset of moderate-to-high fever, extreme exhaustion (prostration), muscle pain, severe headache, chills, conjunctival infection, and maculopapular rash on extremities on about the third day, which spreads to the palms, soles, and much of the body (Fig. 19-8). In about 4 days, small purplish areas (petechiae) develop as a result of bleeding in the skin. Although uncommon, death can result. Spotted fever rickettsiosis occurs in all parts of the United States, especially the Atlantic seaboard. **Patient Care.** Use Standard Precautions for hospitalized patients.	**Pathogen.** The etiologic agent of spotted fever rickettsiosis is *Rickettsia rickettsii*, a Gram-negative bacterium. Like all rickettsias, *R. rickettsii* is an obligate intracellular pathogen; it invades endothelial cells (cells that line blood vessels). **Reservoirs and Mode of Transmission.** Reservoirs include infected ticks on dogs, rodents, and other animals. Transmission occurs via the bite of an infected tick. Person-to-person transmission rarely occurs—through blood transfusion. **Laboratory Diagnosis.** Immunodiagnostic procedures are used to diagnose this disease.
Endemic Typhus Fever. Endemic typhus fever, also known as murine typhus fever and flea-borne typhus, is an acute febrile disease that is similar to, but milder than, epidemic typhus, which is described next. Symptoms include shaking chills, headache, fever, and a faint, pink rash. Endemic typhus has a worldwide occurrence, but is rare in the United States. **Patient Care.** Use Standard Precautions for hospitalized patients.	**Pathogen.** The etiologic agent of endemic typhus is *Rickettsia typhi*, a Gram-negative bacterium and obligate intracellular pathogen. **Reservoirs and Mode of Transmission.** Reservoirs include rats, mice, possibly other mammals, and infected rat fleas. Transmission occurs from rat to flea to human. Infected fleas defecate while feeding, and the rickettsiae in the feces are rubbed into the bite wound or other superficial abrasions. Person-to-person transmission does not occur. **Laboratory Diagnosis.** Immunodiagnostic procedures are used to diagnose endemic typhus.
Epidemic Typhus Fever. Epidemic typhus or louse-borne typhus is an acute rickettsial disease, often with sudden onset of headache, chills, prostration, fever, and general pains. A rash appears on the fifth or sixth day, initially on the upper trunk, followed by spread to the entire body, but usually not to the face, palms, or soles. Epidemic typhus fever may be fatal if untreated. It occurs in cold climates in areas where people live under unhygienic conditions and are louse infested. In World War I, the body lice that transmitted epidemic typhus were referred to as "cooties" by soldiers. **Patient Care.** Use Standard Precautions for hospitalized patients.	**Pathogen.** The etiologic agent of epidemic typhus is *Rickettsia prowazekii*, a Gram-negative bacterium and obligate intracellular pathogen. **Reservoirs and Mode of Transmission.** Reservoirs include infected humans and body lice (*Pediculus humanus*; see Fig. 21–14 in Chapter 21). Transmission occurs from human to louse to human. Infected lice defecate while feeding, and the rickettsiae in the feces are rubbed into the bite wound or other superficial abrasions. **Laboratory Diagnosis.** Immunodiagnostic procedures are used to diagnose epidemic typhus.
Ehrlichiosis. Ehrlichiosis is an acute, febrile illness ranging from asymptomatic to mild to severe and life threatening. Patients usually present with acute influenza-like illness with fever, headache, and generalized malaise. Ehrlichiosis is reminiscent of spotted fever rickettsiosis, without the rash. The estimated fatality rate is about 5%. There are two types of ehrlichiosis: human monocytic ehrlichiosis (HME) and human granulocytic ehrlichiosis (HGE). Cases of HME are more common than HGE cases. Most HME cases have occurred in the southeast and mid-Atlantic states, whereas most HGE cases have occurred in states with high rates of Lyme disease (particularly Connecticut, Minnesota, New York, and Wisconsin). In these states, the tick that transmits the HGE agent is the same tick that transmits *Borrelia burgdorferi*, the etiologic agent of Lyme disease. **Patient Care.** Use Standard Precautions for hospitalized patients.	**Pathogens.** The etiologic agents of ehrlichiosis are Gram- negative coccobacilli that are closely related to rickettsias. They are obligate intraleukocytic pathogens. *Ehrlichia chaffeensis* invades human monocytes, causing HME. *Anaplasma phagocytophilum* invades human granulocytes, causing HGE. A canine species, *Ehrlichia ewingii*, has caused a small number of human cases. **Reservoirs and Mode of Transmission.** Reservoirs are unknown. Transmission occurs via tick bite. The two different types of ehrlichiosis seem to be transmitted by different species of ticks. **Laboratory Diagnosis.** Ehrlichiosis is diagnosed using immunodiagnostic procedures and nucleic acid assays.

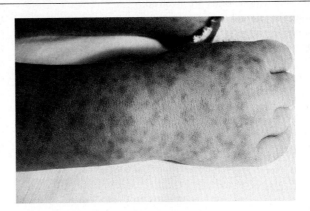

Figure 19-8. ▶ Rash of spotted fever rickettsiosis (formerly called Rocky Mountain spotted fever.) (Courtesy of the CDC.)

375

can break loose and be transported to vital organs, where they can block arterial blood flow. Obviously, such obstructions are very serious, possibly leading to strokes, heart attacks, and death.

The two most common types of infective endocarditis are acute bacterial endocarditis and subacute bacterial endocarditis (SBE). Acute bacterial endocarditis is usually caused by colonization of heart valves by virulent bacteria such as *Staphylococcus aureus* (the most common cause), *Streptococcus pneumoniae*, *Neisseria gonorrhoeae*, *Streptococcus pyogenes*, and *Enterococcus faecalis*. In SBE, heart valves are infected by less virulent organisms such as α-hemolytic streptococci of oral origin (viridans streptococci), *Staphylococcus epidermidis*, *Enterococcus* spp., and *Haemophilus* spp. Fungal endocarditis is rare, but cases of *Candida* and *Aspergillus* endocarditis do occur.

Oral streptococci can enter the bloodstream following minor or major dental procedures, oral surgery, and aggressive tooth brushing. Phlebotomy procedures and insertion of intravenous (IV) lines sometimes force organisms from the skin into the bloodstream. IV drug users are at high risk of developing infective endocarditis as a result of contaminated needles, syringes, and drug solutions.

Blood cultures are required for diagnosis of infective endocarditis. Treatment will depend on the specific pathogen involved and the antimicrobial susceptibility results.

Additional information pertaining to bacterial infections of the cardiovascular system is contained in Table 19-11.

> Lyme disease is the most common arthropod-borne disease in the United States.

Table 19-11 Other Bacterial Infections of the Cardiovascular System

Disease	Additional Information
Lyme Disease. Lyme disease or Lyme borreliosis is a tick-borne disease characterized by three stages: (a) an early, distinctive, target-like, red skin lesion, usually at the site of the tick bite, expanding to a diameter of 15 cm, often with a central clearing (Fig. 19-9); (b) early systemic manifestations that may include fatigue, chills, fever, headache, stiff neck, muscle pain, joint aches, with or without lymphadenopathy; and (c) neurologic abnormalities (e.g., aseptic meningitis, facial paralysis, myelitis, and encephalitis) and cardiac abnormalities (e.g., arrhythmias, pericarditis) several weeks or months after the initial symptoms appear. The disease gets its name from the fact that the first U.S. cases occurred in Lyme, Connecticut. Although Lyme disease is the most common arthropod-borne disease in the United States, it does not occur nationwide. In 2011, 96% of cases were reported from 13 states, primarily in the northeast and upper Midwest. **Patient Care.** Use Standard Precautions for hospitalized patients.	**Pathogen.** The etiologic agent of Lyme disease is *Borrelia burgdorferi*, a loosely coiled Gram-negative, spirochete (refer back to Fig. 4-30 in Chapter 4). **Reservoirs and Mode of Transmission.** Ticks, rodents (especially deer mice), and mammals (especially deer) serve as reservoirs. Transmission occurs via tick bite. Person-to-person transmission does not occur. **Laboratory Diagnosis.** Lyme disease is usually diagnosed by observation of the characteristic target-like skin lesion, plus immunodiagnostic and molecular diagnostic procedures. *B. burgdorferi* can be grown in the laboratory on a special medium (Barbour-Stoenner-Kelley [BSK] medium at 33°C).
Plague. Plague is an acute, often severe zoonosis. Initial signs and symptoms may include fever, chills, malaise, myalgia, nausea, prostration, sore throat, and headache. **Bubonic plague** is named for the swollen, inflamed, and tender lymph nodes (buboes) that develop. Usually, the lymph nodes affected are those receiving drainage from the site of the bite of an infected flea. In about 90% of cases, the inguinal (groin area) lymph nodes are involved. **Pneumonic plague,** which is highly communicable, involves the lungs. It can result in localized outbreaks or devastating epidemics. **Septicemic plague** may lead to septic shock, meningitis, and death. **Patient Care.** Use Standard Precautions for hospitalized patients with bubonic and septicemic plague. Add Droplet Precautions for pneumonic plague patients, until 48 hours after initiation of effective therapy.	**Pathogen.** The etiologic agent of plague is *Yersinia pestis*, a nonmotile, bipolar-staining, Gram-negative coccobacillus, sometimes referred to as the plague bacillus. **Reservoirs and Mode of Transmission.** Reservoirs include wild rodents (especially ground squirrels in the United States) and their fleas, and, rarely, rabbits, wild carnivores, and domestic cats. Transmission is usually via flea bite (from rodent to flea to human). Transmission may also occur as a result of handling tissues of infected rodents, rabbits, and other animals, as well as droplet transmission from person to person (in pneumonic plague). **Laboratory Diagnosis.** Plague is diagnosed by observation of the typical appearance of *Y. pestis* (bipolar-staining bacilli that resemble safety pins) in Gram-stained or Wright-Giemsa–stained sputum, cerebrospinal fluid, or material aspirated from a bubo (Fig. 19-10). Diagnosis can also be made by culture, biochemical tests, and immunodiagnostic tests.

Table 19-11 Other Bacterial Infections of the Cardiovascular System (continued)

Disease	Additional Information
Tularemia. Tularemia, also known as rabbit fever, is an acute zoonosis with a variety of clinical manifestations, depending on the portal of entry of the pathogen into the body. Tularemia most often presents as a skin ulcer (Fig. 19-11) and regional lymphadenitis. Ingestion of the pathogen results in pharyngitis, abdominal pain, diarrhea, and vomiting. Inhalation of the pathogen results in pneumonia and septicemia, with a 30%–60% fatality rate. **Patient Care.** Use Standard Precautions for hospitalized patients.	**Pathogen.** The etiologic agent of tularemia is *Francisella tularensis*, a small, pleomorphic Gram-negative coccobacillus. Some strains are more virulent than others. **Reservoirs and Mode of Transmission.** Reservoirs include wild animals (especially rabbits, muskrats, and beavers), some domestic animals, and hard ticks. Transmission occurs via tick bite; ingestion of contaminated meat or drinking water, entry of organisms into a wound while skinning infected animals, inhalation of dust, or animal bites. Person-to-person transmission does not occur. **Laboratory Diagnosis.** Diagnosis of tularemia is by culture, biochemical tests, and immunodiagnostic procedures.

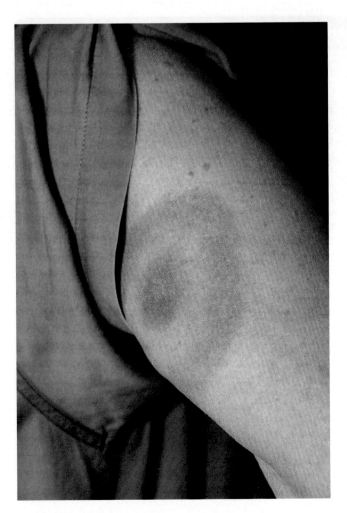

Figure 19-9. Bull's eye rash of Lyme disease, technically known as erythema migrans. Recognition of this characteristic rash is a key component in the early diagnosis of Lyme disease. (Courtesy of James Gathany and the CDC.)

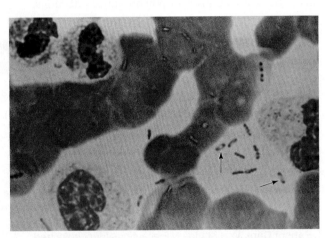

Figure 19-10. *Yersinia pestis*, the etiologic agent of plague, in a Wright-stained blood smear. Note the safety-pin appearance of the bacterial cells that results from bipolar staining (*arrows*). (Courtesy of the CDC.)

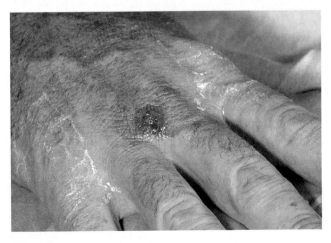

Figure 19-11. Lesion of tularemia caused by *Francisella tularensis*. (Courtesy of Dr. Brachman and the CDC.)

Bacterial Infections of the Central Nervous System

Bacteria that can cause meningitis were discussed under "Infections of the CNS Having Multiple Causes" in Chapter 17. Additional information pertaining to bacterial infections of the CNS is contained in Table 19-12.

Diseases Caused by Anaerobic Bacteria

Some of the human diseases caused by anaerobic bacteria (usually referred to as "anaerobes") are shown in Figure 19-12 and Table 19-13. Many infections that involve anaerobes are synergistic or polymicrobial infections.

Diseases Associated with Biofilms

Recall from Chapter 10 that biofilms are complex and persistent communities of assorted microbes. Biofilms exist in many environments, including certain anatomical sites within the human body. Listed here are some of the human diseases that are known to or thought to be associated with biofilms:

Bacterial endocarditis
Central venous catheter infection
Chronic wounds
Cystic fibrosis lung infections
Gingivitis
Infection of prosthetic joints, heart valves, and intrauterine devices
Infectious kidney stones
Middle ear infections

Table 19-12 Bacterial Infections of the Central Nervous System

Disease	Additional Information
Botulism (see Appendix 1 on thePoint: "Microbial Intoxications").	
Listeriosis. Generally, listeriosis is only a mild febrile illness in healthy, immunocompetent individuals. However, the disease can be manifested as meningoencephalitis and/or septicemia in newborns and elderly and/or immunosuppressed adults, with fever, intense headache, nausea, vomiting, delirium, coma, occasionally collapse, shock, and death. Listeriosis causes fever and spontaneous abortion in pregnant women. **Patient Care.** Use Standard Precautions for hospitalized patients.	**Pathogen.** Listeriosis is caused by *Listeria monocytogenes*, a Gram-positive coccobacillus. **Reservoirs and Mode of Transmission.** Reservoirs include soil, water, mud, silage, infected mammals, humans, and soft cheeses (*Listeria* multiplies in contaminated refrigerated foods.) Transmission occurs via ingestion of raw or contaminated milk, soft cheeses, or vegetables. Listeriosis can also be transmitted from mother to fetus in utero or during passage through an infected birth canal. **Laboratory Diagnosis.** Listeriosis is diagnosed by isolation and identification of the pathogen from cerebrospinal fluid (CSF), blood, amniotic fluid, placenta, and other specimens. Gram-positive coccobacilli can be observed in Gram-stained smears of neonatal CSF.
Tetanus (Lockjaw). Tetanus is an acute neuromuscular disease induced by a bacterial exotoxin called tetanospasmin, with painful muscular contractions, primarily of the masseter (the muscle that closes the jaw) and neck muscles, spasms, and rigid paralysis (refer back to Fig. 14-9 in Chapter 14). Respiratory failure and death may result. **Patient Care.** Use Standard Precautions for hospitalized patients.	**Pathogen.** Tetanus is caused by *Clostridium tetani*, a motile, Gram-positive, anaerobic, spore-forming bacillus (refer back to Fig. 4-27 in Chapter 4) that produces a potent neurotoxin called tetanospasmin. **Reservoirs and Mode of Transmission.** Reservoirs include soil contaminated with human, horse, or other animal feces (*C. tetani* is a member of the indigenous intestinal microbes of humans and animals.) Spores of *C. tetani* are introduced into a puncture wound, burn, or needlestick by contamination with soil, dust, or feces. Under anaerobic conditions in the wound, spores germinate into vegetative *C. tetani* cells, which produce the exotoxin in vivo. Person-to-person transmission does not occur. **Laboratory Diagnosis.** Diagnosis of tetanus is usually made on clinical and epidemiologic grounds. Attempts to isolate *C. tetani* from wounds or demonstrate antibody production are rarely successful.

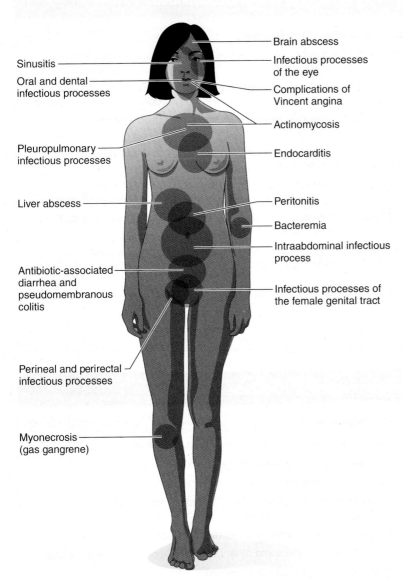

Necrotizing fasciitis
Osteomyelitis
Periodontitis
Prostatitis
Sinusitis
Tooth decay
Urinary catheters
UTIs

Figure 19-12. Human diseases that commonly involve anaerobes.

Recap of Major Bacterial Infections of Humans

Table 19-14 provides a recap of some major bacterial infections of humans.

Recap of Major Bacterial Pathogens of Humans

Table 19-15 and Figure 19-13 provide a recap of some major bacterial pathogens of humans.

Appropriate Therapy for Bacterial Infections

Recommendations for the treatment of infectious diseases change frequently. The bacterial infections described in this chapter must be

Table 19-13 Some Human Diseases Caused by Anaerobic Bacteria	
Disease	**Anaerobe(s) That Cause(s) the Disease**
Acne	*Propionibacterium acnes*
Actinomycosis	Various *Actinomyces* spp. and *Propionibacterium propionicus*
Acute necrotizing ulcerative gingivitis (also known as Vincent's angina and trench mouth)	*Fusobacterium necrophorum* and anaerobic spirochetes
Antibiotic-associated diarrhea and pseudomembranous colitis	*Clostridium difficile*
Botulism	*Clostridium botulinum*
Brain abscess	Most often caused by *Bacteroides* and *Fusobacterium* spp. and anaerobic Gram-negative cocci; often polymicrobial
Gas gangrene (myonecrosis)	*Clostridium perfringens* (usually), *Clostridium novyi*, *Clostridium septicum*

(continued)

Disease	Anaerobe(s) That Cause(s) the Disease
Gynecologic and obstetric infectious processes	Many different types of anaerobes, including *Bacteroides* spp., clostridia, and anaerobic Gram-positive cocci
Intra-abdominal infectious processes	Many different types of anaerobes, including *Bacteroides* and *Fusobacterium* spp., *C. perfringens*, other clostridia, and anaerobic Gram-positive cocci; usually polymicrobial
Liver abscess	Many different types of anaerobes, including *Bacteroides*, *Fusobacterium*, *Clostridium*, and *Actinomyces* spp.
Oral/dental infectious processes (periodontitis)	Many different types of anaerobes, including *Porphyromonas*, *Wolinella*, and *Fusobacterium* spp. and anaerobic Gram-positive cocci
Perineal and perirectal infectious processes	Many different types of anaerobes, including *Bacteroides*, *Fusobacterium*, *Clostridium*, *Eubacterium*, and *Actinomyces* spp. and anaerobic Gram-positive cocci
Peritonitis	Many different types of anaerobes, including *Bacteroides* and *Clostridium* spp., *F. necrophorum*, and anaerobic Gram-positive cocci
Pleuropulmonary infectious processes	Many different types of anaerobes, including *Bacteroides*, *Porphyromonas*, *Actinomyces*, and *Eubacterium* spp., *Fusobacterium nucleatum*, and anaerobic Gram-positive cocci
Sinusitis	*Bacteroides* and *Fusobacterium* spp. and anaerobic Gram-positive cocci; often polymicrobial
Tetanus	*Clostridium tetani*

Table 19-14 Recap of Some Major Bacterial Infections of Humans

Disease	Bacterial Pathogen
Anthrax	*Bacillus anthracis* (a spore-forming, Gram-positive bacillus)
Cholera	*Vibrio cholerae* (comma-shaped Gram-negative bacilli)
Diphtheria	*Coynebacterium diphtheriae* (a Gram-positive bacillus)
Gas gangrene	*Clostridium perfringens* and some other *Clostridium* spp. (anaerobic, spore-forming, Gram-positive bacilli)
Gonorrhea	*Neisseria gonorrhoeae* (a Gram-negative diplococcus)
Legionellosis (Legionnaire disease)	*Legionella pneumophila* and some other *Legionella* spp. (Gram-negative bacilli)
Leprosy (Hansen disease)	*Mycobacterium leprae* (an acid-fast bacillus)
Listeriosis	*Listeria monocytogenes* (a Gram-negative bacillus)
Lyme disease	*Borrelia burgdorferi* (a Gram-negative spirochete)
Plague	*Yersinia pestis* (a Gram-negative bacillus)
Spotted fever rickettsiosis (formerly called Rocky Mountain spotted fever)	*Rickettsia rickettsii* (a Gram-negative bacillus; an obligate intracellular pathogen)
Salmonellosis	*Salmonella enteritidis* and *Salmonella typhimurium* (Gram-negative bacilli)
Shigellosis	*Shigella dysenteriae*, *Shigella flexneri*, *Shigella boydii*, and *Shigella sonnei* (Gram-negative bacilli)
Strep throat	*Streptococcus pyogenes* (a Gram-positive coccus)
Syphilis	*Treponema pallidum* (a tightly coiled spirochete)
Tetanus	*Clostridium tetani* (an anaerobic, spore-forming, Gram-positive bacillus)
Trachoma	Certain serotypes of *Chlamydia trachomatis* (a Gram-negative bacillus; an obligate intracellular pathogen)
Tuberculosis	Most cases are caused by *Mycobacterium tuberculosis* (an acid-fast bacillus)
Tularemia	*Francisella tularensis* (a Gram-negative bacillus)
Typhoid fever	*Salmonella typhi* (a Gram-negative bacillus)
Whooping cough (pertussis)	*Bordetella pertussis* (a Gram-negative coccobacillus)
Wound botulism	*Clostridium botulinum* (an anaerobic, spore-forming, Gram-positive bacillus)

Table 19-15 Recap of Some Major Bacterial Pathogens of Humans

Gram-Positive Cocci:

Enterococcus (en-ter-oh-kok'-us) species	Gram-positive cocci; common members of the indigenous microbiota of the gastrointestinal tract; opportunistic pathogens; a fairly common cause of cystitis and healthcare-associated infections; some strains, called vancomycin-resistant enterococci (VRE), are multidrug resistant.
Staphylococcus aureus (staf'-ih-low-kok'-us aw'-ree-us)	A catalase-positive (meaning that it produces the enzyme catalase), Gram-positive coccus, usually arranged in clusters (refer back to Figure 4-18A in Chapter 4). In the laboratory, *S. aureus* can be differentiated from other *Staphylococcus* species of human origin by using the coagulase test; *S. aureus* is coagulase-positive (meaning that it produces the enzyme coagulase), whereas other *Staphylococcus* spp. are coagulase-negative. *S. aureus* is a facultative anaerobe and opportunistic pathogen that is often found in low numbers as indigenous microbiota of the skin. Approximately 20% to 30% of the general population are "staph carriers," their nasal passages being colonized with *S. aureus*. Infections caused by *S. aureus* are often referred to as "staph infections" (see Fig. 19-1). It is a major cause of skin, soft tissue, respiratory, bone, joint, endovascular, and wound infections. Most pimples, boils, carbuncles, and styes involve *S. aureus*. It is a less common cause of pneumonia and UTIs. *S. aureus* is one of the four most common causes of healthcare-associated infections, often causing surgical site infections. Strains of *S. aureus* produce a variety of exotoxins, including cytotoxins, exfoliative toxin, and leukocidin. Some strains produce TSS-1 toxin, the cause of TSS. Some strains (those that produce an enterotoxin) are the cause of staphylococcal food poisoning, one of the most common types of food poisoning. Strains of *S. aureus* produce a variety of exoenzymes, including protease, lipase, and hyaluronidase that destroy tissues; coagulase that causes clot formation; and staphylokinase that dissolves clots. Especially troublesome strains of *S. aureus* are methicillin-resistant *S. aureus* (MRSA) strains (which are resistant to most of the drugs used to treat staph infections) and vancomycin-intermediate *S. aureus* (VISA) strains (which are resistant to the dosages of vancomycin usually used to treat staph infections).
Streptococcus agalactiae (strep-toh-kok'-us ay-guh-lak'-tee-ee)	Also known as group B streptococcus; a β-hemolytic, Gram-positive coccus; often colonizes the vagina; a frequent cause of neonatal meningitis.
Streptococcus pneumoniae (strep-toh-kok'-us new-moh'-nee-ee)	Also known as pneumococcus (pl., pneumococci). It is an encapsulated, α-hemolytic, catalase-negative, Gram-positive coccus, usually arranged in pairs (diplococci) (refer to Figures 4-25 and 19-4). In the laboratory, *S. pneumoniae* can be differentiated from other α-hemolytic *Streptococcus* species of human origin by using the P-disk (Optochin sensitivity) test; *S. pneumoniae* is Optochin-sensitive (killed by Optochin), whereas other α-hemolytic streptococci are Optochin-resistant. *S. pneumoniae* is a facultative anaerobe and opportunistic pathogen, found in low numbers as indigenous microbiota of the upper respiratory tract. It is the most common cause of bacterial pneumonia in the world; the pneumonia it causes is often referred to as pneumococcal pneumonia. *S. pneumoniae* is also a common cause of meningitis (especially in the elderly) and sinusitis, and causes about one-third of U.S. cases of otitis media. Many strains of *S. pneumoniae* are penicillin resistant and some strains are multidrug-resistant. A vaccine is available to prevent pneumococcal infections in the elderly.
Streptococcus pyogenes (strep-toh-kok'-us py-oj'-uh-nees)	Also known as group A strep, GAS, and Strep A. It is a β-hemolytic, catalase-negative, Gram-positive coccus, usually arranged in chains (refer back to Figure 4-24 in Chapter 4). In the laboratory, *S. pyogenes* can be differentiated from other β-hemolytic *Streptococcus* species of human origin by using the A-disk (bacitracin sensitivity) test; *S. pyogenes* is bacitracin-sensitive (killed by bacitracin), whereas the other β-hemolytic streptococci are bacitracin-resistant. It is a facultative anaerobe and opportunistic pathogen that is infrequently found in low numbers as indigenous microbiota of the upper respiratory tract. *S. pyogenes* is the cause of streptococcal pharyngitis (strep throat) and a frequent cause of skin infections (e.g., impetigo and erysipelas) and wound infections. Untreated strep throat or other *S. pyogenes* infections can lead to a variety of sequelae (complications), including scarlet fever, TSS, rheumatic fever (sometimes referred to as rheumatic heart disease because it includes myocarditis and endocarditis), rheumatoid arthritis, and glomerulonephritis. Scarlet fever is caused by strains that produce erythrogenic toxin. Some strains of *S. pyogenes* produce a toxin that causes TSS, although most cases of TSS are caused by *S. aureus*. Some strains of *S. pyogenes* (referred to as the "flesh-eating bacteria") produce necrotizing enzymes that cause rapid and extensive destruction of tissue (a condition known as necrotizing fasciitis). Necrotizing fasciitis has a mortality rate of approximately 20% to 30%.

(continued)

Recap of Some Major Bacterial Pathogens of Humans (continued)

Gram-Negative Cocci

Neisseria gonorrhoeae (ny-see'-ree-uh gon-or-ree'-ee)
Also known as gonococcus or GC; a fastidious, Gram-negative diplococcus; microaerophilic and capnophilic; always a pathogen; causes gonorrhea; many strains are penicillin resistant.

Neisseria meningitidis (ny-see'-ree-uh men-in-jih'-tid-is)
Also known as meningococcus; an aerobic, Gram-negative diplococcus; found as indigenous microbiota of the upper respiratory tract of some people (referred to as carriers); a common cause of bacterial meningitis; also causes respiratory infections.

Gram-Positive Bacilli

Bacillus anthracis (buh-sil'-us an'-thray-sis)
An aerobic, spore-forming, Gram-positive bacillus; the causative agent of anthrax in humans, cattle, swine, sheep, rabbits, guinea pigs, and mice; causes a cutaneous, respiratory, or gastrointestinal disease, depending on the portal of entry.

Corynebacterium diphtheriae (kuh'-ry-nee-bak-teer'-ee-um dif-thee'-ree-ee)
A pleomorphic, Gram-positive bacillus; toxigenic (toxin-producing) strains cause diphtheria, whereas nontoxigenic strains do not.

Lactobacillus (lak-toh-buh-sil'-us) species
Gram-positive bacilli; some species are found in foods (e.g., yogurt, cheese); other species are common members of the indigenous microbiota of the vagina and gastrointestinal tract; rarely pathogenic.

Listeria monocytogenes (lis-teer'-ee-uh mon-oh-sigh-toj'-uh-nees)
A Gram-positive bacillus; the causative agent of listeriosis; can cause meningitis, encephalitis, septicemia, endocarditis, abortion, and abscesses; enters the body via ingestion of contaminated foods (e.g., cheese).

Gram-Negative Bacilli

Acinetobacter baumannii (as-i-ne'-toe-bak'-ter bow-man'-e-eye)
A strictly aerobic, Gram-negative, coccobacillus; a common cause of hospital-acquired infections; often multidrug resistant.

Bordetella pertussis (bor-duh-tel'-uh per-tus'-sis).
A fastidious, Gram-negative coccobacillus; the causative agent of whooping cough, which is also called pertussis.

Campylobacter jejuni (kam'-pih-low-bak'-ter juh-ju'-nee)
A curved, Gram-negative bacillus, having a characteristic corkscrew-like motility; often seen in pairs (described as a gull-wing morphology because a pair of curved bacilli resembles a bird); microaerophilic and capnophilic; a common cause of gastroenteritis with malaise, myalgia, arthralgia, headache, and cramping abdominal pain.

Escherichia coli (esh-er-ick'-ee-uh koh'-ly)
A member of the family *Enterobacteriaceae*; a Gram-negative bacillus; a facultative anaerobe; a lactose fermenter (thus, it produces pink colonies on MacConkey agar); a very common member of the indigenous microbiota of the colon; an opportunistic pathogen; the most common cause of septicemia and urinary tract and healthcare-associated infections; some serotypes (called the enterovirulent *E. coli*) are always pathogens.

Francisella tularensis (fran'-suh-sel-luh tool-uh-ren'-sis)
A Gram-negative bacillus; the causative agent of tularemia; may enter the body by inhalation, ingestion, tick bite, or penetration of broken or unbroken skin; tularemia frequently follows contact with infected animals (e.g., rabbits).

Haemophilus influenzae (he-mof'-uh-lus in-flu-en'-zee)
A fastidious, Gram-negative bacillus; a facultative anaerobe; encapsulated; found in low numbers as indigenous microbiota of the upper respiratory tract; an opportunistic pathogen; a cause of bacterial meningitis, ear infections, and respiratory infections, but is *not* the cause of influenza (which is caused by influenza viruses); some strains are ampicillin resistant.

Helicobacter pylori (hee'-luh-ko-bak-ter py-lor'-ee)
A curved, Gram-negative bacillus; capable of colonizing the stomach; a common cause of stomach and duodenal ulcers.

Klebsiella pneumoniae (kleb-see-el'-uh new-moh'-nee-ee)
A member of the family *Enterobacteriaceae*; a Gram-negative bacillus; a facultative anaerobe; a common member of the indigenous microbiota of the colon; an opportunistic pathogen; a fairly common cause of pneumonia and cystitis.

Legionella pneumophila (lee-juh-nel'-luh new-mah'-fill-uh)
An aerobic, Gram-negative bacillus; common in soil and water; the causative agent of legionellosis (a type of pneumonia); can contaminate water tanks and pipes; has caused epidemics in hotels, hospitals, and cruise ships.

Proteus (pro'-tee-us) species
Members of the family *Enterobacteriaceae*; Gram-negative bacilli; facultative anaerobes; common members of the indigenous microbiota of the colon; opportunistic pathogens; a fairly common cause of cystitis.

Table 19-15 Recap of Some Major Bacterial Pathogens of Humans (continued)

Pseudomonas aeruginosa (su-doh-moh'-nas air-uj-in-oh'-suh)	An aerobic, Gram-negative bacillus; produces a characteristic blue-green pigment (pyocyanin); has a characteristic fruity odor; causes burn wound, ear, urinary tract, and respiratory infections; one of the major causes of healthcare-associated infections; most strains are multidrug resistant and resistant to some disinfectants.
Salmonella (sal'-moh-nel'-uh) species	Members of the family *Enterobacteriaceae*; Gram-negative bacilli; facultative anaerobes; a fairly common cause of food poisoning, especially cases caused by contaminated poultry; *Salmonella typhi* is the causative agent of typhoid fever.
Shigella (she-gel'-uh) species	Members of the family *Enterobacteriaceae*; Gram-negative bacilli; facultative anaerobes; a major cause of gastroenteritis and child mortality in the developing nations of the world.
Vibrio cholerae (vib'-ree-oh khol'-er-ee)	An aerobic, curved (comma-shaped), Gram-negative bacillus; halophilic; lives in salt water; the causative agent of cholera.
Yersinia pestis (yer-sin'-ee-uh pes'-tis)	A Gram-negative bacillus; the causative agent of plague in humans, rodents, and other mammals; transmitted from rat to rat and rat to human by the rat flea.
Acid-Fast Bacilli	
Mycobacterium leprae (my'-koh-bak-teer'-ee-um lep'-ree)	An aerobic, acid-fast, Gram-variable bacillus; referred to as the leprosy bacillus or Hansen bacillus; the causative agent of leprosy (Hansen's disease); transmitted from person to person; has been found in wild armadillos, which are now used as laboratory animals to propagate this organism.
Mycobacterium tuberculosis (my'-koh-bak-teer'-ee-um tu-ber'-kyu-loh-sis)	An acid-fast, Gram-variable bacillus; causes tuberculosis; many strains are multidrug resistant.
Nocardia (no-kar'-dee-uh) species	Aerobic, acid-fast, Gram-positive bacilli; the causative agents of nocardiosis (a respiratory disease) and mycetoma (a tumor-like disease, most often involving the feet).
Anaerobes	
Bacteroides (bak-ter-oy'-dez) species	Anaerobic, Gram-negative bacilli; common members of the indigenous microbiota of the oral cavity, gastrointestinal tract, and vagina; opportunistic pathogens that cause various infections, including appendicitis, peritonitis, abscesses, and postsurgical wound infections.
Clostridium botulinum (klos-trid'-ee-um bot-yu-ly'-num)	An anaerobic, spore-forming, Gram-positive bacillus; common in soil; produces a neurotoxin called botulinum toxin, which causes botulism, a very serious and sometimes fatal type of food poisoning.
Clostridium difficile (klos-trid'-ee-um dif'-fuh-seal)	An anaerobic, spore-forming, Gram-positive bacillus; it can colonize the intestinal tract, where overgrowth (superinfection) commonly occurs after ingestion of oral antibiotics; this organism produces two toxins—an enterotoxin that causes AAD and a cytotoxin that causes pseudomembranous colitis (PMC); a common cause of healthcare-associated infections.
Clostridium perfringens (klos-trid'-ee-um purr-frin'-jens)	An anaerobic, spore-forming, Gram-positive bacillus; common in feces and soil; the most common cause of gas gangrene (myonecrosis); produces an enterotoxin that produces a relatively mild type of food poisoning.
Clostridium tetani (klos-trid'-ee-um tet'-an-eye)	An anaerobic, spore-forming, Gram-positive bacillus; common in soil; produces a neurotoxin called tetanospasmin, which causes tetanus.
Fusobacterium (few'-zoh-bak-teer'-ee-um) species	Anaerobic, Gram-negative bacilli; common members of the indigenous microbiota of the oral cavity, gastrointestinal tract, and vagina; opportunistic pathogens that cause various infections, including oral and respiratory infections.
Peptostreptococcus (pep'-toh-strep-toh-kok'-us) species	Anaerobic, Gram-positive cocci; common members of the indigenous microbiota of the gastrointestinal tract, vagina, and oral cavity; opportunistic pathogens that cause various infections, including abscesses, oral infections, and appendicitis.
Porphyromonas (porf'-uh-row-mow'-nus) species	Anaerobic, Gram-negative bacilli; common members of the indigenous microbiota of the oral cavity and gastrointestinal tract; opportunistic pathogens that cause various infections, including abscesses, oral infections, and bite wound infections.
Prevotella (pree'-voh-tel'-luh) species	Anaerobic, Gram-negative bacilli; common members of the indigenous microbiota of the vagina and gastrointestinal tract; opportunistic pathogens that cause various infections, including abscesses.
Veillonella (vy-low-nel'-uh) species	Very small, anaerobic, Gram-negative cocci; indigenous microbiota of the oral cavity; sometimes encountered in head, neck, dental, pulmonary, and bite wound infections.

(continued)

Table 19-15 Recap of Some Major Bacterial Pathogens of Humans (continued)

Unique Bacteria

Chlamydia (kluh-mid'-ee-uh) and Chlamydiophila species	Pleomorphic, Gram-negative bacteria that are obligate intracellular pathogens; unable to grow on artificial media; etiologic agents of nongonococcal urethritis (NGU), trachoma, inclusion conjunctivitis, lymphogranuloma venereum, pneumonia, and psittacosis (ornithosis); different serotypes of Chlamydia trachomatis cause different diseases.
Mycoplasma pneumoniae (my'-koh-plaz-muh new-moh'-nee-ee)	A small, pleomorphic, Gram-negative bacterium; lacks a cell wall; the causative agent of atypical pneumonia.
Rickettsia (rih-ket'-see-uh) species	Gram-negative bacilli that are obligate intracellular pathogens; unable to grow on artificial media; the causative agents of typhus and typhus-like diseases (e.g., spotted fever rickettsiosis); all rickettsial diseases are transmitted by arthropods (ticks, fleas, mites, lice).

Spirochetes

Borrelia burgdorferi (boh-ree'-lee-uh burg-door'-fur-eye)	A Gram-negative, loosely coiled spirochete; the causative agent of Lyme disease; transmitted from infected deer and mice to humans by tick bite.
Treponema pallidum (trep-oh-nee'-muh pal'-luh-dum)	A very thin, tightly coiled spirochete; the causative agent of syphilis.

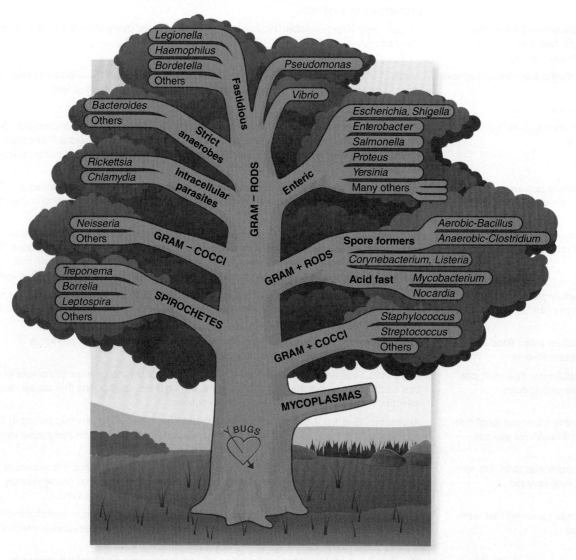

Figure 19-13. Recap of major groups of medically important bacteria. Please note that this illustration is presented merely as a study aid. It is not a taxonomic or phylogenetic tree. (Redrawn from Engleberg NC, et al. *Schaechter's Mechanisms of Microbial Disease.* 5th ed. Philadelphia, PA: Lippincott Williams & Wilkins; 2013.)

treated using appropriate antibacterial drugs. For certain bacterial diseases, antisera (e.g., for botulism and tetanus) are available for treatment. Additional information about antibacterial agents can be found in Chapter 9 and at en.wikipedia.org/wiki/Antibiotics.

ON thePoint

- Terms Introduced in This Chapter
- Review of Key Points
- Increase Your Knowledge
- Critical Thinking
- Additional Self-Assessment Exercises

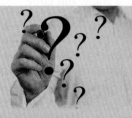

Self-Assessment Exercises

After you have read this chapter, answer the following multiple-choice questions.

1. The most common STD in the United States is caused by:
   a. *Candida albicans.*
   b. *Chlamydia trachomatis.*
   c. *Neisseria gonorrhoeae.*
   d. *Trichomonas vaginalis.*

2. _____ is the most common cause of pneumonia in the world.
   a. *Chlamydophila pneumoniae*
   b. *Legionella pneumophila*
   c. *Mycoplasma pneumoniae*
   d. *Streptococcus pneumoniae*

3. Gas gangrene is always caused by:
   a. *Bacillus anthracis.*
   b. *Clostridium* spp.
   c. *Staphylococcus aureus.*
   d. *Streptococcus pyogenes.*

4. The bacterial species most frequently associated with necrotizing fasciitis is:
   a. *Francisella tularensis*
   b. *S. aureus*
   c. *S. pneumoniae*
   d. *S. pyogenes*

5. Which of the following diseases may be caused by *C. trachomatis*?
   a. Inclusion conjunctivitis
   b. Nongonococcal urethritis (NGU)
   c. Trachoma
   d. All of the above

6. Which of the following organisms is the most common cause of urethritis?
   a. *C. albicans*
   b. *C. trachomatis*
   c. *N. gonorrhoeae*
   d. *T. vaginalis*

7. Which of the following organisms is the most common cause of cystitis?
   a. *C. trachomatis*
   b. *E. coli*
   c. *N. gonorrhoeae*
   d. *T. vaginalis*

8. Which of the following is the most common arthropod-borne disease in the United States?
   a. Lyme disease
   b. Plague
   c. Spotted fever rickettsiosis (formerly, Rocky Mountain spotted fever)
   d. Tularemia

9. Which of the following diseases is not caused by a spirochete?
   a. Lyme disease
   b. Plague
   c. Relapsing fever
   d. Syphilis

10. Which of the following associations is incorrect?
    a. Lyme disease ... tick
    b. Plague ... rat flea
    c. Spotted fever rickettsiosis ... tick
    d. Typhoid fever ... mosquito

Case Studies

Case 1. A 19-year-old woman visits the clinic complaining of a frequent, urgent desire to urinate, a burning sensation during urination, and pain above her pubic bone. The physician suspects cystitis and arranges for the patient to collect a clean-catch, midstream urine specimen. The urine is cloudy and tinged with blood. In the laboratory, a colony count confirms that the patient does have a urinary tract infection. The pathogen causing the infection is producing pink colonies on MacConkey agar.

A. Which one of the following pathogens do you suspect is causing this patient's cystitis?

1. *Chlamydia trachomatis*
2. *Escherichia coli*
3. *Neisseria gonorrhoeae*
4. *Proteus mirabilis*
5. *Staphylococcus saprophyticus*

Case 2. A 2-year-old girl is admitted to the hospital with massive tissue destruction along her right arm. The skin is a violet color, and large fluid-filled blisters are present. The patient has a fever, a rapid heart rate, and low blood pressure, and seems confused. Her mother informs the physician that the child had been recovering from chickenpox, and, for the past 2 days, had frequently been scratching at chickenpox lesions on that area of her arm. Once the area appeared to have become infected, the infection spread very rapidly. A Gram-stain of exudate from the infected tissue reveals Gram-positive cocci in chains.

A. The physician suspects that her infection is being caused by _____.

1. *Clostridium perfringens*
2. *Clostridium tetani*
3. *Staphylococcus aureus*
4. *Streptococcus pneumoniae*
5. *Streptococcus pyogenes* (Group A strep)

Case 3. A 16-year-old girl is admitted to the hospital with severe abdominal cramps and bloody diarrhea. She has a fever of 102°F. She has been experiencing her symptoms for the past 3 days, since several hours after eating at a fast-food restaurant with a group of her friends. She recalls that the hamburger she ate was not very well cooked. (It is later learned that the meat being used in that restaurant to prepare hamburgers has been recalled because of bacterial contamination.)

A. All of the following organisms can cause diarrhea, but which is the most likely cause of her illness?

1. A species of *Salmonella*
2. A species of *Shigella*
3. *Escherichia coli* O157:H7
4. *Staphylococcus aureus*
5. *Vibrio cholerae*

Case Studies

Case 4. A 20-year-old man is admitted to the hospital with fever, headache, stiff neck, sore throat, and vomiting. The attending physician suspects that the patient has meningitis and immediately performs a lumbar puncture. A cerebrospinal fluid (CSF) specimen is rushed to the laboratory, where it is processed immediately. After centrifuging an aliquot of the specimen, the sediment is spread onto a microscope slide, fixed, and Gram-stained. Microscopic examination of the Gram-stained specimen reveals numerous WBCs and numerous Gram-negative diplococci.

A. This information is telephoned to the attending physician, who will now treat the patient for a meningitis caused by _____.

1. *Haemophilus influenzae*
2. *Neisseria meningitidis*
3. *Streptococcus agalactiae* (Group B strep)
4. *Streptococcus pneumoniae*
5. *Streptococcus pyogenes* (Group A strep)

Case 5. An 80-year-old woman is transferred from a nursing home to the hospital because she is suspected of having pneumonia. She is experiencing chest pain, chills, fever, and shortness of breath. She has a productive cough (meaning that she is coughing up sputum). A Gram-stain of the sputum reveals numerous WBCs and numerous Gram-positive diplococci.

A. On receipt of the Gram-stain report, the physician treats the patient for a pneumonia caused by _____.

1. *Haemophilus influenzae*
2. *Staphylococcus aureus*
3. *Streptococcus agalactiae* (Group B strep)
4. *Streptococcus pneumoniae*
5. *Streptococcus pyogenes* (Group A strep)

(Answers to Case Studies are in Appendix B.)

20

Fungal Infections of Humans

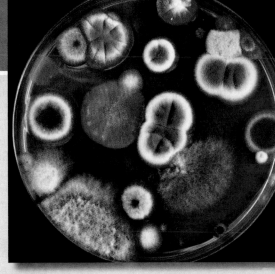

Various types of fungi growing on a solid culture medium.

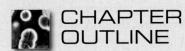

CHAPTER OUTLINE

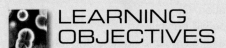

LEARNING OBJECTIVES

After studying this chapter, you should be able to:

- Define the following terms: mycosis, dimorphic, cutaneous, systemic
- Categorize various fungal diseases by body system (e.g., respiratory system, circulatory system)
- Correlate a particular fungal disease with its major characteristics, etiologic agent, reservoir(s), mode(s) of transmission, and diagnostic laboratory procedures
- Briefly explain how fungi cause disease
- Classify a given fungal infection as being a superficial, cutaneous, subcutaneous, or systemic mycosis
- State several diseases caused by dimorphic fungi

Introduction

It would be impossible in a book of this size to describe *all* of the human infectious diseases caused by fungi. Thus, only selected fungal diseases (mycoses) are described in this chapter. Readers should keep in mind that, although a certain fungal disease is described in one particular section of the chapter (e.g., under cardiovascular infections or respiratory infections), many fungal diseases have various clinical manifestations, affecting more than one anatomical site.

> Fungal infections are also known as mycoses (sing., mycosis).

Human mycoses are caused by fungi within three fungal categories: yeasts, moulds, and dimorphic fungi. Recall that dimorphic fungi are fungi that may grow as yeasts *or* moulds, depending on the temperature at which they are growing. Some fungi can also cause microbial intoxications, which are discussed in Appendix 1 on thePoint.

> Mycoses are caused by certain yeasts, moulds, and dimorphic fungi.

What to Learn?

This chapter contains a large amount of information. Of primary importance will be your ability to later recall the type and name of the fungus that causes a particular fungal disease and the manner in which the disease is transmitted. For example, if your teacher says "cryptococcosis," you should be able to state the type and name of the fungus that causes the disease (an encapsulated yeast named *Cryptococcus neoformans*), and the manner in which cryptococcosis is transmitted (inhalation of yeasts).

How Do Fungi Cause Disease?

Unlike bacteria, fungi do not secrete toxins that cause damage to the host. Rather, the tissue damage associated with fungal infections results primarily from direct invasion of tissue, with subsequent displacement and destruction of vital structures, coupled with toxic effects of the inflammatory response. Masses of fungal cells can cause obstruction of bronchi in the lungs and tubules and ureters in the kidneys, leading to obstruction of the flow of bodily fluids. Certain fungi, such as *Aspergillus* and *Mucor spp.*, can grow in the walls of the arteries and veins, leading to occlusion and tissue necrosis resulting from a lack of oxygen.

> Fungal pathogens cause disease by invasion and mechanical destruction of tissues and/or obstruction of the flow of bodily fluids.

Classification of Fungal Diseases

Fungal infections (mycoses) can be classified into the following four categories:

- **Superficial mycoses.** These are fungal infections of the outermost areas of the human body, including the outer surfaces of hair shafts and the outermost, nonliving layer of the skin (the epidermis). Superficial mycoses include otomycosis,[a] black piedra, white piedra, tinea (or pityriasis) versicolor, and tinea nigra. All are caused by moulds. Black piedra, caused by *Piedraia hortae*, is a fungal infection of scalp hair and, less commonly, eyebrows and eyelashes. White piedra, usually caused by *Trichosporon beigelii*, is a fungal infection of moustache, beard, pubic, and axilla hair. Tinea versicolor, caused by *Malassezia furfur*, is a ringworm infection that affects the skin of the chest or back and, less commonly, the arms, thighs, neck, and face. Tinea nigra, caused by *Hortaea werneckii*, is a ringworm infection of the palms of the hands and, less commonly, the neck and feet.

> Superficial mycoses are fungal infections of the outer surfaces of hair shafts and the outermost, nonliving layer of the skin (the epidermis).

- **Cutaneous, hair, and nail mycoses.** Fungal infections of the living layers of skin (the dermis), hair shafts, and nails—commonly called tinea infections or ringworm infections—are caused by a group of moulds collectively referred to as dermatophytes. Tinea infections are named in accordance with the part of the anatomy infected (Fig. 20-1).

> Fungal infections of the living layers of skin (the dermis), hair shafts, and nails are commonly called tinea or ringworm infections. They are caused by moulds collectively referred to as dermatophytes.

Ringworm

The term *ringworm* is used in reference to some of the superficial and cutaneous mycoses, which, more correctly, are known as tinea infections. Be aware that diseases referred to as ringworm have absolutely *nothing* to do with worms. The term most likely arose long before fungi were known to be the cause of these lesions. Some of the lesions are circular and raised, prompting speculation that a worm lay coiled beneath the skin surface.

- **Subcutaneous mycoses.** These are fungal infections of the dermis and underlying tissues. They are more severe than superficial and cutaneous mycoses. Examples of subcutaneous mycoses are sporotrichosis, chromomycosis (chromoblastomycosis), and mycetomas

---

[a]Otomycosis is a fungal infection of the outer ear canal, most often caused by a mould.

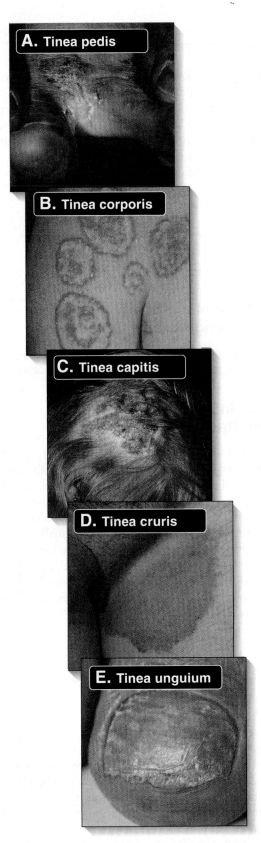

(Fig. 20-2). Sporotrichosis is caused by *Sporothrix schenckii*, a dimorphic fungus, and typically affects the skin of an extremity. Chromomycosis, caused by various species of moulds, is a chronic, spreading infection of the skin and subcutaneous tissues, usually affecting a lower extremity (Fig. 20-3). Mycetomas, caused by various moulds, are chronic granulomatous infections that involve the feet (usually), hands, or other areas of the body. Some of these subcutaneous mycoses can be quite grotesque in appearance.

> Subcutaneous mycoses, such as sporotrichosis, chromomycosis, and mycetomas, are fungal infections of the dermis and underlying tissues.

- **Systemic mycoses** (also known as generalized or deep-seated mycoses). These are the most serious types of fungal infections. They are fungal infections of internal organs of the body, sometimes affecting two or more

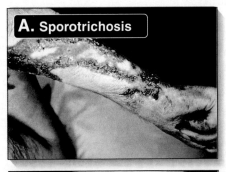

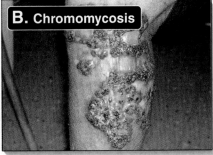

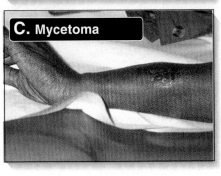

Figure 20-1. Various types of tinea infections. (A) Tinea pedis (athlete's foot), **(B)** tinea corporis (ringworm of the trunk, shown here on the shoulder), **(C)** tinea capitis (ringworm of the head), **(D)** tinea cruris (ringworm of the groin area), and **(E)** tinea unguium (ringworm of the nails). (From Harvey RA, et al. *Lippincott's Illustrated Reviews: Microbiology*. 3rd ed. Philadelphia, PA: Lippincott Williams & Wilkins; 2013.)

Figure 20-2. Subcutaneous mycoses. (A) The cutaneous–lymphatic form of sporotrichosis on a patient's arm, **(B)** chromomycosis on a patient's leg, **(C)** mycetoma on a patient's arm. (From Harvey RA, et al. *Lippincott's Illustrated Reviews: Microbiology*. 3rd ed. Philadelphia, PA: Lippincott Williams & Wilkins; 2013.)

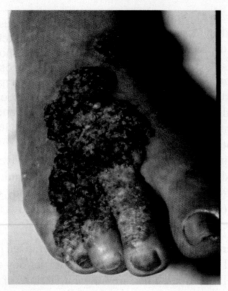

Figure 20-3. Chromoblastomycosis of the foot. (From Engleberg NC, et al. *Schaechter's Mechanisms of Microbial Disease*. 5th ed. Philadelphia, PA: Lippincott Williams & Wilkins; 2013.)

> Systemic mycoses—also known as generalized or deep-seated mycoses—are the most serious types of fungal infections.

organ systems simultaneously—for example, simultaneous infection of the respiratory system and the bloodstream, or simultaneous infection of the respiratory tract and the central nervous system.

Fungal Infections of the Skin

Dermatophytoses

Dermatophytoses are also known as *tinea* (ringworm) infections and *dermatomycoses.*

> Ringworm infections are fungal infections and have nothing to do with worms.

Diseases. (See preceding sections on superficial and cutaneous mycoses.) Some of the dermatomycoses cause only limited irritation, scaling, and redness. Others cause itching, swelling, blisters, and severe scaling.

Patient Care. Use Standard Precautions.

Pathogens. Dermatomycoses are caused by various filamentous fungi (moulds), collectively referred to as dermatophytes. Examples include species of *Microsporum, Epidermophyton,* and *Trichophyton.*

Reservoirs and Mode of Transmission. Infected humans and animals and soil serve as reservoirs. Transmission is by direct or indirect contact with lesions of humans or animals; or contact with contaminated floors,

shower stalls, or locker room benches; barbers' clippers, combs, and hairbrushes; or clothing.

Laboratory Diagnosis. Microscopic examination of potassium hydroxide (KOH) preparations of skin scrapings or hair or nail clippings can reveal the presence of fungal hyphae. (The KOH preparation is described in Appendix 5 on thePoint.) Dermatophytes can be cultured on various media, including Sabouraud dextrose agar. Moulds are identified using a combination of macroscopic and microscopic observations (refer back to Chapter 13).

Fungal Infections of the Respiratory System

Infections of the Lower Respiratory Tract Having Multiple Causes

Information pertaining to infections of the lower respiratory tract having multiple causes is contained in Chapter 19.

Fungal Infections of the Lower Respiratory Tract

Table 20-1 contains information pertaining to fungal infections of the lower respiratory tract. Although they are not included in Table 20-1, moulds in the genera *Aspergillus* (Fig. 20-4) and *Penicillium* are also common causes of lower respiratory infections, especially in immunosuppressed patients. Infection is usually the result of inhalation of spores. In addition to the lungs, invasive aspergillosis can affect the sinuses, eyes, heart, kidneys, skin, and other organs. Infection with *Penicillium* spp.—penicilliosis—is usually a disseminated disease, involving the lungs, liver, and skin.

Fungal Infections of the Oral Region

Thrush

Disease. Thrush is a yeast infection of the oral cavity. It is common in infants, elderly patients, and immunosuppressed individuals. White, creamy patches occur on the tongue, mucous membranes, and the corners of the mouth (Fig. 20-5). Thrush can be a manifestation of disseminated *Candida* infection (candidiasis). *Candida albicans* is the yeast and the fungus most commonly isolated from clinical specimens—sometimes isolated as a pathogen and sometimes as a contaminant.

> *Candida albicans* is the yeast and the fungus most commonly isolated from clinical specimens.

Table 20-1 Fungal Infections of the Lower Respiratory Tract

Disease	Additional Information
Coccidioidomycosis (Valley Fever). Coccidioidomycosis starts as a respiratory infection, with fever, chills, cough, and, rarely, pain. The primary infection may heal completely or may progress to the disseminated form of the disease, which is often fatal. Disseminated coccidioidomycosis may include lung lesions and abscesses throughout the body, especially in subcutaneous tissues, skin, bone, and the central nervous system. Other tissues and organs, such as inguinal lymph nodes, kidneys, thyroid gland, heart, pituitary gland, esophagus, and pancreas, may also be involved. **Patient Care.** Use Standard Precautions for hospitalized patients with draining lesions or pneumonia.	**Pathogen.** Coccidioidomycosis is caused by *Coccidioides immitis*, a dimorphic fungus. It exists as a mould in soil and on culture media (25°C), where it produces arthrospores (arthroconidia). In tissues, it appears as spherical yeast cells called spherules that reproduce by endospore formation. *C. immitis* arthrospores have potential use as a bioterrorist agent. **Reservoirs and Mode of Transmission.** Arthrospores are present in soil in arid and semiarid areas of the Western Hemisphere; in the United States, from California to southern Texas; and in Mexico, Central America, and South America. Transmission occurs by inhalation of arthrospores, especially during wind and dust storms. It is not directly transmissible person to person or animal to person. **Laboratory Diagnosis.** Coccidioidomycosis is diagnosed by direct examination and culturing of sputum, pus, urine, cerebrospinal fluid, or biopsy materials. The mould form is highly infectious. All work must be performed in a biosafety level (BSL)-2 or BSL-3 facility (refer to Appendix 4 on thePoint). Skin tests, molecular diagnostic procedures, and immunodiagnostic procedures are also available.
Cryptococcosis. Cryptococcosis starts as a lung infection, but usually spreads via the bloodstream to the brain. The disease is described later in the chapter, in the section entitled "Fungal Infections of the Central Nervous System."	
Histoplasmosis. Histoplasmosis is a systemic mycosis of varying severity, ranging from asymptomatic to acute to chronic. The primary lesion is usually in the lungs. The acute disease involves malaise, fever, chills, headache, myalgia, chest pains, and a nonproductive cough (i.e., sputum is not produced). Histoplasmosis is the most common systemic fungal infection in AIDS patients. **Patient Care.** Use Standard Precautions for hospitalized patients.	**Pathogen.** Histoplasmosis is caused by *Histoplasma capsulatum* var. *capsulatum*, a dimorphic fungus that grows as a mould in soil and as a yeast in animal and human hosts (refer back to Fig. 5-18 in Chapter 5). **Reservoirs and Mode of Transmission.** Reservoirs include warm, moist soil containing a high organic content and bird droppings, especially chicken droppings, but also bat droppings in caves and around starling, blackbird, and pigeon roosts. Transmission occurs via inhalation of conidia (asexual spores) from soil. Bulldozing and excavation may produce aerosols of spores. Histoplasmosis is the most common systemic fungal disease in the United States, occurring primarily in the Ohio, Mississippi, and Missouri River valleys. Histoplasmosis is not transmitted from person to person. **Laboratory Diagnosis.** *H. capsulatum* yeasts may be observed in Giemsa- or Wright-stained smears of ulcer exudates, bone marrow, sputum, and blood. *H. capsulatum* produces mould colonies when incubated at room temperature and yeast colonies when incubated at body temperature. Conversion from the mould form to the yeast form can sometimes be accomplished in the laboratory. Skin tests and immunodiagnostic procedures are available.

(continued)

Table 20-1 Fungal Infections of the Lower Respiratory Tract (Continued)

Disease	Additional Information
Pneumocystis Carinii Pneumonia (PCP, Interstitial Plasma-Cell Pneumonia). PCP is an acute-to-subacute pulmonary disease found in malnourished, chronically ill children; premature infants; and immunosuppressed patients, such as those with AIDS. Patients have fever, difficulty in breathing, rapid breathing, dry cough, cyanosis, and pulmonary infiltration of alveoli with frothy exudate. PCP is usually fatal in untreated immunosuppressed patients. It is a common contributory cause of death in AIDS patients. *Pneumocystis* causes an asymptomatic infection in immunocompetent people. **Patient Care.** Use Standard Precautions for hospitalized patients. Do not place PCP patients in the same room with an immunocompromised patient.	**Pathogen.** The etiologic agent of PCP is *Pneumocystis jiroveci* (formerly *P. carinii*). This organism has both protozoal and fungal properties. It was classified as a protozoan for many years, but is currently classified as a nonfilamentous fungus. **Reservoirs and Mode of Transmission.** Infected humans serve as reservoirs. The mode of transmission is unknown—perhaps direct contact, perhaps transfer of pulmonary secretions from infected to susceptible persons, perhaps airborne. **Laboratory Diagnosis.** Diagnosis of PCP is made by demonstration of *Pneumocystis* in material from bronchial brushings, open lung biopsy, lung aspirates, or smears of tracheobronchial mucus by various staining methods. *P. jiroveci* cannot be cultured.
Pulmonary Zygomycosis. The term *zygomycosis* (formerly mucormycosis or phycomycosis) refers to a disease caused by one of the many fungi in the class Zygomycetes. These fungi are widely distributed in soil and vegetative matter. Although being discussed in the section on lower respiratory diseases, these fungi cause diseases with a wide range of clinical manifestations. Other clinical syndromes caused by members of the Zygomycetes class include sinusitis, cerebral infection, cutaneous disease, gastrointestinal disease, and disseminated disease, which involve virtually every organ. **Patient Care.** Use Standard Precautions.	**Pathogens.** Many different fungi can cause zygomycosis, including some that are often referred to as bread moulds. These fungi, which include species of *Mucor*, *Rhizopus*, and *Absidia*, are responsible for the white or gray fuzzy growth seen on foods such as bread and cheese. The fuzziness is the result of aerial hyphae. **Reservoirs and Modes of Transmission.** Most commonly, humans become infected with zygomycetes by inhaling airborne spores, although ingestion and direct inoculation through traumatic breaks in the skin and mucous membranes can also lead to infection. Zygomycosis is not transmitted from person to person. **Laboratory Diagnosis.** Diagnosis of zygomycosis can be made by microscopic observation of distinctive, ribbon-like, broad, aseptate hyphae in tissue sections and by culture of biopsy tissue (see Fig. 13-16 in Chapter 13).

- Coccidioidomycosis is caused by a dimorphic fungus named *C. immitis*.
- Histoplasmosis is caused by a dimorphic fungus named *H. capsulatum*.
- Pneumocystis pneumonia is caused by a nonfilamentous fungus named *P. jiroveci*.

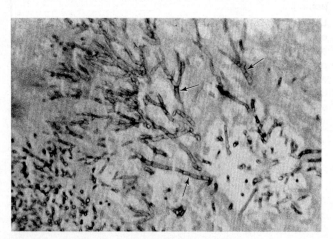

Figure 20-4. Tissue invasion by an *Aspergillus* species, showing many branching septate hyphae (arrows). (From Engleberg NC, et al. *Schaechter's Mechanisms of Microbial Disease*. 5th ed. Philadelphia, PA: Lippincott Williams & Wilkins; 2013.)

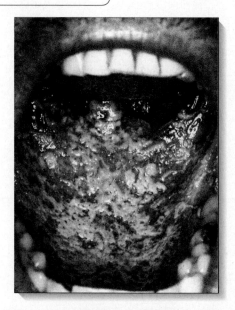

Figure 20-5. Oral candidiasis (thrush). (From Harvey RA, et al. *Lippincott's Illustrated Reviews: Microbiology*. 3rd ed. Philadelphia, PA: Lippincott Williams & Wilkins; 2013.)

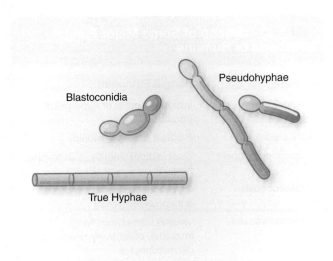

Figure 20-6. Various forms of *Candida* yeasts that can be seen in clinical specimens and cultures.

Pathogens. The yeast, *C. albicans* and related species.

Reservoir and Mode of Transmission. Infected humans serve as reservoirs. Transmission occurs by contact with secretions or excretions of mouth, skin, vagina, or feces of patients or carriers; also by passage from mother to neonate during childbirth and by endogenous spread (i.e., from one area of the body to another).

Laboratory Diagnosis. Thrush can be diagnosed by

> Thrush is a yeast infection (most often a *Candida* infection) of the oral cavity.

observation of yeast cells (blastoconidia) and pseudohyphae (strings of elongated buds) in microscopic examination of wet mounts, and by culture confirmation (Fig. 20-6).

Fungal Infections of the Genitourinary System

Yeast Vaginitis
Disease. The three most common causes of vaginitis in the United States, each causing about one-third of the cases, are *Candida albicans* (a yeast), *Trichomonas vaginalis* (a protozoan), and a mixture

> *Candida albicans* causes approximately one-third of the cases of vaginitis in the United States.

of bacteria (including bacteria in the genera *Mobiluncus* and *Gardnerella*). A saline wet mount preparation is usually used to diagnose vaginitis; this test procedure is described in Appendix 5 on thePoint. Typical symptoms of yeast vaginitis are vulvar pruritis (itching), a burning sensation, dysuria, and a white discharge. Vulvar erythema (redness) and rash sometimes occur.

Pathogens. The yeast, *C. albicans*, causes about 85% to 90% of yeast vaginitis; other *Candida* spp. can also cause this disease.

Reservoir and Mode of Transmission. (See previous section on "Thrush.")

Laboratory Diagnosis. Yeast vaginitis can be diagnosed by microscopic examination of a saline wet mount of vaginal discharge material, in which yeasts and hyphae may be observed. The vaginal discharge material should also be cultured. *Candida* spp. grow well on blood agar and Sabouraud dextrose agar. *Candida* spp. can usually be identified using a commercial yeast identification minisystem. It is important to keep in mind that the vaginal microbiota of up to 25% of healthy women can contain *Candida* spp.

Fungal Infections of the Circulatory System

Fungal endocarditis is rare, but cases of *Candida* and *Aspergillus* endocarditis do occur.

Fungal Infections of the Central Nervous System

Cryptococcosis (Cryptococcal Meningitis)
Disease. Cryptococcosis starts as a lung infection, but spreads via the bloodstream to the brain. It usually presents as a subacute or chronic meningitis. Infection of the lungs, kidneys, prostate, skin, and bone may also occur. Cryptococcosis is a common infection in acquired immunodeficiency syndrome (AIDS) patients.

Patient Care. Use Standard Precautions for hospitalized patients.

Pathogens. Cryptococcosis can be caused by three subspecies of *Cryptococcus neoformans*, an encapsulated yeast (refer back to Fig. 5-12 in Chapter 5). The capsule enables *C. neoformans* to adhere to mucosal surfaces and avoid phagocytosis by white blood cells.

> Cryptococcosis is caused by an encapsulated yeast named *Cryptococcus neoformans*.

Reservoirs and Modes of Transmission. Reservoirs include pigeon nests; pigeon, chicken, turkey, and bat droppings; and soil contaminated with bird droppings. Growth of *C. neoformans* is stimulated by the alkaline pH and high nitrogen content of bird droppings. Transmission occurs by inhalation of yeasts, often projected into the air by sweeping or excavation. *Cryptococcus* is not transmitted from person to person or animal to person.

Laboratory Diagnosis. Cryptococcal meningitis is often diagnosed by observing encapsulated, budding yeasts in cerebrospinal fluid specimens examined by an India ink preparation. (Details of the India ink preparation can be found in Appendix 5 on thePoint; "Clinical Microbiology Laboratory Procedures.") Yeasts may also be observed in sputum, urine, and pus examined by an India ink preparation or Gram stain (refer back to Fig. 5-15). *C. neoformans* can be cultured on routine media used in the Mycology Section. A sensitive cryptococcal antigen detection test is available.

STUDY AID

Beware of Similar Sounding Names

Do not confuse *Cryptococcus neoformans* (a yeast) with *Cryptosporidium parvum* (a protozoan). Likewise, do not confuse **cryptococcosis** (a yeast infection) with **cryptosporidiosis** (a protozoan infection). *C. parvum* and cryptosporidiosis are described in Chapter 21.

Recap of Major Fungal Infections of Humans

Table 20-2 provides a recap of some major fungal infections of humans.

Appropriate Therapy for Fungal Infections

Recommendations for the treatment of infectious diseases change frequently. The fungal diseases described in this chapter must be treated using appropriate antifungal drugs. Additional information about antifungal agents can be found in Chapter 9 and at en.wikipedia.org/wiki/Antifungal_medication.

Table 20-2 Recap of Some Major Fungal Infections of Humans

Disease	Fungal Pathogen
Aspergillosis	Various species of *Aspergillus* (moulds)
Black piedra	*Piedraia hortae* (a mould)
Coccidioidomycosis	*Coccidioides immitis* (a dimorphic fungus)
Cryptococcosis	*Cryptococcus neoformans* (an encapsulated yeast)
Dermatomycoses	Various filamentous fungi (moulds), collectively referred to as dermatophytes
Histoplasmosis	*Histoplasma capsulatum* (a dimorphic fungus)
Penicilliosis	Various species of *Penicillium* (moulds)
Pneumocystis pneumonia	*Pneumocystis jiroveci* (formerly *Pneumocystis carinii*) (a nonfilamentous fungus having both protozoal and fungal properties)
Sporotrichosis	*Sporothrix schenckii* (a dimorphic fungus)
Tinea nigra	*Hortaea werneckii* (a mould)
Tinea versicolor (pityriasis versicolor)	*Malassezia furfur* (a mould)
Thrush	*Candida albicans* (a yeast)
White piedra	Usually caused by *Trichosporon beigelii* (a mould)
Yeast vaginitis	*C. albicans* (a yeast)
Zygomycosis (mucormycosis, phycomycosis)	Various zygomycetes, including bread moulds

ON thePoint

- Terms Introduced in this Chapter
- Review of Key Points
- Increase Your Knowledge
- Additional Self-Assessment Exercises

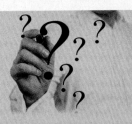

Self-Assessment Exercises

After you have read this chapter, answer the following multiple-choice questions.

1. Which of the following diseases is caused by an encapsulated yeast?

    a. Coccidioidomycosis
    b. Cryptococcosis
    c. Histoplasmosis
    d. Pneumocystis pneumonia

2. Which of the following diseases is *not* caused by a dimorphic fungus?

    a. Coccidioidomycosis
    b. Cryptococcosis
    c. Histoplasmosis
    d. Sporotrichosis

3. Which of the following diseases is a synonym for ringworm infection of the nails?

    a. Tinea barbae
    b. Tinea cruris
    c. Tinea nigra
    d. Tinea unguium

4. Which of the following is the most common systemic fungal disease in the United States?

    a. Cryptococcosis
    b. Coccidioidomycosis
    c. Histoplasmosis
    d. Pneumocystis pneumonia

5. One should associate the India ink preparation with diagnosis of which of the following?

    a. Cryptococcal meningitis
    b. Thrush
    c. Tinea pedis
    d. Yeast vaginitis

6. Bread moulds are most commonly associated with which of the following diseases?

    a. Thrush
    b. Tinea versicolor
    c. Vaginitis
    d. Zygomycosis

7. Which of the following is the fungus most often isolated from human clinical specimens?

    a. *Candida albicans*
    b. *C. neoformans*
    c. *Histoplasma capsulatum*
    d. *Pneumocystis jiroveci*

8. Which of the following methods is the quickest and most common way to diagnose yeast vaginitis?

    a. Culture
    b. India ink preparation
    c. KOH preparation
    d. Saline wet mount

9. In the United States, *C. albicans* causes approximately _____ of the cases of vaginitis.

    a. 10%
    b. 25%
    c. 33%
    d. 50%

10. Tinea cruris is a ringworm infection of which of these body sites?

    a. Feet
    b. Groin area
    c. Nails
    d. Palms of the hands

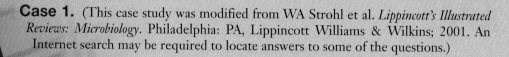

Case 1. (This case study was modified from WA Strohl et al. *Lippincott's Illustrated Reviews: Microbiology*. Philadelphia: PA, Lippincott Williams & Wilkins; 2001. An Internet search may be required to locate answers to some of the questions.)

A 68-year-old woman was admitted because of headaches of about one month's duration. She also complained of vertigo, photophobia, drowsiness, and forgetfulness. Physical examination revealed a slight fever, stiff neck, crackles (a crackling noise) in her lungs, and a tendency to overreach objects. Because of the signs of meningeal irritation, a lumbar puncture was performed. The patient was also found to have malignant lymphoma. She had an elevated peripheral white blood cell (WBC) count. A chest X-ray revealed diffuse interstitial infiltrates of both lower lungs. The CSF examination revealed the presence of WBCs, a decreased glucose level, and a slightly increased protein level. While performing the WBC count, the technician noticed spherical objects that did not resemble WBCs. These objects ranged from 10 to 20 µm in diameter.

A. Based upon the available information, which of the following causes of meningitis should be suspected?

1. *Cryptococcus neoformans*
2. *Haemophilus influenzae*
3. *Neisseria meningitidis*
4. *Streptococcus pneumoniae*
5. *Escherichia coli*

B. If this pathogen is suspected of being the cause of the patient's meningitis, what test should be performed next on the CSF?

C. If this pathogen is the cause of the patient's meningitis, what should be observed when an India ink preparation is examined?

D. Should this pathogen also be suspected of being the cause of the patient's pulmonary infection?

Case 2. A 14-year-old, immunosuppressed, female patient presents with white, creamy patches on her tongue, oral mucous membranes, and the corners of her mouth.

A. What is the most likely name of her condition?

1. White piedra
2. Tinea versicolor
3. Thrush
4. Zygomycosis
5. Coccidioidomycosis

B. Of the fungi listed below, which one is the most likely cause?

1. *Cryptococcus neoformans*
2. *Histoplasma capsulatum*
3. *Pneumocystis jiroveci*
4. *Candida albicans*
5. *Trichosporon beigelii*

Case 3. A 40-year-old, male, AIDS patient, who spends a great deal of his time exploring caves, presents with malaise, fever, chills, headache, myalgia, chest pains, and a nonproductive cough.

A. Based upon this limited information, which of the following fungal diseases does this patient most likely have?

1. Coccidioidomycosis
2. Histoplasmosis
3. Cryptococcosis
4. Sporotrichosis
5. Zygomycosis

B. If your preliminary diagnosis is correct, what would most likely be observed in a sputum specimen from this patient?

1. Broad, aseptate hyphae
2. Encapsulated, budding yeasts
3. Nonencapsulated, budding yeasts
4. Pseudohyphae
5. Thin, septate hyphae

(Answers to Case Studies can be found in Appendix B.)

21

Parasitic Infections of Humans

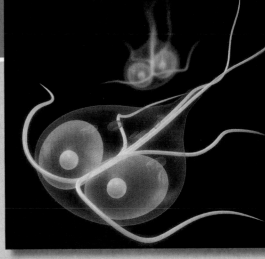

Artist rendering of *Giardia lamblia*, a pathogenic protozoan.

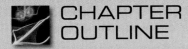

CHAPTER OUTLINE

Introduction

Definitions

How Parasites Cause Disease

Parasitic Protozoa

Protozoal Infections of Humans

Protozoal Infections of the Skin
  Leishmaniasis
Protozoal Infections of the Eyes
Protozoal Infections of the Gastrointestinal Tract
Protozoal Infections of the Genitourinary Tract
  Trichomoniasis
Protozoal Infections of the Circulatory System
Protozoal Infections of the Central Nervous System
  Primary Amebic Meningoencephalitis

Helminths

Helminth Infections of Humans

Appropriate Therapy for Parasitic Infections

Medically Important Arthropods

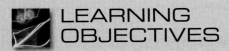

LEARNING OBJECTIVES

After studying this chapter, you should be able to:

- Differentiate between the following: ectoparasites versus endoparasites; definitive hosts versus intermediate hosts; facultative parasites versus obligate parasites; and mechanical vectors versus biologic vectors

- Classify a particular parasitic infection as a protozoal or helminth disease
- Categorize various parasitic infections by body system (e.g., respiratory system, gastrointestinal tract, circulatory system)
- Correlate a particular parasitic infection (e.g., giardiasis) with its major characteristics, causative agent, reservoir(s), mode(s) of transmission, and diagnostic laboratory procedures

> *So, naturalists observe, a flea*
> *Hath smaller fleas that on him prey*
> *And these have smaller still to bite 'em;*
> *And so proceed ad infinitum.*

from Poetry, a Rhapsody, 1733
by Jonathan Swift (1667–1745)

Introduction

Although parasitology (the study of parasites) is considered a branch of microbiology, not all organisms studied in a parasitology course are microbes. In fact, of the three categories of organisms (parasitic protozoa, helminths, and arthropods) that are studied in a parasitology course, only one category—parasitic protozoa—contains microbes. Therefore, in this chapter, parasitic protozoa are discussed in greater detail than are helminths and arthropods.

It would be impossible in a book of this size to describe *all* of the human infectious diseases caused by parasites. Thus, only selected parasitic diseases are described in this chapter. Although these diseases are described in one particular section of the chapter (e.g., under gastrointestinal infections), readers should keep in mind that some parasitic diseases have various clinical manifestations, affecting several body systems simultaneously, and that the pathogens may move from one body site to another.

Nationally Notifiable Parasitic Diseases

Parasitic Disease	No. of New U.S. Cases Reported to the CDC in 2010[a]
Cryptosporidiosis	8,944
Cyclosporiasis	179
Giardiasis	19,811
Malaria	1,773
Trichinellosis	7

Source: http://www.cdc.gov.

[a]These figures provide insight regarding how common or rare these diseases are in the United States. For updated information, go to the CDC web site; click on "Morbidity & Mortality Weekly Report"; then click on "Notifiable Diseases"; then click on the most recent year that is listed.

Certain of the parasitic diseases described in this chapter are nationally notifiable infectious diseases, meaning that when a patient is diagnosed with one of these diseases in the United States, the information must be reported to the Centers for Disease Control and Prevention (CDC). As of 2010, there were five nationally notifiable parasitic diseases–four protozoal diseases and one helminth disease (see Table 21-1). These diseases are described in this chapter, as are some parasitic diseases that are not nationally notifiable.

Definitions

Parasitism is a symbiotic relationship that is of benefit to one party or symbiont (the parasite) at the expense of the other party (the **host**). Although many parasites cause disease, some do not. Even if a parasite is not causing disease, it is depriving the host of nutrients; therefore, parasitic relationships are always considered detrimental to the host.

Parasites are defined as organisms that live *on* or *in* other living organisms (hosts), at whose expense they gain some advantage. In addition to parasites of humans, there are many types of plant parasites (i.e., parasites of plants) and many types of animal parasites (i.e., parasites of animals).

Parasites that live outside the host's body are referred to as **ectoparasites**, whereas those living inside the host are called **endoparasites**. Arthropods such as mites, ticks, and lice are examples of ectoparasites. Parasitic protozoa and helminths are examples of endoparasites.

> Parasites are organisms that live on or in other living organisms, at whose expense they gain some advantage.

> Parasites that live outside the host's body are ectoparasites; those that live inside the host are endoparasites.

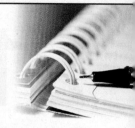
The life cycle of a particular parasite may involve one or more hosts. If more than one host is involved, the **definitive host** is the one that harbors the adult or sexual stage of the parasite or the sexual phase of the life cycle. The **intermediate host** harbors the larval or asexual stage of the parasite or the asexual phase of the life cycle. Parasite life cycles range from simple to complex. There are one-, two-, and three-host parasites. Knowing the life cycle of a particular parasite enables epidemiologists and other healthcare professionals to control the parasitic infection through intervention at some point in the life cycle. In addition, parasitic infections are most often diagnosed by observing and recognizing a particular life cycle stage in a clinical specimen.

> The definitive host harbors the adult or sexual stage of the parasite or the sexual phase of the parasite's life cycle. The intermediate host harbors the larval or asexual stage of the parasite or the asexual phase of its life cycle.

An **accidental host** is a living organism that can serve as a host in a particular parasite's life cycle, but is not a *usual* host in that life cycle. Some accidental hosts are **dead-end hosts**, from which the parasite cannot continue its life cycle.

A **facultative parasite** is an organism that can be parasitic but does not have to live as a parasite. It is capable of living an independent life, apart from a host. The free-living amebae that can cause keratoconjunctivitis and primary amebic meningoencephalitis (PAM) are examples of facultative parasites. An **obligate parasite**, on the

> Facultative parasites are organisms that can be parasitic but are also capable of a free-living existence. Obligate parasites have no choice; to survive, they must be parasitic.

other hand, has no choice; to survive, it must be a parasite. Most parasites that infect humans are obligate parasites.

Parasitology is the study of parasites, and a **parasitologist** is someone who studies parasites. As previously stated, any upper-division or graduate-level parasitology course would be divided into three areas of study: the study of parasitic protozoa, of helminths, and of arthropods.

Medical parasitology is the study of parasites that cause human disease. The overall responsibility of the Parasitology Section of the Clinical Microbiology Laboratory is to assist clinicians in the diagnosis of parasitic diseases—primarily, parasitic diseases caused by endoparasites such as parasitic protozoa and helminths.

In general, parasitic infections are diagnosed by observing and recognizing various parasite life cycle stages in clinical specimens. Some life cycle stages (e.g., amebic cysts and *Cryptosporidium* oocysts) are extremely small. Finding them in specimens represents one of the greatest challenges faced by clinical microbiologists.

> In general, parasitic infections are diagnosed by observing and recognizing various parasite life cycle stages in clinical specimens.

How Parasites Cause Disease

The manner in which parasites cause damage to their host varies from one species of parasite to another, and often depends on the number of parasites that are present. For helminths, the number that are present is often referred to as the "worm burden." Some parasites produce toxins, some produce harmful enzymes, some invasive and migratory parasites cause physical damage to tissues and organs, some cause the destruction of individual cells, and some cause occlusion of blood vessels and other tubular structures. Some parasites interfere with vital processes of the host, whereas others deprive their host of essential nutrients. In some cases, the host immune response to the presence of parasites or their products causes more injury than do the parasites themselves.

Parasitic Protozoa

In the five-kingdom system of classification of living organisms, protozoa are in the kingdom Protista, together with algae. Some taxonomists prefer to place them in a kingdom by themselves—the kingdom Protozoa. Most protozoa are unicellular, but some are multicellular (colonial). Protozoa can be classified taxonomically by their mode of locomotion. **Amebas** (amebae) move by means of pseudopodia

> Protozoa can be classified taxonomically by their mode of locomotion. Some move by pseudopodia, others by flagella, others by cilia, and some are nonmotile.

(literally, "false feet"). **Flagellates** move by means of whiplike flagella. **Ciliates** move by means of hairlike cilia. Protozoa classified as *Sporozoa* (sporozoans) have no pseudopodia, flagella, or cilia, and therefore exhibit no motility.

Not all protozoa are parasitic. For example, many of the pond water protozoa (e.g., *Paramecium* and *Stentor* spp.) studied in introductory biology and microbiology courses are not parasites; some are pictured in Chapter 5. Although most protozoal parasites of humans are obligate parasites, some are facultative parasites—capable of a free-living, nonparasitic existence, but also able to become parasites when they accidentally gain entrance to the body. *Acanthamoeba* spp. and *Naegleria fowleri* are examples of facultative parasites. These free-living amebas normally reside in soil or water, but can cause serious diseases when they gain entrance to the eyes or the nasal mucosa. From the nasal mucosa, they travel via the olfactory nerve into the brain and cause diseases affecting the central nervous system (CNS).

Because protozoa are tiny, protozoal infections are most often diagnosed by microscopic examination of body fluids, tissue specimens, or feces. Peripheral blood smears are usually stained with Giemsa stain, whereas fecal specimens are stained with trichrome, iron hematoxylin, or acid-fast stains. Most parasitic protozoal infections are diagnosed by observing trophozoites, cysts, oocysts, or spores in the specimen.

The *trophozoite* is the motile, feeding, dividing stage in a protozoan's life cycle, whereas cysts, oocysts, and spores are dormant stages (much like bacterial spores). Protozoal infections are primarily acquired by ingestion or inhalation of cysts, oocysts, or spores, or injection via the bite of an infected arthropod. Because of their fragile nature, only rarely do trophozoites serve as the infective stages.

> The trophozoite is the motile, feeding, dividing stage in the protozoal life cycle, and the cyst, oocyst, and spore are dormant stages. Protozoal infections are most often acquired by ingestion or inhalation of dormant stages or by injection via the bite of an infected arthropod.

Protozoal Infections of Humans

Protozoal Infections of the Skin

Leishmaniasis
Disease. There are three forms of leishmaniasis: cutaneous, mucocutaneous (or mucosal), and visceral. The cutaneous form starts with a papule that enlarges into a craterlike ulcer (Fig. 21-1). Individual ulcers may coalesce, causing severe tissue destruction and disfigurement. Visceral leishmaniasis, also known as kala-azar, is characterized by fever, enlarged liver and spleen, lymphadenopathy, anemia, leukopenia, and progressive emaciation and weakness. Death may result in untreated cases.

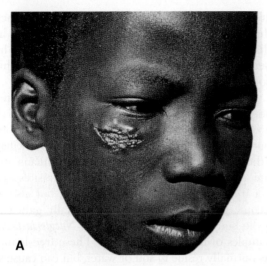
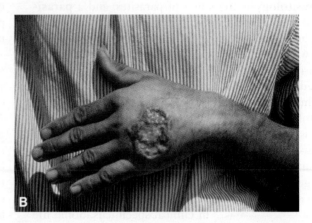

Figure 21-1. Patients with cutaneous leishmaniasis. ([A] From Binford CH, Connor DH. *Pathology of Tropical and Extraordinary Diseases*. vol. 1. Washington, DC: Armed Forces Institute of Pathology; 1976. **[B]** Courtesy of Dr. DS Martin and the CDC.)

Patient Care. Use Standard Precautions for hospitalized patients.

Geographic Occurrence. Leishmaniasis occurs in many regions of the world, including Pakistan, India, China, the Middle East, Africa, South and Central America, and Mexico. Cases have also occurred in south central Texas. It is estimated that between 1.5 and 2 million people have leishmaniasis and that about 57,000 people die each year of the disease.

> Leishmaniasis is caused by various species of flagellated protozoa and is usually transmitted via the bite of an infected sand fly.

Parasites. Leishmaniasis is caused by various species of flagellated protozoa in the genus *Leishmania*. The nonmotile, intracellular form of the parasite is called an *amastigote*. The motile, extracellular form of the parasite is called a *promastigote*.

Reservoirs and Mode of Transmission. Reservoirs include infected humans, domestic dogs, and various wild animals. Leishmaniasis is principally a zoonosis and is usually transmitted via the bite of an infected sand fly. Transmission by blood transfusion and person-to-person contact have been reported.

Laboratory Diagnosis. Diagnosis of cutaneous and mucocutaneous leishmaniasis is made by microscopic identification of the amastigote form in stained preparations from lesions or by culture of the extracellular promastigote form on suitable media. Culture is rarely performed in clinical microbiology laboratories. In stained preparations, amastigotes are seen within macrophages and close to disrupted cells. An intradermal test,

called the Montenegro test, and immunodiagnostic and molecular diagnostic procedures are also available. In the Montenegro test, an antigen derived from promastigotes is injected into the skin.

Protozoal Infections of the Eyes

Protozoal infections of the eyes include conjunctivitis and keratoconjunctivitis (inflammation of the cornea and conjunctiva), caused by amebas in the genus *Acanthamoeba*, and toxoplasmosis, caused by the sporozoan, *Toxoplasma gondii*. Although toxoplasmosis is described in this section of the chapter, there are many manifestations of toxoplasmosis in addition to ocular disease. Ocular manifestations of toxoplasmosis occur primarily in immunosuppressed patients, in whom the infection can lead to removal of the infected eyeball (enucleation). Amebic conjunctivitis and keratoconjunctivitis can also result in enucleation. Table 21-2 contains information about these diseases.

Protozoal Infections of the Gastrointestinal Tract

Of the many protozoal infections of the gastrointestinal tract, only amebiasis, balantidiasis, cryptosporidiosis, cyclosporiasis, and giardiasis are discussed here. As previously mentioned, the latter three diseases are nationally notifiable infectious diseases in the United States. Figure 21-2 and Table 21-3 contain information about protozoal infections of the gastrointestinal tract.

> The largest waterborne outbreak ever to occur in the United States was caused by *Cryptosporidium parvum*, a protozoan parasite.

Table 21-2 Protozoal Infections of the Eyes

Disease	Additional Information
Ambic Eye Infections. Amebic conjunctivitis and keratoconjunctivitis are amebic infections causing inflammation of the conjunctiva, corneal ulcers, pus formation, and severe pain. These infections can lead to loss of vision. The disease process is more rapid if corneal abrasions are present. **Patient Care.** Use Standard Precautions for hospitalized patients. **Geographic Occurrence.** Amebic eye infections occur in many countries on all continents.	**Parasites.** Amebic eye infections are caused by several species of amebas in the genus *Acanthamoeba*. Because these amebas are capable of either a free-living or a parasitic existence, they are referred to as facultative parasites. **Reservoirs and Mode of Transmission.** The amebas enter the eye from ameba-contaminated waters. Infections have occurred primarily in people who wear soft contact lenses and have used nonsterile, homemade cleaning or wetting solutions, or have become infected in ameba-contaminated spas or hot tubs. **Laboratory Diagnosis.** Amebic eye infections are diagnosed by microscopic examination of scrapings, swabs, or aspirates of the eye, or by culture on media seeded with *Escherichia coli* or another member of the family *Enterobacteriaceae*. The bacteria on the media serve as food for the amebas.
Toxoplasmosis. Toxoplasmosis is a systemic sporozoan infection that, in immunocompetent persons, may be asymptomatic or resemble infectious mononucleosis. However, serious disease, even death, may occur in immunodeficient persons. Disease typically involves the CNS, eyes (chorioretinitis), lungs, muscles, or heart. Cerebral toxoplasmosis is common in AIDS patients. Infection during early pregnancy may lead to fetal infection, causing death of the fetus or serious birth defects (e.g., brain damage). **Patient Care.** Use Standard Precautions for hospitalized patients. **Geographic Occurrence.** Toxoplasmosis occurs worldwide.	**Parasite.** Toxoplasmosis is caused by *Toxoplasma gondii*, an intracellular sporozoan. **Reservoirs and Mode of Transmission.** Definitive hosts include cats and other felines that usually acquire infection by eating infected rodents or birds. Intermediate hosts include rodents, birds, sheep, goats, swine, and cattle. Humans usually become infected by eating infected raw or undercooked meat (usually pork or mutton) containing the cyst form of the parasite or by ingesting oocysts that have been shed in the feces of infected cats. Oocysts may be present in food or water contaminated by feline feces. Children may ingest oocysts from sand boxes containing cat feces. Infection can also be acquired transplacentally, by blood transfusion, or by organ transplantation. **Laboratory Diagnosis.** Toxoplasmosis is typically diagnosed using immunodiagnostic procedures. Other diagnostic methods include demonstration of the parasite in stained body tissues or fluids obtained by biopsy or necropsy; and isolation of *T. gondii* using laboratory animals or cell culture.

Protozoal Infections of the Genitourinary Tract

Trichomoniasis

Disease. Trichomoniasis is a sexually transmitted protozoal disease affecting both men and women. The disease is usually symptomatic in women, causing vaginitis with a profuse, thin, foamy, malodorous, greenish-yellowish discharge. It has been estimated that trichomoniasis accounts for approximately one-third of the cases of vaginitis in the United States (another third

> Trichomoniasis is caused by a flagellated protozoan named *Trichomonas vaginalis* and is transmitted by direct contact with vaginal and urethral discharges of infected people. Trichomoniasis is usually symptomatic in females and asymptomatic in males.

is caused by *Candida albicans*, and another third by bacteria). In women, trichomoniasis may also present as urethritis or cystitis. Although rarely symptomatic in men, trichomoniasis may lead to prostatitis, urethritis, or infection of the seminal vesicles. Persons with trichomoniasis often also have other sexually transmitted diseases, especially gonorrhea.

Patient Care. Use Standard Precautions.

Geographic Occurrence. Trichomoniasis occurs worldwide.

Parasite. Trichomoniasis is caused by *Trichomonas vaginalis*, a flagellate.

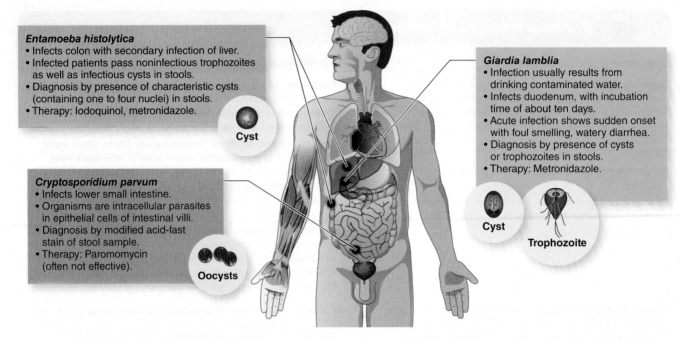

Entamoeba histolytica
- Infects colon with secondary infection of liver.
- Infected patients pass noninfectious trophozoites as well as infectious cysts in stools.
- Diagnosis by presence of characteristic cysts (containing one to four nuclei) in stools.
- Therapy: Iodoquinol, metronidazole.

Cyst

Giardia lamblia
- Infection usually results from drinking contaminated water.
- Infects duodenum, with incubation time of about ten days.
- Acute infection shows sudden onset with foul smelling, watery diarrhea.
- Diagnosis by presence of cysts or trophozoites in stools.
- Therapy: Metronidazole.

Cyst   Trophozoite

Cryptosporidium parvum
- Infects lower small intestine.
- Organisms are intracellular parasites in epithelial cells of intestinal villi.
- Diagnosis by modified acid-fast stain of stool sample.
- Therapy: Paromomycin (often not effective).

Oocysts

Figure 21-2. Three protozoal infections of the gastrointestinal tract. (Redrawn from Harvey RA, et al. *Lippincott's Illustrated Reviews: Microbiology*. 2nd ed. Philadelphia, PA: Lippincott Williams & Wilkins; 2007.)

Table 21-3 Protozoal Infections of the Gastrointestinal Tract

Disease	Additional Information
Amebiasis. Amebiasis or amebic dysentery is a protozoal gastrointestinal infection that may be asymptomatic, mild, or severe and is often accompanied by dysentery, fever, chills, bloody or mucoid diarrhea or constipation, and colitis. The amebas may invade mucous membranes of the colon, forming abscesses and amebomas, which are granulomas that are sometimes mistaken for carcinoma. Amebas may also be disseminated via the bloodstream to extraintestinal sites, leading to abscesses of the liver, lung, brain, and other organs. Depending on their location, untreated extraintestinal amebic abscesses can be fatal. **Patient Care.** Use Standard Precautions for hospitalized patients. **Geographic Occurrence.** Amebiasis occurs worldwide.	**Parasite.** Amebiasis is caused by *Entamoeba histolytica*. Like all amebas, *E. histolytica* has two stages: the cyst stage, which is the dormant, infective stage, and the motile, metabolically active, reproducing trophozoite stage. **Reservoirs and Mode of Transmission.** Reservoirs include symptomatic and asymptomatic humans and fecally contaminated food or water. Transmission occurs in one of several ways: (a) via ingestion of fecally contaminated food or water containing cysts, (b) by flies transporting cysts from feces to food, (c) via the fecally soiled hands of infected food handlers, (d) by oral–anal sexual contact, or (e) by anal intercourse involving multiple sex partners. **Laboratory Diagnosis.** Amebic dysentery is diagnosed by microscopic observation of *E. histolytica* trophozoites and/or cysts in stained smears of fecal specimens. Amebic trophozoites and cysts are only 1 or 2 μm in diameter and are thus difficult to find in permanent stained smears of fecal material. It is also necessary for microbiology professionals to be able to differentiate *E. histolytica* from other pathogenic and nonpathogenic intestinal amebas. The presence of red blood cells within trophozoites indicates invasive amebiasis.
Balantidiasis. Balantidiasis is a protozoal gastrointestinal infection of the colon causing diarrhea or dysentery, colic, nausea, and vomiting. **Patient Care.** Use Standard Precautions for hospitalized patients. **Geographic Occurrence.** Although seen worldwide, balantidiasis is rare in the United States.	**Parasite.** Balantidiasis is caused by *Balantidium coli*, a ciliated protozoan (refer back to Fig. 5-7 in Chapter 5). *B. coli* is the only ciliate that causes disease in humans. Balantidiasis occurs more commonly in pigs than in humans. **Reservoirs and Mode of Transmission.** Reservoirs include pigs and anything that might be contaminated with pig feces (e.g., drinking water). Transmission most often occurs via ingestion of *B. coli* cysts in fecally contaminated food or water.

Table 21-3   Protozoal Infections of the Gastrointestinal Tract (continued)

Disease	Additional Information
	Laboratory Diagnosis. Balantidiasis is diagnosed by observing and identifying *B. coli* trophozoites or cysts in fecal specimens, which may also contain blood and mucus. *B. coli* is the largest of the protozoa that infect humans.
Cryptosporidiosis. Cryptosporidiosis is a gastrointestinal infection caused by a coccidial protozoan. Coccidia are sporozoa. Cryptosporidiosis may be asymptomatic or may cause diarrhea, cramping, and abdominal pain. Less common symptoms include malaise, fever, anorexia, nausea, and vomiting. The disease may be prolonged, fulminant, and fatal in immunosuppressed patients. Children younger than 2 years of age, animal handlers, travelers, homosexuals, and day care center workers are particularly likely to be infected. Outbreaks in day care centers are common. Outbreaks have also been associated with drinking water, recreational use water, and drinking unpasteurized apple cider contaminated with cattle feces. **Patient Care.** Use Standard Precautions for hospitalized patients. Add Contact Precautions for diapered or incontinent patients. **Geographic Occurrence.** This disease has been reported worldwide. The largest waterborne outbreak that has ever occurred in the United States was the 1993 cryptosporidiosis outbreak in Milwaukee, WI, which affected more than 400,000 people.	**Parasite.** Cryptosporidiosis results from ingestion of oocysts of *Cryptosporidium parvum*, a coccidian (Other coccidial parasites of humans are in the genera *Cyclospora*, *Isospora*, and *Sarcocystis*.) **Reservoirs and Mode of Transmission.** Reservoirs include infected humans, cattle, and other domestic animals. Fecal–oral transmission; from person to person, from animal to person, or via ingestion of contaminated water or food. **Laboratory Diagnosis.** Cryptosporidiosis can be diagnosed by microscopic observation of small (4–6 μm-diameter) acid-fast oocysts in stained smears of fecal specimens. Sensitive and specific immunodiagnostic procedures are also available.
Cyclosporiasis. Cyclosporiasis is a coccidial gastrointestinal infection, causing watery diarrhea (6 or more stools per day), nausea, anorexia, abdominal cramping, fatigue, and weight loss. The diarrhea lasts between 9 and 43 days in immunocompetent patients, and months in immunocompromised patients. **Patient Care.** Use Standard Precautions for hospitalized patients. **Geographic Occurrence.** Cyclosporiasis has been diagnosed in Asia, the Caribbean, Mexico, Peru, and the United States.	**Parasite.** Cyclosporiasis results from ingestion of oocysts of *Cyclospora cayetanensis*, a coccidian. **Reservoirs and Mode of Transmission.** Reservoirs include fecally contaminated water sources and produce that has been rinsed with fecally contaminated water. Transmission is primarily waterborne, but outbreaks have involved contaminated raspberries, basil, and lettuce. **Laboratory Diagnosis.** Diagnosis of cyclosporiasis is made by microscopic observation of the 8- to 9-μm-diameter acid-fast oocysts, which are about twice the size of *Cryptosporidium* oocysts. The oocysts autofluoresce a bright green to intense blue under ultraviolet fluorescence, when examined using appropriate filters.
Giardiasis. Giardiasis is a protozoal infection of the duodenum (the uppermost portion of the small intestine) and may be asymptomatic, mild, or severe. Patients experience diarrhea, steatorrhea (loose, pale, malodorous, fatty stools), abdominal cramps, bloating, abdominal gas, fatigue, and possibly weight loss. **Patient Care.** Use Standard Precautions for hospitalized patients. Add Contact Precautions for diapered or incontinent patients. **Geographic Occurrence.** This disease occurs worldwide.	**Pathogen.** Giardiasis is caused by *Giardia lamblia* (also called *Giardia intestinalis*), a flagellated protozoan (Fig. 21-3). Trophozoites attach by means of a ventral sucker to the mucosal lining of the duodenum. Trophozoites and/or cysts are expelled in feces. **Reservoirs and Mode of Transmission.** Reservoirs include infected humans, possibly beavers and other wild and domestic animals that have consumed water containing *Giardia* cysts; and fecally contaminated drinking water and recreational water. The disease commonly occurs in day care centers. Transmission occurs via the fecal–oral route, usually by ingestion of cysts in fecally contaminated water or foods, or from person to person by soiled hands to mouth (as occurs in day care centers). Large community outbreaks have resulted from drinking treated but unfiltered water. Filtration is necessary because the concentrations of chlorine used in routine water treatment do not kill *Giardia* cysts, especially in cold water. Smaller outbreaks have involved contaminated food, person-to-person transmission in day care centers, and fecally contaminated recreational water (e.g., swimming and wading pools).

(continued)

Disease	Additional Information
	Laboratory Diagnosis. Giardiasis is usually diagnosed by microscopic observation of trophozoites and/or cysts in stained smears of fecal specimens or duodenal aspirates. The characteristic teardrop-shaped *Giardia* trophozoite contains two nuclei, giving it the appearance of a face (Fig. 21-3). It appears to be looking up at the person observing it microscopically. The *Giardia* trophozoite has been described as resembling an owl face, a clown face, or an old man with glasses. Immunodiagnostic procedures are also available. Other photographs of *Giardia* can be found in Chapters 5 and 15.

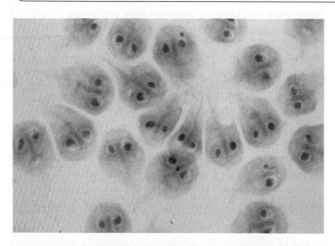

Figure 21-3. Stained *Giardia lamblia* trophozoites, which were cultured in a research laboratory. *G. lamblia* trophozoites, 10 to 20 μm long by 5 to 15 μm wide, are easy to recognize in microscopically examined fecal specimens. Their two oval nuclei resemble eyes. As you observe a *Giardia* trophozoite through the microscope, it appears to be looking up at you. (Courtesy of Biomed Ed., Round Rock, TX.)

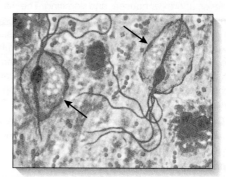

Figure 21-4. *Trichomonas vaginalis* and Gram-positive cocci, for size comparison. *T. vaginalis* trophozoites (*arrows*) are easy to recognize in a saline wet mount preparation of a freshly collected specimen. Their flagella and undulating membrane cause them to be constantly in motion. When they die, however, they become spherical and cannot be distinguished from white blood cells. (From Harvey RA, et al. *Lippincott's Illustrated Reviews: Microbiology*. 3rd ed. Philadelphia, PA: Lippincott Williams & Wilkins; 2013.)

Reservoirs and Mode of Transmission. Infected humans serve as reservoirs. Transmission occurs by direct contact with vaginal and urethral discharges of infected people during sexual intercourse. Because this organism exists only in the fragile trophozoite stage (there is no cyst stage), it cannot survive very long outside the human body.

Laboratory Diagnosis. Vaginitis caused by *T. vaginalis* can be diagnosed by performing a saline wet mount examination (described in Appendix 5 on thePoint) of freshly collected vaginal discharge material and observing the motile trophozoites (Fig. 21-4). Culture procedures are also available, but are rarely performed in clinical microbiology laboratories. *T. vaginalis* trophozoites are sometimes seen in urine and Papanicolaou (Pap) smears. Diagnosis of trichomoniasis in men can be accomplished by performing a saline wet mount of urethral discharge material or prostatic secretions.

Protozoal Infections of the Circulatory System

Table 21-4 contains information about protozoal infections of the circulatory system.

Protozoal Infections of the Central Nervous System

Protozoal infections of the CNS include African trypanosomiasis, amebic abscesses, PAM, and toxoplasmosis. Each of these diseases, except PAM, was discussed earlier in this chapter.

> Malaria is one of the most important infectious diseases in the world. Humans become infected following the injection of male and female gametocytes into the bloodstream by a female *Anopheles* mosquito.

STUDY AID

"Bugs"

Some people refer to all, or most, insects as bugs, but only one category of insects—class Insecta—actually contains bugs. Technically, true bugs are in the order Hemiptera. Included in this order are bed bugs, reduviid bugs, several types of water bugs, and many plant bugs.

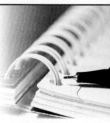

Table 21-4 Protozoal Infections of the Circulatory System

Disease	Additional Information
African Trypanosomiasis (African Sleeping Sickness). African trypanosomiasis is a systemic disease caused by flagellated protozoa in the bloodstream, known as hemoflagellates. Early stages of the disease include a painful chancre at the site of a tsetse fly bite, fever, intense headache, insomnia, lymphadenitis, anemia, local edema, and rash. Later stages of the disease include body wasting, falling asleep, coma, and death if untreated. The latter stages of the disease have given rise to the name African sleeping sickness or simply sleeping sickness. **Patient Care.** Use Standard Precautions for hospitalized patients. **Geographic Occurrence.** African trypanosomiasis is transmitted by the tsetse fly (Genus *Glossina*), so the disease occurs only in tropical Africa, where tsetse flies are found. It is estimated that more than 300,000 people have African trypanosomiasis and that about 66,000 people die each year of the disease.	**Pathogens.** Two subspecies of *Trypanosoma brucei* cause African trypanosomiasis. *T. brucei* ssp. *gambiense*, in western and central Africa, causes most cases of sleeping sickness; the disease may last several years. *T. brucei* ssp. *rhodesiense*, in eastern Africa, causes a more rapidly fatal form of African trypanosomiasis, usually lethal within weeks or a few months without treatment. **Reservoirs and Mode of Transmission.** Infected humans serve as reservoirs of *T. brucei* ssp. *gambiense*, whereas wild animals and domestic cattle are the primary reservoirs of *T. brucei* ssp. *rhodesiense*. Tsetse flies become infected when they ingest blood that contains the trypanosomes. The parasites then multiply and mature within the infected tsetse flies. Humans become infected when mature trypanosomes (trypomastigotes) are injected into the bloodstream as the infected tsetse flies take blood meals. **Laboratory Diagnosis.** African trypanosomiasis is diagnosed by observing and identifying trypomastigotes in blood, lymph node aspirates, or CSF (Fig. 21-5). Immunodiagnostic procedures are also available.)
American Trypanosomiasis (Chagas' Disease). American trypanosomiasis is also known as Chagas' disease, in honor of Carlos Chagas, who described the entire life cycle of *Trypanosoma cruzi* in 1909. In the acute stage of the disease, patients may present with an inflammatory response at the site of the reduviid bug bite, fever, malaise, lymphadenopathy, **hepatomegaly** (enlarged liver), and **splenomegaly** (enlarged spleen), although it may be asymptomatic. Chronic irreversible complications include heart damage, arrhythmias, enlarged esophagus (megaesophagus), and enlarged colon (megacolon). Life-threatening meningoencephalitis may occur. **Patient Care.** Use Standard Precautions for hospitalized patients. **Geographical Occurrence.** Chagas' disease occurs primarily in South America, Central America, and Mexico, although a few cases have been reported in the United States (by bug bite or blood transfusion). As increasing numbers of infected people enter the country from endemic areas, concern is growing in the United States about the safety of the blood supply. It is estimated that between 16 million and 18 million people have Chagas' disease and that about 50,000 people die each year from the disease.	**Parasite.** The etiologic agent of American trypanosomiasis is *T. cruzi*, which occurs in two stages: a hemoflagellate (the trypomastigote form) and a nonmotile, intracellular parasite (the amastigote form). **Reservoirs and Mode of Transmission.** Reservoirs include infected humans and more than 150 species of domestic and wild animals, including dogs, cats, rodents, carnivores, and primates. The vectors of American trypanosomiasis are rather large bugs (see "Study Aid: Bugs" on page 408). They are known by many names, including reduviid bugs, triatome bugs, kissing bugs, and cone-nosed bugs. A bug becomes infected when it takes a blood meal from an infected animal. Later, when the bug takes a blood meal or feeds at the corner of a sleeping person's eye, the bug defecates. The person becomes infected by rubbing the insect feces—which contain the parasite—into the bite wound or eye. The characteristic unilateral swelling of the eyelid that occurs after *T. cruzi* is rubbed into the eye is called Romaña sign. Transmission by blood transfusion and organ transplantation also occurs. **Laboratory Diagnosis.** American trypanosomiasis is diagnosed by observation of trypomastigotes in blood (Fig. 21-6) or amastigotes in tissue (especially cardiac tissue) or lymph node biopsies. Immunodiagnostic procedures are also available. Xenodiagnosis is performed in endemic countries. In this procedure, sterile (uninfected), laboratory-raised reduviid bugs are allowed to take blood meals from persons suspected of having Chagas' disease. (The bite is painless.) The bugs are then taken to a laboratory, where their feces are periodically checked microscopically for the presence of the parasite.

(continued)

Protozoal Infections of the Circulatory System (continued)

Disease	Additional Information
Babesiosis. Babesiosis is a sporozoan disease that may include fever, chills, myalgia, fatigue, jaundice, and anemia. It is potentially severe and sometimes fatal, especially in splenectomized and elderly people. Patients may be simultaneously infected with *Borrelia burgdorferi*, the bacterium that causes Lyme disease, which is transmitted by the same species of tick. **Patient Care.** Use Standard Precautions for hospitalized patients. **Geographic Occurrence.** Babesiosis is an endemic disease in many parts of the world, including Europe, Mexico, and the United States. Most U.S. cases occur in New York and New England.	**Parasites.** Babesiosis is caused by *Babesia microti* and other *Babesia* spp., including *Babesia divergens* in Europe. Like the malaria parasites, *Babesia* spp. are intraerythrocytic sporozoa (i.e., they live within erythrocytes). **Reservoirs and Mode of Transmission.** Reservoirs include rodents for *B. microti* and cattle for *B. divergens*. Transmission occurs by tick bite and, rarely, by blood transfusion. **Laboratory Diagnosis.** Babesiosis is diagnosed by observation and identification of intraerythrocytic *Babesia* parasites in Giemsa-stained blood smears. They resemble the early "ring forms" of malarial parasites—particularly *Plasmodium falciparum*—and thus must be differentiated from malarial parasites. Immunodiagnostic and molecular diagnostic procedures are also available.
Malaria. Malaria is a systemic sporozoan infection with malaise, fever, chills, sweating, headache, and nausea. The frequency with which the cycle of chills, fever, and sweating is repeated is referred to as periodicity, which depends on the particular species of malarial parasite that is causing the infection. The intermittent bouts of chills and fever are sometimes referred to as paroxysms. In addition to these symptoms, falciparum malaria may be accompanied by cough, diarrhea, respiratory distress, shock, renal and liver failure, pulmonary and cerebral edema, coma, and death. **Patient Care.** Use Standard Precautions for hospitalized patients. **Geographic Occurrence.** Malaria is one of the most important infectious diseases in the world. It is a major health problem in many tropical and subtropical countries, with an estimated 300–500 million cases and 1.5–2.7 million deaths annually. About 90% of all malaria cases occur in Africa, where approximately 1 million children die from malaria each year. Malaria is a nationally notifiable infectious disease in the United States. Most U.S. cases are imported, meaning that the disease was acquired outside of the country. A few nonimported, mosquito-transmitted cases of malaria occur in the United States each year.	**Parasites.** Human malaria is caused by four species in the genus *Plasmodium*: *Plasmodium vivax* (the most common species), *P. falciparum* (the most deadly), *Plasmodium malariae*, and *Plasmodium ovale*. These are intraerythrocytic sporozoan parasites. Infection with *P. vivax* and *P. ovale* results in chills and fever every 48 hours, and is referred to as tertian malaria. *P. malariae* infection causes chills and fever every 72 hours, and is referred to as quartan malaria. *P. falciparum* periodicity varies from 36–48 hours. Mixed infections—that is, infections involving more than one *Plasmodium* species—occur in certain geographic areas. Drug-resistant strains of *P. vivax* and *P. falciparum* are common. *Plasmodium* spp. have a complex life cycle involving a female *Anopheles* mosquito, the liver and erythrocytes of an infected human, and many life cycle stages (Fig. 21-7). **Reservoirs and Mode of Transmission.** Infected humans and infected mosquitoes serve as reservoirs. Most human infections occur as a result of injection of sporozoites into the bloodstream by an infected female *Anopheles* mosquito while taking a blood meal. Infection may also occur as a result of blood transfusion or the use of blood-contaminated needles and syringes. **Laboratory Diagnosis.** Malaria is diagnosed by observation and identification of intraerythrocytic *Plasmodium* parasites in Giemsa-stained blood smears (Fig. 21-8). Immunodiagnostic and molecular diagnostic procedures are being tested.

Primary Amebic Meningoencephalitis

Disease. PAM is an amebic disease causing inflammation of the brain and meninges, sore throat, severe frontal headache, hallucinations, nausea, vomiting, high fever, and stiff neck. Unless diagnosed and treated promptly, death occurs within 10 days, usually on the fifth or sixth day.

Patient Care. Use Standard Precautions for hospitalized patients.

Geographic Occurrence. PAM has been reported worldwide.

Parasite. PAM is caused by *N. fowleri*, an ameboflagellate.[a] Amebas in the genera *Acanthamoeba* and *Balamuthia* can cause similar conditions.

> PAM is caused by an ameboflagellate named *Naegleria fowleri*.

Reservoirs and Mode of Transmission. Water and soil serve as reservoirs. The amebas usually enter the

---

[a] *Naegleria fowleri* is classified as an ameboflagellate because its life cycle consists of three stages: trophozoite, a temporary flagellar stage known as an ameboflagellate, and cyst.

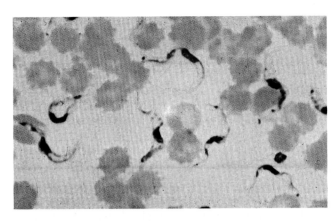

Figure 21-5. *Trypanosoma brucei* trypomastigotes in a stained peripheral blood smear from a patient with African trypanosomiasis. *T. brucei* trypomastigotes are 14 to 33 μm long by 1.5 to 3.5 μm wide. (From Winn WC Jr., et al. *Koneman's Color Atlas and Textbook of Diagnostic Microbiology*. 6th ed. Philadelphia, PA: Lippincott Williams & Wilkins; 2006.)

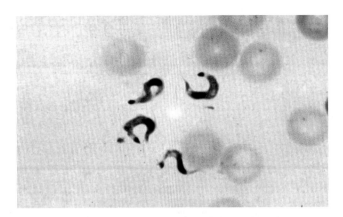

Figure 21-6. *Trypanosoma cruzi* trypomastigotes in a stained peripheral blood smear from a patient with **American trypanosomiasis (Chagas' disease).** Several trypomastigotes of *T. cruzi*, with their typical "C" shape, can be seen among the red blood cells. (From Winn WC Jr., et al. *Koneman's Color Atlas and Textbook of Diagnostic Microbiology*. 6th ed. Philadelphia, PA: Lippincott Williams & Wilkins, 2006.)

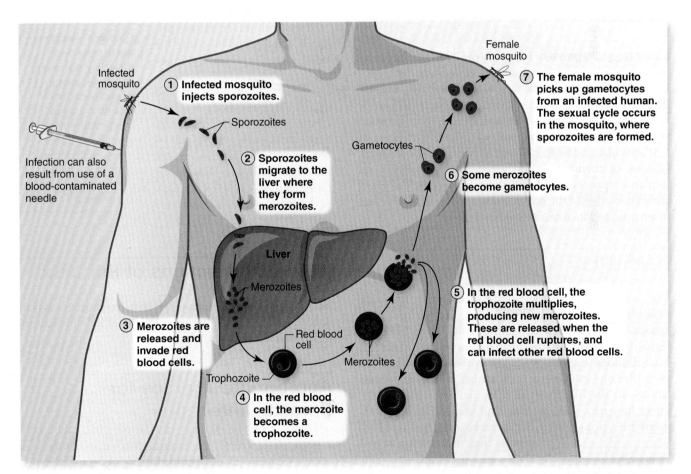

Figure 21-7. Life cycle of malarial parasites. Note that humans become infected when a female *Anopheles* mosquito injects sporozoites while taking a blood meal. Mosquitoes become infected when they ingest male and female gametocytes (at least one of each) while taking a blood meal. (Redrawn from Harvey RA, et al. *Lippincott's Illustrated Reviews: Microbiology*. 3rd ed. Philadelphia, PA: Lippincott Williams & Wilkins; 2013.)

nasal passages of a person diving and/or swimming in ameba-contaminated water, such as ponds, lakes, "the old swimming hole," thermal springs, hot tubs, spas, and public swimming pools. After the amebas colonize the nasal tissues, they invade the brain and meninges by traveling along the olfactory nerves.

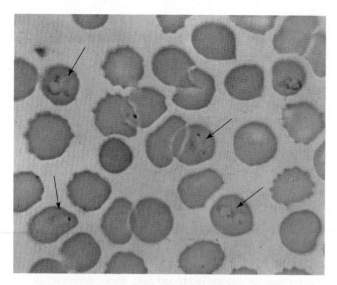

Figure 21-8. Giemsa-stained peripheral blood smear showing *Plasmodium falciparum* trophozoites (*arrows*) within red blood cells. (From Binford CH, Connor DH. *Pathology of Tropical and Extraordinary Diseases.* vol. 1. Washington, DC: Armed Forces Institute of Pathology; 1976.)

Laboratory Diagnosis. Diagnosis of PAM can sometimes be made by microscopic examination of wet mount preparations of fresh cerebrospinal fluid (CSF). However, because they are colorless and transparent, amebas are difficult to see in wet mounts, unless the microscope light is turned very low. Phase-contrast microscopy is helpful. Smears of CSF sediment can be stained with Wright, Wright-Giemsa, Giemsa, or trichrome stain. Leukocytes and amebas are similar in appearance. Unfortunately, most cases of PAM are diagnosed after the patient's death through observation of amebas in stained sections of brain tissue.

Helminths

The word **helminth** means parasitic worm. Although helminths are not microorganisms, the various procedures used to diagnose helminth infections are performed in the Parasitology Section of the Clinical Microbiology Laboratory. These procedures often involve the observation of microscopic stages—eggs and larvae—in the life cycles of these parasites. Helminths infect humans, other animals, and plants, but only helminth infections of humans are discussed here. The helminths that infect humans are always endoparasites.

Helminths are multicellular, eukaryotic organisms in the Kingdom Animalia. The two major divisions of helminths are roundworms (**nematodes**) and flatworms. The flatworms are further divided into tapeworms (**cestodes**) and flukes (**trematodes**).

> Helminths (parasitic worms) are divided into roundworms (nematodes) and flatworms. Flatworms are further divided into tapeworms (cestodes) and flukes (trematodes).

The typical helminth life cycle includes three stages: the *egg*, the *larva*, and the *adult worm*. Adults produce eggs, from which larvae emerge, and the larvae mature into adult worms.

> The stages of the typical helminth life cycle are the egg, the larva, and the adult worm.

Adult nematodes are either male or female. Cestodes and many trematodes are hermaphroditic, meaning that adult worms contain both male and female reproductive organs. Thus, it only takes one worm to produce fertile eggs.

The host that harbors the larval stage is called the *intermediate host*, whereas the host that harbors the adult worm is called the *definitive host*. Sometimes helminths have more than one intermediate host or more than one definitive host. The fish tapeworm, for example, is what is known as a three-host parasite, having one definitive host (human) and two intermediate hosts (a freshwater crustacean called a *Cyclops* and a freshwater fish) in its life cycle (Fig. 21-9). Fleas serve as intermediate hosts in the life cycle of the dog tapeworm, whereas dogs, cats, or humans can serve as definitive hosts.

Helminth infections are primarily acquired by ingesting the larval stage, although some larvae are injected into the body via the bite of infected insects, and others enter the body by penetrating skin. Helminth infections are usually diagnosed by observing whole worms or segments of worms in clinical specimens (usually, fecal specimens), or larvae or eggs in stained or unstained clinical specimens.

> Helminth infections are usually diagnosed by observing (a) whole worms or segments of worms in clinical specimens—most often, fecal specimens, or (b) larvae or eggs in stained or unstained clinical specimens.

Helminth Infections of Humans

The major helminth infections of humans are shown in Table 21-5. Additional information about helminth infections can be found on thePoint.

Appropriate Therapy for Parasitic Infections

Recommendations for the treatment of infectious diseases change frequently. The parasitic infections described in this chapter must be treated using appropriate antiprotozoal or antihelminth drugs.

Additional information about antiprotozoal agents can be found in Chapter 9 and at www.courses.ahc.umn.edu/pharmacy/6124/remel_notes/antiparasitic.pdf. Drugs used to treat helminth infections are also known as anthelmintics, anthelminthics, antihelmintics, and antihelminthics.

Medically Important Arthropods

There are many classes of arthropods, but only three are studied in a parasitology course: *insects* (class Insecta), *arachnids* (class Arachnida), and certain *crustaceans* (class Crustacea). The insects studied include lice, fleas, flies, mosquitoes, and reduviid bugs. Arachnids include mites and ticks. Crustaceans include crabs, crayfish, and certain *Cyclops* species. Arthropods may be involved in human diseases in any of four ways, as shown in Table 21-6.

Arthropods may serve as mechanical or biologic vectors in the transmission of certain infectious diseases. **Mechanical vectors** merely pick up the parasite at point A and drop it off at point B, similar to an overnight delivery service. For example, a housefly could pick up parasite cysts on the sticky hairs of its legs while walking around on animal feces in a meadow. The fly might then come through an open kitchen window and drop off the parasite cysts while walking on a pie cooling on the counter. A **biologic vector**, on the other hand, is an arthropod in whose body the pathogen multiplies or matures (or both). Many arthropod vectors of human diseases are biologic vectors. A particular arthropod may serve as both a host and a biologic vector. Refer back to Table 11-3 in Chapter 11 for a list of arthropods that serve as vectors of human

infectious diseases. Several arthropods that serve as vectors of human diseases are shown in Figure. 21-14.

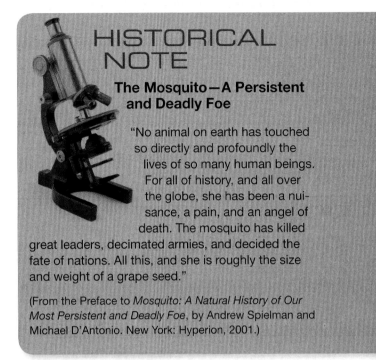

HISTORICAL NOTE

The Mosquito—A Persistent and Deadly Foe

"No animal on earth has touched so directly and profoundly the lives of so many human beings. For all of history, and all over the globe, she has been a nuisance, a pain, and an angel of death. The mosquito has killed great leaders, decimated armies, and decided the fate of nations. All this, and she is roughly the size and weight of a grape seed."

(From the Preface to *Mosquito: A Natural History of Our Most Persistent and Deadly Foe*, by Andrew Spielman and Michael D'Antonio. New York: Hyperion, 2001.)

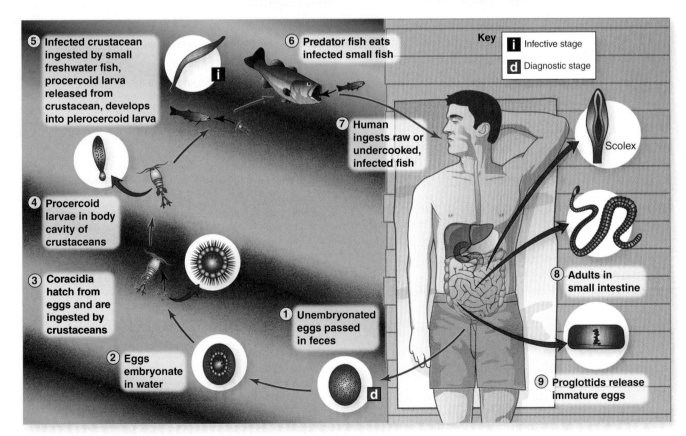

Figure 21-9. Fish tapeworm life cycle—an example of a three-host life cycle. A human serves as the definitive host, harboring the adult worm. A *Cyclops* species (a crustacean) serves as the first intermediate host, harboring the procercoid larva stage. A freshwater fish serves as the second intermediate host, harboring the plerocercoid larva (the infective stage). Humans become infected by ingesting the plerocercoid larva in raw or undercooked fish.

Table 21-5 Helminth Infections of Humans

Anatomic Location	Helminth Disease	Helminth that Causes The Disease
Skin	Onchocerciasis (also known as "river blindness")	*Onchocerca volvulus* (N); microfilariae (tiny prelarval stages of these helminths) are found in the skin
Muscle and Subcutaneous Tissues	Trichinellosis	*Trichinella spiralis* (N)
	Dracunculiasis	*Dracunculus medinensis* (N); also known as the guinea worm
Eyes	Onchocerciasis	*Onchocerca volvulus* (N); microfilariae enter the eyes, causing an intense inflammatory reaction
	Loiasis	*Loa loa* (N); also known as the African eyeworm
Respiratory System	Paragonimiasis	*Paragonimus westermani* (T); the lung fluke
Gastrointestinal Tract	Ascariasis infection (See Fig. 21-10)	*Ascaris lumbricoides* (N); the large intestinal roundworm of humans
	Hookworm infection	*Ancylostoma duodenale* (N) or *Necator americanus* (N)
	Pinworm infection (enterobiasis)[a] (See Fig. 21-11)	*Enterobius vermicularis* (N)
	Whipworm infection (trichuriasis)	*Trichuris trichiura* (N)
	Strongyloidiasis	*Strongyloides stercoralis* (N)
	Beef tapeworm infection	*Taenia saginata* (C)
	Dog tapeworm infection	*Dipylidium caninum* (C)
	Dwarf tapeworm infection	*Hymenolepis nana* (C)
	Fish tapeworm infection	*Diphyllobothrium latum* (C)
	Pork tapeworm infection	*Taenia solium* (C)
	Rat tapeworm infection	*Hymenolepis diminuta* (C)
	Fasciolopsiasis	*Fasciolopsis buski* (T); an intestinal fluke
	Fascioliasis	*Fasciola hepatica* (T); a liver fluke
	Clonorchiasis	*Clonorchis sinensis* (T); also known as the Chinese or Oriental liver fluke
Circulatory System	Filariasis (See Fig. 21-12)	*Wuchereria bancrofti* (N) and *Brugia malayi* (N); microfilariae of these helminths are found in the bloodstream
	Schistosomiasis (also known as bilharzia) (See Fig. 21-13)	Trematodes in the genus *Schistosoma*
Central Nervous System	Cysticercosis	Cysts (the larval stage) of the pork tapeworm (*Taenia solium*) are found in the brain
	Hydatid cyst disease	*Echinococcus granulosis* (C) or *Echinococcus multilocularis* (C); in addition to the brain, hydatid cysts (the larval form of these helminths) can form in many other locations in the body

N, nematode; *C*, cestode; *T*, trematode.

[a] Enterobiasis (pinworm infection) is the most common nematode infection in the United States.

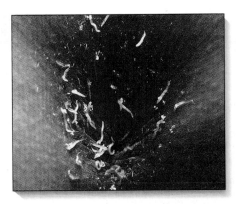

Figure 21-10. Pinworms, having migrated from the colon, are seen here on the perianal skin of a five-year-old child. Each female worm, measuring approximately 8 to 13 by 0.3 to 0.5 mm, may deposit as many as 10,000 or more eggs on the perianal and perineal skin. See thePoint for additional information. (From Harvey RA, et al. *Lippincott's Illustrated Reviews: Microbiology*. 3rd ed. Philadelphia, PA: Lippincott Williams & Wilkins; 2013.)

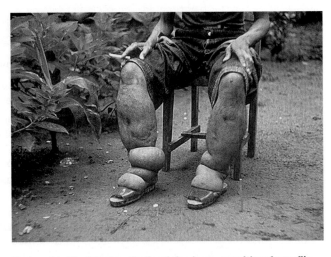

Figure 21-12. Elephantiasis of the legs, resulting from filariasis. In filariasis, long, threadlike adult worms live in lymph nodes, where they block the flow of lymph. Chronic filariasis leads to enlargement of legs, breasts, and genitalia—a condition known as elephantiasis. (Courtesy of the CDC.)

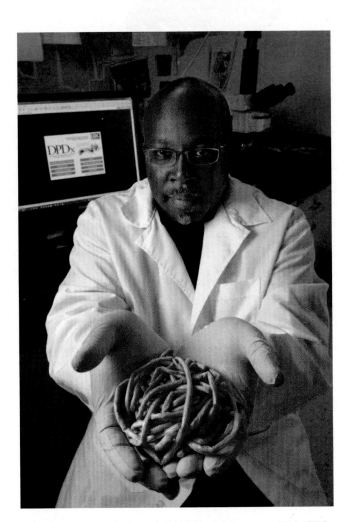

Figure 21-11. Adult *Ascaris lumbricoides* worms. This CDC technician is holding *Ascaris* worms that had been passed with the feces of a 5-year-old child in Kenya, Africa. Adult female worms may reach 20 to 35 cm in length, whereas adult male worms are usually 15 to 31 cm in length. (Courtesy of Henry Bishop, James Gathany, and the CDC.)

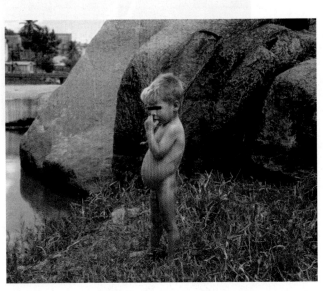

Figure 21-13. Young Puerto Rican boy with a swollen abdomen due to schistosomiasis. Chronic inflammation in the patient's liver has led to scarification, which has caused obstructed blood flow through that organ. This, in turn, has led to a condition known as ascites (a buildup of fluid in the abdominal cavity). (Courtesy of the CDC.)

Table 21-6 How Arthropods May Be Involved in Human Diseases

Type of Involvement	Example(s)
The arthropod may actually be the *cause* of the disease.	Scabies, a disease in which microscopic mites live in subcutaneous tunnels and cause intense itching.
The arthropod may serve as the *intermediate host* in the life cycle of a parasite.	Flea in the life cycle of the dog tapeworm. Beetle in the life cycle of the rat tapeworm. *Cyclops* sp. in the life cycle of the fish tapeworm. Tsetse fly in the life cycle of African trypanosomiasis. *Simulium* black fly in the life cycle of onchocerciasis. Mosquito in the life cycle of filariasis.
The arthropod may serve as the *definitive host* in the life cycle of a parasite.	Female *Anopheles* mosquito in the life cycle of malarial parasites.
The arthropod may serve as a *vector* in the transmission of an infectious disease.	Oriental rat flea in the transmission of plague. Tick in the transmission of spotted fever rickettsiosis and Lyme disease. Louse in the transmission of epidemic typhus.

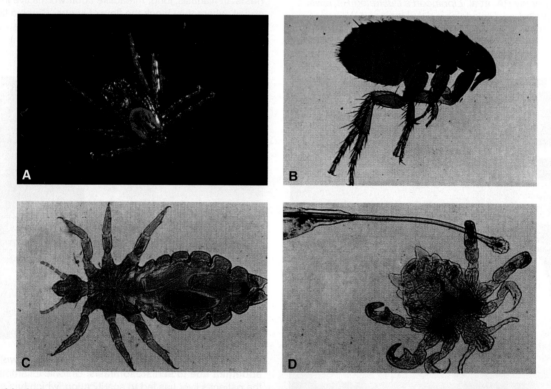

Figure 21-14. Arthropod ectoparasites and vectors of human infectious diseases. A. *Dermacentor andersoni*, the wood tick; one of the tick vectors of spotted fever rickettsiosis (formerly Rocky Mountain spotted fever). **B.** *Xenopsylla cheopis*, the oriental rat flea; the vector of plague and endemic typhus. **C.** *Pediculus humanus*, the human body louse; a vector of epidemic typhus. **D.** *Phthirus pubis*, the pubic louse; because of its appearance, it is also known as the crab louse. (From Winn WC Jr., et al. *Koneman's Color Atlas and Textbook of Diagnostic Microbiology.* 6th ed. Philadelphia, PA: Lippincott Williams & Wilkins; 2006.)

ON thePoint

- Terms Introduced in This Chapter
- Review of Key Points
- A Closer Look at Helminth Infections
- Increase Your Knowledge
- Critical Thinking
- Additional Self-Assessment Exercises

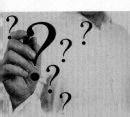

Self-Assessment Exercises

After studying this chapter, answer the following multiple-choice questions.

1. Humans develop malaria after the injection of *Plasmodium* _____ into the bloodstream by an infected female *Anopheles* mosquito when she takes a blood meal.
   a. male and female gametocytes
   b. schizonts
   c. sporozoites
   d. trophozoites

2. These *Plasmodium* life cycle stages must be ingested by a female *Anopheles* mosquito for the *Plasmodium* life cycle to continue in the mosquito.
   a. Male and female gametocytes
   b. Schizonts
   c. Sporozoites
   d. Trophozoites

3. Which of the following protozoal diseases is *not* transmitted via an arthropod vector?
   a. African trypanosomiasis
   b. American trypanosomiasis
   c. babesiosis
   d. giardiasis

4. Which of the following protozoal diseases is *least* likely to be transmitted via blood transfusion?
   a. American trypanosomiasis
   b. babesiosis
   c. malaria
   d. trichomoniasis

5. Which of the following protozoal diseases is *least* likely to be transmitted via an infected food handler who fails to wash his or her hands after using the bathroom?
   a. Amebiasis
   b. Cryptosporidiosis
   c. Giardiasis
   d. Toxoplasmosis

6. You are visiting a friend whose parents raise pigs. Which of the following diseases are you *most* likely to acquire by drinking well water at their farm?
   a. Amebiasis
   b. Balantidiasis
   c. Cryptosporidiosis
   d. Giardiasis

7. You are working on a cattle ranch. Which of the following diseases are you *most* apt to acquire as you perform your duties at the ranch?
   a. Amebiasis
   b. Balantidiasis
   c. Cryptosporidiosis
   d. Giardiasis

8. Which of the following protozoal diseases are you *most* likely to acquire by eating a rare hamburger?
   a. Amebiasis
   b. Balantidiasis
   c. Giardiasis
   d. Toxoplasmosis

9. Which of the following associations is incorrect?
   a. African trypanosomiasis… tsetse fly
   b. amebiasis… fecally contaminated water
   c. Chagas' disease… mosquito
   d. toxoplasmosis… cats

10. Which of the following is an example of an infectious disease that is caused by a facultative parasite?
    a. African trypanosomiasis
    b. giardiasis
    c. malaria
    d. PAM

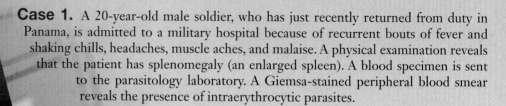

Case 1. A 20-year-old male soldier, who has just recently returned from duty in Panama, is admitted to a military hospital because of recurrent bouts of fever and shaking chills, headaches, muscle aches, and malaise. A physical examination reveals that the patient has splenomegaly (an enlarged spleen). A blood specimen is sent to the parasitology laboratory. A Giemsa-stained peripheral blood smear reveals the presence of intraerythrocytic parasites.

A. Which one of the following pathogens do you suspect is causing this patient's disease?

1. *Ehrlichia*
2. *Plasmodium*
3. *Toxoplasma*
4. *Trypanosoma cruzi*

Case 2. A 19-year-old pregnant woman is visiting the clinic for a routine prenatal examination. Included in the advice that she is given are the following statements: (1) "Wash your hands thoroughly after handling raw meat." (2) "Never eat raw or rare meat." (3) "If you have a cat, wear latex gloves when changing the kitty litter, and wash your hands thoroughly afterward. Better yet, have someone else change the kitty litter." (4) "Avoid contact with sand in sandboxes."

A. All of these precautions are necessary to avoid infection with which one of the following parasites?

1. *Balantidium coli*
2. *Cryptosporidium parvum*
3. *Toxoplasma gondii*
4. *Trichomonas vaginalis*

Case 3. A 24-year-old man visits the clinic complaining of persistent diarrhea, crampy abdominal pain, and foul-smelling flatulence. He has not had any fever or chills, but often feels nauseous after a meal. He states that the diarrhea has lasted for more than 2 weeks, and started about a week to 10 days after he returned from a backpacking trip high in the Colorado Rockies. When asked if he drank any stream or lake water on the trip, he replies, "Sure, all the time! That water sure is pure!" Perhaps the water is not as pure as he thinks! The laboratory reports the presence of trophozoites and cysts of a flagellated protozoan in his stool specimens.

A. Which one of the following parasites, all of which cause diarrheal illness, do you suspect?

1. *Balantidium coli*
2. *Cryptosporidium parvum*
3. *Entamoeba histolytica*
4. *Giardia lamblia*

Case 4. A 26-year-old woman visits a public health clinic, concerned that she might have contracted some type of sexually transmitted disease. She states that she has experienced a greenish-yellow, frothy vaginal discharge and mild pain in her genital area. Physical examination reveals inflamed and swollen labia. Specimens of the discharge material are sent to the laboratory for a wet mount examination and culture and sensitivity. The wet mount examination reveals the presence of actively moving flagellated protozoa.

A. Which one of the following pathogens is causing her vaginitis?
1. *Chlamydia trachomatis*
2. *Neisseria gonorrhoeae*
3. *Treponema pallidum*
4. *Trichomonas vaginalis*

Case 5. A 53-year-old man is admitted to the hospital with severe dysentery. Other symptoms that he reports include nausea, vomiting, anorexia, headache, insomnia, muscle weakness, and weight loss. The patient states that he is a farmer, and that his illness has made it impossible for him to care for his crops and animals. He also mentions that most of his pigs are experiencing a diarrheal illness. Examination of a trichrome-stained stool specimen reveals the presence of trophozoites and cysts of a ciliated protozoan.

A. Which one of the following parasites, all of which cause diarrheal illness, do you suspect?
1. *Balantidium coli*
2. *Cryptosporidium parvum*
3. *Entamoeba histolytica*
4. *Giardia lamblia*

(Answers to Case Studies can be found in Appendix B.)

Answers to Self-Assessment Exercises

Chapter 1

1. a
2. b
3. d
4. d
5. b
6. b
7. d
8. b
9. b
10. b

Chapter 2

1. d
2. b
3. a
4. d
5. d
6. b
7. a
8. d
9. b
10. b

Chapter 3

1. c
2. c
3. b
4. c
5. c
6. c
7. b
8. c
9. a
10. c

Chapter 4

1. d
2. a

3. a
4. c
5. a
6. b
7. c
8. a
9. d
10. a

Chapter 5

1. d
2. d
3. b
4. c
5. d
6. c
7. d
8. a
9. d
10. d

Chapter 6

1. a
2. a
3. c
4. a
5. a
6. d
7. d
8. d
9. d
10. c

Chapter 7

1. c
2. a
3. d
4. a
5. c

6. d
7. b
8. b
9. c
10. a

Chapter 8

1. b
2. b
3. b
4. d
5. c
6. c
7. a
8. d
9. b
10. a

Chapter 9

1. c
2. d
3. b
4. d
5. b
6. c
7. a
8. b
9. b
10. c

Chapter 10

1. d
2. a
3. d
4. a
5. a
6. b
7. c
8. a

9. d
10. c

Chapter 11

1. b
2. d
3. a
4. d
5. a
6. b
7. a
8. c
9. c
10. d

Chapter 12

1. a
2. d
3. b
4. b
5. b
6. b
7. a
8. d
9. a
10. d

Chapter 13

1. d
2. c
3. c
4. d
5. c
6. c
7. c
8. d
9. d
10. d

Chapter 14

1. d
2. a
3. d
4. b
5. c
6. b
7. c
8. b
9. a
10. d

Chapter 15

1. b
2. a
3. d
4. d
5. d
6. a
7. d
8. d
9. a
10. c

Chapter 16

1. a
2. c
3. c
4. c
5. c
6. d
7. b
8. d
9. d
10. c

Chapter 17

1. a
2. b
3. d
4. c
5. a
6. b
7. a
8. a
9. a
10. a

Chapter 18

1. c
2. a
3. d
4. a
5. b
6. a
7. b
8. a
9. c
10. a

Chapter 19

1. b
2. d
3. b
4. d
5. d
6. b
7. b
8. a
9. b
10. d

Chapter 20

1. b
2. b
3. d
4. c
5. a
6. d
7. a
8. d
9. c
10. b

Chapter 21

1. c
2. a
3. d
4. d
5. d
6. b
7. c
8. d
9. c
10. d

B
Answers to the Case Studies

Chapter 18

Case 1

A. The fact that the rash occurred in June caused the clinician to think of spotted fever rickettsiosis, which is transmitted by ticks. In many areas of the country, ticks are quite active in June.
B. Measles
C. Rubeola virus (measles virus)
D. Koplik spots; in the setting of a compatible febrile illness with rash, Koplik spots are very good evidence of measles.
E. An immunodiagnostic procedure to detect anti-rubeola virus antibodies; viral culture could also be used, but it is a more expensive procedure

Case 2

A. (4) Human papillomavirus
B. (3) Cervical cancer

Case 3

A. (2) Varicella-zoster virus (the patient is experiencing shingles)
B. (5) Chickenpox

Chapter 19

Case 1

A. (2) *Escherichia coli*

Case 2

A. (5) *Streptococcus pyogenes* - Group A strep

Case 3

A. (3) *Escherichia coli* O157:H7

Case 4

A. (2) *Neisseria meningitidis*

Case 5

A. (4) *Streptococcus pneumoniae*

Chapter 20

Case 1

A. (1) *Cryptococcus neoformans*; the other pathogens listed are as much as 20 μm in diameter
B. An India ink preparation
C. The India ink preparation would reveal encapsulated yeast cells, some of which would be in the process of budding; the capsules would appear as clear halos around the yeast particles, against the dark background of India ink particles.
D. Yes, although pulmonary cryptococcosis can occur in immunocompetent people, it occurs primarily in people who are immunosuppressed; lymphomas are accompanied by defects in cell-mediated immunity.

Case 2

A. (3) Thrush
B. (4) *Candida albicans*

Case 3

A. (2) Histoplasmosis
B. (3) Nonencapsulated, budding yeasts

Chapter 21

Case 1

A. (2) *Plasmodium*

Case 2

A. (3) *Toxoplasma gondii*

Case 3

A. (4) *Giardia lamblia*

Case 4

A. (4) *Trichomonas vaginalis*

Case 5

A. (1) *Balantidium coli*

C

Useful Conversions

Length Conversions

To convert inches into centimeters, multiply by 2.54.
To convert centimeters into inches, multiply by 0.39.
To convert yards into meters, multiply by 0.91.
To convert meters into yards, multiply by 1.09.
1 mile (mi) = 1.609 kilometers
1 yard (yd) = 0.914 meter
1 foot (ft) = 30.48 centimeters
1 inch (in) = 2.54 centimeters
1 kilometer (km) = 0.62 mile
1 meter (m) = 39.37 inches
1 centimeter (cm) = 0.39 inch
1 millimeter (mm) = 0.039 inch

Note: Information about micrometers and nanometers can be found in Figure 2-1 in Chapter 2.

Volume Conversions

To convert gallons into liters, multiply by 3.78.
To convert liters into gallons, multiply by 0.26.
To convert fluid ounces into milliliters, multiply by 29.6.
To convert milliliters into fluid ounces, multiply by 0.034.
1 gallon (gal) = 3.785 liters
1 quart (qt) = 0.946 liter
1 pint (pt) = 0.473 liter
1 fluid ounce (fl oz) = 29.573 milliliters
1 liter (L) = 1.057 quarts
1 milliliter (mL) = 0.0338 fluid ounce

Weight Conversions

To convert ounces into grams, multiply by 28.4.
To convert grams into ounces, multiply by 0.035.
To convert pounds into kilograms, multiply by 0.45.
To convert kilograms into pounds, multiply by 2.2.
1 pound (lb) = 0.454 kilogram
1 ounce (oz) = 28.35 grams
1 kilogram (kg) = 2.2 pounds
1 gram (g) = 0.035 ounce
1 gram = 1,000 milligrams (mg)
1 gram = 1,000,000 micrograms (µg)

Temperature Conversions

To convert Celsius (°C) into Fahrenheit (°F), use
°F = (°C × 1.8) + 32.
To convert Fahrenheit (°F) into Celsius (°C), use
°C = (°F − 32) × 0.556.

D

Greek Alphabet

GREEK LETTER		Name	Pronunciation
Uppercase	**Lowercase**		
A	α	Alpha	al-fah
B	β	Beta	bay-tah
Γ	γ	Gamma	gam-ah
Δ	δ	Delta	del-tah
E	ε	Epsilon	ep-si-lon
Z	ζ	Zeta	zay-tah
H	η	Eta	ay-tah
Θ	θ	Theta	thay-tah
I	ι	Iota	eye-o-tah
K	κ	Kappa	cap-ah
Λ	λ	Lambda	lamb-dah
M	μ	Mu	mew
N	ν	Nu	new
Ξ	ξ	Xi	zzEye
O	ο	Omicron	om-ah-cron
Π	π	Pi	pie
P	ρ	Rho	row
Σ	σ	Sigma	sig-ma
T	τ	Tau	tawh
Y	υ	Upsilon	oop-si-lon
Φ	φ	Phi	figh or fie
X	χ	Chi	kigh
Ψ	ψ	Psi	sigh
Ω	ω	Omega	o-may-gah

A

Abiogenesis (ab'-ee-oh-jen-uh-sis). The theory that life can arise from nonliving matter; also known as spontaneous generation (Chap. 1).

Acellular Microbe. A microbe that is not composed of cells (e.g., viruses, prions, viroids) (Chap. 1).

Acid-Fast Stain. A differential staining procedure that differentiates acid-fast bacteria from non–acid-fast bacteria; primarily used in the presumptive diagnosis of tuberculosis (Chap. 4).

Acidophile (uh-sid'-oh-file). An organism that prefers acidic environments; such an organism is said to be *acidophilic* (Chap. 8).

Acquired Immunodeficiency Syndrome (AIDS). A disease characterized by a variety of opportunistic infections and malignancies; caused by human immunodeficiency virus (HIV) (Chap. 18).

Acquired Immunity. Immunity or resistance acquired at some point in an individual's lifetime (Chap. 16).

Acquired Resistance. When bacteria become resistant to a drug that they were once susceptible to (Chap. 9).

Active Acquired Immunity. Immunity or resistance acquired as a result of the active production of antibodies (Chap. 16).

Active Carrier. A person who has recovered from an infectious disease but continues to harbor and transmit the causative agent of that disease (Chap. 11).

Acute Coryza (kuh-rye'-zuh). A synonym for the common cold (Chap. 18).

Acute Disease. A disease having a sudden onset and short duration (Chap. 14).

Adenosine Triphosphate (uh-den'-oh-seen try-fos'-fate). The major energy-carrying (energy-storing) molecule in a cell (Chap. 7).

Adhesins (ad-hee'-zinz). Molecules on the surface of a pathogen that enable the pathogen to recognize and bind to a particular receptor on the surface of a host cell; also known as *ligands* (Chap. 14).

Aerial Hyphae (high'-fee). Mycelial hyphae extending above the surface (of the soil, agar, skin, or wherever the mycelium is growing); where spores are produced; also called *reproductive hyphae* (Chap. 5).

Aerotolerant Anaerobe (air-oh-tol'-er-ant an'-air-obe). An organism that can live in the presence of oxygen but grows best in an anaerobic environment (an environment containing no oxygen) (Chap. 4).

Agammaglobulinemia (ay-gam'-uh-glob'-yu-luh-nee'-me-uh). Absence of, or extremely low levels of, the gamma fraction of serum globulin; the absence of immunoglobulins in the bloodstream (Chap. 16).

AIDS. See *acquired immunodeficiency syndrome.*

Airborne Infection Isolation Room (AIIR). A hospital room for placement for patients who require Airborne Precautions; AIIRs are under negative pressure, and air that is evacuated from these rooms passes through high-efficiency particulate air (HEPA) filters (Chap. 12).

Airborne Precautions. Standardized safety precautions that are practiced in a healthcare setting to prevent infections transmitted by the airborne route (Chap. 12).

Algae (al'-gee), sing. *alga.* Eukaryotic, photosynthetic organisms that range in size from unicellular to multicellular; includes many seaweeds (Chap. 5).

Algicidal (al'-juh-side-ul) **Agent.** A disinfectant or chemical that specifically kills algae (Chap. 8).

Alkaliphile (al'-kuh-luh-file). An organism that prefers alkaline (basic) environments; such an organism is said to be *alkaliphilic* (Chap. 8).

Allergen (al'-ur-jin). An antigen to which some people become allergic (Chap. 16).

Ameba (uh-me'-bah), pl. *amebae.* A type of protozoan that moves by means of pseudopodia; in the phylum Sarcodina (which is a subphylum in some classification schemes) (Chap. 5).

Ames Test. A method of testing compounds to determine whether they are mutagenic (i.e., to see whether they cause mutations in bacteria); uses a mutant strain of *Salmonella* (Chap. 7).

Amino (uh-me'-no) **Acids.** The basic units or building blocks of proteins (Chap. 6).

Ammonification (uh-mon'-uh-fuh-kay'-shun). Conversion of nitrogenous compounds (e.g., proteins) into ammonia (Chap. 10).

Amphitrichous (am-fit'-ri-kus) **Bacterium.** A bacterium that possesses one flagellum or more than one flagellum at each end (pole) of the cell (Chap. 3).

Anabolic Reactions. Metabolic reactions that require energy for the creation of chemical bonds; also known as *biosynthetic reactions* (Chap. 7).

Anabolism (uh-nab'-oh-lizm). Term referring to all of the anabolic reactions that occur within a cell (Chap. 7).

Anaerobe (an'-air-obe). An organism that does not require oxygen for survival; can exist in the absence of oxygen (Chap. 4).

Anaphylactic (an-uh-fuh-lak'-tick) **Reactions.** Allergic reactions; may be localized or systemic; also known as *type I hypersensitivity reactions* (Chap. 16).

Anaphylactic (an-uh-fuh-lak'-tick) **Shock.** Shock after anaphylaxis; may lead to death (Chap. 16).

Anaphylaxis (an-uh-fuh-lak'-sis). An immediate, severe, sometimes fatal, systemic allergic reaction (Chap. 16).

Anoxygenic Photosynthesis (an'-ox-uh-gen'-ik foe-toe-sin'-thuh-sis). A type of photosynthesis in which oxygen is not produced (Chap. 4).

Antagonism (an-tag'-ohn-izm). As the term relates to the use of drugs, the use of two drugs that work against each other; also see *microbial antagonism* (Chap. 9).

Anthrax. A bacterial disease caused by *Bacillus anthracis*, a spore-forming Gram-positive bacillus (Chap. 19).

Antibacterial Agents. Technically, any physical or chemical agents that kill or inhibit the growth of bacteria; in this book, the term is reserved for drugs that are used to treat bacterial diseases (Chap. 9).

Antibiogram (an-tee-by'-oh-gram). The pattern of susceptible (S) and resistant (R) results obtained when antimicrobial susceptibility testing is performed on a particular microorganism (Chap. 12).

Antibiotic (an'-tee-by-ot'-tik). A substance produced by a microorganism that kills or inhibits the growth of other microorganisms (Chap. 1).

Antibiotic-Associated Diarrhea. A diarrheal disease that follows antibiotic therapy; usually caused by *Clostridium difficile*, a spore-forming, anaerobic, Gram-positive bacillus (Chap. 19).

Antibody (an'-tee-bod-ee). A glycoprotein produced by lymphocytes in response to an antigen; if it protects the host in some manner, it is referred to as a *protective antibody* (Chap. 15).

Anticodon (an-tee-ko'-don). A trinucleotide sequence that is complementary to a codon; found on a transfer RNA molecule (Chap. 6).

Antifungal Agents. Technically, any physical or chemical agents that kill or inhibit the growth of fungi; in this book, the term is reserved for drugs that are used to treat fungal diseases (Chap. 9).

Antigen (an'-tuh-jen). A substance, usually foreign, that stimulates the production of antibodies; an *anti*body *gen*erating substance; also known as an *immunogen* (Chap. 15).

Antigen–Antibody Complex. The structure produced as a result of the binding of an antibody to an antigen; also known as an *immune complex* (Chap. 16).

Antigen-Presenting Cell (APC). A macrophage that is displaying antigenic determinants on its surface (Chap. 16).

Antigenic (an-tuh-jen'-ick). If a molecule is antigenic, it stimulates the immune system to produce antibodies; such a molecule is also said to be *immunogenic* (Chap. 16).

Antigenic Determinant. The smallest part of an antigen capable of stimulating the production of antibodies; an antigenic molecule; also known as an *epitope* (Chap. 16).

Antigenic Variation. The ability of a microorganism to change its surface antigens (Chap. 16).

Antimicrobial (an'-tee-my-kro'-be-ul) **Agents.** Technically, any physical or chemical agents that kill or inhibit the growth of microorganisms; in this book, the term is reserved for drugs that are used to treat infectious diseases (Chap. 9).

Antiprotozoal Agents. Technically, any physical or chemical agents that kill or inhibit the growth of protozoa; in this book, the term is reserved for drugs that are used to treat protozoal diseases (Chap. 9).

Antisepsis (an-tee-sep'-sis). Prevention of infection by inhibiting the growth of pathogens (Chap. 8).

Antiseptic (an-tee-sep'-tick). An agent or substance capable of effecting antisepsis; usually refers to a chemical disinfectant that is safe to use on skin and other living tissues (Chap. 8).

Antiseptic Technique. Procedures followed to effect antisepsis; the use of antiseptics (Chap. 8).

Antiserum (an-tee-see'-rum). A serum containing specific antibodies; also known as an *immune serum* (Chap. 16).

Antitoxins (an-tee-tok'-sinz). Antibodies produced in response to a toxin; often capable of neutralizing the toxin that stimulated their production (Chap. 16).

Antiviral Agents. Technically, any physical or chemical agents that inactivate viruses; in this book, the term is reserved for drugs that are used to treat viral diseases (Chap. 9).

Apoenzyme. A protein that cannot function as an enzyme (i.e., cannot catalyze a chemical reaction) until it attaches to a cofactor (Chap. 6).

Arbovirus (are'-boh-vy'-rus). A virus that is transmitted by an arthropod; an arthropod-borne virus (Chap. 18).

Arthropod-borne Virus. See *arbovirus*.

Artificial Active Acquired Immunity. Active acquired immunity that is induced artificially (e.g., by injecting a vaccine into an individual) (Chap. 16).

Artificial Media. Culture media that are prepared in the laboratory; they do not occur naturally; also known as *synthetic media* (Chap. 8).

Artificial Passive Acquired Immunity. Passive acquired immunity that is induced artificially (e.g., by injecting antibodies into an individual) (Chap. 16).

Asepsis (a-sep'-sis). Literally, "without infection"; a condition in which living pathogens are absent (Chap. 8).

Aseptate Hyphae. Fungal hyphae that do not contain septa (cross-walls) (Chap. 5).

Aseptic Meningitis (ay-sep'-tick men-in-ji'-tis). A type of meningitis that is not caused by a pathogen or where the etiologic agent will not grow on standard bacteriological culture media; often used as a synonym for viral meningitis.

Aseptic (ay-sep'-tick) **Techniques.** Measures taken to ensure that living pathogens are absent (Chap. 8).

Asexual Reproduction. A type of reproduction in which a single organism is the sole parent; it passes copies of its entire genome to its offspring (Chap. 3).

Asymptomatic (ay'-simp-tow-mat'-ick) **Disease.** A disease having no symptoms; also referred to as a *subclinical disease* (Chap. 14).

Asymptomatic Infection. The presence of a pathogen in or on the body, without any clinical symptoms of disease; also referred to as a *subclinical infection* (Chap. 14).

Atopic (ay-tope'-ick) **Person.** Allergic person; one who suffers from allergies (Chap. 16).

Attenuated (uh-ten'-yu-ay-ted). An adjective meaning weakened, less pathogenic; used to describe certain microorganisms (Chap. 16).

Attenuated Vaccine. A vaccine prepared from an attenuated microorganism (Chap. 16).

Attenuation (uh-ten-yu-ay-'shun). The process by which microorganisms are attenuated (Chap. 16).

Autoclave (aw'-toe-klav). An apparatus used for sterilization by steam under pressure (Chap. 8).

Autogenous (aw-toj'-uh-nus) **Vaccine.** A vaccine prepared from microorganisms or cells obtained from the person's own body (Chap. 16).

Autoimmune (aw-toh-uh-myun') **Disease.** A disease in which the body produces antibodies directed against its own tissues (Chap. 16).

Autolysis (aw-tol'-uh-sis). Autodigestion; self-digestion (Chap. 3).

Autotroph (aw'-toe-trof). An organism that uses carbon dioxide as its sole carbon source (Chap. 7).

Avirulent (ay-veer'-yu-lent) **Strains.** Strains that are not virulent; not pathogenic; not capable of causing disease (Chap. 14).

Axial Filaments. Flagella-like fibrils that enable spirochetes to move in a spiral, helical, or inchworm manner.

B

B Cells (B Lymphocytes). The leukocytes that produce antibodies (Chap. 16).

Bacillus (bah-sil'-us), pl. *bacilli*. A rod-shaped bacterium; there is also a bacterial genus named *Bacillus*, made up of aerobic, Gram-positive, spore-forming bacilli (Chap. 2).

Bacteremia (bak-ter-ee'-me-uh). The presence of bacteria in the bloodstream (Chap. 13).

Bacteria (back-teer'-ee-uh). Microorganisms in the Domain *Bacteria* (Chap. 3).

Bacterial Vaginosis (BV). A vaginal infection caused by a variety of bacteria; an example of a *synergistic infection* (Chap. 17).

Bactericidal (bak-tear'-eh-sigh'-dull) **Agent.** A chemical agent or drug that kills bacteria; a *bactericide* (Chap. 8).

Bacteriocins (bak-teer'-ee-oh-sinz). Proteins produced by certain bacteria (those possessing bacteriocinogenic plasmids) that can kill other bacteria (Chap. 10).

Bacteriologist (back'-tier-ee-ol'-oh-jist). One who specializes in the science of bacteriology (Chap. 1).

Bacteriology (back'-tier-ee-ol'-oh-gee). The study of bacteria (Chap. 1).

Bacteriophage (back-tier'-ee-oh-faj). A virus that infects a bacterium; also known simply as a *phage* (Chap. 4).

Bacteriostatic (bak-tear'-ee-oh-stat'-ick) **Agent.** A chemical agent or drug that inhibits the growth of bacteria (Chap. 8).

Bacteriuria (bak-ter-ee'-yu'-ree-uh). The presence of bacteria in the urine (Chap. 13).

Barometric Pressure. The pressure of the atmosphere as indicated by an instrument called a barometer (Chap. 8).

Bartholinitis (bar-toe-lin-eye'-tis). Inflammation of the Bartholin's gland in women (Chap. 17).

Basophil (bay'-so-fil). A type of granulocyte found in blood; its granules contain acidic substances (e.g., histamine) that attract basic dyes (Chap. 15).

Beneficial Mutation. A mutation that is of benefit to the mutant organism (Chap. 7).

Binary (by'-nare-ee) **Fission.** A method of reproduction whereby one cell divides to become two cells; the method by which bacteria reproduce (Chap. 3).

Biochemistry (by-oh-kem'-is-tree). The chemistry of living organisms; the chemistry of life (Chap. 6).

Biocidal (by-o-sigh'-dull) **Agent.** A chemical agent that destroys living organisms, especially microorganisms (Chap. 8).

Biofilms. Complex and persistent communities of assorted microorganisms (Chap. 10).

Biogenesis (by-oh-gen'-uh-sis). The theory that life originates only from preexisting life and never from nonliving matter (Chap. 1).

Biologic Catalysts. Enzymes; biologic molecules that catalyze chemical reactions (Chap. 6).

Biologic Warfare (BW) Agents. Pathogens used as weapons in warfare (Chap. 11).

Biological Vector. An arthropod vector (such as a flea or tick) within which a pathogen multiplies or matures (Chap. 21).

Biology. The study of living organisms; the study of life (Chap. 1).

Biomass. The total mass or number of living organisms in a particular area or volume (Chap. 1).

Bioremediation (by'-oh-ruh-meed'-ee-a-shun). The use of microorganisms to clean up industrial and toxic wastes (Chap. 1).

Biotechnology (by'-oh-tek-nol'-oh-gee). The use of living organisms or their derivatives to make or modify products or processes (Chap. 1).

Bioterrorist Agents. Pathogens used by terrorists (Chap. 11).

Biotherapeutic (by'-oh-ther-uh-pu'-tik) **Agents.** Microorganisms used for therapeutic purposes (to treat various diseases or conditions) (Chap. 10).

Biotype. The pattern of positive and negative biochemical test results obtained when a particular microorganism is tested; in some biochemical test systems (e.g., minisystems), biotype refers to the specific code number generated by the test results (Chap. 12).

Black Piedra (pee-a'-druh). A hair infection caused by the mould *Piedraia hortae* (Chap. 20).

Blocking Antibodies. Immunoglobulin G (IgG) antibodies produced by the body in response to allergy shots; they combine with allergens, thus preventing the allergens from attaching to IgE antibodies on the surface of basophils and mast cells (Chap. 16).

Botulinal (bot'-you-ly-nal) **Toxin.** The neurotoxin produced by *Clostridium botulinum*; causes botulism; known by various other names such as botulin and botulinum toxin (Chap. 14).

Botulism. A neurological disease caused by a neurotoxin (botulinal toxin) produced by *C. botulinum*, a spore-forming, anaerobic, Gram-positive bacillus (Chap. 19).

Brightfield Microscope. Alternate name for a compound light microscope; refers to the fact that objects are observed against a bright background (or bright field) (Chap. 2).

Broad-Spectrum Antibiotics. Antibiotics that are effective against a wide range of bacteria; they are effective against both Gram-positive and Gram-negative bacteria (Chap. 9).

Bronchitis (brong-ky'-tis). Inflammation of the mucous membrane lining of the bronchial tubes (Chap. 17).

Bronchopneumonia (brong'-ko-new-mow'-nee-uh). Combination of bronchitis and pneumonia (Chap. 17).

C

Calibrated Loop. A bacteriologic loop manufactured to contain a precise volume of liquid (usually 0.01 or 0.001 mL) (Chap. 13).

Candidiasis (kan-duh-dy'-uh-sis). Infection with, or disease caused by, a yeast in the genus *Candida*—usually *Candida albicans*; also known as *moniliasis* (Chap. 10).

Capnophile (cap'-no-file). An organism that grows best in the presence of increased concentrations of carbon dioxide; such an organism is said to be *capnophilic* (Chap. 4).

Capsid (kap'-syd). The external protein coat or covering of a virion (Chap. 4).

Capsomeres (kap'-so-meers). The individual protein subunits that make up the capsid of some virions (Chap. 4).

Capsule (kap'-sool). An organized layer of glycocalyx, firmly attached to the outer surface of a bacterial cell wall; some yeasts are also encapsulated (Chap. 3).

Carbohydrates (kar-boh-high'-drates). Organic compounds containing carbon, hydrogen, and oxygen in a ratio of 1:2:1; also known as *saccharides* (Chap. 6).

Carbuncle (kar'-bung-kul). A deep-seated pyogenic (pus-producing) infection of the skin, usually arising from a coalescence of furuncles (Chap. 17).

Carrier (keh'-ree-er). An individual having an asymptomatic infection that can be transmitted to other susceptible individuals (Chap. 10).

Catabolic (cat-uh-bohl'-ik) **Reactions.** Metabolic reactions that involve the breaking of chemical bonds and the release of energy; also known as *degradative reactions* (Chap. 7).

Catabolism (kuh-tab'-oh-lizm). Term referring to all the catabolic reactions that occur within a cell (Chap. 7).

Catalyst (kat'-uh-list). A substance (usually an enzyme) that speeds up a chemical reaction but is not itself consumed or permanently changed in the process (Chap. 6).

Catalyze (cat'-uh-lyz). To act as a catalyst; to speed up a reaction (Chap. 6).

Cell (sell). The smallest unit of living structure capable of independent existence (Chap. 3).

Cell-Mediated Immunity. A type of immunity involving many different cell types (e.g., macrophages, various types of lymphocytes), but where antibodies play only a minor role, if any; also known as *delayed hypersensitivity* (Chap. 16).

Cell Membrane (sell mem'-brain). The protoplasmic boundary of all cells; provides selective permeability and serves other important functions (Chap. 3).

Cell Theory. The theory stating that all living organisms are composed of cells (Chap. 3).

Cell Wall. The outermost layer of many types of cells (e.g., algal, bacterial, fungal, and plant cells); it serves to protect the cell (Chap. 3).

Cellular Microbe. A microbe that is composed of cells (e.g., bacteria, algae, protozoa) (Chap. 1).

Cellulose (sell'-you-los). A polysaccharide found in the cell walls of algae and plants (Chap. 3).

Centimeter (sen'-tuh-me-ter). One hundredth of a meter (Chap. 2).

Central Dogma. The flow of genetic information within a cell; from DNA to an mRNA molecule to a protein molecule (Chap. 6).

Cephalosporinase (sef'-uh-low-spore'-uh-nase). An enzyme that destroys the β-lactam ring in cephalosporin antibiotics; a type of β-lactamase (Chap. 9).

Cerebrospinal (sir-ee'-broh-spy'-nul) **Fluid (CSF).** The fluid within the spinal cord and the ventricles and cavities of the brain; also referred to simply as *spinal fluid* (Chap. 13).

Cervicitis (sir-vuh-sigh'-tis). Inflammation of the cervix (the part of the uterus that opens into the vagina) (Chap. 17).

Cestodes (sess'-toadz). A subcategory of flatworms; includes tapeworms (Chap. 21).

Chemically Defined Media. Types of culture media where the exact chemical composition is known (Chap. 8).

Chemoautotroph (keem'-oh-awe'-toe-trof). An organism that uses chemicals as an energy source and carbon dioxide as a carbon source; a type of autotroph (Chap. 7).

Chemoheterotroph (keem'-oh-het'-er-oh-trof). An organism that uses chemicals as an energy source and organic chemicals as a carbon source; a type of heterotroph (Chap. 7).

Chemokines. Chemotactic agents produced by various types of cells in the body (Chap. 15).

Chemolithotroph (keem'-oh-lith'-oh-trof). A type of chemotroph that uses inorganic compounds as a source of energy; also referred to as a *lithotroph* (Chap. 7).

Chemoorganotroph (keem'-oh-or-gan'-oh-trof). A type of chemotroph that uses organic compounds as a source of energy; also referred to as an *organotroph* (Chap. 7).

Chemosynthesis (keem'-oh-syn'-thuh-sis). The process of obtaining energy and synthesizing organic compounds from simple inorganic reactions; carried out by some chemoautotrophic bacteria (Chap. 7).

Chemotactic (keem'-oh-tack'-tick) **Agents.** Chemical substances that attract leukocytes; also referred to as *chemotactic factors*, *chemotactic substances*, and *chemoattractants* (Chap. 15).

Chemotaxis (keem'-oh-tack'-sis). The movement of cells in response to a chemical (e.g., the attraction of phagocytes to an area of injury) (Chap. 15).

Chemotherapeutic (keem'-oh-ther-uh-pyu'-tik) **Agent.** Any chemical used to treat any disease or medical condition (Chap. 9).

Chemotherapy (keem'-oh-ther'-uh-pee). The treatment of a disease (including an infectious disease) using chemical substances or drugs (Chap. 9).

Chemotroph (keem'-oh-trof). An organism that uses chemicals as an energy source (Chap. 7).

Chitin (ky'-tin). A polysaccharide found in fungal cell walls but not found in the cell walls of other microorganisms; also found in the exoskeleton of beetles and crabs (Chap. 3).

Chloroplast (klor'-oh-plast). A membrane-bound organelle found in the cytoplasm of algal and plant cells; a *plastid* that contains chlorophyll (Chap. 3).

Cholera. A diarrheal disease caused by *Vibrio cholerae*, a curved Gram-negative bacillus (Chap. 19).

Choleragin (kol'-er-uh-jen). The enterotoxin that causes cholera; produced by *V. cholerae* (Chap. 19).

Chromosomes (kro'-mow-soamz). Cellular structures where most (sometimes all) of the cell's genes are located; eukaryotic chromosomes consist of linear double-stranded DNA molecules and proteins (histones and nonhistone proteins); a prokaryotic chromosome usually consists of a single, long, supercoiled, circular, double-stranded DNA molecule (Chap. 3).

Chronic Disease. A disease having an insidious (slow) onset and a long duration (Chap. 14).

Ciliates (sil'-ee-itz), sing. *ciliate*. Ciliated protozoa (Chap. 5).

Cilium (sil'-ee-um), pl. *cilia*. A thin, usually short, hairlike organelle of motility (Chap. 3).

Clean-Catch, Midstream Urine (CCMS urine). A urine specimen that has been collected in a manner that minimizes contamination with indigenous microflora; the proper type of specimen for a urine culture (Chap. 13).

Clinical Specimens. Various types of specimens (e.g., blood, urine, cerebrospinal fluid) collected from patients (Chap. 13).

Clinically Relevant Laboratory Results. Laboratory results that provide the physician with useful, accurate information about a patient's disease (Chap. 13).

Coagulase (ko-ag'-yu-lace). A bacterial enzyme that causes plasma to clot; converts fibrinogen (a plasma protein) to fibrin (Chap. 14).

Coccidioidomycosis (kok-sid-ee-oy'-doe-my-ko'-sis). A systemic mycosis caused by *Coccidioides immitis*, a dimorphic fungus (Chap. 20).

Coccobacillus (kok'-ko-buh-sil'-us), pl. *coccobacilli*. A very short bacillus (Chap. 4).

Coccus (kok'-us), pl. *cocci*. A spherical bacterium (Chap. 2).

Codon (koh'-don). A sequence of three consecutive nucleotides in a strand of mRNA that provides the genetic information (code) for a certain amino acid to be incorporated into a growing protein chain (Chap. 6).

Coenzyme (koh'-en-zym). A type of cofactor; several vitamins are coenzymes (Chap. 6).

Cofactor (koh'-fak'-tor). An ion or molecule essential for the enzymatic action of certain proteins (called apoenzymes) (Chap. 6).

Colicin (kol'-uh-sin). A type of bacteriocin produced by *Escherichia coli* and other closely related bacteria (Chap. 10).

Coliforms (ko'-lee-forms). *E. coli* and other lactose-fermenting members of the Family *Enterobacteriaceae* (Chap. 11).

Colitis (ko-ly'-tis). Inflammation of the colon (the large intestine) (Chap. 17).

Collagen (kol'-luh-jen). The major protein in the white fibers of connective tissue, cartilage, and bone (Chap. 14).

Collagenase (kol'-uh-juh-nace). A bacterial enzyme that causes the breakdown of collagen (Chap. 14).

Commensalism (ko-men'-sul-izm). A symbiotic relationship in which one party derives benefit and the other party is unaffected; many members of the indigenous microflora are commensals (Chap. 10).

Communicable (kuh-myun'-uh-kuh-bul) **Disease.** A disease capable of being transmitted from person to person (Chap. 11).

Community-Acquired Infection. Any infection acquired outside a healthcare setting (Chap. 12).

Competence (kom'-puh-tense). As used in this book, the ability of a bacterial cell to take up (absorb) free (naked) DNA from the environment; may lead to transformation (Chap. 7).

Competent Bacteria. Bacteria capable of taking up (absorbing) free (naked) DNA from the environment (Chap. 7).

Complement (kom'-pluh-ment). A protein complex of 25 to 30 components (including proteins designated C1 through C9) found in blood; involved in inflammation, chemotaxis, phagocytosis, and lysis of bacteria (Chap. 15).

Complement Cascade. The stepwise manner in which proteins of the complement system (complement components) interact with each other (Chap. 15).

Complex Media. Culture media, the exact chemical composition of which is unknown; often contain ground-up animal organs (e.g., brain, heart, liver) or yeast extract (Chap. 8).

Compound Light Microscope. A compound microscope that uses visible light as its source of illumination (Chap. 2).

Compound Microscope. A microscope containing more than one magnifying lens (Chap. 2).

Conidium (ko-nid'-ee-um), pl. *conidia*. An asexual fungal spore (Chap. 5).

Conjugate (kon'-ju-git) **Vaccine.** A vaccine prepared by linking a weakly antigenic molecule (e.g., bacterial capsule material) to a powerful antigen (Chap. 16).

Conjugation (kon-ju-gay'-shun). As used in this book, the union of two bacterial cells for the purpose of genetic transfer; *not* a reproductive process (Chap. 3).

Conjunctiva (kon-junk-ty'vuh). The mucous membrane that lines the eyelids and covers the anterior portion of the eyeball (Chap. 17).

Conjunctivitis (kon-junk'-tuh-vi'-tis). Inflammation of the conjunctiva (Chap. 17).

Constitutive Genes. Genes that are expressed at all times (Chap. 6).

Contact Precautions. Standardized safety precautions that are practiced in a healthcare setting to prevent infections transmitted by contact (Chap. 12).

Contagious Disease. A disease easily transmitted from one person to another; a type of communicable disease (Chap. 11).

Contamination (kon-tam-uh-nay'-shun). As used in this book, a condition indicating the presence of undesirable or accidentally introduced microorganisms (which would be referred to as *contaminants*) (Chap. 8).

Contractile Vacuole. An organelle that pumps water out of a protozoal cell (Chap. 5).

Convalescent (kon-vuh-less'-ent) **Carrier.** A person who no longer shows the signs or symptoms of a particular infectious disease but continues to harbor and transmit the causative agent during the convalescence period (Chap. 11).

Covalent (koh-vayl'-ent) **Bond.** A type of chemical bond in which two atoms share a pair of electrons (Chap. 6).

Crenated (kree'-nay-ted). Wrinkled, shriveled; (e.g., the appearance of erythrocytes placed into a hypertonic solution) (Chap. 8).

Crenation (kree-nay'-shun). The process of becoming, or state of being, crenated (Chap. 8).

Cryptococcosis (krip'-toe-kok-oh'-sis). A fungal infection caused by *Cryptococcus neoformans*, an encapsulated yeast (Chap. 20).

Cutaneous Anaphylaxis. Swelling and redness at the site where an antigen is injected intradermally or subcutaneously; also known as a *wheal-and-flare reaction* (Chap. 16).

Cyanobacteria (sigh'-an-oh-bak-tier'-ee-uh). A group of photosynthetic bacteria (Chap. 4).

Cyst. As the term applies to parasitology, the dormant, survival stage in a protozoan's life cycle; its tough wall enables the cyst to resist desiccation and temperature extremes (Chap. 5).

Cystitis (sis-ty'-tis). Inflammation or infection of the urinary bladder (Chap. 17).

Cytokines (sigh'-toe-kynz). Soluble chemical messages released by cells of the body; the manner in which different types of cells communicate with each other; examples include *lymphokines* (produced by lymphocytes) and *monokines* (produced by monocytes) (Chap. 16).

Cytokinesis (sigh'-toe-kuh-knee'-sis). Division of the cytoplasm, resulting in two daughter cells; follows mitosis (Chap. 3).

Cytology (sigh-tol'-oh-gee). The study of cells (Chap. 3).

Cytoplasm (sigh'-toe-plazm). A type of protoplasm; lies outside the nucleus of a eukaryotic cell (Chap. 3).

Cytoskeleton. A system of fibers (microtubules, microfilaments, and intermediate filaments) running throughout the cytoplasm of eukaryotic cells (Chap. 3).

Cytostome (sigh'-toe-stoam). A primitive mouth possessed by some protozoa (Chap. 5).

Cytotoxins (sigh'-tow-tok'-sinz). Toxic substances that inhibit or destroy cells (Chap. 14).

D

Darkfield Microscope. A compound light microscope that has been fitted with a darkfield condenser; refers to the fact that objects are observed against a dark background (or dark field) (Chap. 2).

Death Phase. The part of a bacterial growth curve during which no multiplication occurs and organisms are dying; the fourth and final phase in a bacterial growth curve (Chap. 8).

Decimeter (des'-uh-me-ter). One tenth of a meter (Chap. 2).

Decomposers. Microorganisms that decompose or break down substances (Chap. 1).

Decomposition. The breaking up or separation of something into basic components or parts (Chap. 1).

Definitive Host. In a parasitic relationship, the host that harbors the adult or sexual stage of a parasite, or the sexual phase of the parasite's life cycle (Chap. 21).

Dehydration Synthesis Reaction. An anabolic reaction in which two molecules are bonded together as a result of the loss of a water molecule; also called a *dehydrolysis reaction* (Chap. 6).

Dehydrogenation (dee-hy'-drah-jen-ay'-shun) **Reactions.** Chemical reactions in which a pair of hydrogen atoms is removed from a compound, usually by the action of enzymes called *dehydrogenases* (Chap. 7).

Delayed-Type Hypersensitivity (DTH) Reactions. Hypersensitivity reactions that usually take more than 24 hours to manifest themselves; also known as *cell-mediated immune reactions* and *type IV hypersensitivity reactions* (Chap. 16).

Denitrifying (dee'-ni-truh-fy-ing) **Bacteria.** Bacteria capable of converting nitrates into nitrogen gas; the process is known as *denitrification* (Chap. 10).

Dental Caries (kay'-reez). Tooth decay (Chap. 17).

Deoxyribonucleic (dee-ox'-ee-ry'-bow-new-clay'-ick) **Acid (DNA).** A macromolecule containing the genetic code in the form of genes (Chap. 3).

Dermatitis (der-muh-ty'-tis). Inflammation of the skin (Chap. 17).

Dermatophytes (der-mah'-toh-fytes). Fungi that cause superficial mycoses of the skin, hair, and nails; the cause of tinea infections (ringworm infections) (Chap. 20).

Dermis (der'-mis). The layer of skin containing blood and lymphatic vessels, nerves and nerve endings, glands, and hair follicles (Chap. 17).

Desiccation (des-uh-kay'-shun). The process of being desiccated (thoroughly dried) (Chap. 8).

Diarrhea (die-uh-ree'-uh). An abnormally frequent discharge of semisolid or fluid fecal matter (Chap. 17).

Differential (dif-er-en'-shul) **Media.** Culture media that enable microbiologists to readily differentiate one organism or group of organisms from another (Chap. 8).

Differential Staining Procedures. Bacterial staining procedures that enable differentiation of two groups of bacteria; (e.g., the Gram stain enables differentiation of Gram-positive bacteria from Gram-negative bacteria) (Chap. 4).

Dimorphic (dy-more'-fik) **Fungus.** A fungus that can exist either as a yeast or a mould (Chap. 5).

Dimorphism (dy-more'-fizm). A phenomenon whereby an organism can exist in two shapes or forms (e.g., dimorphic fungi can exist either as yeasts or moulds) (Chap. 5).

Dipeptide (dy-pep'-tide). A protein consisting of two amino acids held together by a peptide bond (Chap. 6).

Diphtheria. A bacterial disease caused by toxigenic (diphtheria toxin-producing) strains of *Corynebacterium diphtheriae*, Gram-positive bacilli (Chap. 19).

Diplobacilli (dip'-low-bah-sill'-eye). Bacilli arranged in pairs (Chap. 4).

Diplococci (dip'-low-kok'-sigh). Cocci arranged in pairs (Chap. 4).

Diploid (dip'-loyd) **Cells.** Eukaryotic cells containing two sets of chromosomes (Chap. 3).

Disaccharide (die-sack'-uh-ride). A carbohydrate consisting of two monosaccharides; examples include sucrose (table sugar), lactose (milk sugar), and maltose (malt sugar) (Chap. 6).

Disinfectant (dis-in-fek'-tent). A chemical agent used to destroy pathogens or inhibit their growth and vital activity; usually refers to a chemical agent used on nonliving materials (Chap. 8).

Disinfection (dis-in-fek'-shun). The process of destroying pathogens and their toxins (Chap. 8).

DNA Nucleotides. The building blocks of DNA; each DNA nucleotide consists of a nitrogenous base, deoxyribose, and a phosphate group (Chap. 6).

DNA Polymerase (poh-lim'-er-ace). The most important enzyme required in DNA replication (Chap. 6).

DNA Replication (rep-luh-kay'-shun). Production of two new DNA molecules (called *daughter molecules*) from one parent DNA molecule (Chap. 6).

DNA Vaccine. An experimental type of vaccine that stimulates host cells to produce numerous copies of a harmless microbial protein (antigen); the host's immune system then produces antibodies directed against the protein, and these antibodies protect the person from infection with the pathogen that possesses the protein; also known as a *gene vaccine* (Chap. 16).

Domain *Archaea*. One of the domains in the Three-Domain System of Classification of living organisms; members of this domain are prokaryotes; the other two domains are *Bacteria* and *Eucarya* (Chap. 3).

Domain *Bacteria*. One of the domains in the Three-Domain System of Classification of living organisms; members of this domain are prokaryotes; the other two domains are *Archaea* and *Eucarya* (Chap. 3).

Double Bond. A type of chemical bond, containing two pairs of shared electrons (Chap. 6).

Droplet Precautions. Standardized safety precautions that are practiced in a healthcare setting to prevent infections transmitted by droplets (Chap. 12).

Drug-Binding Site. A specific molecule on the surface of a cell that a particular drug attaches to (Chap. 9).

Dysentery (dis'-en-tay-ree). Frequent watery stools, accompanied by abdominal pain, fever, and dehydration; the stool specimens may contain blood or mucus (Chap. 17).

E

Ebola (ee-bow'-luh) **Virus.** An especially large virus that causes viral hemorrhagic fever. (Chap. 18).

Ecology (ee-kol'-oh-jee). The branch of biology concerned with the total complex of interrelationships among living organisms; encompassing the relationships of organisms to each other, to the environment, and to the entire energy balance within a given ecosystem (Chap. 7).

Ecosystem (ee'-koh-sis-tem). An ecologic system that includes all the organisms and the environment within which they occur naturally (Chap. 7).

Ectoparasite (ek'-toh-par'-uh-site). A parasite that lives on the external surface of its host (Chap. 21).

Edema (uh-dee'-muh). Swelling caused by an accumulation of watery fluid in cells, tissues, or body cavities; swollen areas are described as being *edematous* (Chap. 15).

Ehrlichiosis. A bacterial disease caused by *Ehrlichia* spp., Gram-negative bacilli that are obligate intracellular pathogens (Chap. 19).

Electron (ee-lek'-tron) **Micrograph.** Photograph taken through the lens system of an electron microscope (Chap. 2).

Electron Microscope. A type of microscope that uses electrons as a source of illumination (Chap. 2).

Electron Transport Chain. A series of biochemical reactions by which energy is transferred in a stepwise manner; a major source of energy in some cells (Chap. 7).

Empiric (em-peer'-uh-kul) **Therapy.** Treatment or therapy that is initiated by a physician (or other healthcare professional) before receipt of test results (Chap. 9).

Empty Magnification. Microscopy term meaning an increase in magnification without any concurrent increase in resolving power (Chap. 2).

Encephalitis (en-sef-uh-ly'-tis). Inflammation or infection of the brain (Chap. 13).

Encephalomyelitis (en-sef-uh-low-my'-uh-ly'-tis). Inflammation or infection of the brain and spinal cord (Chap. 17).

Endemic (en-dem'-ick) **Disease.** A disease that is always present in a community or geographic area (Chap. 11).

Endemic Typhus. Synonym for fleaborne typhus fever; caused by *Rickettsia typhi*, a Gram-negative bacillus that is an obligate intracellular pathogen (Chap. 19).

Endocarditis (en'-doh-kar-dy'-tis). Inflammation of the endocardium (the innermost lining of the heart) (Chap. 17).

Endoenzyme (en'-doh-en'-zym). An enzyme produced by a cell that remains within the cell; an intracellular enzyme (Chap. 7).

Endometritis (en'-dough-me-try'-tis). Inflammation of the endometrium (the inner layer of the uterine wall) (Chap. 17).

Endoparasite (en-doh-par'-uh-site). A parasite that lives within the body of its host (Chap. 21).

Endoplasmic Reticulum (end-oh-plaz'-mick re-tick'-you-lum) **(ER).** A network of membranous tubules and flattened sacs in the cytoplasm of a eukaryotic cell; ER with attached ribosomes is called *rough ER (RER)* or *granular ER*; ER having no attached ribosomes is called *smooth ER (SER)* (Chap. 3).

Endospore (en'-dough-spore). Thick-walled, resistant body formed within a bacterial cell for the purpose of survival; a bacterial cell produces only one endospore, and from that endospore emerges (a process known as *germination*) one bacterial cell; also referred to as a *bacterial spore* (Chap. 3).

Endosymbiont (en'-doh-sym'-be-ont). The party in a symbiotic relationship that lives within the body of the other symbiont (Chap. 10).

Endotoxin (en-doh-tok'-sin). The lipid portion of the lipopolysaccharide found in the cell walls of Gram-negative bacteria; intracellular toxin (Chap. 14).

Enriched Media. Culture media that enable microbiologists to isolate fastidious organisms from samples or specimens and grow them in the laboratory (Chap. 8).

Enteric (en-tare'-ik) **Bacilli.** Gram-negative bacilli in the Family *Enterobacteriaceae* (Chap. 10).

Enteritis (en-ter-eye'-tis). Inflammation of the intestines, usually referring to the small intestine (Chap. 17).

Enterohemorrhagic *E. Coli*. Strains of *E. coli* that produce enterotoxins that cause bloody diarrhea and hemolytic uremic syndrome (Chap. 19).

Enterotoxigenic *E. Coli*. Strains of *E. coli* that produce toxins that cause diarrhea (Chap. 19).

Enterotoxin (en-ter-oh-tok'-sin). A bacterial exotoxin specific for cells of the intestinal mucosa (Chap. 14).

Enterovirulent *E. Coli*. Strains of *E. coli* that produce toxins that cause gastrointestinal diseases; examples include enterohemorrhagic *E. coli* and enterotoxigenic *E. coli* (Chap. 19).

Enzyme (en'-zyme). A protein molecule that catalyzes (causes or speeds up) a chemical reaction; remains unchanged in the process; a biologic catalyst (Chap. 6).

Eosinophil (ee-oh-sin'-oh-fil). A type of granulocyte found in blood; its granules contain basic substances (e.g., major basic protein) that attract acidic dyes (Chap. 15).

Eosinophilia (ee'-oh-sin-oh-fil'-ee-uh). An abnormally high number of eosinophils in the bloodstream (Chap. 15).

Epidemic (ep-uh-dem'-ick) **Disease.** A disease occurring in a higher than usual number of cases in a population during a given time interval (Chap. 11).

Epidemic Typhus. Synonym for louseborne typhus fever; caused by *Rickettsia prowazekii*, a Gram-negative bacillus that is an obligate intracellular pathogen (Chap. 19).

Epidemiology (ep-uh-dee-me-ol'-oh-jee). The study of relationships between the various factors that determine the frequency and distribution of diseases (Chap. 11).

Epidermis (ep-ee-derm'-is). The superficial epithelial portion of the skin (Chap. 17).

Epididymitis (ep-uh-did-uh-my'-tis). Inflammation of the epididymis (a tubular structure within the testis) (Chap. 17).

Epiglottitis (ep-ee-glot-eye-tis). Inflammation of the epiglottis (the mouth of the windpipe) (Chap. 17).

Episome (ep'-eh-som). An extrachromosomal element (plasmid) that may either integrate into the host bacterium's chromosome or replicate and function stably when physically separated from the chromosome (Chap. 7).

Epstein-Barr Virus. The virus that causes infectious mononucleosis; an oncogenic virus that causes several types of cancer. (Chap. 18).

Erysipelis (err-eh-sip'-uh-lis). An acute cutaneous cellulitis caused by *Streptococcus pyogenes* (Chap. 19).

Erythema (air-uh-thee'-muh). Redness of the skin; a reddened area of skin is described as being *erythematous* (Chap. 16).

Erythrocytes (ee-rith'-roh-sites). Red blood cells (Chap. 13).

Erythrogenic (ee-rith-roh-jen'-ick) **Toxin.** The exotoxin produced by *S. pyogenes* that causes scarlet fever; *erythrogenic* means "produces redness," referring to the red rash of scarlet fever (Chap. 14).

Essential Amino Acids. Amino acids that must be provided to an organism because the organism is unable to synthesize them (Chap. 6).

Essential Fatty Acids. Fatty acids that must be provided to an organism because the organism is unable to synthesize them (Chap. 6).

Essential Nutrients. Any nutrients that must be provided to an organism because the organism is unable to synthesize them (Chap. 7).

Etiologic (e'-tee-oh-loj'-ik) **Agent.** The causative agent of an infectious disease (i.e., the pathogen that causes the disease) (Chap. 1).

Etiology. Cause; as in the etiology of a disease (Chap. 1).

Eucarya (you-ker'-ee-uh). One of the three domains in the three-domain system of classification; alternate spelling = *Eukarya*; members of this domain are eukaryotes; the other two domains are *Archaea* and *Bacteria* (Chap. 3).

Eukaryotic (you'-kar-ee-ah'-tick) **Cells.** Cells containing a true nucleus; organisms possessing such cells are

referred to as *eukaryotes*; can also be spelled eucaryotic (Chap. 3).

Exfoliative (eks-foh'-lee-uh-tiv) **Toxin.** The exotoxin produced by *Staphylococcus aureus* that causes staphylococcal scalded skin syndrome (SSSS); also known as *epidermolytic toxin* (Chap. 14).

Exoenzyme (ek-soh-en'-zyme). An enzyme produced by a cell that is released from the cell; an extracellular enzyme (Chap. 7).

Exotoxin (ek-soh-tok'-sin). A toxin that is released from the cell; an extracellular toxin (Chap. 14).

Exudate (eks'-yu-date). Any fluid (e.g., pus) that exudes (oozes) from tissue, often as a result of injury, infection, or inflammation (Chap. 17).

F

Facultative (fak'-ul-tay-tive) **Anaerobe.** An organism that can live either in the presence or absence of oxygen (Chap. 4).

Facultative Intracellular Pathogen. A pathogen that can live either intracellularly or extracellularly (Chap. 14).

Facultative Parasite. An organism that is capable of being a parasite but is also capable of a free-living existence (Chap. 21).

Fascia (fash'-ee-uh). A sheet of fibrous tissue that envelops the body beneath the skin; also encloses muscles and groups of muscles (Chap. 19).

Fasciitis (fas-ee-eye'-tis). Inflammation in fascia (Chap. 19).

Fastidious (fas-tid'-ee-us) **Microbes.** Microbes that are difficult to isolate from specimens and grow in the laboratory, owing to their complex nutritional requirements (Chap. 1).

Fatty Acid. Any acid derived from fats by hydrolysis; fatty acids are the building blocks of lipids (Chap. 6).

Fermentation (fer-men-tay'-shun). An anaerobic biochemical pathway in which substances are broken down, and energy and reduced compounds are produced; oxygen does not participate in the process (Chap. 7).

Fermentative Pathways. Metabolic pathways in which oxygen does not participate (Chap. 7).

Fimbriae (fim'-bree-ee), sing. *fimbria* (fim'-bree-uh). See *pili* (Chap. 3).

Fixed Macrophages. Macrophages that remain localized within certain organs and tissues; also known as *histocytes* or *histiocytes* (Chap. 15).

Flagella (fluh-jel'-uh), sing. *flagellum.* Whiplike organelles of motility; prokaryotic and eukaryotic flagella differ in structure; prokaryotic flagella are composed of a protein called *flagellin*; eukaryotic flagella contain nine doublet microtubules arranged around two central microtubules (a 9 + 2 arrangement) (Chap. 3).

Flagellates (flaj'-eh-letz). Flagellated protozoa (Chap. 5).

Flagellin (flaj'-eh-lin). The protein of which bacterial flagella are composed (Chap. 3).

Fluorescence (floor'-es-ence) **Microscope.** A type of compound light microscope that uses an ultraviolet (UV) light source (Chap. 2).

Folliculitis (foh-lick-you-ly'-tis). Inflammation of a hair follicle, the sac that contains a hair shaft (Chap. 17).

Fomites (foh'-mitz). Inanimate objects or substances capable of absorbing and transmitting a pathogen (e.g., clothing, bed linens, towels, eating utensils) (Chap. 11).

Fungemia (fun-gee'-me-uh). The presence of fungi in the bloodstream (Chap. 13).

Fungi (fun'-ji), sing. *fungus*. Eukaryotic, nonphotosynthetic microorganisms that can be either saprophytic or parasitic (Chap. 5).

Fungicidal (fun-juh-sigh'-dull) **Agent.** A chemical agent or drug that kills fungi; a *fungicide* or *mycocide* (Chap. 8).

Furuncle (few'-rung-kul). A localized pyogenic (pus-producing) infection of the skin, usually resulting from folliculitis; often referred to as a *boil* (Chap. 17).

G

Gangrene (gang'-green). Necrosis (cell death) as a result of ischemia (lack of blood flow) (Chap. 19).

Gas Gangrene. Gangrene caused by *Clostridium* spp.; the gas that forms in the necrotic tissue is the result of bacterial fermentations; also known as *myonecrosis* (Chap. 19).

Gastritis (gas-try'-tis). Inflammation of the mucosal lining of the stomach (Chap. 17).

Gastroenteritis (gas'-tro-en-ter-eye'-tis). Inflammation of the mucosal linings of the stomach and intestines (Chap. 17).

Gene (jeen). A functional unit of heredity that occupies a specific space (locus) on a chromosome; contains the genetic information that will enable a cell to produce a protein (usually), an rRNA molecule, or a tRNA molecule (Chap. 3).

Gene Product. The molecule (usually a protein) that is coded for by a gene (Chap. 3).

Gene Therapy. The insertion of normally functioning genes into a cell to correct problems associated with abnormally functioning genes (Chap. 7).

Generation Time. The time required for a cell to split into two cells; also called the *doubling time* (Chap. 3).

Genetic (juh-net'-ick) **Code.** The sequence of nucleotide bases on a DNA molecule that provides the information necessary for cells to produce gene products (Chap. 6).

Genetic Engineering. The insertion of foreign genes into microorganisms to enable the microorganisms to produce specific gene products or to enable them to be used for other purposes (Chap. 1).

Genetics (juh-net'-iks). The branch of science concerned with heredity (Chap. 7).

Genotype (jeen'-oh-type). The complete genetic constitution of an individual (i.e., all of that individual's genes); also known as the *genome* (Chap. 3).

Genus (jee'-nus), pl. *genera*. The first name in binomial nomenclature; a genus contains closely related species (Chap. 3).

Germ. Slang term for pathogen (Chap. 1).

Germicidal (jer-muh-sigh'-dull) **Agent.** A chemical agent or drug that kills pathogens; a *germicide* (Chap. 8).

Gingivitis (jin-juh-vy'-tis). Inflammation or infection of the gingiva (gums) (Chap. 17).

Glucose (glue'-kohs). A biologically important, six-carbon monosaccharide; a hexose; $C_6H_{12}O_6$; also called *dextrose*; the product of complete hydrolysis of polysaccharides such as cellulose, starch, and glycogen (Chap. 6).

Glycocalyx (gly-ko-kay'-licks). Extracellular material that may or may not be firmly attached to the outer surface of a bacterial cell wall; capsules and slime layers are examples (Chap. 3).

Glycogen (gly'-koh-jen). A polysaccharide stored by animal cells as a food reserve; composed of numerous glucose molecules (Chap. 6).

Glycolysis (gly-kol'-eh-sis). The anaerobic, energy-producing breakdown of glucose into two molecules of pyruvic acid via a series of chemical reactions; an example of a biochemical pathway; also called *anaerobic glycolysis* (Chap. 7).

Glycosidic (gly'-ko-sid'-ik) **Bond.** The covalent bond that holds monosaccharides together in carbohydrate molecules (Chap. 6).

Golgi (goal'-jee **Complex.** A membranous system located within the cytoplasm of a eukaryotic cell; associated with the transport and packaging of secretory proteins; also known as *Golgi apparatus* or *Golgi body* (Chap. 3).

Gonococcal (gon-oh-kok'-ul) **Ophthalmia** (of-thal'-me-uh) **Neonatorum** (ne'-oh-nay-tor'-um). A bacterial eye disease of newborns caused by *Neisseria gonorrhoeae*, a Gram-negative diplococcus (Chap. 19).

Gonococcus (gon-oh-kok'-us), pl. *gonococci*. A slang term for *N. gonorrhoeae*; abbreviated GC (Chap. 13).

Gonorrhea (gon-oh-ree'-uh). A sexually transmitted bacterial disease caused by *N. gonorrhoeae*, a Gram-negative diplococcus (Chap. 19).

Gram Stain. A differential staining procedure named for its developer, Hans Christian Gram, a Danish bacteriologist; differentiates bacteria into those that stain blue to purple (called *Gram-positive bacteria*) and those that stain pink to red (called *Gram-negative bacteria*) (Chap. 4).

Granulocytes (gran'-yu-loh-sites). A category of leukocytes having prominent cytoplasmic granules; neutrophils, eosinophils, and basophils are examples (Chap. 15).

Growth Curve. As used in this book, a graphic representation of the change in size of a bacterial population over a period of time; includes a lag phase, a log phase, a stationary phase, and a death phase (Chap. 8).

H

Haloduric (hail-oh-dur'-ick) **Organisms.** Organisms capable of surviving in a salty environment (Chap. 8).

Halophiles (hail'-oh-file). Organisms whose growth is enhanced by a high salt concentration; such an organism is said to be *halophilic* (Chap. 8).

Hantavirus (hon'-tuh-vi-rus) **Pulmonary Syndrome (HPS).** A pulmonary disease caused by various hantaviruses. (Chap. 18).

Haploid (hap'-loyd) **Cells.** Eukaryotic cells containing only one set of chromosomes (Chap. 3).

Hapten (hap'-ten). A small, nonantigenic molecule that becomes antigenic when combined with a larger molecule (e.g., a carrier protein) (Chap. 16).

Harmful Mutation. A mutation that causes harm to the mutant organism (Chap. 7).

HBV. Hepatitis B virus; the causative agent of serum hepatitis (Chap. 18).

Helminth (hel'-minth). A parasitic worm (Chap. 21).

Hemolysin (he-moll'-uh-sin). A bacterial enzyme capable of lysing erythrocytes (Chap. 14).

Hemolysis (he-moll'-uh-sis). Destruction of erythrocytes in such a manner that hemoglobin is liberated into the surrounding environment (Chap. 8).

Hepatitis (hep-uh-ty'-tis). Inflammation of the liver (Chap. 17).

Heptose. A monosaccharide containing seven carbon atoms (Chap. 6).

Herpes Labialis (her'-peez lay-bee-al-us). A cold sore (fever blister) caused by herpes simplex viruses (Chap. 18).

Herpes Simplex Viruses. Viruses that cause a variety of infections, including cold sores (fever blisters), genital herpes, and shingles (Chap. 18).

Heterotroph (het'-er-oh-trof). An organism that uses organic chemicals as a source of carbon (Chap. 7).

Hexose. A monosaccharide containing six carbon atoms (Chap. 6).

Histamine (his'-tuh-meen). Potent chemical released from basophils and mast cells during allergic reactions; causes constriction of bronchial smooth muscles and vasodilation (Chap. 16).

HIV. Human immunodeficiency virus; the causative agent of AIDS (Chap. 4).

Holoenzyme. Apoenzyme plus cofactor; a whole (functional) enzyme (Chap. 6).

Healthcare-Associated Infection. Any infection acquired while one is hospitalized (or while a patient in some other healthcare facility) (Chap. 12).

Host. In a parasitic relationship, the organism on or in which a parasite lives (Chap. 10).

Host Defense Mechanisms. Mechanisms that serve to protect the body from pathogens and the infections they cause (Chap. 15).

Humoral Immunity. A type of immunity in which antibodies play a major role; also known as *antibody-mediated immunity* (*AMI*) (Chap. 16).

Hyaluronic (high'-uh-lu-ron'-ick) **Acid.** A gelatinous mucopolysaccharide that acts as an intracellular cement in body tissue (Chap. 14).

Hyaluronidase (high'-uh-lu-ron'-uh-dase). A bacterial enzyme that breaks down hyaluronic acid; sometimes called *diffusing* or *spreading factor*, because it enables bacteria to invade deeper into tissue (Chap. 14).

Hybridoma (high-brid-oh'-muh). A tumor produced in vitro by fusion of mouse tumor cells and specific antibody-producing cells; used in the production of monoclonal antibodies (Chap. 16).

Hydrocarbon (high-droh-kar'-bun). An organic compound consisting of only hydrogen and carbon atoms (Chap. 6).

Hydrolysis (hi-drol'-eh-sis) **Reaction.** A chemical process whereby a compound is cleaved into two or more simpler compounds with the uptake of the H and OH parts of a water molecule on either side of the chemical bond that is cleaved (Chap. 6).

Hypersensitivity (high'-per-sen-suh-tiv'-uh-tee) **Reactions.** Exaggerated immunologic reactions that result from an overly sensitive immune system (Chap. 16).

Hypertonic (hi-per-tahn'-ick) **Solution.** A solution having a greater osmotic pressure than cells placed into that solution; a higher concentration of solutes exists outside the cell (Chap. 8).

Hyphae (hy'-fee), sing. *hypha.* Long, thin, intertwined, cytoplasmic filaments that make up a mould colony (*mycelium*) (Chap. 5).

Hypogammaglobulinemia (high'-poh-gam'-uh-glob-yu-luh-nee'-me-uh). Decreased quantity of the gamma fraction of serum globulin, including a decreased quantity of immunoglobulins (Chap. 16).

Hypotonic (hi-poh-tahn'-ick) **Solution.** A solution having a lower osmotic pressure than cells placed into that solution; a lower concentration of solutes exists outside the cell (Chap. 8).

I

Iatrogenic (eye-at-roh-jen'-ick) **Infection.** An infection caused by medical treatment; literally, "physician induced," but could be caused by any healthcare professional (Chap. 12).

Immediate-Type Hypersensitivity Reactions. Hypersensitivity reactions that occur from within a few minutes to 24 hours after contact with a particular antigen (Chap. 16).

Immune (im-myun'). To be free from the possibility of acquiring a particular infectious disease; to be resistant to an infectious disease (Chap. 16).

Immunity (im-myu'-nuh-tee). The status of being immune or resistant to an infectious disease (Chap. 16).

Immunocompetent (im'-you-no-kom'-puh-tent) **Person.** A person who is able to mount a normal immune response; a person whose immune system is functioning properly (Chap. 16).

Immunodiagnostic (im'-yu-noh-dy-ag-nos'-tick**) Procedures.** Laboratory procedures used to diagnose infectious diseases by using the principles of immunology; used to detect either antigen or antibody in patients' specimens (Chap. 16).

Immunoglobulins (im'-yu-noh-glob'-yu-lin). A class of glycoproteins, which contains antibodies (Chap. 16).

Immunohematology Laboratory. The laboratory where donor blood is collected, tested, and stored; often referred to as the *Blood Bank* (Chap. 13).

Immunologist (im-you-nol'-oh-jist). One who specializes in the science of immunology (Chap. 16).

Immunology (im-you-nol'-oh-je). The study of immunity and the immune system (Chap. 16).

Immunosuppressed (im'-you-no-sue-pressed) **Person.** A person whose immune system is not functioning properly; such persons are also said to be *immunodepressed* or *immunocompromised* (Chap. 16).

Impetigo (im-peh-ty'-go). A bacterial skin disease caused by *S. aureus* and/or *S. pyogenes* (Chap. 19).

In Vitro (in vee'-trow). In an artificial environment, as in a laboratory setting; used in reference to what occurs *outside* an organism (Chap. 1).

In Vivo (in vee'-voh). Used in reference to what occurs *within* a living organism (Chap. 1).

Inactivated Vaccine. A vaccine prepared from inactivated (killed) microorganisms (Chap. 16).

Incidence. The number of new cases of a particular disease in a defined population during a specific period of time (Chap. 11).

Inclusion Bodies. Distinctive clusters of virions, frequently formed in the nucleus or cytoplasm of cells infected with certain viruses (Chap. 4).

Incubation. In microbiology, refers to holding a culture at a particular temperature for a certain length of time (Chap. 8).

Incubator. In microbiology, the chamber within which cultures are held at a particular temperature for a certain length of time (Chap. 8).

Incubatory (in'-kyu-buh-tor'-ee) **Carrier.** A person capable of transmitting a pathogen during the incubation period of a particular infectious disease (Chap. 11).

India Ink Preparation. A laboratory procedure primarily used to presumptively diagnose cryptococcal meningitis (Chap. 20).

Indigenous Microbiota (in-dij'-uh-nus my-crow-by-oh-tuh). Microbes that live on and in the healthy body; also called the human *microbiome*; referred to in the past as indigenous microflora and normal flora (Chap. 1).

Inducible Genes. Genes that are not expressed all the time (Chap. 6).

Infection (in-fek'-shun). The presence and multiplication of a pathogen on or within the body; often used as a synonym for infectious disease (Chap. 14).

Infectious Disease (in-fek'-shus di-zeez'). Any disease caused by a microbe that follows colonization of the body by that microbe (Chap. 1).

Infestation (in-fes-tay'-shun). The presence of ectoparasites (e.g., lice) on the body (Chap. 21).

Inflammation (in-fluh-may'-shun). A nonspecific pathologic process consisting of a dynamic complex of cytologic and histologic reactions that occur in response to an injury or abnormal stimulation by a physical, chemical, or biologic agent (Chap. 15).

Inflammatory Exudate. An accumulation of fluid, cells, and cellular debris at a site of inflammation (Chap. 15).

Inoculation. In microbiology, refers to adding a specimen to some type of culture medium (Chap. 8).

Inorganic (in-or-gan'-ick) **Chemistry.** The science dealing with all types of chemicals except those classified as organic compounds (Chap. 6).

Inorganic Compounds. Chemical compounds in which the atoms or radicals consist of elements other than carbon. (Chap. 6).

Interferons (in-ter-fear'-onz). Small, antiviral glycoproteins produced by cells infected with an animal virus; interferons are cell-specific and species-specific, but not virus-specific (Chap. 15).

Interleukins (in-ter-lu'-kinz). Lymphokines and polypeptide hormones; interleukin 1 is produced by monocytes; interleukin 2 is produced by lymphocytes; a category of cytokines (Chap. 15).

Intermediate Host. In a parasitic relationship, the host that harbors the larval or asexual stage of a parasite, or the asexual phase of the parasite's life cycle (Chap. 21).

Intraerythrocytic Pathogen. A pathogen that lives within erythrocytes (Chap. 14).

Intraleukocytic Pathogen. A pathogen that lives within leukocytes (Chap. 14).

Intrinsic Resistance. Resistance to a particular drug that is the result of some naturally occurring property of a bacterial cell (Chap. 9).

Ischemia (is-key'-me-uh). Localized anemia as a result of mechanical obstruction of the blood supply (Chap. 19).

Isotonic (eye-soh-tahn'-ick) **Solution.** A solution having the same osmotic pressure as cells placed into that solution; when the concentration of solutes outside the cell equals the concentration of solutes inside the cell (Chap. 8).

K

Keratitis (ker-uh-ty'-tis). Inflammation of the cornea (Chap. 17).

Keratoconjunctivitis (ker'-at-oh-kon-junk'-tuh-vi'-tis). Inflammation of the cornea and conjunctiva (Chap. 17).

Killer Cell. A type of cytotoxic T cell involved in cell-mediated immune responses (Chap. 16).

Kinase (ky'-nace). A bacterial enzyme capable of dissolving clots; also known as *fibrinolysin* (Chap. 14).

Koch's Postulates. A series of scientific steps, proposed by Robert Koch, that must be fulfilled to prove that a specific microorganism is the cause of a particular disease (Chap. 1).

KOH Prep. See *potassium hydroxide preparation*.

Koplik Spots. Small red spots containing a minute bluish white speck; they appear on the buccal mucosa early in measles. (Chap. 18).

Krebs Cycle. A biochemical pathway that is part of aerobic respiration; also known as the *citric acid cycle*, *tricarboxylic acid*, and *TCA cycle* (Chap. 7).

L

L-Forms. Abnormal forms of bacteria that have lost part or all of their rigid cell walls; sometimes the result of exposure of an organism to an antimicrobial agent; also called *L-phase variants*; the "L" is derived from Lister Institute (Chap. 4).

β-Lactam Ring. One of the two double-ringed structures found in penicillin and cephalosporin molecules (Chap. 9).

β-Lactamases. Enzymes that destroy the β-lactam ring in antibiotics such as penicillin and cephalosporins (Chap. 9).

Lag Phase. The part of a bacterial growth curve during which multiplication of the organisms is very slow or scarcely appreciable; the first phase in a bacterial growth curve (Chap. 8).

Laryngitis (lar-in-ji'-tis). Inflammation of the mucous membrane of the larynx (voice box) (Chap. 17).

Latent Infection. An asymptomatic infection capable of manifesting symptoms under particular circumstances or if activated (Chap. 14).

Lecithin (less'-uh-thin). A name given to several types of phospholipids that are essential constituents of animal and plant cells (Chap. 14).

Lecithinase (less'-uh-thuh-nace). A bacterial enzyme capable of breaking down lecithin (Chap. 14).

Legionellosis (lee-juh-nel-oh'-sis). A bacterial respiratory disease caused by Gram-negative bacilli in the genus *Legionella* (Chap. 19).

Leprosy (lep-roh-see). A bacterial disease of the skin, peripheral nerves, and testes caused by the acid-fast bacillus *Mycobacterium leprae*; Hansen disease is a synonym for leprosy (Chap. 19).

Lethal Mutation. A mutation that causes death of the organism possessing the mutation (Chap. 7).

Leukemia (lew-key'-me-uh). A type of cancer in which there is a proliferation of abnormal leukocytes in the blood (Chap. 13).

Leukocidin (lu-koh-sigh'-din). A bacterial exotoxin capable of destroying leukocytes (Chap. 14).

Leukocytes (lu'-koh-sites). White blood cells (Chap. 13).

Leukocytosis (lu'-koh-sigh-toe'-sis). An increased number of leukocytes in the blood (Chap. 15).

Leukopenia (lu-koh-pea'-nee-uh). A decreased number of leukocytes in the blood (Chap. 15).

Lichen (like'-in). An organism composed of a green alga (or a cyanobacterium) and a fungus; an example of a symbiotic relationship known as *mutualism* (Chap. 5).

Life Cycle. The generation-to-generation sequence of stages that occur in the history of an organism (Chap. 3).

Light Microscope. A type of microscope that uses visible light as a source of illumination; also called a *brightfield microscope* (Chap. 2).

Lipids (lip'-ids). Organic compounds containing carbon, hydrogen, and oxygen that are insoluble in water but soluble in so-called fat solvents such as diethyl ether and carbon tetrachloride (Chap. 6).

Lipopolysaccharide (lip'-oh-pol-ee-sack'-a-ride). A macromolecule of combined lipid and polysaccharide, found in the cell walls of Gram-negative bacteria (Chap. 4).

Listeriosis (lis-tear'-ee-oh'-sis). A bacterial disease caused by *Listeria monocytogenes*, a Gram-positive bacillus (Chap. 19).

Lithotroph (lith'-oh-trof). An organism that uses inorganic molecules as a source of energy; a type of chemotroph (Chap. 7).

Localized Infection. An infection that remains localized; that does not spread; also known as a *local infection* or *focal infection* (Chap. 14).

Logarithmic (log'-uh-rith-mik) **Growth Phase.** The part of a bacterial growth phase during which maximal multiplication is occurring by geometric progression; the second phase in a bacterial growth curve; also known as the *log phase* or *exponential growth phase* (Chap. 8).

Logarithmic (log'-uh-ryth-mik) **Scale.** A scale (as on graph paper) in which the values of a variable (e.g., number of organisms at a particular point in time) are expressed as logarithms (Chap. 8).

Lophotrichous (low-fot'-ri-kus) **Bacterium.** A bacterium that possesses two or more flagella at one end (pole) of the cell (Chap. 3).

Lyme Disease. A bacterial disease caused by *Borrelia burgdorferi*, a loosely coiled spirochete; transmitted by tick bite (Chap. 19).

Lymphadenitis (lim'-fad-uh-ny'-tis). Inflammation of a lymph node or lymph nodes (Chap. 17).

Lymphadenopathy (lim-fad-uh-nop'-uh-thee). A disease process affecting a lymph node or lymph nodes (Chap. 17).

Lymphangitis (lim-fan-ji'-tis). Inflammation of lymphatic vessels (Chap. 17).

Lymphokines (lim'-foh-kinz). Soluble proteins released by sensitized lymphocytes; examples include chemotactic factors and interleukins; lymphokines represent one category of *cytokines* (Chap. 16).

Lyophilization (ly-ahf'-eh-leh-zay'-shun). Freeze-drying; a method of preserving microorganisms and foods (Chap. 8).

Lysogenic (lye-so-jen'-ick) **Bacterium.** A bacterium in the state of lysogeny (Chap. 7).

Lysogenic Conversion. Alteration of the genetic constitution of a bacterial cell due to lysogeny (Chap. 7).

Lysogeny (lye-soj'-eh-nee). A situation in which viral genetic material is integrated into the genome of the host cell (Chap. 7).

Lysosome (lye'-so-som). A membrane-bound vesicle found in the cytoplasm of eukaryotic cells; contains a variety of digestive enzymes, including lysozyme (Chap. 3).

Lysozyme (lye'-so-zyme). A digestive enzyme found in lysosomes, tears, and other body fluids; especially destructive to bacterial cell walls (Chap. 15).

Lytic Cycle. When a virus takes over the metabolic machinery of the host cell, reproduces itself, and ruptures (lyses) the host cell so that the newly assembled virions can escape (Chap. 4).

M

Macrophage (mak'-roh-faj). A large phagocytic leukocyte that arises from a monocyte (Chap. 15).

Malaise (muh-laz'). A generalized feeling of discomfort or uneasiness (Chap. 17).

Mast Cell. A tissue cell that closely resembles a basophil (Chap. 16).

Mechanical Vector. An arthropod vector (e.g., a housefly) that merely transports a pathogen from "point A" to "point B," and within which the pathogen neither multiplies nor matures (Chap. 21).

Medical Asepsis (ay-sep'-sis). The absence of pathogens in a patient's environment (Chap. 12).

Medical Aseptic (ay-sep'-tick) **techniques.** Procedures followed and steps taken to ensure medical asepsis (Chap. 12).

Medical Laboratory Scientists. Laboratory professionals possessing a baccalaureate degree in medical laboratory science (medical technology); also known as *medical technologists* or *MTs* (Chap. 13).

Medical Laboratory Technicians. Laboratory professionals possessing an associate degree in medical laboratory technology; also known as *MLTs* (Chap. 13).

Meiosis (my-oh'-sis). The type of cell division that results in the formation of haploid gametes; also known as *meiotic division* (Chap. 3).

Meninges (muh-nin'-jez), sing. *meninx*. As used in this book, the membranes that surround the brain and spinal cord (Chap. 17).

Meningitis (men-in-ji'-tis). Inflammation or infection of the meninges (Chap. 13).

Meningococcemia (meh-ninge'-oh-kok-see'-me-uh). The presence of *Neisseria meningitidis* in the blood (Chap. 13).

Meningococcus (meh-ninge'-oh-kok-us), pl. *meningococci*. A slang term for *N. meningitidis* (Chap. 13).

Meningoencephalitis (muh-ning'-go-en-sef-uh-ly'-tis). Inflammation or infection of the brain and its surrounding membranes (Chap. 13).

Mesophile (meez'-oh-file). A microorganism having an optimum growth temperature between 25°C and 40°C; such an organism is said to be *mesophilic* (Chap. 8).

Messenger RNA (mRNA). The type of RNA that contains exactly the same genetic information as a single gene on a DNA molecule; also called *informational RNA* (Chap. 6).

Metabolic (met-uh-bol'-ik) **Reactions.** Chemical reactions that occur within cells; of two types—catabolic and anabolic reactions (Chap. 7).

Metabolism (muh-tab'-oh-lizm). The sum of all the chemical reactions occurring in a cell; consists of *anabolism* and *catabolism* (Chap. 3).

Metabolite (muh-tab'-oh-lite). Any chemical product of metabolism (Chap. 7).

Methanogens. Prokaryotic microbes that live on carbon dioxide and and hydrogen and produce methane gas (Chap. 4).

Microaerophiles (my-krow-air'-oh-files). Organisms requiring oxygen, but in concentrations lower than the 20% to 21% found in air; they usually require around 5% oxygen (Chap. 4).

Microbes. All-encompassing term that includes acellular viruses and prions as well as cellular microorganisms (e.g., bacteria, protozoa, some algae, some fungi) (Chap. 1).

Microbial (my-krow'-be-ul). Pertaining to microorganisms (Chap. 1).

Microbial Antagonism (an-tag'-un-izm). The killing, injury, or inhibition of one microbe by substances produced by another (Chap. 10).

Microbial Ecology. Study of the interrelationships among microbes and the world around them (other microbes, other living organisms, and the nonliving environment) (Chap. 1).

Microbial Intoxication. A disease that results from ingestion of a toxin that was produced by a pathogen in vitro (outside the body) (Chap. 1).

Microbial Physiology. The study of the vital life processes of microbes (Chap. 7).

Microbicidal (my-krow'-buh-sigh'-dull) **Agent.** A chemical or drug that kills microorganisms; a *microbicide* (Chap. 8).

Microbiologist (my'-crow-by-ol'-oh-jist). One who specializes in the science of microbiology (Chap. 1).

Microbiology (my'-crow-by-ol'-oh-je). The study of microbes (Chap. 1).

Microbistatic (my-krow'-buh-stat'-ick) **Agent.** A chemical agent or drug that inhibits the growth of microorganisms (Chap. 8).

Microcolonies. Tiny clusters of bacteria within biofilms (Chap. 10).

Micrometer (my-crow'-me-ter). A unit of length, equal to one millionth of a meter and one thousandth of a millimeter (Chap. 2).

Microorganisms (my'-crow-or'-gan-izms). Very small organisms; usually microscopic; also called *cellular microbes*; includes bacteria, archaea, certain algae, protozoa, and certain fungi (Chap. 1).

Microscope (my'-crow-skope). An optical instrument that permits one to observe a small object by producing an enlarged image of the object (Chap. 1).

Microscopic (my-crow-skop'-ik). If an object is microscopic, it is so small that it can only be seen using a microscope (Chap. 2).

Microtubules (my-kro'-two-bules). Cylindrical, cytoplasmic tubules found in the cytoskeleton of eukaryotic cells; may be related to the movement of chromosomes during nuclear division (Chap. 3).

Millimeter (mill'-uh-me-ter). A unit of length equal to one thousandth of a meter (Chap. 2).

Mimivirus. An extremely large double-stranded DNA virus that has been recovered from amebas.

Minisystems. Miniaturized biochemical test systems; often used when attempting to speciate microorganisms that have been isolated from clinical specimens (Chap. 13).

Mitochondria (my-toe-kon'-dree-uh), sing. *mitochondrion*. Eukaryotic organelles involved in cellular respiration for the production of energy; energy factories of the cell (Chap. 3).

Mitosis (my-toe'-sis). The type of cell division that results in the formation of two daughter cells, each of which contains exactly the same number of chromosomes as the parent cell; also known as *mitotic division* (Chap. 3).

Molecular Epidemiology. Determining relatedness of two microbial isolates in a healthcare setting by genotypic methods (Chap. 12).

Monoclonal (mon-oh-klo'-nul) **Antibodies.** Antibodies produced by a clone of genetically identical hybrid cells (Chap. 16).

Monocyte (mon'-oh-site). A relatively large mononuclear leukocyte (Chap. 15).

Monosaccharides (mon-oh-sak'-uh-rides). Carbohydrates that cannot be broken down into any simpler sugar by simple hydrolysis; simple sugars containing three to nine carbon atoms (usually three to seven); the basic units or building blocks of polysaccharides (Chap. 6).

Monotrichous (mah-not'-ri-kus) **Bacterium.** A bacterium that possesses only one flagellum (Chap. 3).

Monounsaturated Fatty Acid. A fatty acid containing only one double bond (Chap. 6).

Morbidity Rate. The number of new cases of a particular disease that occurred during a specified time period per a specifically defined population (e.g., per 100,000) (Chap. 11).

Mortality Rate. The ratio of the number of people who died of a particular disease during a specified time period per a specified population (e.g., per 100,000); also known as the *death rate* (Chap. 11).

Mucormycosis (mew'-kor-my-koh'-sis). Infection caused by a bread mould; also known as *zygomycosis* (Chap. 20).

Mutagen (myu'-tah-jen). Any agent that can cause a mutation to occur (e.g., radioactive substances, x-rays, or certain chemicals); such an agent is said to be *mutagenic* (Chap. 7).

Mutant (myu'-tant). A phenotype in which a mutation is manifested (Chap. 7).

Mutation (myu-tay'-shun). An inheritable change in the character of a gene; a change in the sequence of base pairs in a DNA molecule (Chap. 7).

Mutualism (myu'-chew-ul-izm). A symbiotic relationship in which both parties derive benefit (Chap. 10).

Mycelium (my-see'-lee-um), pl. *mycelia*. A fungal colony; composed of a mass of intertwined hyphae (Chap. 5).

Mycologist (my-kol'-oh-jist). One who specializes in the science of mycology (Chap. 1).

Mycology (my-kol'-oh-gee). The study of fungi (Chap. 1).

Mycosis (my-ko'-sis), pl. *mycoses*. A fungal disease (Chap. 5).

Mycotoxicosis (my'-ko-tox'-uh-ko-sis), pl. *mycotoxicoses*. A microbial intoxication caused by a mycotoxin (Chap. 5).

Mycotoxins (my'-ko-tox-inz). Toxins produced by fungi (Chap. 5).

Myelitis (my-uh-ly'-tis). Inflammation or infection of the spinal cord (Chap. 17).

Myocarditis (my'-oh-kar-dy'-tis). Inflammation of the myocardium (the muscular walls of the heart) (Chap. 17).

N

Nanobacteria (nah'-no-back-teer'-ee-uh). Especially small bacteria; less than 1 μm in diameter; the sizes of these bacteria are expressed in nanometers (Chap. 4).

Nanometer (nan'-oh-me'-ter). A unit of length, equal to one billionth of a meter and one thousandth of a micrometer (Chap. 2).

Narrow-Spectrum Antibiotics. Antibiotics that are effective only against a narrow range of bacteria (e.g., perhaps only effective against certain Gram-positive bacteria, or only effective against certain Gram-negative bacteria) (Chap. 9).

Natural Active Acquired Immunity. Active acquired immunity that is acquired naturally (e.g., by being infected with a particular pathogen) (Chap. 16).

Natural Killer (NK) Cell. A type of cytotoxic human blood lymphocyte (Chap. 16).

Natural Passive Acquired Immunity. Passive acquired immunity that is acquired in a natural manner (e.g., when a fetus receives the mother's antibodies in utero) (Chap. 16).

Necrosis (nuh-kro'-sis). Cell death (Chap. 19).

Negative Stain. A staining procedure in which unstained objects can be seen against a stained background (Chap. 3).

Nematodes (nem'-uh-toadz'). Roundworms (Chap. 21).

Nephritis (nef-ry'-tis). Inflammation of the kidneys (Chap. 17).

Neurotoxin (new'-roh-tok'-sin). A bacterial exotoxin that attacks the nervous system (Chap. 14).

Neutralism (new'-trul-izm). A symbiotic relationship in which organisms occupy the same niche but do not affect one another (Chap. 10).

Neutrophil (nu'-tro-fil). A type of granulocyte found in blood; its granules contain neutral substances that attract neither acidic nor basic dyes; also called a *polymorphonuclear cell*, *poly*, or *PMN* (Chap. 15).

Nitrifying Bacteria. Bacteria capable of converting ammonia to nitrites and nitrites to nitrates; the process is known as *nitrification* (Chap. 10).

Nitrogen Fixation. The process by which atmospheric nitrogen gas is converted into ammonia (Chap. 4).

Nitrogen-Fixing Bacteria. Bacteria capable of converting nitrogen gas into ammonia; the process is known as *nitrogen fixation* (Chap. 10).

Nonpathogen (non'-path'-oh-jen). A microbe that does not cause disease; such a microbe is said to be *nonpathogenic* (Chap. 1).

Nonspecific Host Defense Mechanisms. Host defense mechanisms directed against all types of invading pathogens and other foreign substances (Chap. 15).

Nuclear (new'-klee-er) **Membrane.** The membrane that surrounds the chromosomes and nucleoplasm of a eukaryotic cell (Chap. 3).

Nucleic (new-klay'-ick) **Acids.** Macromolecules consisting of linear chains of nucleotides; DNA, mRNA, tRNA, and rRNA are examples (Chap. 6).

Nucleolus (new-klee'-oh-lus). A dense portion of the nucleus of a eukaryotic cell; where ribosomal RNA (rRNA) is produced (Chap. 3).

Nucleoplasm (new'-klee-oh-plazm). That portion of a eukaryotic cell's protoplasm that lies within the nucleus (Chap. 3).

Nucleotides (new'-klee-oh-tides). The basic units or building blocks of nucleic acids, each consisting of a purine or pyrimidine combined with a pentose (either ribose or deoxyribose) and a phosphate group (Chap. 6).

Nucleus (new'-klee-us), pl. *nuclei*. That portion of a eukaryotic cell that contains the nucleoplasm and chromosomes (Chap. 3).

O

Obligate Aerobe (air'-obe). An organism that requires 20% to 21% oxygen (the amount found in the air we breathe) to survive (Chap. 4).

Obligate Anaerobe (an'-air-obe). An organism that cannot survive in oxygen (Chap. 4).

Obligate Intracellular Pathogen. A pathogen that must reside within another living cell; examples include viruses, chlamydias, and rickettsias (Chap. 1).

Obligate Parasite. An organism that can exist only as a parasite; incapable of a free-living existence (Chap. 21).

Octad. A packet of eight cocci (Chap. 4).

Oncogenic (ong-koh-jen'-ick). An adjective meaning cancer-causing (Chap. 17).

Oncogenic Viruses. Viruses capable of causing cancer; also known as *oncoviruses* (Chap. 4).

Oophoritis (oh-of-or-eye'-tis). Inflammation or infection on an ovary (Chap. 17).

Opportunistic Pathogen (op-poor-tune'-is-tick path'-oh-jen). A microbe with the potential to cause disease, but that does not do so under ordinary circumstances; may cause disease in susceptible persons with lowered resistance; also called an *opportunist* (Chap. 1).

Opsonins (op'-soh-ninz). Substances (such as antibodies or complement fragments) that enhance phagocytosis (Chap. 15).

Opsonization (op'-suh-nuh-zay'-shun). The process by which bacteria (or other particles) are altered so that they may be more readily and more efficiently engulfed by phagocytes; often involves coating the bacteria with antibodies or complement fragments (Chap. 15).

Orchitis (or-ky'-tis). Inflammation or infection of the testes (Chap. 17).

Organelles (or'-guh-nelz). General term for the various and diverse structures contained within a eukaryotic cell (e.g., mitochondria, Golgi complex, nucleus, endoplasmic reticulum, and lysosomes) (Chap. 3).

Organic (or-gan'-ick) **Chemistry.** The study of organic compounds; the study of carbon and its covalent bonds (Chap. 6).

Organic Compounds. Chemical compounds composed of atoms (some of which are carbon) held together by covalent bonds (Chap. 6).

Osmosis (oz-moh'-sis). The process by which a solvent (e.g., water) moves through a semipermeable membrane from a solution having a lower concentration of solutes (dissolved substances) to a solution having a higher concentration of solutes (Chap. 8).

Osmotic (oz-maht'-ick) **Pressure.** A measure of the tendency for water to move into a solution by osmosis; always a positive value (Chap. 8).

Otitis (oh-ty'-tis) **Externa.** Inflammation or infection of the outer ear canal (Chap. 17).

Otitis Media. Inflammation or infection of the middle ear (Chap. 17).

Otomycosis. A fungal ear infection (Chap. 20).

Oxidation (ok-seh-day'-shun). As used in this book, the loss of one or more electrons, thus making the atom more electropositive (Chap. 7).

Oxidation–Reduction Reactions. Paired chemical reactions involving the transfer of one or more electrons from one compound to another; reactions that involve both oxidation and reduction; also known as *redox reactions* (Chap. 7).

Oxidative Pathways. Metabolic pathways requiring the participation of oxygen (Chap. 7).

Oxygenic Photosynthesis (ox'-uh-gen'-ik foe-toe-sin'-thuh-sis). A type of photosynthesis in which oxygen is produced (Chap. 4).

P

Paleomicrobiology(pay'-ee-oh-my'-crow-by-ol'-oh-je). The study of ancient microbes (Chap. 1).

Pandemic (pan-dem'-ick) **Disease.** A disease occurring in epidemic proportions in several to many countries; sometimes occurring worldwide (Chap. 11).

Papillomaviruses. Viruses that cause human warts and some types of carcinoma. (Chap. 18).

Parasite (par'-uh-sight). An organism that lives on or in another living organism (called the *host*) and derives benefit from the host (usually in the form of nutrients) (Chap. 1).

Parasitemia (par'-uh-suh-tee'-me-uh). The presence of parasites in the blood (Chap. 13).

Parasitism (par'-uh-suh-tizm). A symbiotic relationship that is beneficial to one party (the parasite) and detrimental to the other party (the host) (Chap. 10).

Parasitologist (par'-uh-suh-tol'-oh-jist). One who specializes in the science of parasitology (Chap. 1).

Parasitology (par'-uh-suh-tol'-oh-jee). The study of parasites (Chap. 1).

Parenteral (puh-ren'-ter-ul) **Injection.** Injection of substances directly into the bloodstream (Chap. 11).

Parotitis (par-oh-ty'-tis). Inflammation of the parotid gland (a salivary gland located near the ear); also known as *parotiditis*; epidemic parotitis is a synonym for mumps (Chap. 18).

Passive Acquired Immunity. Immunity or resistance acquired as a result of receipt of antibodies produced by another person or by an animal (Chap. 16).

Passive Carrier. A person who harbors a particular pathogen without ever having had the infectious disease it causes (Chap. 11).

Pasteurization (pas'-tour-i-zay'-shun). A heating process that kills pathogens in milk, wines, and other beverages (Chap. 1).

Pathogen (path'-oh-jen). Disease-causing microorganism; such an organism is said to be *pathogenic* (Chap. 1).

Pathogenesis (path-oh-jen-uh-sis). The steps or mechanisms involved in the development of a disease (Chap. 14).

Pathogenicity (path'-oh-juh-nis'-uh-tee). The ability to cause disease (Chap. 14).

Pathologist (pah-thol'-oh-jist). A physician who is a specialist in pathology (Chap. 13).

Pathology (pah-thol'-oh-gee). The study of disease, especially structural and functional changes that result from disease processes (Chap. 13).

Pellicle (pel'-uh-kul). As used in this book, a thickened outer membrane possessed by certain protozoa (Chap. 5).

Pelvic Inflammatory Disease (PID). Acute or chronic inflammation in the pelvic cavity, usually referring to infection of the female genital tract (Chap. 17).

Penicillinase. An enzyme that destroys the β-lactam ring in penicillin molecules; a type of β-lactamase (Chap. 9).

Pentose. A monosaccharide containing five carbon atoms (Chap. 6).

Peptide Bond. The name given to the covalent bond that holds amino acids together in protein molecules (Chap. 6).

Peptidoglycan (pep'-tuh-doh-gly'-kan). A complex structure found in the cell walls of bacteria, consisting of carbohydrates and proteins (Chap. 3).

Pericarditis (per'-ee-kar-dy'-tis)**.** Inflammation of the pericardium (the membrane or sac around the heart) (Chap. 17).

Periodontal (purr'-ee-oh-don'-tul) **Disease.** Disease around the teeth (Chap. 17).

Periodontitis (purr'-ee-oh-don-ty'-tis). Inflammation or infection of the *periodontium* (tissues that surround and support the teeth) (Chap. 17).

Peritrichous (peh-rit'-ri-kus) **Bacterium.** A bacterium that possesses flagella over its entire surface (Chap. 3).

Peroxisome (per-ok'-suh-some). A membrane-bound organelle found in eukaryotic cells, within which hydrogen peroxide is both produced and degraded (Chap. 3).

Pertussis (purr-tus'-is). Synonym for whooping cough; a bacterial respiratory disease caused by *Bordetella pertussis*, a Gram-negative bacillus (Chap. 19).

Petri (pea'-tree) **Dish.** A shallow, circular container made of thin glass or clear plastic, with a loosely fitting, overlapping cover; used in microbiology laboratories for cultivation of microorganisms on solid media (Chap. 1).

pH. The degree of acidity or alkalinity of a solution (Chap. 8).

Phagocyte (fag'-oh-site). A cell capable of ingesting bacteria, yeasts, and other particulate matter by phagocytosis; amebae and certain leukocytes are examples of phagocytic cells (Chap. 3).

Phagocytosis (fag'-oh-sigh-toe'-sis). Ingestion of particulate matter involving the use of pseudopodia to surround the particle (Chap. 3).

Phagolysosome (fag-oh-ly'-soh-sohm). A membrane-bound vesicle formed by the fusion of a phagosome and a lysosome (Chap. 15).

Phagosome (fag'-oh-sohm). A membrane-bound vesicle containing an ingested particle (e.g., a bacterial cell); found in phagocytic cells (Chap. 15).

Pharyngitis (far-in-ji'-tis). Inflammation or infection of the throat; sore throat (Chap. 17).

Phase-Contrast Microscope. A type of compound light microscope that can be used to observe unstained living microorganisms (Chap. 2).

Phenotype (fee'-no-type). Manifestation of a genotype; all the attributes or characteristics of an individual (Chap. 7).

Phospholipid (fos'-foh-lip'-id). A lipid containing glycerol, fatty acids, a phosphate group, and an alcohol; glycerophospholipids (also called *phosphoglycerides*) and sphingolipids are examples (Chap. 6).

Photoautotroph (foh'-toe-aw'-toe-trof). An organism that uses light as an energy source and carbon dioxide as a carbon source; a type of autotroph (Chap. 7).

Photoheterotroph (foh'-toe-het'-er-oh-trof). An organism that uses light as an energy source and organic compounds as a carbon source; a type of heterotroph (Chap. 7).

Photomicrograph. Photograph taken through the lens system of a compound light microscope (Chap. 2).

Photosynthesis (foe-toe-sin'-thuh-sis). Chemical process by which light energy is converted into chemical energy; an organism that produces organic substances in this manner is said to be *photosynthetic* (Chap. 3).

Phototroph (foh'-toe-trof). An organism that uses light as an energy source (Chap. 7).

Phycologist (fy-kol'-oh-jist). One who specializes in the science of phycology (Chap. 1).

Phycology (fy-kol'-oh-gee). The study of algae (Chap. 1).

Phycotoxicosis (fy'-koh-tox-uh-coh-sis), pl. *phycotoxicoses*. A microbial intoxication caused by a phycotoxin (Chap. 5).

Phycotoxins (fy'-ko-tox-inz). Toxins produced by algae (Chap. 5).

Phytoplankton (fy'-toh-plank'-ton). Microscopic marine plants and algae that are components of plankton (Chap. 1).

Piezophile (peez'-oh-file). An organism that thrives under high environmental pressure; such an organism is said to be *piezophilic* (Chap. 8).

Pili (py'-ly), sing. *pilus*. Hairlike surface projections possessed by some bacteria (called *piliated bacteria*); most are organelles of attachment; also called *fimbriae*; certain specialized pili are called *sex pili*, (Chap. 3).

Pinocytosis (pin'-oh-sigh-toe'-sis). A process resembling phagocytosis but used to engulf and ingest liquids rather than solid matter (Chap. 5).

Plague (playg). A bacterial disease caused by *Yersinia pestis*, a Gram-negative bacillus; transmitted by rodent fleas (Chap. 19).

Plankton (plank'-ton). Microscopic organisms in the ocean that serve as the starting point of many food chains (Chap. 1).

Plasma (plaz'-muh). The liquid portion of circulating blood (Chap. 13).

Plasma (plaz'-muh) **Cell.** An antibody-secreting cell produced by a stimulated B cell (Chap. 16).

Plasmid (plaz'-mid). An extrachromosomal genetic element; a molecule of DNA that can function and replicate while physically separate from the bacterial chromosome (Chap. 3).

Plasmolysis (plaz-moll'-uh-sis). Cell shrinkage as a result of a loss of water from the cell's cytoplasm (Chap. 8).

Plasmoptysis (plaz-mop'-tuh-sis). The escape of cytoplasm from a ruptured cell (Chap. 8).

Plastid. A membrane-bound organelle containing photosynthetic pigment; plastids are the sites of photosynthesis; a *chloroplast* is a plastid that contains chlorophyll (Chap. 3).

Pleomorphism (plee-oh-more'-fizm). Existing in more than one form; also known as *polymorphism*; an organism that exhibits pleomorphism is said to be *pleomorphic* (Chap. 4).

Pneumonia (new-mow'-nee-uh). Inflammation of one or both lungs (Chap. 17).

Polymer (pol'-uh-mer). A large molecule consisting of repeating subunits; nucleic acids, polypeptides, and polysaccharides are examples (Chap. 6).

Polymicrobial Infection. An infection caused by the correlated action of two or more microorganisms;

also known as a *synergistic infection*; examples include trench mouth and bacterial vaginosis (Chap. 10).

Polypeptide (pol-ee-pep'-tide). A protein consisting of more than three amino acids held together by peptide bonds (Chap. 6).

Polyribosomes (pol-ee-ry'-boh-somz). Two or more ribosomes connected by a molecule of messenger RNA (mRNA) (Chap. 3).

Polysaccharide (pol-ee-sack'-uh-ride). Carbohydrate consisting of many sugar units; glycogen, cellulose, and starch are examples (Chap. 6).

Polyunsaturated Fatty Acid. A fatty acid containing more than one double bond (Chap. 6).

Population Growth Curve. A graph that represents changes in the number of viable bacteria in a population over time; constructed by plotting the logarithm ($\log_{10}$) of the number of viable bacteria (on the vertical or *y* axis) against the incubation time (on the horizontal or *x* axis) (Chap. 8).

Potassium Hydroxide Preparation. A laboratory procedure primarily used to observe fungal elements in skin scrapings, hair clippings, and nail clippings; usually referred to as the KOH prep (Chap. 20).

Preliminary Report. Any report furnished by the laboratory before publication of the final report (Chap. 13).

Prevalence. The number of cases of a particular disease existing in a given population during a specific period of time (period prevalence) or at a particular moment in time (point prevalence) (Chap. 11).

Primary Atypical Pneumonia. An older term for mycoplasmal pneumonia; caused by the bacterium, *Mycoplasma pneumoniae* (Chap. 19).

Primary Disease. The initial disease; often creates the conditions that lead to a secondary disease; if the primary disease is an infection, it is referred to as a *primary infection* (Chap. 14).

Primary Response. The immune response that occurs the first time an antigen enters a person's body (Chap. 16).

Prions (pree'-onz). Infectious protein molecules (i.e., proteins capable of causing certain diseases of animals and humans) (Chap. 4).

Prokaryotic (pro'-kar-ee-ah'-tick) **Cells.** Cells lacking a true nucleus; organisms consisting of such cells are referred to as *prokaryotes*; can also be spelled procaryotic (Chap. 3).

Prophage (pro'-faj). During lysogeny, all that remains of the infecting bacteriophage is its DNA; in this form, the bacteriophage is referred to as a prophage (Chap. 7).

Prophylactic (pro'-fuh-lak'-tick) **Agent.** A drug used to prevent a disease (Chap. 17).

Prophylaxis (pro-fuh-lak'-sis). Prevention of a disease or a process that can lead to a disease (e.g., taking antimalarial medication in a malarious area) (Chap. 17).

Prostaglandins (pros-tuh-glan'-dinz). Physiologically active tissue substances that cause many effects, including vasodilation, vasoconstriction, and stimulation of smooth muscle (Chap. 15).

Prostatitis (pros-tuh-ty'-tis). Inflammation or infection of the prostate (Chap. 17).

Prostration (pros-tray'-shun). Significant loss of strength; the patient is prostrate (lying flat) (Chap. 13).

Protective Antibodies. Antibodies that protect an individual from infection or reinfection (Chap. 16).

Protective Environments. Hospital rooms for placement of patients who are especially vulnerable to infection; Protective Environments are under positive pressure, and vented air that enters these rooms passes through HEPA filters. (Chap. 12).

Proteins (pro'-teens). Macromolecules consisting of two, three, or more amino acids (Chap. 6).

Protists (pro'-tists). Members of the Kingdom Protista; includes algae and protozoa (Chap. 3).

Protoplasm (pro'-toe-plazm). The semifluid matter within living cells; *cytoplasm* and *nucleoplasm* are two types of protoplasm (Chap. 3).

Protozoa (pro-toe-zoe'-uh), sing. *protozoan*. Eukaryotic microorganisms frequently found in water and soil; some are pathogens; usually unicellular (Chap. 5).

Protozoologist (pro'-toe-zoe-ol'-oh-jist). One who specializes in protozoology (Chap. 1).

Protozoology (pro'-toe-zoe-ol'-oh-gee). The study of protozoa (Chap. 1).

Pseudohypha (su-doh-hy-fuh), pl. *pseudohyphae*. An elongated string of yeast buds (Chap. 5).

Pseudomembranous (soo-doe-mem'-bran-us) **Colitis** (koh-ly'-tis). Inflammation of the intestinal mucosa, with the formation and passage of pseudomembranous material in the stools; often a consequence of antibiotic therapy; most often caused by a cytotoxin produced by *C. difficile*, an anaerobic, spore-forming Gram-positive bacillus; also called *pseudomembranous enterocolitis* (Chap. 19).

Pseudomonicidal (su'-doh-moan-uh-side'-ul) **Agent.** A drug or disinfectant that kills *Pseudomonas* spp. (Chap. 8).

Pseudopodium (su-doe-poh'-dee-um), pl. *pseudopodia*. A temporary extension of protoplasm that is extended by an ameba or leukocyte for locomotion or the engulfment of particulate matter; also called a *pseudopod* (Chap. 5).

Psychroduric (sigh-krow-dur'-ick) **Organisms.** Organisms able to endure very cold temperatures (Chap. 8).

Psychrophile (sigh'-krow-file). An organism that grows best at a low temperature (0°C–32°C), with optimum growth occurring at 15°C to 20°C; such an organism is said to be *psychrophilic* (Chap. 8).

Psychrotroph (sigh'-krow-trof). A psychrophile that grows best at refrigerator temperature (4°C); such an organism is said to be *psychrotrophic* (Chap. 8).

Pure Culture. When only one type of organism is growing on or in a culture medium in the laboratory; no other types of organisms are present (Chap. 1).

Purine (pure'-een). A double-ringed nitrogenous base found in certain nucleotides and, therefore, in nucleic acids; adenine and guanine are purines found in both DNA and RNA (Chap. 6).

Purulent Exudate. A thick, greenish yellow exudate that contains many live and dead leukocytes; also known as *pus* (Chap. 15).

Pustule (pus'-chul). A small rounded elevation of the skin that contains purulent material (pus) (Chap. 17).

Pyelonephritis (py'-uh-low-nef-ry'-tis). Inflammation of certain areas of the kidneys, most often the result of bacterial infection (Chap. 17).

Pyogenic (py-oh-jen'-ick). Pus-producing; causing the production of pus (Chap. 15).

Pyogenic Microorganisms. Pathogens that cause pus-containing infectious processes (Chap. 15).

Pyrimidine (pi-rim'-uh-deen). A single-ringed nitrogenous base found in certain nucleotides and, therefore, in nucleic acids; thymine and cytosine are pyrimidines found in DNA; cytosine and uracil are pyrimidines found in RNA (Chap. 6).

Pyrogen (py'-roh-jen). A fever-producing substance; also referred to as a *pyrogenic substance* (Chap. 14).

R

R-Factor. A plasmid that contains multiple drug resistance genes; a bacterium that possesses an R-factor is multidrug-resistant (i.e., it is a "superbug"); the "R" stands for resistance (Chap. 7).

Receptors. Molecules on the surface of a host cell that a particular pathogen is able to recognize and attach to; also known as *integrins* (Chap. 14).

Reduction (ree-duk'-shun). As used in this book, the gain of one or more electrons, thus making the atom more electronegative (Chap. 7).

Regulatory T Cells. T cells that regulate various aspects of immune responses; helper T cells and suppressor T cells are examples (Chap. 16).

Reservoirs (rez'-ev-wars) **of Infection.** Places where pathogens are living and from which they can be transmitted to humans; reservoirs of infection may be living or nonliving; sometimes simply referred to as *reservoirs* (Chap. 11).

Resident Microflora. Members of the indigenous microflora that are more or less permanent residents (Chap. 10).

Resistance Factor. See *R-factor*.

Resolving Power. The ability of the eye or an optical instrument to distinguish detail, such as the separation of closely adjacent objects; also called *resolution* (Chap. 2).

Reticuloendothelial (ree-tick'-yu-loh-en-doh-thee'-lee-ul) **System (RES).** A collection of phagocytic cells that includes macrophages and cells that line the sinusoids of the spleen, lymph nodes, and bone marrow (Chap. 15).

Ribonucleic (ry-boe-new-klee'-ick) **Acid (RNA).** A macromolecule of which there are three main types: messenger RNA (mRNA), ribosomal RNA (rRNA), and transfer RNA (tRNA); found in all cells but only in certain viruses (called *RNA viruses*) (Chap. 3).

Ribosomal (rye-boh-so'-mul) **RNA (rRNA).** The type of RNA molecule found within ribosomes (Chap. 6).

Ribosomes (ry'-boh-soams). Organelles that are the sites of protein synthesis in both prokaryotic and eukaryotic cells (Chap. 3).

Ringworm Infections. See *tinea infections.*

RNA Nucleotides. The building blocks of RNA; each RNA nucleotide consists of a nitrogenous base, ribose, and a phosphate group (Chap. 6).

RNA Polymerase (poh-lim'-er-ace). The enzyme required for transcription (Chap. 6).

Rough Endoplasmic Reticulum (RER). See *endoplasmic reticulum* (Chap. 3).

Rubella (roo-bell'-uh) **Virus.** The virus that causes rubella (German measles) (Chap.18).

Rubeola (roo-bee-oh'-luh) **Virus.** The virus that causes measles (Chap. 18).

S

Salmonellosis (sal'-moh-nel-oh'-sis). A diarrheal disease caused by Gram-negative bacilli in the genus *Salmonella* (Chap. 19).

Salpingitis (sal-pin-jy'-tis). As used in this book, inflammation of the fallopian tube (Chap. 17).

Sanitization (san'-uh-tuh-zay'-shun). The process of making something sanitary (healthful); usually involves reducing the number of microbes present to a safe level (Chap. 8).

Saprophyte (sap'-row-fight). An organism that lives on dead or decaying organic matter; such an organism is said to be *saprophytic* (Chap. 1).

Saturated Fatty Acid. A fatty acid containing no double bonds (Chap. 6).

Scanning Electron Micrograph. Photograph taken through the lens system of a scanning electron microscope (Chap. 2).

Scanning Electron Microscope. A type of electron microscope; enables the operator to observe the outer surfaces of specimens (i.e., to observe surface detail) (Chap. 2).

Sebaceous (seb-ay'-shous) **Gland.** An oil gland located in the dermis (Chap. 17).

Sebum (see'-bum). The oily secretion produced by sebaceous glands of the skin (Chap. 17).

Secondary Disease. A disease that follows an initial disease; if the secondary disease is an infection, it is referred to as a *secondary infection* (Chap. 14).

Secondary Response. The immune response that occurs the second time an antigen enters a person's body; also known as a *memory response* or an *anaphylactic response* (Chap. 16).

Selective Medium. A culture medium that allows a certain organism or group of organisms to grow while inhibiting growth of all other organisms (Chap. 8).

Selective Permeability. An attribute of membranes whereby only certain substances are able to cross the membranes (Chap. 3).

Semisynthetic Antibiotic. An antibiotic that has been chemically altered, usually to increase the drug's spectrum of activity (Chap. 9).

Sepsis. The presence of pathogens or their toxins in the bloodstream; often used as a synonym for *septicemia* (Chap. 8).

Septate Hyphae. Hyphae that contain septa (crosswalls) (Chap. 5).

Septic Shock. A type of shock resulting from sepsis or septicemia (Chap. 14).

Septicemia (sep-tuh-see'-me-uh). A serious disease consisting of chills, fever, prostration, and the presence of pathogens or their toxins in the blood (Chap. 13).

Serologic (ser-oh-loj'-ick) **Procedures.** Immunodiagnostic test procedures performed on serum (Chap. 16).

Serology (suh-rol'-oh-jee). That branch of science concerned with serum and serologic procedures (Chap. 13).

Serum (seer'-um), pl. *sera*. The liquid portion of blood that remains after coagulation (clotting) (Chap. 13).

Severe Acute Respiratory Syndrome (SARS). A pulmonary disease caused by SARS coronavirus (SARS-CoV) (Chap. 18).

Sex Pilus. A specialized pilus that plays a role in bacterial conjugation (Chap. 3).

Sexual Reproduction. In this type of reproduction, two parents give rise to offspring that have unique combinations of genes inherited from both parents (Chap. 3).

Shigellosis (shig-uh-loh'-sis). A diarrheal disease caused by Gram-negative bacilli in the genus *Shigella* (Chap. 19).

Shingles. A painful nerve disease caused by reactivation of varicella virus (chickenpox virus) (Chap. 18).

Shock. A sudden, often severe, physical or mental disturbance, usually resulting from low blood pressure and a lack of oxygen in organs (Chap. 14).

Signs of a disease. Abnormalities indicative of disease that are discovered on examination of a patient; objective findings; examples include abnormal laboratory results; abnormal heart or breath sounds; lumps; abnormalities revealed by radiographs, computed tomographic scans, magnetic resonance imaging, electrocardiography, and ultrasound (Chap. 14).

Silent Mutation. A mutation that is neither beneficial nor harmful to the mutant organism; the organism is unaware of the mutation; also called a *neutral mutation* (Chap. 7).

Simple Microscope. A microscope containing only one magnifying lens (Chap. 2).

Simple Stain. A single dye that is used to stain objects (e.g., bacterial cells), enabling scientists to gain information about the objects (e.g., size, shape) (Chap. 4).

Single Bond. A type of chemical bond containing one pair of shared electrons (Chap. 6).

Sinusitis (sigh-neu-sigh'-tis). Inflammation of the lining of one or more of the paranasal sinuses (Chap. 17).

Slime Layer. An unorganized, loosely attached layer of glycocalyx surrounding a bacterial cell (Chap. 3).

Slime Mould. A eukaryotic organism having characteristics of protozoa and fungi; there are two types: cellular and acellular slime moulds (Chap. 5).

Smooth Endoplasmic Reticulum (SER). See *endoplasmic reticulum*.

Solute (sol'-yute). The dissolved substance in a solution; for example, sucrose (table sugar) when it is dissolved in water (Chap. 8).

Solution (soh-loo'-shun). A homogeneous molecular mixture; generally, a substance dissolved in water (referred to as an aqueous solution); solute plus solvent (Chap. 8).

Solvent (sol'-vent). A liquid in which another substance dissolves (Chap. 8).

Species (spe'-shez), pl. *species*. A specific member of a given genus; (e.g., *E. coli* is a species in the genus *Escherichia*); the name of a particular species consists of two parts—the generic name ("the first name") and the specific epithet ("the second name"); singular species is abbreviated sp., and plural species is abbreviated spp. (Chap. 3).

Specific Epithet. The second part ("second name") is the name of a species; the specific epithet cannot be used alone (Chap. 3).

Specific Host Defense Mechanisms. Host defense mechanisms directed against a specific invading pathogen; synonym for the immune system or the third line of defense (Chap. 15).

Spirochetes (spy'-roh-keets). Spiral-shaped bacteria; (e.g., *Treponema pallidum*, the causative agent of syphilis) (Chap. 3).

Splenomegaly (splen-oh-meg'-uh-lee). Enlargement of the spleen (Chap. 17).

Sporadic (spoh-rad'-ick) **Disease.** A disease that occurs occasionally, usually affecting only one person; neither endemic nor epidemic (Chap. 11).

Sporicidal (spor-uh-sigh'-dull) **Agent.** A chemical agent that kills spores; a *sporicide* (Chap. 8).

Sporulation (spor'-you-lay'-shun). Production of spores (Chap. 3).

Spotted Fever Rickettsiosis. Formerly called Rocky Mountain spotted fever; a bacterial disease caused by *Rickettsia rickettsii*, an obligate intracellular pathogen (Chap. 19).

Sputum. Pus that accumulates in the lungs of patients with lower respiratory tract infections such as pneumonia and tuberculosis (Chap. 13).

Standard Precautions. Safety precautions taken by healthcare workers to protect themselves and their patients from infection; these precautions are taken for *all* patients and *all* patient specimens (body substances); includes safety precautions previously referred to as universal precautions or universal body substance precautions (Chap. 12).

Staphylococci (staff"-eh-low-kok'-sigh). Cocci arranged in clusters, such as in the genus *Staphylococcus* (Chap. 4).

Staphylokinase (staf'-uh-low-ky'-nace). A kinase produced by *S. aureus* (Chap. 14).

Starch. A polysaccharide storage material found in plants (Chap. 6).

Stationary Phase. The part of a bacterial growth phase during which organisms are dying at the same rate at which new organisms are being produced; the third phase in a bacterial growth curve (Chap. 8).

STD. Sexually transmitted disease (Chap. 17).

Sterile (stir'-ill). Free of all living microorganisms, including spores (Chap. 8).

Sterile Techniques. Techniques used in an attempt to create an environment that is sterile (devoid of microbes) (Chap. 8).

Sterilization (stir'-uh-luh-zay'-shun). The destruction of *all* microbes in or on something (e.g., on surgical instruments) (Chap. 8).

Stigma. A photosensing (light sensing) organelle; also known as an *eyespot* (Chap. 5).

Streptobacilli (strep'-toh-bah-sill'-eye). Bacilli arranged in chains of varying lengths (Chap. 4).

Streptococci (strep'-toh-kok'-sigh). Cocci arranged in chains of varying lengths, such as in the genus *Streptococcus* (Chap. 4).

Streptokinase (strep'-toh-ky'-nace). A kinase produced by streptococci (Chap. 14).

Structural Staining Procedures. Staining procedures used to stain bacterial structures such as capsules, flagella, and endospores (Chap. 4).

Sty (Stye). Inflammation of a sebaceous gland that opens into a follicle of an eyelash (Chap. 17).

Syphilis (sif'-uh-lis). A sexually transmitted bacterial disease, caused by the spirochete *T. pallidum* (Chap. 19).

Subclinical Disease. See *asymptomatic disease*.

Substrate (sub'-strayt). The chemical substance that is acted upon or changed by an enzyme (Chap. 6).

Subunit Vaccine. A vaccine that uses antigenic (antibody-stimulating) portions of a pathogen, rather than using the whole pathogen; also known as an *acellular vaccine* (Chap. 16).

"Superbugs." Term originated by the press referring to especially drug-resistant or multidrug-resistant microbes (Chap. 9).

Superinfection (sue'-per-in-fek'-shun). An overgrowth or population explosion of one or more particular pathogens; often pathogens that are resistant to an antimicrobial agent that a patient is receiving (Chap. 9).

Surgical Asepsis. The absence of microorganisms in a surgical environment (e.g., an operating room) (Chap. 12).

Surgical Aseptic Techniques. Procedures followed and steps taken to ensure surgical asepsis (Chap. 12).

Symbionts (sim'-bee-ontz). The parties in a symbiotic relationship (Chap. 10).

Symbiosis (sim-bee-oh'-sis). The living together or close association of two dissimilar organisms (usually two different species) (Chap. 10).

Symptomatic Disease. A disease in which the patient experiences symptoms (Chap. 14).

Symptoms of a Disease. Indications of disease that are experienced by the patient; subjective; examples include aches and pains, chills, blurred vision, nausea (Chap. 14).

Synergism (sin'-er-jiz-um). When two or more drugs work together to accomplish a cure rate that is greater than either drug could accomplish by itself (Chap. 9).

Synergistic (sin-er-jis'-tik) **Infection.** An infection caused by the correlated action of two or more microorganisms; also known as a *polymicrobial infection*; examples include trench mouth and bacterial vaginosis (Chap. 10).

Synergistic Relationship. A symbiotic relationship in which two or more microorganisms work together to accomplish a task (e.g., to cause a synergistic infection) (Chap. 10).

Systemic Infection. An infection that has spread throughout the body; also known as a *generalized infection* (Chap. 14).

T

T Cells (T Lymphocytes). A category of leukocytes that play a variety of important roles in the immune system (Chap. 16).

T-Dependent Antigens. Antigens that require T-helper cells for their processing in the body (Chap. 16).

T-Independent Antigens. Antigens that do not require T-helper cells for their processing in the body (Chap. 16).

Taxa, sing. *taxon.* The names given to various groups in taxonomy; the usual taxa are kingdoms, phyla (or divisions), classes, orders, families, genera, species, and subspecies (Chap. 3).

Taxonomy (tak-sawn'-oh-me). The systematic classification of living things (Chap. 3).

Teichoic (tie-ko'-ick) **Acids.** Polymers found in the cell walls of Gram-positive bacteria (Chap. 4).

Temperate Bacteriophage. A bacteriophage whose genome incorporates into and replicates with the genome of the host bacterium; also known as a *lysogenic bacteriophage* (Chap. 4).

Tetanospasmin (tet'-uh-noh-spaz'-min). The neurotoxin produced by *Clostridium tetani* that causes tetanus (Chap. 14).

Tetanus (tet'-uh-nus). A bacterial disease of the central nervous system caused by a neurotoxin produced by *C. tetani*, an anaerobic, spore-forming Gram-positive bacillus (Chap. 19).

Tetrad. A packet of four cocci (Chap. 4).

Tetrose. A monosaccharide containing four carbon atoms (Chap. 6).

Thermal Death Point (TDP). The temperature required to kill all microorganisms in a liquid culture in 10 minutes at pH 7 (Chap. 8).

Thermal Death Time (TDT). The length of time required to kill all microorganisms in a liquid culture at a given temperature (Chap. 8).

Thermophile (ther'-mow-file). An organism that thrives at a temperature of 50°C or higher; such an organism is said to be *thermophilic* (Chap. 8).

Thrush. An oral infection caused by the yeast *C. albicans* (Chap. 20).

Tinea (tin'-ee-uh) **Barbae.** A fungal infection of the beard and moustache (Chap. 20).

Tinea Capitis. A fungal infection of the scalp, eyebrows, and eyelashes (Chap. 20).

Tinea Corporis. A fungal infection of the face, trunk, and major limbs (Chap. 20).

Tinea Cruris. A fungal infection of the groin and perineal and perianal areas (Chap. 20).

Tinea Infections. Fungal infections of the skin, hair, and nails; also called *ringworm infections*; named for the part of the body that is affected (Chap. 20).

Tinea Pedis. Also called *athlete's foot*; a fungal infection of the soles of the feet and between the toes (Chap. 20).

Tinea Unguium. A fungal infection of the nails; also called *onychomycosis* (Chap. 20).

Toxemia (tok-see'-me-uh). The presence of toxins in the blood (Chap. 13).

Toxigenicity (tok'-suh-juh-nis'-uh-tee) **or Toxinogenic-ity** (tok'-suh-no-juh-nisv-uh-tee). The ability to produce toxin; a microorganism capable of producing a toxin is said to be *toxigenic* (or *toxinogenic*) (Chap. 14).

Toxin (tok'-sin). As used in this book, a poisonous substance produced by a microorganism (Chap. 1).

Toxoid (tok'-soyd). A toxin that has been altered in such a way as to destroy its toxicity but retain its antigenicity; certain toxoids are used as vaccines (Chap. 16).

Toxoid Vaccine. A vaccine prepared from a toxoid (Chap. 16).

Trachoma (truh-koh'-muh). A bacterial eye disease caused by *Chlamydia trachomatis*, an obligate intracellular pathogen (Chap. 19).

Transcription (tran-skrip'-shun). Transfer of the genetic code from one type of nucleic acid to another; usually, the synthesis of an mRNA molecule using a DNA template (Chap. 6).

Transduction (trans-duk'-shun). Transfer of genetic material (and its phenotypic expression) from one bacterial cell to another via bacteriophages; in *generalized transduction*, the transducing bacteriophage is able to transfer any gene of the donor bacterium; in *specialized transduction*, the bacteriophage is able to transfer only one or some of the donor bacterium's genes (Chap. 7).

Transfer RNA (tRNA). The type of RNA molecule that is capable of combining with (and thus activating) a specific amino acid; involved in protein synthesis (translation); the anticodon on a tRNA molecule recognizes the codon on an mRNA molecule (Chap. 6).

Transferrin (trans-fer'-in). A glycoprotein, synthesized in the liver, used to store iron and deliver it to host cells (Chap. 15).

Transformation (trans-for-may'-shun). In microbial genetics, transfer of genetic information between bacteria via uptake or absorption of naked DNA; bacteria capable of absorbing naked DNA from their environment are said to be *competent* (Chap. 7).

Transient Bacteremia. A temporary bacteremia (Chap. 17).

Transient Microflora. Temporary members of the indigenous microflora (Chap. 10).

Translation (trans-lay'-shun). The process by which mRNA, tRNA, and ribosomes effect the production of proteins from amino acids; translation is also known as *protein synthesis* (Chap. 6).

Transmission-Based Precautions. Safety precautions taken by healthcare workers, in addition to standard precautions, to protect themselves and their patients from infection via airborne, contact, or droplet routes of transmission (Chap. 12).

Transmission Electron Micrograph. Photograph taken through the lens system of a transmission electron microscope (Chap. 2).

Transmission Electron Microscope. A type of electron microscope in which electrons are transmitted through very thin sections of specimens; enables the operator to observe internal detail (Chap. 2).

Trematodes (trem'-uh-toadz). A category of flatworms; often referred to as *flukes* (Chap. 21).

Trench Mouth. Synonym for acute necrotizing ulcerative gingivitis (ANUG); also called *Vincent's angina*; involves painful, bleeding gums and tonsils, erosion of gum tissue, and swollen lymph nodes beneath the jaw; a synergistic infection involving two or more species of anaerobic bacteria of the indigenous oral microflora (Chap. 19).

Triglyceride (try-glis'-er-ide). A lipid that is composed of glycerol (a three-carbon alcohol) and three fatty acids; fats and oils are examples (Chap. 6).

Triose. A monosaccharide containing three carbon atoms (Chap. 6).

Tripeptide (try-pep'-tide). A protein consisting of three amino acids held together by peptide bonds (Chap. 6).

Triple Bond. A type of chemical bond containing three pairs of shared electrons (Chap. 6).

Trophozoite (trof-oh-zoe'-ite). The motile, feeding, dividing stage in a protozoan's life cycle (Chap. 5).

Tuberculocidal (too-bur'-kyu-low-sigh'-dull) **Agent.** A chemical or drug that kills the bacterium that causes tuberculosis (*Mycobacterium tuberculosis*); also known as a *tuberculocide* (Chap. 8).

Tularemia (too-luh-ree'-me-uh). A bacterial disease caused by *Francisella tularensis*, a Gram-negative bacillus (Chap. 19).

Tyndallization (tin-dull-uh-zay'-shun). A process of boiling and cooling in which spores are allowed to germinate and then the vegetative bacteria are killed by boiling again (Chap. 3).

Typhoid Fever. A bacterial disease caused by *Salmonella typhi*, a Gram-negative bacillus (Chap. 19).

U

Ubiquitous (you-bik'-wah-tus). Present everywhere (Chap. 1).

Ureteritis (you-ree-ter-eye'-tis). Inflammation or infection of a ureter (Chap. 17).

Urethritis (you-ree-thry'-tis). Inflammation or infection of the urethra (Chap. 17).

V

Vaccine (vak'-seen). Any preparation that, after injection (or ingestion, in some cases), produces active acquired immunity (Chap. 16).

Vaccinia (vak-sin'-ee-uh) **Virus.** The virus that causes cowpox (also known as *vaccinia*); used in a vaccine to convey resistance to smallpox (Chap. 18).

Vaginitis (vaj-uh-ny'-tis). Inflammation of the vagina (Chap. 10).

Vaginosis (vag-uh-no'-sis). Infection of the vagina, with no influx of leukocytes (Chap. 10).

Varicella (var-uh-sell'-uh) **Virus.** The virus that causes chickenpox (also known as *varicella*) and shingles (Chap. 18).

Variola (var-ee'-oh-luh) **Virus.** The virus that causes smallpox (also known as *variola*). (Chap. 18).

Vasoconstriction (vay'-so-kon-strik'-shun). A decrease in the diameter of blood vessels (Chap. 15).

Vasodilation (vay'-soh-die-lay'-shun). An increase in the diameter of blood vessels (Chap. 15).

Vectors (vek'-tour). As used in this book, invertebrate animals (e.g., ticks, mites, mosquitoes, fleas) capable of transmitting pathogens among vertebrates (Chap. 4).

Vegetative Hyphae. Hyphae that lie below the surface of whatever a fungal mycelium is growing on (Chap. 5).

Viable Plate Count. A laboratory technique used to determine the number of living bacteria in a milliliter of liquid; involves the use of plated media (Chap. 8).

Viral Rhinitis (rye-ny'-tis). A synonym for the common cold (Chap. 18).

Viremia (vy-ree'-me-uh). The presence of viruses in the blood (Chap. 13).

Viricidal (vy-ruh-sigh'-dull) **Agent.** A chemical or drug that inactivates a virus, rendering it noninfectious; can also be spelled *virucidal agent*; also known as a *viricide* or a *virucide* (Chap. 8).

Virion (veer'-ee-on). A complete, infectious viral particle (i.e., a virus that contains all of its parts) (Chap. 4).

Viroids (vi'-roydz). Infectious RNA molecules (i.e., RNA molecules capable of causing certain plant diseases) (Chap. 4).

Virologist (vi-rol'-oh-jist). One who studies or works with viruses (Chap. 1).

Virology (vi-rol'-oh-gee). That branch of science concerned with the study of viruses (Chap. 1).

Virulence (veer'-u-lenz). A measure of pathogenicity (i.e., some pathogens are more or less *virulent* than others) (Chap. 14).

Virulence Factors. Attributes or properties of a microorganism that contribute to its virulence or pathogenicity (e.g., certain exoenzymes and toxins produced by pathogenic bacteria) (Chap. 14).

Virulent Bacteriophage. A bacteriophage that regularly causes lysis of the bacteria it infects; causes the lytic cycle to occur (Chap. 4).

Virulent (veer'-yu-lent) **Strains.** Strains that are pathogenic; capable of causing disease (Chap. 14).

Viruses (vi'-rus-ez), sing. *virus*. Acellular microbes that are smaller than bacteria; obligate intracellular parasites; sometimes referred to as *infectious particles* rather than microbes (Chap. 4).

Vulvovaginitis (vul'-voh-vaj-uh-ny'-tis). Inflammation of the vulva (the external genitalia of women) and the vagina (Chap. 17).

W

Wandering Macrophages. Macrophages that migrate in the bloodstream and tissues; sometimes called *free macrophages* (Chap. 15).

Waxes. Lipids consisting of a saturated fatty acid and a long-chain alcohol (Chap. 6).

White Piedra. A fungal hair infection usually caused by the mould *Trichosporon beigelii* (Chap. 20).

Z

Zoonoses (zoh-oh-no'-seez), sing. *zoonosis*. Infectious diseases transmissible from animals to humans; also known as *zoonotic diseases* (Chap. 1).

Zooplankton (zoh'-oh-plank'-ton). Microscopic marine animals that are components of plankton (Chap. 1).

Page numbers in *italics* denote figures; those followed by an n or t indicate material in notes or tables, respectively.

Glutamine, 102
Glutaraldehyde, 222t
Glycerophospholipids, *99*, 100
Glycine, 102
Glycocalyx, 33
Glycogen, 96, 98
Glycolipids, 99, *99*, 101
Glycolysis, 120, *120*, 121t
Glycolytic pathway, 120
Glycopeptide, 158t, 160
Glycosidic bond, 97
Goggles, 229
Golden algae, 76, 77t
Golgi apparatus/Golgi body (*See* Golgi complex)
Golgi complex
  of algae, 76
  of eukaryotic cells, 27, 29
  as packaging plant, 29
  of protozoa, 79
Gonococcal conjunctivitis, 364t, *365*
Gonococcal ophthalmia neonatorum, *365*
Gonococcal urethritis, 267
Gonococci, 39 (*See also* Neisseria *gonorrhoeae*)
  cultures, 251, *251*
Gonorrhea, 329, 374t
  causative agent of, 39t, 374t (*See also* Neisseria *gonorrhoeae*)
  diagnosis of, 251, *251*, *374*
  reporting of, 205t, 359t
  symptomatic *vs.* asymptomatic, 263–264
  transmission of, 202, 374t
Gonorrheal ophthalmia neonatorum, 364t, *365*
Gonyaulax, 332
Gowns, 145, 223, *223–224*, 228
Gram, Christian, 61–62
Gram-negative bacteria, 32, *33*, 58, 61–62, 63t, 64t, *65*, 100
  antibacterial action on, 160
  cultures of, 139–140, *140*
  healthcare-associated infections of, 217
  in indigenous microbiota, 177t
Gram-positive bacteria, 32, *33*, 58, 62, 63t, 64t, *65*
  antibacterial action on, 160
  healthcare-associated infections of, 217
  in indigenous microbiota, 177t
Gram stain, 61–66, *64–65*
  color differences in, 62, 63t
  of important pathogenic bacteria, 64t
  remembering reactions in, method for, 62
  shapes observed in, 62, *65*
  steps in, *63*
Gram-variable bacteria, 62
Granulocytes, 245, 283–284, 305
Granuloma inguinale, 373
Graphite, 95
Great Potato Famine, 86, 185
Greek alphabets, 424
Green algae, 76, 77–78, 77t, *78*
Green bacteria, 72, 123
Griffith, Frederick, 105, 127
Griseofulvin, 161, 162t
Growth (*See also* Microbial growth (in vitro))
  hormone, genetically engineered, 130

GSS disease (*See* Gerstmann–Sträussler–Scheinker disease)
Guanine, 105, *106*, 107–108
Guarnieri bodies, 54
Guinea worm infection, 204
Gynecologic infectious processes, 380t

H

H1N1, 194
Haemophilus
  atmospheric requirements of, 68–69
  cardiovascular infection of, 376
  in indigenous microbiota, 177t, 179
  transformation in, 127
Haemophilus ducreyi, 64t, 373
Haemophilus influenzae, 160
  antibody
    destruction by, 273
    testing for, 315
  capsule of, 33, 269
  CNS infection of, 332
  cultures of, 139
  diseases caused by, *363*
  ear infection of, 363t
  eye infection of, 364t
  Gram stain of, 64t
  infections caused by, *363*
  morphology of, 60
  multidrug-resistant, 165t
  nomenclature for, 39
  pneumonia with, 323, 366
  reporting of, 359t
  sinus infection of, 322
  vaccine against, 33
Haemophilus influenzae type b (Hib), 297, 332, 332n
Hair clippings, 242t, 256
Hair mycoses, 390
HAIs (*See* Healthcare-associated infections)
Haloduric organisms, 136
Halofantrine, 162t
Halophiles, 72t, 137
Halophilic organisms, 136
Hand hygiene, 145, 202, 220
  in dental healthcare, 236
  proper technique for, *226–227*
  Semmelweis as father of, 227
  in Standard Precautions, 225, 226
Hanging-drop technique, of determining motility, 66, *67*
Hansen disease (*See* Leprosy)
Hantavirus pulmonary syndrome (HPS), 191, 192, 199t, 333, 338t, 344t
Haptens, 300, 308
Hard measles (*See* Measles)
Harmful mutations, 124
HBIG (*See* Hepatitis B immune globulin)
Health and Human Services, Department of, 204
Healthcare-associated infections (HAIs), 164t, 216–220
  antimicrobial resistance in, 217–218, 219
  frequency of, 216
  iatrogenic infections *vs.*, 216
  major factors contributing to, 219, *219*

modes of transmission, 217
  most common types of, 217–218
  pathogens involved in, 216–217
  patients most likely to develop, 218–219
  pneumonia, 218, 366–367
  prevention of, 216, 219–220
  urinary tract, 217, 372–373
Healthcare epidemiology, 216–240
  definition of, 216
  health care-associated infections, 216–220
  infection control, 220–239
  regulations pertaining to, 224
  role of clinical microbiology laboratory in, 238
Heart
  anatomy of, 329, *330*
  infectious diseases of, 329
Heart-lung machine, 223
Heat
  fixation, 61
  in inflammation, 281, 281n
  sterilization
    dry, 144, 146, *146*
    moist, 146–148
Helicobacter pylori, 179, 369t
Helminth(s), 412
  definition of, 412
  infections, 200t, 401, 403, 412, 414t
  life cycle of, 412, *413*
Helper T cells, 55, 267, 299, 305
Hematology, 245, 252
Hemoglobin, 102–103
Hemolysins, 269, 270–271
Hemolysis, 136, *137*, 256, *257*, 271
Hemolytic uremic syndrome (HUS), 192, 359t
Hemorrhagic conjunctivitis, 342t
Hemorrhagic diseases, viral, 349t
Hendra virus infection, 333
HEPA filters (*See* High-efficiency particulate air filters)
Hepatitis (hepatitis virus), 326, 345–346, 346t
  as oncogenic virus, 55
  reservoirs of, 201
Hepatitis A, 201, 345–346, 346t
  reporting of, 338t
  vaccine against, 297, 346
Hepatitis B, 345–346, 346t
  immune globulin, 298
  reporting of, 338t
  transmission of, 329, 346t
  vaccine against, 297, 346
Hepatitis C, 338t, 345, 346t
Hepatitis D, 345, 346t
Hepatitis E, 345, 346
Hepatitis G, 346t, 354
Hepatitis GB virus A, 345
Hepatitis GB virus B, 345
Hepatitis GB virus C, 345
Hepatocellular carcinoma, 55
Hepatotoxins, 72
Heptose, 96, 96t
Herbal medicine, 154
Herbicidal agents, 186

RES (*See* Reticuloendothelial system)
Reservoirs of infection, 197–201, *197*
   animals, 198, 199–200t
   arthropods, 200
   definition of, 197
   fomites, 200, 201
   human carriers, 197–198
   living, 197–200
   nonliving, 200–201
Resident microbiota, 177–178
Resistance, antimicrobial, 163–168,
   163–171
   antimicrobial use/misuse and,
      151–152, 167
   bacterial acquisition of, 164–165, 167t
   bacteriophage research
      prompted by, 51–52
   biofilms and, 182
   conjugation and, 128, 165
   to disinfectants, 150, 150t
   in healthcare-associated infections,
      217–218, 219
   intrinsic, 164
   in mycoplasmas, 71
   prevention, among hospitalized adults,
      217, 218t
   selection for, 170, *170*
   strategies in war against, 167–168
   "superbugs" and, 163–164
Resistance factor, 128, 165
Resistant organisms, selection of, 170, *170*
Resistant, use of term, 294
Resolving power (resolution), 15, 15t
   of compound light microscope, 17–20
   of electron microscope, 17–19
Respiratory chain (*See* Electron
   transport chain)
Respiratory infections, healthcare-
   associated, 217
Respiratory protection, 229, *229*
Respiratory syncytial virus (RSV), 323,
   342, 343t, 363t, 366
Respiratory system
   anatomy of, 322, *324*
   bacterial infections of, 362, 365t,
      366–367, 368–369t
   fungal infections of, 392, 393–394t
   host defense mechanisms of, 277–278
   infectious diseases of, 322–324
   microbiota of, *176*, 177t, 178, 322
   transmission via, 203, 203t
   viral infections of, 342–343, 343–344t
Respiratory therapists, 324
Reticuloendothelial system (RES), 284
Retrograde evolution theory, of viruses, 48
Retroviruses, 49t, 55, 130
R (resistance) factor, 128, 165
Rheostat, of compound microscope,
   17, *18*, 18t
Rhinitis, acute viral, 342
Rhinovirus, 342, 343t
Rhizobium, 183, *184*
Rhizopus, *84*, 87t, 88, 394t
Riboflavin, production of, 186
Ribose, 96, 105
Ribosomal RNA (rRNA), 28, 105, 110, 123
   (*See also* RNA)
   identification by, 42

relatedness determined by, 41–42
sequencing, 41–42, 69, 72–73
Ribosome(s)
   of algae, 75–76
   antimicrobial action on, 161
   of eukaryotic cells, 27, 29, 37t, 109
   of prokaryotic cells, 30, *31*, 32, 37t, 109
Ricketts, Howard T., 69
Rickettsia, 69, 70t
Rickettsia akari, 70t
Rickettsial pox, 199t
Rickettsia prowazekii, 70t, 375t
Rickettsia rickettsii, 70t
   cardiovascular infection of, 375t
   Gram stain of, 64t
   intracellular survival mechanisms of,
      268–269, 287
Rickettsias, 38, 69–70, 70t
   antibacterial action on, 161
   cardiovascular infection of, 373, 375t
   cultures of, 139, 143
   intracellular survival mechanisms of,
      268–269, 269t, 287
   virulence of, 269t
Rickettsia typhi, 70t, 375t
Rifampin, 161, 165t
Rifamycins, 158t
Rift Valley fever, 333
RIG (*See* Rabies immune globulin)
Rings (cyclic compounds), 95, *95*
Ringworm, 87t, 199t, 390, *391*, 392
"River blindness," 204, 414t
RNA (ribonucleic acid)
   bacterial, 69
   bacteriophage, 50
   Central Dogma and, 108
   DNA *vs.*, 107
   eukaryotic, 28
   as macromolecule, 94
   mRNA, 29, 105
   nucleotides, 104–105
   polymerase, 109, 116
   rRNA, 28, 41–42, 69, 72–73,
      105, 110, 123
   transcription of, 108–109, 123
   translation by, 109–110, *109–110*
   tRNA, 28, 105, 109–110, 123
   types of, 105
   viral, 46, *47*, 52–53
Rochalimaea quintana, 69
Rocky Mountain spotted fever, 69, 199t,
   375t, *375*, *416*
Roquefort cheese, 86, 186
Rosaniline, 154
Rotaviruses, 297, 345
Rough endoplasmic reticulum
   (RER), 27, 28
Roundworms, 412
RSV (*See* Respiratory syncytial virus)
Rubella, 338t, 339–340t, *341*
Rubeola virus, 354, 422 (*See also* Measles)
Rudimentary bacteria, 69–71
Rusts, 86–87, 185, 185t

S

Sabouraud dextrose agar (SDA), 144, 256
Saccharomyces, 121, 181

Saccharomyces cerevisiae, 84
Salinity
   and indigenous microbiota, 178
   and microbial growth, 135–136, *137*
Saliva, as host defense mechanism,
   278, 325
Salivary transmission, 203t
Salmon, Daniel Elmer, 39
Salmonella, *35*, 39, 60
   in Ames test, 124
   CNS infection of, 332
   diagnosis of infection, 251–252
   fimbriae or pili of, 268–269
   foodborne infections of, 193, 202t, 370t
   gastrointestinal infection of, 199t, 205t,
      359t, 370t
   in gene therapy, 130
   Gram stain of, 64t
   multidrug-resistant, 151, 165t
   phagocytosis evasion by, 287
   radiation and, 148
   reservoirs of, 198
   toxin of, 271
   virulence of, 267–269, 271
Salmonella enterica, 370t
Salmonella enteritidis, 202t, 370t
Salmonella paratyphi, 370t
Salmonella typhi, 370t
   Gram stain of, 64t
   phenol coefficient test with, 151
   reservoirs of, 201
   Typhoid Mary as carrier of, 198
Salmonella typhimurium, 370t
Salmonella typhimurium DT-104, 202t
Salmonellosis, 199t, 205t, 359t, 370t
Salpingitis, 327
Salton, M. R. J., 62
Salvarsan (arsphenamine), 154
Sand flies, 201t
Sanitization, definition of, 144
Saprobe (*See* Saprophytes)
Saprophytes, 3, *4*, 81, 98, 116, 183
Sarcina ventriculi, 59
SARS (*See* Severe acute respiratory
   syndrome)
Saturated fatty acids, 98–99
SBE (*See* Subacute bacterial
   endocarditis)
Scabies, 416t
Scalded skin syndrome, 271, 361t
Scanning electron micrographs, 22
Scanning electron microscope (SEM), 15t,
   19–22, *21*, *22*
Scarlet fever, 126, 271–272, 361t
Schistosome, 272–273
Schistosomiasis, 272–273, 414t, *415*
Schoenlein, K., 367
Schroeter, Joseph, 138
SCID (*See* Severe combined immune
   deficiency)
S-colonies, 33
Scopulariopsis, *83*
"Scotch tape prep," 242t
Scrapie, 57
Scrub typhus, 199t
SDA (*See* Sabouraud dextrose agar)
Sebaceous glands, 277, *320*, 321
Sebum, 277, 321